Neoplastic Hematopathology

CONTEMPORARY HEMATOLOGY

Judith E. Karp, MD, SERIES EDITOR

For other titles published in the series, go to
www.springer.com/series/7681

Neoplastic Hematopathology

Experimental and Clinical Approaches

Edited by

Dan Jones, MD, PhD

Department of Hematopathology
M. D. Anderson Cancer Center
The University of Texas
Houston, TX
USA

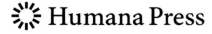 Humana Press

Editor
Dan Jones
Department of Hematopathology
M. D. Anderson Cancer Center
The University of Texas
Houston, TX
USA
dajones@mdanderson.org

ISBN 978-1-60761-383-1   e-ISBN 978-1-60761-384-8
DOI 10.1007/978-1-60761-384-8
Springer New York Dordrecht Heidelberg London

Library of Congress Control Number: 2009932414

Printed on acid-free paper

Humana Press is part of Springer Science+Business Media (www.springer.com)

Preface

My goal for this textbook is to provide an overview of the discipline of hematopathology that connects the field with recent advances in immunology research and with current clinical practice in the treatment of lymphomas and leukemias. With separate sections on laboratory techniques, diagnostic hematopathology, treatment, and stem cell transplantation, this book is designed to be useful for both trainees and specialists in pathology and hematology-oncology. We have also summarized the current directions in translational research that will be of most interest to experienced hematopathologists and scientists working in lymphoma and leukemia biology.

The terminology and diagnostic categories used are those of the 4th World Health Organization (WHO) Classification of Tumors of Hematopoietic and Lymphoid Tissues, which was released in late 2008. However, the chapter authors also provide a clinical and experimental context for this classification and point out areas where improvements are needed. A study guide is provided which highlights central concepts from each chapter to make the book suitable for boards review in hematopathology and hematology-oncology. The concluding chapter attempts to connect broad swaths of cancer biology and immunology with the trend towards individualized risk prediction and therapeutics (i.e. personalized medicine).

No area of pathology currently encompasses as many disparate disciplines as hematopathology, including laboratory medicine, molecular diagnostics, surgical pathology, clinical hematology and translational science. For this reason, I believe there is a need for a broader approach to the diagnostic endeavor that encompasses other approaches and concerns. My reasons for taking this more multidisciplinary approach arise out of my interactions over the last 10 years with my clinical colleagues at M. D. Anderson Cancer Center in the departments of Leukemia, Lymphoma, and Stem Cell Transplantation, all of whom have helped me focus on the elements of diagnosis that most impact clinical care. I am grateful to have some of those colleagues joining me as coauthors to provide their insights into treatment. My interest in linking diagnostics more closely with clinical management was also shaped by my training at Brigham and Women's Hospital in Boston where I had three terrific role models in this regard in Geraldine Pinkus, Chris Fletcher, and Ramzi Cotran.

For their constant support of my work, I dedicate this book to my parents, Bernice Katz Jones and Professor Richard Victor Jones, whose boundless intellectual curiosity remains a continuing source of inspiration for me. I thank all the authors for their outstanding contributions and for their willingness to participate in this type of multi-disciplinary project. I also greatly appreciate the editorial assistance of Frances Louie at Humana Press and Sundardevadoss Dharmendra at SPi, as well as Brian Stewart, Jenna Boatright, Lakisha Rodgers, Orelia Kelly, and Steven Reyes at M.D. Anderson. Finally, I am greatly indebted to Roberto Miranda for his expert assistance with chapter review and editing.

Houston, TX   Dan Jones, MD, PhD

Contents

Preface v

Contributors xi

How to Use This Book xv

Section 1   Introduction to Diagnosis and Laboratory Techniques

1   Approaches to Classification of Lymphoma and Leukemia 3
    Dan Jones

2   Immunohistochemical Profiling of Lymphoma 21
    Matthew W. Anderson and Yasodha Natkunam

3   Flow Cytometry in the Evaluation of Hematologic Malignancies 45
    Jeffrey L. Jorgensen

4   Molecular Diagnostics and Cytogenetic Testing 61
    Su Chen, Zhuang Zuo, and Dan Jones

Section 2   Neoplasms of the Bone Marrow

5   The Bone Marrow in Normal and Disease States 99
    Dan Jones and Roberto N. Miranda

6   Myelodysplastic Syndromes and Myelodysplastic/Myeloproliferative
    Neoplasms 123
    Sa A. Wang

7   Acute Myeloid Leukemia 145
    Carlos E. Bueso-Ramos

8   Treatment of Acute Myeloid Leukemia and Myelodysplastic Syndromes 165
    Farhad Ravandi

9   Myeloproliferative Neoplasms 177
    C. Cameron Yin and Dan Jones

10   Chronic Myelogenous Leukemia 193
     Robert P. Hasserjian

11   Treatment of Myeloproliferative Neoplasms 213
     Starla Sweany and Elias Jabbour

Section 3   Tumors of the Lymph Node and Extranodal Tissues

12   Lymph Node Biology and Lymphadenitis 223
     Roberto N. Miranda

13   Lymphoblastic Leukemia and Lymphoma 239
     Andrea M. Sheehan

14   Chronic Lymphocytic Leukemia and Small Lymphocytic Lymphoma 251
     Ellen Schlette

15   Marginal Zone Lymphomas 263
     Rachel L. Sargent

16   Follicular Lymphoma and Mantle Cell Lymphoma 279
     Dan Jones

17   Aggressive B-cell Lymphomas: Diffuse Large B-cell Lymphoma
     and Burkitt Lymphoma 303
     Henry Y. Dong

18   Therapy of B-cell Lymphoproliferative Disorders 323
     Nathan Fowler, Sandra Horowitz, and Peter McLaughlin

19   Plasma Cell Myeloma and Other Plasma Cell Dyscrasias 333
     Marwan A. Yared

20   Hodgkin Lymphoma 349
     Robert Lin, Dan Jones, and Sherif Ibrahim

21   Treatment of Hodgkin Lymphoma 367
     Samer A. Srour and Luis E. Fayad

22   Classification of T-cell and NK-cell Malignancies 391
     Dan Jones

23   Clinical Management of Non-cutaneous T-cell and NK-cell Malignancies 413
     Marco Herling

24   Cutaneous T-cell Lymphomas 427
     Pranil Chandra, Mauricio P. Oyarzo, and Dan Jones

25   Treatment of Cutaneous T-cell Lymphomas 449
     Katherine M. Cox and Madeleine Duvic

26   Histiocytic and Dendritic Cell Neoplasms 459
     Kedar V. Inamdar and Dan Jones

27 Extranodal Lymphomas and Tumors of the Thymus............................. 477
    Brian D. Stewart, John T. Manning, and Dan Jones

Section 4   Stem Cell Transplantation

28 Clinical Aspects of Hematopoietic Stem Cell Transplantation 505
    Elizabeth J. Shpall and Marcos de Lima

29 Post-transplant Molecular Monitoring... 513
    Dan Jones

30 Post-transplant Immune Function and the Development of Lymphoma 521
    Deqin Ma and Dan Jones

Section 5   Experimental Hematopathology

31 Hematopoiesis and Stem Cell Biology 531
    Claudiu Cotta

32 Role of Host Genetics in Lymphoma... 545
    Ahmet Dogan

33 Developing Prognostic Models for Diffuse Large B-cell Lymphoma.................... 553
    Izidore S. Lossos

34 Growth Signaling and Survival Pathways in Aggressive B-cell Lymphoma.......... 563
    Lan V. Pham and Richard J. Ford

35 Proteomic Profiling and Target Identification in Lymphoma 573
    Megan S. Lim

36 Mouse Models of Lymphoma and Lymphoid Leukemia.. 583
    M. James You

37 Mouse Models of Myeloid Leukemia... 597
    Robert B. Lorsbach

38 Designing Targeted Therapies for Lymphomas and Leukemias............................ 611
    Dan Jones

Study Guide 627

Index 635

Contributors

Matthew W. Anderson, MD, PhD
Department of Pathology, Stanford University School of Medicine, Stanford, CA, USA

Carlos E. Bueso-Ramos, MD, PhD
Department of Hematopahology, M. D. Anderson Cancer Center, The University of Texas, Houston, TX, USA

Pranil Chandra, DO
ACL Laboratories, Great Lakes Pathology, Milwaukee, WI

Su Chen, MD, PhD
Department of Hematopahology, M. D. Anderson Cancer Center, The University of Texas, Houston, TX, USA

Claudiu Cotta, MD, PhD
Department of Clinical Pathology, Cleveland Clinic, Cleveland, OH, USA

Katherine M. Cox, MD
Department of Dermatology, University of Texas Medical School at Houston, Houston, TX, USA

Marcos de Lima, MD
Department of Stem Cell Transplantation and Cell Therapy, M. D. Anderson Cancer Center, The University of Texas, Houston, TX, USA

Ahmet Dogan, MD, PhD
Departments of Anatomic Pathology and Laboratory Medicine and Pathology, Mayo Clinic, Rochester, MN, USA

Henry Y. Dong, MD, PhD
Molecular Pathology, Genzyme Genetics, New York, NY, USA

Madeleine Duvic, MD
Department of Dermatology, M. D. Anderson Cancer Center, The University of Texas, Houston, TX, USA

Luis E. Fayad, MD
Department of Lymphoma & Myeloma, M. D. Anderson Cancer Center,
The University of Texas, Houston, TX, USA

Richard J. Ford, MD, PhD
Department of Hematopathology, M. D. Anderson Cancer Center,
The University of Texas, Houston, TX, USA

Nathan Fowler, MD
Department of Lymphoma & Myeloma, M. D. Anderson Cancer Center,
The University of Texas, Houston, TX, USA

Robert P. Hasserjian, MD
Department of Pathology, Massachusetts General Hospital, Harvard Medical School,
Boston, MA, USA

Marco Herling, MD
Department of Medicine I, Cologne University, Cologne, Germany

Sandra Horowitz, PharmD
Pharmacy Clinical Programs, M. D. Anderson Cancer Center,
The University of Texas, Houston, TX, USA

Sherif Ibrahim, MD, PhD
Department of Pathology, New York University Medical Center, New York, NY, USA

Kedar V. Inamdar, MD, PhD
Department of Pathology, Henry Ford Hospital, Detroit, MI, USA

Elias Jabbour, MD
Department of Leukemia, M. D. Anderson Cancer Center, The University of Texas,
Houston, TX, USA

Dan Jones, MD, PhD
Department of Hematopathology, M. D. Anderson Cancer Center,
The University of Texas, Houston, TX, USA

Jeffrey L. Jorgensen, MD, PhD
Department of Hematopathology, M. D. Anderson Cancer Center,
The University of Texas, Houston, TX, USA

Megan S. Lim, MD, PhD
Department of Pathology, University of Michigan, Ann Arbor, MI, USA

Robert Lin, MD
Department of Pathology, New York University Medical Center, New York, NY, USA

Robert B. Lorsbach, MD, PhD
Department of Pathology, University of Arkansas for Medical Sciences,
Little Rock, AR, USA

Izidore S. Lossos, MD
Department of Lymphoma, Miller School of Medicine, University of Miami, Miami, FL, USA

Deqin Ma, MD, PhD
Department of Anatomic Pathology, National Institutes of Health, Bethesda, MD, USA

John T. Manning, MD
Department of Hematopathology, M. D. Anderson Cancer Center,
The University of Texas, Houston, TX, USA

Peter McLaughlin, MD
Department of Lymphoma & Myeloma, M. D. Anderson Cancer Center,
The University of Texas, Houston, TX, USA

Roberto N. Miranda, MD
Department of Hematopathology, M. D. Anderson Cancer Center,
The University of Texas, Houston, TX, USA

Yasodha Natkunam, MD, PhD
Department of Pathology, Stanford University School of Medicine, Stanford,
CA, USA

Mauricio P. Oyarzo, MD
Department of Pathology, Clinica Alemana, Santiago, Chile

Lan V. Pham, PhD
Department of Hematopathology, M. D. Anderson Cancer Center,
The University of Texas, Houston, TX, USA

Farhad Ravandi, MD
Department of Leukemia, M. D. Anderson Cancer Center, The University of Texas,
Houston, TX, USA

Rachel L. Sargent, MD
Department of Hematopathology, M. D. Anderson Cancer Center,
The University of Texas, Houston, TX, USA

Ellen Schlette, MD
Department of Hematopathology, M. D. Anderson Cancer Center,
The University of Texas, Houston, TX, USA

Andrea M. Sheehan, MD
Department of Pathology, Texas Children's Hospital, Baylor College of Medicine,
Houston, TX, USA

Elizabeth J. Shpall, MD
Department of Stem Cell Transplantation and Cell Therapy, M. D.
Anderson Cancer Center, The University of Texas, Houston, TX

Samer A. Srour, MB, ChB
Department of Internal Medicine, The University of Oklahoma College of Medicine,
Oklahoma City, OK

Brian D. Stewart, MD
Department of Pathology, The University of Texas Health Sciences Center at Houston,
Houston, TX, USA

Starla Sweany, PharmD, BCOP
Division of Pharmacy, M. D. Anderson Cancer Center, The University of Texas, Houston, TX, USA

Sa A.Wang, MD
Department of Hematopathology, M. D. Anderson Cancer Center,
The University of Texas, Houston, TX, USA

Marwan A. Yared, MD
Department of Pathology, University of Arkansas for Medical Sciences,
Little Rock, AR, USA

Cameron C. Yin, MD, PhD
Department of Hematopathology, M. D. Anderson Cancer Center,
The University of Texas, Houston, TX, USA

M. James You, MD, PhD
Department of Hematopathology, M. D. Anderson Cancer Center,
The University of Texas, Houston, TX, USA

Zhuang Zuo, MD, PhD
Department of Hematopathology, M. D. Anderson Cancer Center,
The University of Texas, Houston, TX, USA

How to Use This Book

As an overview of diagnostic hematopathology for hematologist-oncologists:

- The pathologic overview of each group of tumors is followed by chapters written by experienced clinicians summarizing the current state of diagnosis, staging and treatment for lymphoma, leukemias and related neoplasms.
- The active areas of research that will lead to new therapeutic agents and biomarkers development are summarized in the last section of the text (Chaps. 31–38).

As a reference text for practicing pathologists:

- Chapter 1 lists the current terminology derived from the 2008 WHO Classification of Haematopoietic and Lymphoid Tissues, which should be used for diagnosis whenever possible.
- Diagnostic pitfalls and differential diagnoses that should be considered are highlighted in each of the pathology chapters.
- The treatment overviews (Chaps. 8, 11, 18, 21, 23, 25 and 28) are primarily intended for those pathologists wanting a more in-depth understanding of current treatment issues.

For boards review for pathology and hematopathology trainees:

- Chapters 1 (all lymphoma/leukemia types), 2 (lymph node-based tumors), and 28 (extranodal lymphomas) list the core diagnostic entities and what markers are used for differential diagnosis.
- In addition, the central concepts of each chapter are highlighted in the study guide. Trainees should concentrate their review on those chapters which have the most number of unfamiliar concepts.
- The photomicrographs in each pathology chapter provide the classical appearances of tumor entities.

As a reference for experimental scientists and graduate students working on lymphomas and leukemias:

- The methodology sections (Chaps. 2–4) give helpful hints on the use of immunohisto-chemistry, flow cytometry and molecular techniques.
- The last section (Chaps. 31–38) gives an overview of the main directions of research in stem cell biology, targeted therapy, lymphocyte signaling, and perspective on host genetics and immune function in lymphoma and leukemias.
- The section on prognostic markers in each diagnostic chapter may be particular useful in highlighting outstanding questions in biomarker development which would benefit from additional experimental work.

Section 1

Introduction to Diagnosis and Laboratory Techniques

Chapter 1

Approaches to Classification of Lymphoma and Leukemia

Dan Jones

Abstract/Scope of Chapter The classification of leukemias, lymphomas, and other tumors of the immune system is a constantly changing effort driven by advances in immunology, molecular genetics, and laboratory technologies. Here, we discuss the current 2008 World Health Organization classification and its historical precedents which have resulted in different approaches for myeloid leukemias, plasma cell dyscrasias, and lymphomas. Also discussed are trends in the diagnostic workup for lymphomas including the use of fine needle aspiration and multiparameter flow cytometry, and the increasing use of molecular monitoring in place of morphology for the diagnosis and follow-up of leukemias.

Keywords Lymphoma, classification • Leukemia, classification • Plasma cell neoplasm, classification • Myeloma, classification • Prognostic markers • Therapy response predictors, WHO classification, strengths and weaknesses • FAB (French–American–British), classification • DNA recombination, nonhomologous end-joining, chromosome translocations, mechanism • Mutagens, risk of lymphoma and leukemia • Hematopathology, sample report • Hematopathology, future directions in classification

1.1. History of Classification Efforts in Hematopathology

Progress in hematopathology over the last century has been inextricably linked to the evolution of classification efforts that culminated in the current 2008 World Health Organization (WHO) classification (reviewed in Fig. 1-1). The efforts of lymph node pathologists and leukemia diagnosticians, including clinical hematologists, evolved separately. Beginning with the 1994 Revised European–American Lymphoma (REAL) classification, these efforts have been essentially merged. The latest WHO classification of tumors of haematopoietic and lymphoid tissues (2001, 2008) [1,2] fully reflects this integration. Nonetheless, the current classifications for particular lymphoma and leukemia types have remnants of their respective historical approaches.

1.1.1. Lymphoma Classification: A Histogenetic (Cell of Origin) Focus

Many of the common lymphoma types, including mycosis fungoides (recognized by Jean-Louis-Marc Alibert in 1806), Hodgkin's disease (described by Thomas Hodgkin in 1832), and large cell lymphoma (described by Ewing in 1913, and then codified by Parker and Jackson as reticulum cell sarcoma), have been recognized as distinct entities for over 100 years. Since the nonneoplastic counterparts of the immune system were being recognized

From: *Neoplastic Hematopathology*: Contemporary Hematology,
Edited by: D. Jones, DOI 10.1007/978-1-60761-384-8_1,
© Humana Press, a part of Springer Science+Business Media, LLC 2010

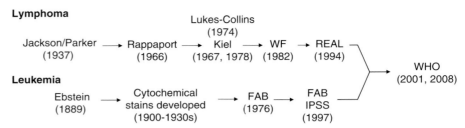

Fig. 1-1. Timeline of classification efforts in leukemia and lymphoma. The WHO brought together efforts to create a broad schema for all hematolymphoid tumors

around the same time, classification efforts inevitably focused on the histogenetic mapping of lymphomas to their normal immune cell counterparts.

For this reason, lymphoma (especially of the B-cell type) was the first tumor type to have a differentiation stage (or histogenetic) classification. Beginning with the work of Henry Rappaport (1956 and 1966) and Drs. Lukes and Collins (1974) [3] in the United States and Karl Lennert and coworkers in Kiel, Germany (1967, 1975), [4] schema were created based on the resemblance of lymphomas to normal populations of lymphocytes. Thus, nodular lymphomas were related to germinal center (GC) B cells and named morphologically as cleaved or noncleaved like the microscopic appearance of the normal GC populations. This type of morphological mapping inevitably lead to great concern and mystery whenever a normal cell counterpart of a lymphoma could not be identified, such as the Reed–Sternberg cell in Hodgkin's lymphoma or the CD5+ B cell in small lymphocytic lymphoma (SLL).

Lymphoma was also the first tumor type to have a widely–used clinicopathological classification, the Working Formulation, which emerged from a National Institutes of Health consensus conference (1982), and divided lymphomas into low, intermediate, and high–grade types based on their clinical behavior [5]. The later REAL classification (1994) attempted, for the first time, to bridge these clinical and morphologic goals [6]. It largely followed the morphologic subtypes identified in the Kiel classification, [4] but added in clinical, molecular, and immunophenotypic data. A parallel effort in cutaneous lymphomas involving dermatologists and pathologists resulted in the European Organization for Research and Treatment of Cancer (EORTC) classification [7,8].

1.1.2. Classification of Leukemias and Plasma Cell Dyscrasias: A Focus on Tumor Progression

In contrast, leukemia classification efforts have focused much more on the evolution of fulminant leukemia from "preneoplastic" states known as myelodysplastic syndromes (MDS). Although acute leukemia was first recognized by J.T. Bennett and Rudolf Virchow in 1845–1846, the important role of bone marrow dysplasia and failure as a precursor to acute myeloid leukemia (AML) was noted only in the early twentieth century when the cell-damaging effects of alkylating agents, such as nitrogen mustard used in chemical warfare, were discovered. The first complete leukemia classification, the French–American–British (FAB) scheme, developed in the 1970s, was focused on the progression of MDS to AML (Fig. 1-2, and Chap. 7). For classification of leukemia, the first FAB system relied on morphology, with cytochemical confirmation, to type the myeloid, monocytic, or lymphoid nature of blasts [9,10]. Clinical progression was also the focus of the classification efforts in the chronic myeloproliferative neoplasms, including chronic myelogenous leukemia (CML, Fig. 1-2).

Because of the ease of obtaining informative chromosomal studies from bone marrow samples and the central role of reciprocal chromosomal translocations in tumor initiation,

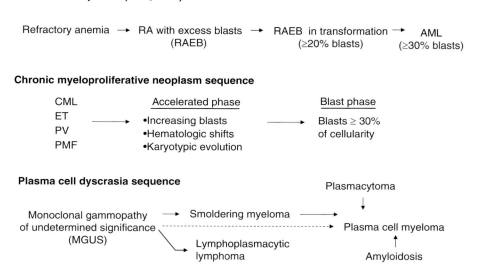

Fig. 1-2. Progression schemas for acute and chronic myeloid leukemias, and for plasma cell dyscrasias

leukemia classifications were the first to routinely integrate genetic findings. Beginning with the discovery of the Philadelphia chromosome as the characteristic feature of CML by Peter Nowell and David Hungerford in 1960, [11] karyotyping has become increasingly integral to the leukemia workup. Cytogenetic data was formally incorporated into the risk stratification classification for MDS in 1997 [12]. The increasing use of cytogenetic and molecular characterization as well as flow cytometry for expanded immunophenotyping was reflected in a move away from the morphologic and cytochemical features of leukemias in the WHO classifications of 2001 and 2008 [13,14].

The evolution of classification efforts in plasma cell dyscrasias greatly resemble those in myeloid leukemia with an emphasis on the progression of low-level monoclonal gammopathy to overt myeloma (Fig. 1-2) [15]. The use of other laboratory data (i.e., level of serum or urine paraprotein) and radiologic findings (i.e., presence of lytic bone lesions) reflects the minimal role of histopathology in diagnosis of this entity. The recent incorporation of specific defining karyotypic abnormalities for subtyping of myeloma parallels the shift in leukemia classification [16].

Acute lymphoblastic leukemia/lymphoblastic lymphoma (ALL/LBL), which was largely ignored in the lymphoma classifications, also did not fare well under the morphology-based FAB system [17]. It has only been with the incorporation of molecular and cytogenetic data that there is now a sophisticated classification for precursor B-cell leukemias in the newest WHO schema. Parallel efforts toward a more sophisticated histogenetic approach to precursor T-cell leukemias are now underway [18,19].

1.2. The Molecular Era: Identification of Tumor–Initiating and Progression Factors

With the possible exception of childhood sarcomas, no other neoplasms have as many tumor-specific reciprocal chromosomal translocations as myeloid and lymphoid leukemias and mature B-cell lymphomas [20]. This is undoubtedly partly because one of the obligate developmental processes for lymphoid progenitors is DNA recombination of the immunoglobulin (B-cell receptor) and T-cell receptor genes to produce a functional receptor through the actions of Rag recombinases [21]. This event and the related lymphocyte-associated DNA recombination processes of immunoglobulin class switch, somatic hypermutation [22, 23] and DNA end-joining (see Chaps 12 and 31) provide mechanisms for generation of chromosome translocations in lymphomas and leukemias [24, 25]. These error-prone normal cellular processes present in lymphocytes and hematopoietic stem cells can produce aberrant chromosomal fusions at some appreciable frequency. Subsequently, these fusions, if unrepaired, can be selected biologically for those that activate genes that block cell differentiation or promote cell growth in a particular cell lineage. In most cases, translocation-bearing cells would need to acquire additional genetic changes before full-blown lymphoma or leukemia would emerge. Support for this multi-step hypothesis of tumorigenesis comes from the finding that cells bearing lymphoma-associated translocations [e.g., t(2;5) or t(14;18)] can be found circulating in the blood of peoples without apparent disease. The effects of DNA-damaging chemotherapy, ionizing radiation, or certain environmental toxins on generating DNA breaks is another possible mechanism for generation of chromosomal fusions, particularly in therapy-related leukemias [26].

Beginning in the early 1980s, Carlo Croce's laboratory and many others began to identify the genes involved in these leukemia- and lymphoma-associated chromosomal translocations by cloning and sequencing the DNA present at the breakpoint between the two partner chromosomes (Table 1-1). A well-known example was the cloning of the t(14;18) breakpoint in follicular lymphoma which demonstrated insertional activation of the antiapoptotic protein BCL2 by its juxtaposition with the immunoglobulin heavy chain (IGH) enhancer [27].

In the 1990s, mouse models of leukemia developed by the laboratories of James Downing, [28] Gary Gilliland, [29] and many others led to an understanding that leukemia-associated translocations usually produce altered transcriptional factors that have dominant–negative roles in suppressing the normal myeloid or lymphoid maturation at specific stages [30]. This has led to a simplified two-step initiation progression model for leukemia. In this scheme, class II genetic alterations, like most of the chromosomal translocations in acute leukemia, involve transcription factors that alter or block the normal maturation, and class I genetic alterations, such as activating mutations in growth factor receptors like FLT3 and KIT, produce a proliferative effect that supports the outgrowth of leukemia. In acute leukemia development, class II alterations usually occur first followed by class I alterations, whereas for chronic myeloid disorders, the reverse is true (e.g., in CML, BCR-ABL is a class I type change, whereas the Ikaros gene deletions that occur with blast transformation are class II).

This simple two-step model has been highly influential in the newest leukemia classifications although it appears too simple to explain the MDS-AML transition in the majority of patients who lack defining chromosomal translocations.

1.3. The 2008 WHO Classification

1.3.1. Overview

The current WHO classification, published in September 2008, is summarized in Tables 1-2 and 1-3. The schema was a group effort by a large number of hematopathologists and hematologist–oncologists worldwide and represents the best consensus on terminology and pathogenesis. It inevitably represents a compromise between the "lumpers" and "splitters", with a different focus for each tumor type reflective of clinical concerns and the historical considerations described above. It introduced relatively few new entities but instead there was an attempt to comprehensively incorporate molecular and immunophenotypic data.

Table 1-1. Chromosomal translocations involved in the initiation of lymphoma types.

Lymphoma type	Initiating chromosomal alterations	Gene(s) involved	of tumor in this group with this change
Follicular lymphoma	t(14;18)(q32;q21)	BCL2 by IGH	85–90% (by FISH)
Mantle cell lymphoma	t(11;14)(q13;q32)	CCND1 by IGH (cyclin D1)	95% (by FISH)
Extranodal marginal zone lymphoma	t(11;18)(q21;q21)	API2-MALT1 fusion	5% (skin)-45% (lung)
	t(1;14)(p22;q32)	BCL10 by IGH	10% (ocular/bowel)
	t(3;14)(p14;q32)	FOXP1 by IGH	20–50% (thyroid/ocular)
	t(14;18)(q32;q21)	MALT1 by IGH	5–14% (skin/salivary)
Plasma cell myeloma	t(11;14)(q13;q32)	CCND1 or MYEOV	15%15%
	t(4;14)(p16.3;q32)	FGFR3 or MMSET	5%
	t(14;16)(q32;q23)	MAF by IGH	3%
	t(6;14)(p21;q32)	CCND3 by IGH	2%
	t(14;20)(q32;q11)	MAFB	
T-cell prolymphocytic leukemia	inv14(q11q32)	TCL1 by TCRA/D	75%
	t(14;14)(q11;q32)		
T lymphoblastic leukemia/lymphoma	t(10;14)(q24;q11)	HOX11 by TCRA/D	5% (childhood)
	t(7;10)(q35;q24)	HOX11 by TCRB	15% (adult)
	t(5;14)(q35;q32)	TLX3/HLX11L2 by BCL11B/CTIP-2	10%
	t(11;14)(p15;q11)	LMO1 by TCRA/D	15–20%
	t(11;14)(p13;q11)	LMO2 by TCRA/D	3–7%
	t(8;14)(q24;q11)	MYC by TCRA/D	<1%
	t(1;14)(p32;q11)	TAL1 by TCRA/D	1–2%
	t(1;7)(p32;q35)	TAL1 by TCRB	3%
	t(7;9)(q35;q31)	TAL2 by TCRB	<1%
			<1%

For translocations involved in B lymphoblastic leukemia/lymphoma and in myeloid disorders see Tables 1-2 and 1-3

1.3.2. What the WHO Classification Says About Myeloid Leukemias

Myeloid disorders are divided into AML and other primitive stem cell leukemias, those with dysplastic features but fewer than 20% blasts (i.e. MDS), (chronic) myeloproliferative neoplasms (MPNs) with a typically indolent course, and disorders with mixed dysplastic and proliferative features, such as chronic myelomonocytic leukemia (CMML). Whenever a defining and recurrent cytogenetic aberration can be identified that is linked to pathogenesis, such as t(9;22) in CML, that genetic alteration is used to separate a neoplasm into its own category.

AML is divided into cases that have characteristic detectable genetic alterations, and others, usually emerging from MDS, in which a defining genetic change is not detected. Therefore, the current schema, in contrast to the FAB system, *requires* the use of often expensive molecular or cytogenetic testing for accurate subtyping of AML, a point which will be discussed further below.

Changes in the 2008 classification that are important to highlight in routine practice are the use of a minimum of 20% blasts (rather than 30%) as the criteria for diagnosing AML; delineation of unilineage vs. multilineage dysplasia in MDS; use of JAK2 mutational analysis as a criteria for the diagnosis of MPNs; and the inclusion of a provisional category of AML with NPM1 mutation as a good prognostic subtype typically having a normal diploid karyotype.

Table 1-2. 2008 WHO classification of hematopoietic tumors of nonlymphoid origin.

Myeloproliferative neoplasms	*Myelodysplastic syndromes*
Mastocytosis, including cutaneous and systemic forms, mast cell leukemia, mast cell sarcoma, and extracutaneous mastocytoma	Refractory cytopenias with unilineage dysplasia, including refractory anemia, neutropenia and thrombocytopenia
Chronic myelogenous leukemia (BCR-ABL1+)	Refractory anemia with ring sideroblasts
Polycythemia vera	Refractory cytopenias with multilineage dysplasia
Essential thrombocythemia	Refractory anemia with excess blasts
Chronic eosinophilic leukemia, NOS	Myelodysplastic syndrome with isolated del(5q)
Myeloproliferative neoplasm, unclassifiable	Myelodysplastic syndrome, unclassifiable
Myeloid and lymphoid neoplasms with eosinophilia and abnormalities of PDGFRA, PDGFRB, and FGFR1	Childhood myelodysplastic syndrome
	Refractory cytopenias of childhood

Acute myeloid leukemia (AML)	*Myelodysplastic/myeloproliferative neoplasms*
AML with recurrent genetic abnormalities	Chronic myelomonocytic leukemia
AML with t(8;21)(q22;q22); RUNX1-RUNX1T1	Atypical chronic myeloid leukemia, BCR-ABL1-negative
AML with inv(16)(p13.1q22) or t(16;16)(p13.1;q22); CBFB-MYH11	Juvenile myelomonocytic leukemia
Acute promyelocytic leukemia with t(15;17)(q22;q12); PML-RARA	MDS/MPN, unclassifiable
AML with t(9;11)(p22;q23); MLLT3-MLL	*Refractory anemia with ring sideroblasts associated with marked thrombocytosis*
AML with t(6;9)(p23;q34); DEK-NUP214	
AML with inv(3)(q21q26.2) or t(3;3)(q21;q26.2); RPN1-EVI1	*Related precursor disorders*
AML (megakaryoblastic) with t(1;22)(p13;q13); RBM15-MKL1	Myeloid proliferations related to Down syndrome
	Transient abnormal myelopoiesis
AML with myelodysplasia-related changes	Myeloid leukemia associated with Down syndrome
Therapy-related myeloid neoplasms	Blastic plasmacytoid dendritic cell neoplasm
	Acute leukemias of ambiguous lineage
AML, not otherwise specified	Acute undifferentiated leukemia
AML with minimal differentiation	Mixed phenotype acute leukemia with t(v;11q23); MLL rearranged
AML without maturation	Mixed phenotype acute leukemia, B/myeloid, NOS
AML with maturation	
Acute myelomonocytic leukemia	Mixed phenotype acute leukemia, T/myeloid
Acute monoblastic and monocytic leukemia	Natural killer (NK) cell lymphoblastic leukemia/lymphoma
Acute erythroid leukemia	
Acute megakaryoblastic leukemia	*Histiocytic and dendritic cell neoplasms*
Acute basophilic leukemia	Histiocytic sarcoma
Acute panmyelosis with myelofibrosis	Langerhans cell histiocytosis
	Langerhans cell sarcoma
Myeloid sarcoma	Interdigitating dendritic cell sarcoma
	Follicular dendritic cell sarcoma
	Fibroblastic reticular cell tumor
	Indeterminate dendritic cell tumor
	Disseminated juvenile xanthogranuloma

Note: Those in italics are provisional entities. Some favor using cytobands t(15;17)(q24;q21) for PML-RARA AML due to the location of the genes

1.3.3. What the WHO Classification Says About B-cell Malignancies

There have been few fundamental changes in the 2008 WHO classification for B-cell tumors when compared to the previous efforts (Table 1-3). At its heart, the schema remains a histogenetic one, mapping tumors according to sequential B-cell maturation stages as precursor lymphoblastic leukemia, mantle cell lymphoma, the pre-GC type of SLL/CLL, follicular lymphoma, the post-GC variant of SLL/CLL, lymphoplasmacytic lymphoma, and plasma cell myeloma. De novo diffuse large B-cell lymphoma is regarded as of GC or post-GC origin in nearly all cases (Fig. 1-3).

Table 1-3. 2008 WHO classification of tumors of lymphoid origin.

Precursor lymphoid neoplasms	*Mature B-cell neoplasms*
B lymphoblastic leukemia/lymphoma (BLBL)	Chronic lymphocytic leukemia/small lymphocytic lymphoma (CLL/SLL)
BLBL, NOS	
BLBL with recurrent genetic abnormalities	B-cell prolymphocytic leukemia
BLBL with t(9;22)(q34;q11.2); BCR-ABL1	Hairy cell leukemia (HCL)
BLBL with t(v;11q23); MLL rearranged	Splenic B-cell marginal zone lymphoma (SMZL)
BLBL with t(12;21)(p13;q22); TEL-AML1	*Splenic B-cell lymphoma/leukemia, NOS*
(ETV6-RUNX1)	*Splenic diffuse red pulp B-cell lymphoma*
BLBL with hyperdiploidy	*Hairy cell leukemia, variant*
BLBL with hypodiploidy	Heavy chain disease (alpha, gamma and mu)
BLBL with t(5;13)(q31;q32); IL3-IGH	Plasma cell myeloma (PCM)
BLBL with t(1;19)(q23;p13.3); E2A-PBX1	Lymphoplasmacytoid lymphoma/Waldenström
(TCF3-PBX1)	macroglobulinemia (LPL/WM)
	Solitary plasmacytoma of bone
T lymphoblastic leukemia/lymphoma	Extraosseous plasmacytoma
	Extranodal marginal zone lymphoma of mucosa-associated lymphoid tissue (MZL of MALT type)
Mature T-cell and NK-cell neoplasms	Nodal marginal zone lymphoma
T-cell prolymphocytic leukemia	Follicular lymphoma (FL)
T-cell large granular lymphocytic (LGL)	
leukemia	Primary cutaneous follicle center lymphoma
Chronic lymphoproliferative disorder	
of NK-cells	
Aggressive NK-cell leukemia	Mantle cell lymphoma (MCL)
Systemic EBV+T-cell lymphoproliferative	Lymphomatoid granulomatosis
disease of childhood	Diffuse large B-cell lymphoma (DLBCL), NOS
Hydroa vacciniforme-like lymphoma	T-cell/histiocyte-rich LBCL
Adult T-cell leukemia/lymphoma (ATLL)	Primary DLBCL of the CNS
Extranodal NK/T-cell lymphoma, nasal type	Primary cutaneous DLBCL, leg-type
Enteropathy-associated T-cell lymphoma	*EBV+DLBCL of the elderly*
Hepatosplenic T-cell lymphoma	DLBCL associated with chronic inflammation
Subcutaneous panniculitits-like	Primary mediastinal (thymic) LBCL
T-cell lymphoma	
Mycosis fungoides (MF)	Intravascular LBCL
Sézary syndrome	ALK+LBCL
Primary cutaneous CD30+ T-cell	Plasmablastic lymphoma
lymphoproliferative disorders	LBCL arising in HHV8+ Castleman's disease
Lymphomatoid papulosis	Primary effusion lymphoma
Primary cutaneous anaplastic large	Burkitt lymphoma
cell lymphoma	
Primary cutaneous CD8+ aggressive	B-cell lymphoma, with features intermediate
epidermotropic cytotoxic T-cell lymphoma	between DLBCL and Burkitt lymphoma
Primary cutaneous CD4+ small/medium	B-cell lymphoma, with features intermediate
T-cell lymphoma	between DLBCL and Hodgkin lymphoma
Primary cutaneous gamma-delta	
T-cell lymphoma	
Angioimmunoblastic T-cell lymphoma	*Hodgkin lymphoma (HL)*
Anaplastic large cell lymphoma, ALK+	Nodular lymphocyte predominant HL
Anaplastic large cell lymphoma, ALK-	Classical HL
Peripheral T-cell lymphoma, NOS	Nodular sclerosis classical HL
	Lymphocyte-rich classical HL
Posttransplant lymphoproliferative disorders	Mixed cellularity classical HL
(early, polymorphic, monomorphic types)	Lymphocyte-depleted classical HL

Note: Those in italics are provisional entities.

However, experimental data has now been incorporated to strongly link the origin of both classical and lymphocyte predominant Hodgkin lymphoma to aberrant/crippled GC B cells. There has also been the introduction of a number of new categories of large B-cell lymphoma, depending on the identification of particular inciting agents (e.g., chronic inflammation

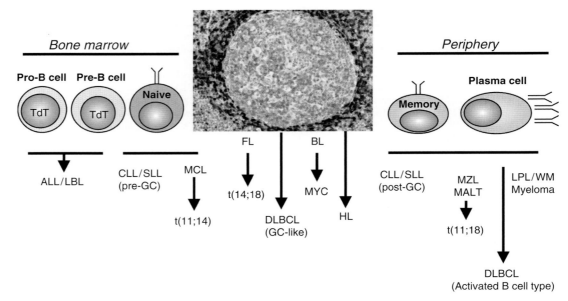

Fig. 1-3. Histogenetic classification of B-cell malignances. The association of each tumor type in relation to the normal B-cell subsets is shown. CLL/SLL has both pre-GC and post-GC subtypes, and DLBCL can arise from GC B cells, post-GC B cells, but only rarely from pre-GC B cells

or human herpesvirus 8 infection). Finally, as discussed in Chap. 15, there has also been a strong recognition that the morphologic category "marginal zone lymphoma" (MZL) actually represents several completely distinct entities, including several primary splenic lymphomas, nodal MZL, and extranodal or MALT-type MZL.

Unlike the myeloid classification, cytogenetic aberrations are mentioned as a common feature of different B-cell neoplasms (e.g., Table 1-1), but are not required for diagnosis if morphologic and immunophenotypic features are characteristic.

1.3.4. What the WHO Classification Says About T-cell and NK-cell Malignancies

As discussed in more detail in Chap. 22, the classification of T-cell and NK-cell malignancies remains incomplete and problematic. Most entities are defined based on the sites of involvement (Fig. 1-4). In the case of systemic anaplastic large cell lymphoma (ALCL), the classical entity is now limited to those tumors which have chromosomal rearrangements involving the ALK locus. However, nearly all other T/NK-cell tumors do not have a molecular definition and are separated based on their site of origin (e.g., mycosis fungoides in skin, intestinal lymphoma, and hepatosplenic lymphoma) or morphology (e.g., large granular lymphocytic leukemia). This approach has proven to have prognostic significance,[31] but lacks an elegant coherence when compared to that of the B-cell and myeloid disorders.

1.4. Weaknesses of the WHO Classification and Alternatives

The beginning student of hematopathology is advised to stop reading the chapter at this point, safe in the knowledge that the 2008 WHO classification represents the full culmination of our understanding of lymphomas and leukemias. For other readers, I close with a discussion of the assumptions, gaps, and weaknesses of the current classification efforts and examine what might be the future directions for the field.

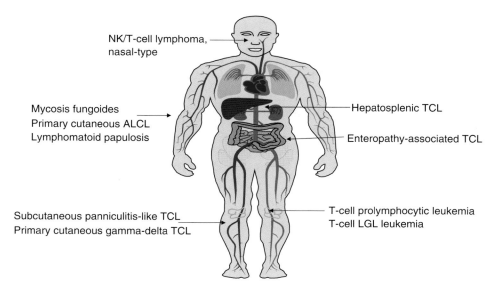

NK/T-cell lymphoma, nasal-type

Mycosis fungoides
Primary cutaneous ALCL
Lymphomatoid papulosis

Hepatosplenic TCL

Enteropathy-associated TCL

Subcutaneous panniculitis-like TCL
Primary cutaneous gamma-delta TCL

T-cell prolymphocytic leukemia
T-cell LGL leukemia

Fig. 1-4. Tissue site-based classification of T-cell and NK-cell malignancies

1.4.1. Nomenclature Dead-Ends: Why Do the Names Keep Changing?

One of the most frequent, if rather petty, criticisms of hematopathology has to do with the subtle shifts in nomenclature that arrive with each new classification. This shortcoming reflects an ongoing desire to further refine our mapping of tumor types onto the normal immune populations and onto the critical initiating genetic aberrations as they are discovered. The renaming of blastic plasmacytoid dendritic cell neoplasm and the introduction of NPM1-mutated AML as a provisional entity are two such recent examples.

However, the histogenetic approach has its limits (these are unpredictable *neoplasms* after all) and does not capture many aspects of tumor biology important for clinical management, such as etiology, risk stratification, or prediction of therapy response.

One major problem in basing diagnoses on specific genetic alterations is that they may not *always* define a particular tumor subtype causing classification headaches. For example, secondary occurrence of MYC-Ig translocations in CLL [32] or in follicular lymphoma [33] or in large B-cell lymphoma [34] has raised diagnostic difficulties with Burkitt lymphoma, which is an entity currently defined by the presence of MYC-Ig translocation. The intersecting and overlapping progression patterns common to lymphoid malignancies (Fig. 1-5) are therefore poorly represented in the WHO classification. Composite/gray-zone lymphoma syndromes such as MZL-HL [35] and ALCL-MF-HL CD30+ cutaneous tumors [36] also present problems.

However, a larger problem with focusing classification on *the* initiating genetic event is that such a two step (initiation-progression) model appears too simple for many neoplasms, including most MDS-derived AML and T/NK-cell malignancies. As described in Chap. 33, even most B-cell lymphomas have complex networks of dysregulated growth signaling at the time of presentation. The argument over whether JAK2 point mutation is the earliest defining event in the development of polycythemia vera, and subsets of myelofibrosis and essential thrombocythemia also reflects a concern over using this approach for grouping of tumors, even within an apparently molecularly homogeneous category. Therefore other approaches to lymphoma/leukemia classification are likely to emerge and are previewed in the following sections.

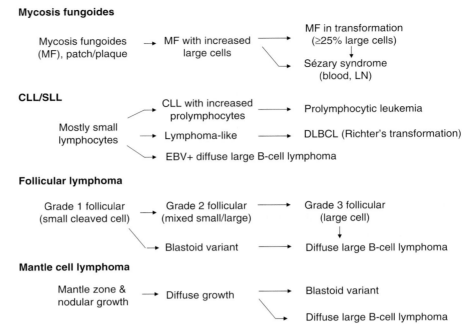

Fig. 1-5. Progression schemes for lymphoproliferative disorders. Missing from this classification scheme is the understanding that all the low-grade and small cell B-cell tumors can transform over time to large cell lymphoma variants

Table 1-4. Classification strategies for tumors.

Classifying factor	Classification based on:	Examples outside hematopathology	Examples in hematopathology
Clinical criteria			
Site of involvement	Organ site	Endocrine (e.g., carotid body, adrenal cortical, pituitary)	T-cell malignancies (e.g., intestinal lymphoma, MF)
Etiologic	External inciting agent	Hepatoma (virus, alcohol)	EBV status of DLBCL
		Medical renal disease	HTLV-I+ATLL
Histologic criteria			
Predominant histologic type	Cell size and/or appearance	Kidney, lung, germ cell, ovary and uterus	ALCL
Histologic grading	Most poorly differentiated area of tumor	Gliomas, prostate (Gleason grade) and cervix	MDS-AML sequence
			Plasma cell dyscrasias
			PTLDs
Pure histogenetic	Cell of origin	Skin and adnexa, bone/cartilage	B-cell lymphomas
			Dendritic cell tumors
Algorithmic	Grouped based on several histologic features	Inflammatory disorders in skin	Chronic myeloproliferative neoplasms
Risk-based	Classifier based on outcome	Undifferentiated sarcomas (mitotic rate)	Thymic tumors (capsular invasion)
Molecular or immunophenotypic findings			
Molecular initiation	Defining genetic event	Soft tissue sarcomas (e.g., EWS-FLI1 in Ewing's sarcoma)	B-cell lymphomas/leukemias
			ALK+ALCL
Pathway-based	Major transforming pathways	Colon (microsatellite stable vs. unstable types)	GC vs. ABC subsets of DLBCL
Therapy response	Targets for treatment	ER/PR and HER2 in breast cancer	BCR-ABL in CML

1.4.2. The Therapy-Response Predictor Approach

Although lymphoma and leukemia classifications were pioneering efforts to link normal cell biology with tumor phenotype, classification efforts in the other tumor types have often taken a different approach. These alternate approaches provide complementary and clinically important strategies to consider (Table 1-4).

For example, in breast cancer, morphogenetic classification has not advanced very far, however, the use of therapy-based classification is a major focus. The estrogen and progesterone receptor status of a breast tumor is determined in all patients at diagnosis to select those who would benefit from adjuvant hormonal therapy. Similarly, HER2 genomic amplification status is assessed by fluorescence in situ hybridization (FISH) to select patients for adjuvant immunotherapy directed against HER2. Finally, proliferative and apoptotic transcriptional signatures (e.g., OncotypeDX) are determined by PCR or by microarrays to guide the use of adjuvant chemotherapy in early-stage breast cancer.

As lymphoma and leukemia therapies move away from the standardized CHOP-based regimens into more individualized therapies with targeted biologic agents and immunotherapy, such a therapy-based classification will become more important in hematopathology.

1.4.3. The Pathway-Based Approach for Risk Modeling

In colorectal cancer (CRC), the early work of Bert Vogelstein and colleagues on the molecular changes that occur along the adenoma to carcinoma sequence [37] led to a CRC classification system that focuses heavily on differential progression pathways in microsatellite stable and unstable tumors [38]. These insights led to the understanding that different patterns of tumor progression are reflected in different histologic and clinical features of CRC and that the particular genetic pathway can influence the outcome and help determine which adjuvant therapy is likely to succeed in advanced/high-stage tumors.

Such an approach is directly applicable to lymphomas and leukemias, such as the linking of genetic subtypes of large B-cell lymphoma to therapeutically relevant pathways and targets (Chap. 32). A challenge for the future will be to determine which testing modality (e.g., genomic profiling, DNA sequencing, transcript panels, microRNA profiling, immunostaining or methylation analysis) is best, and cheapest, for pathway typing.

1.4.4. Algorithmic Classification to Simplify Diagnosis

As discussed, most approaches to lymphoma and leukemia classification have focused on tumor (molecular) histogenesis, sometimes at the expense of diagnostic simplicity (e.g., every "follicular lymphoma" that lacks t(14;18) causes a big headache). In dermatopathology, a purely morphologic or pattern recognition schema has been the standard approach. This may be because there are many more tumor and nonneoplastic entities than in hematopathology and the molecular pathogenesis of most are, as yet, poorly understood.

But such pattern recognition schemes also lend themselves to a strictly algorithmic approach that can be followed either implicitly during histologic examination or explicitly in report checklists to avoid missing possible entities. Such an algorithmic approach may be more useful for lymphoid tumors presenting at extranodal sites, where common inflammatory conditions coexist in the differential diagnosis with common and uncommon lymphoma types (see Chap. 27).

Hematopathology could also learn from the consequences of such an algorithmic approach for dermatopathology reporting. Largely based on tradition, hematopathologists are famous for writing long, anecdotal, text-based reports filled with histologic descriptions. In contrast, the synoptic reporting scheme now used in most centers for malignant melanoma is limited to specific elements of tumor type, depth of invasion, margins, and associated features such as regression and lymphocyte infiltration that have prognostic implications. These types of reports are easier to abstract into databases and then incorporate into complex statistical risk models.

1.4.5. Etiologic Risk Factors and Inciting Causes

The types of external agents which are risk factors for lymphoma development are incompletely understood, as they are for most cancers. The relative importance of occupational exposure to mutagens,[39] and inherited genetic changes have proven difficult to assess (see Chap. 38). The increased risk of lymphoma in some inflammatory conditions (e.g., inflammatory bowel disease or rheumatologic conditions) may be related to the underlying immune dysregulation or to the effects of immnosuppressive therapies [40,41]. The role of Epstein–Barr virus (EBV) in driving B-cell expansion and lymphoma in immunodeficiencies and posttransplant states as well as in senile large B-cell lymphoma and NK/T-cell lymphoma is one notable exception where a pathogenetic factor is clearly established. Other viruses have recognized roles in the outgrowth of much rarer lymphoproliferative disorders (Table 1-5). Playing a larger role in lymphomagenesis are those inflammatory conditions that lead to persistent expansions of B-cell and T-cell populations over many years. These include chronic bacterial infections, which promote B-cell lymphomas of the MALT type, and contact dermatitis, cutaneous infections, and allergies which may drive development of mycosis fungoides through chronic T-cell stimulation.

In contrast to animal models where retroviruses are implicated in leukemogenesis, the role of external agents in human myeloid leukemias are largely unknown. DNA-damaging

Table 1-5. External agents involved in the development of lymphoma.

Agent	Pathogenesis	Tumor types
Directly transforming viruses		
Epstein-Barr virus (EBV)	Early primary infection expands infected B cells	Hodgkin lymphoma Burkitt lymphoma
	Viral LMP1 drives infected B-cell expansion	Posttransplant B-cell lympho-proliferative disorders
	EBNA1 transactivates host genes	NK/T-cell lymphoma
	LMP2a regulates Notch1	Senile large B-cell lymphoma Immunosuppression-related lymphomas
Human herpesvirus 8 (HHV8)	Viral cyclin D homolog, CKR1 chemokine receptor drives angiogenesis	Multicentric Castleman's disease Plasmablastic lymphoma Primary effusion lymphoma
Human T-cell lymphotropic virus, type 1 (HTLV-I)	Viral Tax gene acts as a transcriptional regulator, upregulates IL2R (CD25)	Adult T-cell leukemia/lymphoma
Infections/antigens driving lymphoid expansion through immune response		
Helicobacter pylori	Drives T-cell mediated B-cell expansion	Gastric MZL of MALT type
Campylobacter jejuni	As above	Bowel MZL of MALT type (IPSID)
Borrelia burgdorferi	As above	Skin MZL of MALT type
Hepatitis C virus	As above	Marginal zone lymphomas
Immunosuppressant effects leading to declines in tumor surveillance		
Chemotherapy (particularly fludarabine)	Declines in T cell surveillance	EBV + lymphomas
Use of antimetabolites (e.g., methotrexate, azathioprine) for inflammatory diseases	Altered lymphocyte production	Marginal zone lymphoma
Mutagens		
Pesticide exposure	DNA damage associated with organophosphates and organochlorines	All lymphomas, particularly follicular lymphoma

Table 1-6. Mutagenic agents in the development of MDS, bone marrow cytopenia, and myeloid leukemias.

Agent	Pathogenesis	Tumor types
Chemotherapy with alkylating agents (e.g., cyclophosphamide) or antimetabolites (e.g., cytarabine)	Introduce base pair changes during DNA replication	Secondary AML and MDS
Chemotherapy with topoisomerase inhibitors (e.g. etoposide)	DNA breaks that are fixed by aberrant chromosome fusion	Secondary AML with reciprocal translocations (e.g., translocated MLL)
Occupational exposure to 1,3-butadiene (plastics and rubber industry) [39]	DNA crosslinking agents	High-grade MDS

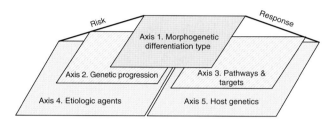

Fig. 1-6. Multidimensional model for tumor classification. A five-level classification approach that integrates the intrinsic tumor qualities (such as Axis 1-histologic/differentiation type, Axis 2-degree of genetic progression, Axis 3-activated pathways and target expression), as well as host genetic factors (Axis 4) and external factors and comorbidities (Axis 5) that may influence response

chemotherapy particularly topoisomerase inhibitors and alkylating agents have an important role in therapy-related myeloid leukemias (Table 1-6). Future progress in this area will likely transform the classification efforts more than any other developments.

1.4.6. Integrated Approaches to Tumor Classification

For practical reasons and cost considerations, it is unlikely that hematopathologists will abandon the histogenetic classification that has been the foundation of diagnosis for the last 50 years. Instead, different models of classification will be integrated that complement the current schema. One model for such a multitiered approach comes from the field of psychiatry where Axes 1–5 are used to connote different aspects of a patient's diagnosis. Such a classification approach, adapted for hematolymphoid malignancies, could include elements such as Axis 1 (histologic/differentiation type), Axis 2 (molecular grade/degree of genetic progression), Axis 3 (pathways and therapy targets expressed by tumor), Axis 4 (coexisting conditions or external etiologic agents), and Axis 5 (host genetic/pharmacogenetic background) as schematized in Fig 1-6. A hypothetical diagnostic report incorporating all of these elements for a case of follicular lymphoma is illustrated in Table 1-7.

Another approach to managing the complex constellation of data available on hematolymphoid tumors could be described as a probabilistic risk model. In this approach, for any given patient's tumor, whatever clinical, radiologic, morphologic, immunophenotypic, or molecular data is available at time of treatment could be mapped onto the wealth of data available from the other patients with similar features. A risk model could then be returned from a database search which would guide therapy. This approach, which could utilize Monte Carlo methods or insights related to the PageRank algorithm of the Google search engine, would

Table 1-7. An integrative hematopathology report of the future in a case of follicular lymphoma.

Summary Report	
Tissue Site:	Lymph node, left axillary
Procedure:	Excisional biopsy
Diagnosis:	Follicular lymphoma, moderate risk (See comment)
Comment:	See detailed report for ancillary studies associated with this neoplasm and this patient's genomic profile. Risk assessments are based on probabilistic risk modeling and are informational and not intended to provide definitive guidance on therapy selection or monitoring for this patient.

Detailed report			
Axis:	Method(s):	Finding:	Interpretation:
1. Morphology	H&E stain	Nodular growth: 75%	WHO grade 2
		Tumor cell size: mixed	
2. Molecular findings	FISH-auto count	IGH-BCL2 fusion: 58%	
	Array CGH	Loss chr 6q12, gain chr 2p13	Genomic grade: 3 of 4
	IHC-image analysis	Ki-67 = 73%	Proliferation grade: 2 of 3
	RQ-PCR, paraffin	11-gene RCHOP panel:	R-CHOP recurrence risk:
		adequate for all genes	Moderate (See ref. 1)
3. Pathway/targets	IHC-quantitative	CD20 density: 2+	Rituximab: ++
	RQ-PCR, paraffin	NF-kB targets: 3+	Bortezomib: +++
4. Coexisting condition(s)	Plasma virus	EBV titer: 100 copies/ml	High risk for viral reactivation
	PCR screen	All other viruses: undetectable	
5. Pharmacogenomic findings	SNP-PCR study	FCGR3A (Locus 158): F/F	Unfavorable: R-CHOP
(See ref. 2)	on PBMCs	C1QA: 276G	Favorable: rituximab

move away from a traditional single integrated diagnostic report and instead resemble the Gestalt thinking that many clinicians already employ.

1.5. Trends in the Workup and Follow-Up Monitoring of Lymphomas and Leukemias

1.5.1. Use of Fine Needle Aspirate to Diagnose Lymphomas

In many centers, there has been a move away from open lymph node biopsy for the diagnosis of lymphadenopathy toward a reliance on fine needle aspiration (FNA, with or without core needle biopsy). If FNA only is used to evaluate lymph node enlargement, flow cytometry is essential to adequately diagnose or exclude lymphoma. However, even with immunophenotyping, diagnosis of Hodgkin lymphoma, T-cell lymphoma, and some cases of large B-cell lymphoma remains problematic by FNA alone. Causes of missed diagnoses include inadequate sampling for technical reasons or fibrosis, and false–negative flow cytometry results due to tumor cell scarcity or loss due to fragmentation in the cytometer because of large tumor cell size.

As discussed in Chap. 12, use of FNA over open LN biopsy also has implications for the loss of information on LN microanatomical features which can be essential in arriving at a particular diagnosis for reactive lymphadenitis. Furthermore, needle aspirates often sample only a small portion of tissue within the node and may miss an occult large cell transformation. Nonetheless, the benefits of cytology in reducing cost, improving speed of diagnosis, and reducing morbidity will likely result in continuing declines in the frequency of open LN biopsy.

1.5.2. Increasing Reliance on Radiologic Studies for Lymphoma Staging

In prior years, following the diagnosis of lymphoma, staging of the spleen and liver in Hodgkin lymphoma and confirmation of pathology of additional enlarged lymph nodes was often done by open biopsy. The advent of routine nuclear medicine studies, particularly gallium scans and now positron emission tomography superimposed on computer tomography (PET/CT), has largely replaced the open biopsy for staging. However, because these scans can detect the enhanced metabolic signal characteristic of more actively replicating large cells, the identification of a "hot spot" may lead to an additional biopsy or needle aspirate to look for evidence of large cell lymphoma. As the resolution and analysis techniques for these imaging modalities improve, reliable radiologic estimates of whole body lymphoma burden will likely become an important measurement in the diagnostic workup and replace more haphazard staging algorithms.

There has also been a move away from the bilateral bone marrow trephine core biopsies for staging lymphoma toward the use of unilateral biopsy or marrow aspirate only in association with flow cytometric and molecular testing. Therefore, it has become increasingly important to integrate all of the diagnostic models into single unified pathology report to help guide therapy.

1.5.3. Sophisticated Flow Cytometric Panels

There is no better technique for analyzing the phenotype of single lymphoid or hematopoietic cells than flow cytometry (FC). Since the development of FC in the late 1970s, there have been progressive improvements in the quality of the antibody reagents, better knowledge on the normal variation in expression patterns of particular markers in different hematopoietic cell types, and increases in the number of antigens that can be tested simultaneously in a single cell. Routine use of "four-color" FC (i.e., four antigens simultaneously assessed) is now being replaced by six to seven or even 11-color in clinical testing, which provides an almost unlimited ability to separate the tumor populations from normal cell subsets.

These technical improvements have led to the development of minimal residual disease (MRD) panels which can routinely detect the presence of one tumor cell among 10,000 cells analyzed in posttherapy samples. Such MRD monitoring has been most widely used in ALL, where complete disease eradication is the treatment goal, but has been increasingly used in CLL and AML as well. One complication of this increased sensitivity of flow cytometry for lymphoma diagnostics has been the "upstaging" of many patients at the time of diagnosis due to the detection of a low-level of circulating lymphoma in blood or bone marrow that would not have been detected by any conventional morphologic examination or immunostaining. The effects of such minimal disease on patient outcomes has not yet been systematically assessed.

A parallel development in FC has been the replacement of simple algorithms for diagnosis (e.g., CD19+CD5+CD23+ cells = CLL) with complex pattern recognition or "cluster analysis," where quantitative and qualitative abnormalities in expression levels of multiple markers are used to separate the tumor cells from normal cells. This has greatly improved the diagnosis of MDS and T-cell lymphomas, where the highly complex patterns of normal BM precursors and T-cell subsets require the use of cluster analysis for an unequivocal discrimination of abnormal neoplastic populations.

1.5.4. Molecular Monitoring in Leukemia

The discovery of the genetic initiating factors in many types of leukemias has led to the widespread use of molecular markers for diagnosis and monitoring. The availability of highly sensitive and specific quantitative reverse transcriptase polymerase chain reaction (RQ-PCR) methodologies (Chap. 4) has allowed the use of routine blood monitoring in place of bone marrow evaluation for patient management. As a result, the importance of morphologic findings, particularly in posttreatment blood and bone marrow, has begun to decline. This model is best developed in CML where the level of BCR-ABL transcripts is measured in blood taken every 3–6 months and used to assess response, patient compliance and to adjust the dose of the kinase inhibitor therapy. The use of RQ-PCR monitoring has also become important in monitoring JAK2-mutated MPNs and AMLs with specific chromosomal translocations. However, even in CML, there has been variability in different approaches and in the speed of adoption of different molecular techniques, which is discussed in Chap 10 [42].

In lymphomas, there has been far less use of molecular studies for routine monitoring following treatment. This is partly because many lymphomas have very low levels of circulating tumor cells which may be difficult to detect by blood or bone marrow monitoring. However, it is also because many lymphoma treatments, such as single-agent rituximab, are not intended to be curative. There is also much less data on what various levels of molecularly detectable residual disease might mean for overall survival and recurrence in most lymphoma types.

1.5.5. Cost and Complexity Considerations in Biomarker Development

A health care economist (or an old school morphologist) would shudder at the prospects of a complex lymphoma workup as outlined in Table 1-7. Nonetheless, as the costs of molecular testing decreases and the push to do germline analysis on all patients for general risk assessment increases, baseline genomic data will be increasingly obtained in cancer patients. A computerized and inter-institutional transferable medical record is an essential component of integration of such complex data into the routine diagnosis of lymphoma and leukemia. Given the anticipated complexity of future diagnostic workups, a critical consideration will be the most cost-effective, fastest, and easiest method for obtaining tumor marker data (Table 1-8). At this moment, transcript profiling by quantitative PCR is the cheapest option, as compared to immunohistochemistry, and the former can now be done routinely in paraffin sections. Because of their ability to type single cells, flow cytometry and FISH, while expensive, will also likely continue to be important methodologies for the forseeable future.

Table 1-8. Cost–benefit comparison of biomarker methodologies.

Marker type	Methodologies	Turn-around time	Advantages	Disadvantages
Tumor-Protein detection	IHC on FFPE sections	1–2 days	High comfort level, histologic correlation	High cost (with professional billing)
Surface markers	Flow cytometry	Hours to days	Single cell profiles, rapid	High cost of reagents and labor
Serum markers	ELISA or other plate methods	Hours to days	Good dynamic ranges	Utility of most markers not yet established
Novel protein identification	Tissue based mass spectrometry	1–2 days	Flexible, expandable, minute samples	Complex, difficult to quantitate
Gene expression panels (RNA)	RQ-PCR from FFPE sections	1–2 days	Flexible, automatable	Requires adequate samples
MicroRNA profiling	PCR from FFPE sections	1–2 days	Flexible, automatable	Quantitative range and prognostic value not yet established
Tumor genomic profiling	aCGH on FFPE	3–4 days	Could be automated	Requires quality/adequate DNA
Chromosomal profiling (tumor)	G-banded karyotype	7–10 days	Whole genomic view, high comfort levels	Expensive, slow, high labor cost, complex
	FISH	1–2 days	Ideal for translocations, easy analysis	Expensive, time consuming if manual count
Host genetic background	Whole genomic SNP typing	3–4 days	One-time test, can be automated	Analysis complex
	DNA sequencing	2–3 weeks	Obtain SNP and CNV data	High cost, analysis complex

Abbreviations: *IHC* immunohistochemistry, *FFPE* formalin-fixed paraffin-embedded tissues, *RQ-PCR* quantitative reverse transcription polymerase chain reaction, *aCGH* array comparative genomic hybridization, *FISH* fluorescence in situ hybridization, *SNP* single nucleotide polymorphism, *CNV* copy number variations

Suggested Readings

Jaffe ES, Harris NL, Stein H, Isaacson PG. Classification of lymphoid neoplasms: the microscope as a tool for disease discovery Blood 2008;112:4384–99.
- A review of the histogenetic classification model for lymphomas by four hematopathologists who were instrumental in creating it.

Stenberg DW, Gilliland DG, The role of signal transducers and activators of transcription factors in leukemogenesis J Clin Oncol 2004: 22: 361–71
- The two step model of acute leukemias summarized.

References

1. Jaffe ES, Harris N, Stein H, Vardiman JW. Tumours of hematopoietic and lymphoid tissues. Lyon, France: IARC Press, 2001.
2. Swerdlow S, Campo E, Harris N, et al. WHO classification of tumors of haematopoietic and lymphoid tissues. Lyon: International Agency for Research on Cancer, 2008.
3. Lukes RJ, Collins RD. Immunologic characterization of human malignant lymphomas. Cancer 1974;34(Suppl):1488–503.
4. Lennert K. Morphology and classification of malignant lymphomas and so-called reticuloses. Acta Neuropathol Suppl 1975;Suppl 6:1–6.
5. National Cancer Institute sponsored study of classifications of non-Hodgkin's lymphomas: summary and description of a working formulation for clinical usage. The Non-Hodgkin's Lymphoma Pathologic Classification Project. Cancer 1982;49:2112–35.
6. Harris NL, Jaffe ES, Stein H, et al. A revised European–American classification of lymphoid neoplasms: a proposal from the International Lymphoma Study Group. Blood 1994;84:1361–92.
7. Willemze R, Kerl H, Sterry W, et al. EORTC classification for primary cutaneous lymphomas: a proposal from the Cutaneous Lymphoma Study Group of the European Organization for Research and Treatment of Cancer. Blood 1997;90:354–71.
8. Willemze R, Meijer CJ. EORTC classification for primary cutaneous lymphomas: a comparison with the R.E.A.L. Classification and the proposed WHO classification. Ann Oncol 2000;11(Suppl 1):11–5.
9. Bennett JM, Catovsky D, Daniel MT, et al. Proposals for the classification of the acute leukaemias French–American-British (FAB) co-operative group. Br J Haematol 1976;33:451–8.
10. Bennett JM, Catovsky D, Daniel MT, et al. Proposed revised criteria for the classification of acute myeloid leukemia. A report of the French–American–British Cooperative Group. Ann Intern Med 1985;103:620–5.
11. Nowell PC. Discovery of the Philadelphia chromosome: a personal perspective. J Clin Invest 2007;117:2033–5.
12. Greenberg P, Cox C, LeBeau MM, et al. International scoring system for evaluating prognosis in myelodysplastic syndromes. Blood 1997;89:2079–88.
13. Jaffe ES, Harris NL, Diebold J, Muller-Hermelink HK. World Health Organization classification of neoplastic diseases of the hematopoietic and lymphoid tissues. A progress report. Am J Clin Pathol 1999;111:S8–12.
14. Harris NL, Jaffe ES, Diebold J, et al. The World Health Organization classification of neoplastic diseases of the haematopoietic and lymphoid tissues: Report of the Clinical Advisory Committee Meeting, Airlie House, Virginia, November 1997. Histopathology 2000;36:69–86.
15. Criteria for the classification of monoclonal gammopathies, multiple myeloma and related disorders: a report of the International Myeloma Working Group. Br J Haematol 2003;121:749–57
16. Stewart AK, Bergsagel PL, Greipp PR, et al. A practical guide to defining high-risk myeloma for clinical trials, patient counseling and choice of therapy. Leukemia 2007;21:529–34.
17. Bennett JM, Catovsky D, Daniel MT, et al. The morphological classification of acute lymphoblastic leukaemia: concordance among observers and clinical correlations. Br J Haematol 1981;47:553–61.
18. Asnafi V, Buzyn A, Thomas X, et al. Impact of TCR status and genotype on outcome in adult T-cell acute lymphoblastic leukemia: a LALA-94 study. Blood 2005;105:3072–8.
19. Baleydier F, Decouvelaere AV, Bergeron J, et al. T cell receptor genotyping and HOXA/TLX1 expression define three T lymphoblastic lymphoma subsets which might affect clinical outcome. Clin Cancer Res 2008;14:692–700.
20. Rowley JD. Chromosomal translocations: revisited yet again. Blood 2008;112:2183–9.

21. Swanson PC, Desiderio S. V(D)J recombination signal recognition: distinct, overlapping DNA–protein contacts in complexes containing RAG1 with and without RAG2. Immunity 1998;9:115–25.
22. Lenz G, Nagel I, Siebert R, et al. Aberrant immunoglobulin class switch recombination and switch translocations in activated B cell-like diffuse large B cell lymphoma. J Exp Med 2007; 204:633–43.
23. Moldenhauer G, Popov SW, Wotschke B, et al. AID expression identifies interfollicular large B cells as putative precursors of mature B-cell malignancies. Blood 2006;107:2470–3.
24. Bassing CH, Ranganath S, Murphy M, Savic V, Gleason M, Alt FW. Aberrant V(D)J recombination is not required for rapid development of H2ax/p53-deficient thymic lymphomas with clonal translocations. Blood 2008;111:2163–9.
25. Gao Y, Ferguson DO, Xie W, et al. Interplay of p53 and DNA-repair protein XRCC4 in tumorigenesis, genomic stability and development. Nature 2000;404:897–900.
26. Super HJ, McCabe NR, Thirman MJ, et al. Rearrangements of the MLL gene in therapy-related acute myeloid leukemia in patients previously treated with agents targeting DNA-topoisomerase II. Blood 1993;82:3705–11.
27. Tsujimoto Y, Finger LR, Yunis J, Nowell PC, Croce CM. Cloning of the chromosome breakpoint of neoplastic B cells with the t(14;18) chromosome translocation. Science 1984;226:1097–9.
28. Downing JR. The core-binding factor leukemias: lessons learned from murine models. Curr Opin Genet Dev 2003;13:48–54.
29. Sternberg DW, Gilliland DG. The role of signal transducer and activator of transcription factors in leukemogenesis. J Clin Oncol 2004;22:361–71.
30. Downing JR, Higuchi M, Lenny N, Yeoh AE. Alterations of the AML1 transcription factor in human leukemia. Semin Cell Dev Biol 2000;11:347–60.
31. Herling M, Khoury JD, Washington LT, Duvic M, Keating MJ, Jones D. A systematic approach to diagnosis of mature T-cell leukemias reveals heterogeneity among WHO categories. Blood 2004;104:328–35.
32. Huh YO, Lin KI, Vega F, et al. MYC translocation in chronic lymphocytic leukaemia is associated with increased prolymphocytes and a poor prognosis. Br J Haematol 2008;142:36–44.
33. De Jong D, Voetdijk BM, Beverstock GC, van Ommen GJ, Willemze R, Kluin PM. Activation of the c-myc oncogene in a precursor-B-cell blast crisis of follicular lymphoma, presenting as composite lymphoma. N Engl J Med 1988;318:1373–8.
34. Hummel M, Bentink S, Berger H, et al. A biologic definition of Burkitt's lymphoma from transcriptional and genomic profiling. N Engl J Med 2006;354:2419–30.
35. Elmahy H, Hawley I, Beard J. Composite splenic marginal zone lymphoma and classic Hodgkin lymphoma – an unusual combination. Int J Lab Hematol 2007;29:461–3.
36. Harris NL. The relationship between Hodgkin's disease and non-Hodgkin's lymphoma. Semin Diagn Pathol 1992;9:304–10.
37. Goldberg DM, Diamandis EP. Models of neoplasia and their diagnostic implications: a historical perspective. Clin Chem 1993;39:2360–74.
38. Eshleman JR, Markowitz SD. Mismatch repair defects in human carcinogenesis. Hum Mol Genet 1996;5 Spec No:1489–94.
39. Clapp RW, Jacobs MM, Loechler EL. Environmental and occupational causes of cancer: new evidence 2005–2007. Rev Environ Health 2008;23:1–37.
40. Jones JL, Loftus EV Jr. Lymphoma risk in inflammatory bowel disease: is it the disease or its treatment? Inflamm Bowel Dis 2007;13:1299–307.
41. Kaiser R. Incidence of lymphoma in patients with rheumatoid arthritis: a systematic review of the literature. Clin Lymphoma Myeloma 2008;8:87–93.
42. Kantarjian H, Schiffer C, Jones D, Cortes J. Monitoring the response and course of chronic myeloid leukemia in the modern era of BCR-ABL tyrosine kinase inhibitors: practical advice on the use and interpretation of monitoring methods. Blood 2008;111:1774–80.

Chapter 2

Immunohistochemical Profiling of Lymphoma

Matthew W. Anderson and Yasodha Natkunam

Abstract/Scope of Chapter This chapter covers the technique of immunostaining for the characterization of lymphoma and hematopoietic tumors in tissues. The range of markers that may be diagnostically useful is discussed, as are the methodologic issues related to new marker identification, reagent validation, standardization and quantitation of staining levels.

Keywords Immunohistochemistry, basic technique • Immunohistochemistry, antigen retrieval • Immunohistochemistry, quantitative • Immunofluorescence, quantum dots

2.1. Historical Developments in the Identification of Tissue-Specific Markers

Immunohistochemistry (IHC) exploits the basic principle of the humoral immune system – specific antigen–antibody recognition and binding – to detect cell- and tissue-based molecules that can be visualized through the light microscope. Attempts to detect the distribution of antigens in tissue cells began as early as 1897 when the Russian microbiologist and Nobel laureate Metchnikoff studied the fixation of tetanus toxin in the tissues of chicken [1,2]. More specific and sensitive methods of detection of tissue antigens followed with the development of immunofluorescently-labeled antibodies using fluorescein isothiocyanate, [1] production of monoclonal antibodies with defined antigen specificity by hybridoma technology, [3] and the generation of enzyme-labeled antibodies that vastly improved the detection sensitivity by means of signal amplification [4,5]. Pioneering work in the early 1980s by Roger Warnke, David Mason, and others demonstrated the diagnostic utility of application of monoclonal antibodies to frozen and formalin-fixed paraffin-embedded (FFPE) tumor tissue sections [6]. Since that time, immunohistologic markers have been critical to the accurate diagnosis of lymphomas and its separation from other tumor types. As stipulated in the 2008 World Health Organization classification of hematopoietic tumors, the immunophenotype is integral to the diagnosis of lymphoid neoplasia [7].

Recent advances in genomic and proteomic technology have provided high throughput tools such as gene expression profiling (GEP) and tissue microarrays (TMA) that have ushered in an era of unprecedented opportunity for biomarker discovery. GEP technology allows for the identification of a clinically relevant 'expression signature' comprised of several to hundreds of different genes from just a few hundred patient-derived tumor cells. Although GEP is too expensive and analysis of the data obtained is too complex for routine use, many molecular targets can be identified that can influence prognosis or the response to

From: *Neoplastic Hematopathology*: Contemporary Hematology,
Edited by: D. Jones, DOI 10.1007/978-1-60761-384-8_2,
© Humana Press, a part of Springer Science+Business Media, LLC 2010

therapy which are then subsequently tested on less costly platforms in validation studies. TMAs are one such tool to assess individual biomarkers across hundreds of tissue samples simultaneously using IHC or RNA/DNA in situ hybridization (ISH) [8]. Validating a new marker in at least one other independent study is a desired benchmark before it can be incorporated into widespread clinical use.

Given the rapidity with which biomarkers can be uncovered using GEP techniques, it is clear that the challenge is not the want of markers but the inability to produce large-scale confirmatory and validation studies that would allow translation of these biomarkers into routine use [9]. A parallel need is for methodologic standardization and assays that are robust enough for widespread clinical use [10,11]. In contrast to the rapidity of GEP discovery, clinical marker development is slow, requiring reagent (antibody) development, establishment of the marker's analytic sensitivity and scoring reproducibility, profiling of many normal and tumor tissues to establish the marker's diagnostic specificity, and evaluation of its clinical impact and cost compared to the other markers already in use [12]. Finally, known prognostic markers must be continually reevaluated in the context of ever-changing therapeutic modalities and the advent of personalized treatment strategies.

2.2. Overview of the Immunohistochemical Technique

The goal of IHC is to reliably detect a specific antigen target in tissue sections at a level that is clearly above the background staining. In most clinical laboratories, IHC is now performed on automated stainers, but the key steps of the technique are identical whether done by hand or machine (Fig. 2-1) [13]. Since there are now a broad range of antibodies that work in FFPE tissue sections, IHC on frozen tissue sections is rarely performed anymore, and will not be discussed.

2.2.1. Antigen Retrieval

For many antibodies, heat-induced antigen retrieval results in marked improvement in staining intensity by allowing renaturation of proteins damaged by tissue fixation such that the surface epitopes recognized by antibodies are regenerated. Antigen retrieval is also capable of mitigating the degenerative effects of long-term FFPE storage by exposing antigen targets in dried-out or poorly preserved tissues. However, it should be noted that detection of some antigens (particularly with polyclonal antisera) is often more robust in unretrieved tissue sections. Antigen retrieval is done by heating the slides in buffer in a microwave oven, vegetable steamer, or pressure cooker with the heating time and the chemical composition and pH of the retrieval buffer determined empirically for each antibody. Common conditions used are

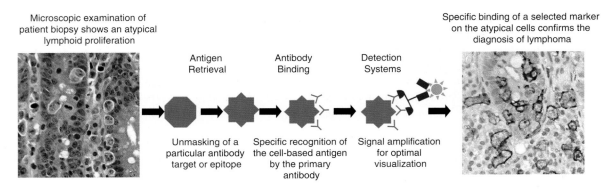

Fig. 2-1. The immunohistochemistry technique. Schematic representation shows the consecutive steps taken in using immunohistochemistry for the diagnosis of a hematolymphoid malignancy. Light microscopic assessment of a patient's stomach biopsy reveals atypical lymphoid cells. This observation then leads to the selection of an antibody panel for interrogation of a FFPE biopsy tissue for expression of specific protein markers that are interpreted in conjunction with the cytomorphologic and clinical features to arrive at a diagnosis

citric acid buffer (10 mM, pH 6.0) for 10 min, Tris buffer (5 mM, pH 10.0) for 20 min, or EDTA buffer (1 mM, pH 8.0) for 15 min. Another method for antigen retrieval is the partial digestion of tissue with proteases (e.g., trypsin).

2.2.2. Blocking Strategies

Pretreatment of sections with a blocking buffer (typically PBS containing 1–5% bovine serum albumin) is important to reduce nonspecific antibody binding; especially when using polyclonal antisera that have multiple antibodies with varied specificities. In some instances, preincubation of the tissue sections with normal serum (from the same species as the tissue or the secondary antibody) is required to further reduce the nonspecific binding. Dilution of the primary antibody will also reduce the effects of background staining but may compromise sensitivity. A short incubation of tissue sections with 0.1% hydrogen peroxide/methanol solution is useful to block endogenous peroxidases that are not easily denatured by fixation and which will otherwise contribute to background staining. When using biotin–avidin reagents, blocking high levels of endogenous biotin in certain tissue types such as pancreas, liver, kidney, and the gastrointestinal tract may be required.

2.2.3. Antigen–antibody Binding (Primary Incubation)

Diagnostic IHC is usually performed using a monoclonal antibody. These are produced by immunizing mice with the target antigen followed by fusion of the responding mouse B cells to a defective plasma cell line to create an antibody-secreting hybridoma, which produces a single clonotypic antibody directed against the target antigen. IHC can also be done with polyclonal antisera, which are usually generated by immunization of rabbits or sheep with the target antigen followed by serial collection of blood over several weeks (known as "bleeds"), with purification of the entire plasma immunoglobulin fraction by chromatography.

Monoclonal antibodies are generally preferred for IHC because they have defined specificity for a single target epitope with reproducible antigen avidity. This also allows for easier titration and reproducibility amongst different preparations of antibody. Polyclonal antibodies may be more sensitive (due to their range of different antibodies recognizing the same target) but are typically less specific (due to binding of off-target proteins) and so have increased background staining. However, with appropriate blocking reagents and careful evaluation of control tissues, polyclonal antibodies can be used with success in clinical applications. Recent strides in generating monoclonal antibodies from rabbits may provide optimal reagents with both higher affinity and defined antigen specificity [14]. The use of rabbit monoclonals have already shown an impact on the detection of specific markers in pathologic diagnosis, [15] and are likely to become increasingly popular as more become available.

The use of control tissues with each run is essential to assess the quality and specificity of staining. Construction of a TMA containing 5–10 different tissue types that would simultaneously assess the reactivity of most or all of the antibodies used in the laboratory is an efficient strategy. A section from this TMA can then be placed on each glass slide along with the diagnostic tissue to provide an internal control for each case. Such TMAs exceed the regulatory standards for controls in the clinical laboratory. At least, one negative control for staining (i.e., one that eliminates the primary antibody incubation step) should also be performed to avoid false-positive results.

2.2.4. Detection Systems

The final steps of IHC involve visualization of the antigen–antibody interactions by attaching tags or labels (e.g., active enzymes, avidin–biotin, fluorescent compounds, or gold particles) to the primary or secondary antibody. Enzymatic methods work by having the antibody-linked enzyme generate a colored product from a substrate, with the converted substrate remaining localized adjacent to the area where the antibody is bound to its target.

Direct conjugation of an antibody to a label has the advantage of rapid one-step detection, but requires a separate conjugation for each antibody and usually shows poor signal-to-noise ratio due to increased nonspecific background staining (particularly when high concentrations of antibody are used) and the lack of a signal amplification step. For these reasons, indirect detection methods in which a labeled secondary antibody is used to detect a primary (unlabeled) antibody bound to the antigen target are favored. This procedure is more efficient, as the same conjugated secondary reagent can be used in combination with many primary antibodies. In addition, higher dilutions of the primary antibody can be used without a commensurate increase in the nonspecific background staining. Many different high-affinity conjugated secondary antibodies that recognize primary antibodies raised in different species are available commercially.

Two such indirect IHC detection systems that are currently in wide use are the peroxidase–antiperoxidase (PAP) and the avidin–biotin conjugate (ABC) methods. The PAP procedure generates a secondary complex composed of rabbit antibodies directed against horseradish peroxidase and the horseradish peroxidase antigen, and generates signal amplification by the presence of many PAP complexes per primary antibody bound. A modification to this system termed APAAP (alkaline phosphatase–anti alkaline phosphatase), which uses a different colorimetric substrate, can be combined with PAP to detect two different markers in the same section (e.g., one antibody developed with a brown PAP substrate, and the other with a red APAAP substrate) [16]. The ABC system utilizes a biotinylated primary or secondary antibody that is recognized by an avidin molecule that is chemically conjugated to horseradish peroxidase and also achieves high-level signal amplification by using multivalent biotin and avidin reagents [17]. A primary limitation of both systems is that the robust signal amplification and nonspecific binding of the secondary reagents can occasionally lead to spurious positive results [13].

Polyvalent cocktails containing both polyclonal and monoclonal antibodies are another approach to enhance signal amplification. More recently, highly efficient polymer-based detection systems that utilize tyramide, dextran, or other synthetic polymers (such as EnVision, Dako, Carpinteria, California) [18–20] have been developed that have not only increased the sensitivity and specificity of detection but also provide more rapid and reliable methods of detection for the routine immunodiagnostic laboratory. These methods have also facilitated labeling of multiple antigen targets simultaneously through the use of double or triple immunoenzymatic [21] or immunofluorescence [22] techniques on FFPE tissue (Fig. 2-2).

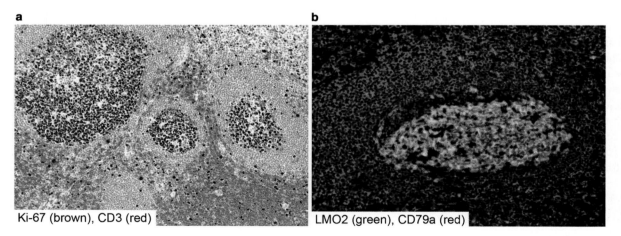

Fig. 2-2. Double labeling protein targets in paraffin-embedded tissue. (**a**) Staining of a FFPE tonsil section shows increased proliferation in germinal centers as highlighted by immunohistochemistry for Ki-67, whereas CD3 highlights T cells. (**b**) Staining of a FFPE tonsil section shows colocalization of the transcription factor LMO2 (*green*) to germinal center B cells but not to mantle or marginal zone B cells or plasma cells. In contrast, CD79a (*red*) shows labeling of all B cells and plasma cells

2.3. Immunohistochemistry Panels in the Differential Diagnosis of Lymphomas

Tumor diagnosis should always be driven by a combination of clinical presentation and morphologic findings, with selection of immunohistochemical stains based on the histologic findings. In the differential diagnosis of lymphoma, tumor cell size, cytologic grade, stage of apparent differentiation, and pattern of lymph node infiltration are the most helpful features in narrowing the selection of appropriate immunostains. In extranodal sites, morphologic clues such as sheet-like proliferations, lymphoepithelial lesions, perivascular or angiodestructive growth and plasmacytoid features can guide the choice of stains.

A workflow diagram summarizing our approach for IHC assisted diagnosis of lymphoma is shown in Fig. 2-3. The IHC panels presented in Tables 2-1, 2-2, 2-3, 2-4, 2-5, 2-6, and 2-7 have been constructed with two goals in mind: first, to allow accurate diagnosis of the lymphocytic, histiocytic, and dendritic cell entities encompassed by most recent WHO classification; [7] and second, to promote the use of cytomorphologic feature(s) to narrow the selection of appropriate immunohistologic markers. First and second tier antibodies are designated to emphasize a focused approach and to avoid the use of an unnecessarily broad panel of markers. The first tier antibodies (i.e., the basic panel) may be sufficient to arrive at a final diagnosis; however, depending on the results of the initial panel, additional markers

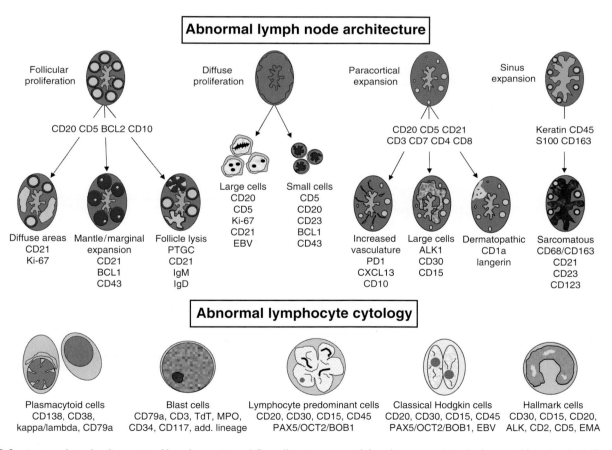

Fig. 2-3. *Approach to the diagnosis of lymphoma.* A workflow diagram summarizing the approach to the immunohistochemical diagnosis of lymphomas based on the morphologic patterns

Table 2-1. Immunodiagnostic panel for small lymphocyte proliferations with a follicular or diffuse growth pattern.

Antibody panels	
1st tier antibodies	2nd tier antibodies
CD20	Follicular dendritic cell (FDC): CD21, CD23
CD5	Additional T-cell markers: CD3, CD43
BCL2	Proliferation: Ki-67
CD10	Immunoglobulins: IgM, IgD, kappa & lambda light chains (IHC or in situ hybridization)
	Cyclins: BCL1, cyclin D2 and D3
	Additional GC B-cell markers: BCL6, HGAL, LMO2
	Plasmacytoid differentiation: CD138, CD38, CD79a
	Special markers: Annexin A1, TRAP, DBA.44, CD25
Specific applications and diagnostic entities	
Follicular lymphoma vs. follicular hyperplasia	Localization of BCL2 staining within follicles, presence of CD20, BCL2 and one or more GC B-cell markers in follicular and interfollicular areas, and the presence of t(14;18) translocation indicates lymphoma.
CLL/SLL	CD5 and CD23 coexpression, absence of CD10
Marginal zone lymphoma	CD43 coexpression, absence of CD5 and CD10
Mantle cell lymphoma	BCL1, CD5 and IgD coexpression
Lymphoplasmacytic lymphoma	CD79a, CD138, kappa or lambda, weak or absent CD20
Hairy cell leukemia	Bone marrow and splenic infiltrates associated with reticulin fibrosis that express CD20, CD25, TRAP, DBA.44 and annexin A1 (most specific)
Progression to large cell lymphoma	CD21 to highlight disrupted FDC meshworks and Ki-67 to assess increased proliferation in more diffuse areas

Table 2-2. Immunodiagnostic panel for nodular or follicular proliferations containing atypical large cells.

Antibody panels	
1st tier antibodies	2nd tier antibodies
CD20	EBV: EBER in situ hybridization
CD3	CD45 (LCA)
CD30	Additional B-cell transcription factors: OCT2, BOB1, PU.1
CD15	
PAX5	GC T cell: CD57, PD-1
Specific applications and diagnostic entities	
Nodular lymphocyte predominant Hodgkin lymphoma	CD20+ large atypical cells within and outside B-cell rich follicles with partial or absent CD30, absent CD15 and EBV, and strong CD45 and B-cell transcription factors; ringing of large cells by CD57+ and PD-1+ T cells
Classical Hodgkin lymphoma	CD30+ large cells with expression of CD15, EBV, partial or absent CD20, and weak or absent expression of B-cell transcription factors and absent CD45

Table 2-3. Immunodiagnostic panels for diffuse large B-cell proliferations.

Antibody panels

1st tier antibodies	2nd tier antibodies
CD20	If mediastinal mass: CD30, CD15, CD23
CD5	If plasmacytoid differentiation: CD138, CD38, CD79a
Ki-67	
CD21	If suspected viral pathogenesis: EBV EBER, HHV8
	B-cell transcription factors: PAX5, OCT2, BOB1, PU.1
	Germinal center (GC) B cells: CD10, BCL6, HGAL, LMO2

Specific applications and diagnostic entities

Burkitt lymphoma	Monomorphic cytology with expression of CD20, CD10, ~ 100% Ki-67, and absence of BCL2.
	EBER + in subset
B-cell lymphoma, unclassifiable, with features intermediate between DLBCL and Burkitt lymphoma	Intermediate cytomorphologic features with expression of CD20 and CD10, variable expression of Ki-67 and BCL2
	Correlate with cytogenetics or FISH for t(14;18), t(8;14) or variants or BCL6 translocations for double-hit or triple-hit cases
DLBCL, NOS	Pleomorphic cytomorphologic features with CD20 expression
	Assess EBV status in ≥ 50 years to distinguish EBV + large B-cell lymphoma of the elderly
Primary mediastinal large B-cell lymphoma	Express CD20 and typically coexpress CD30 and CD23, and lack CD15. Also shows strong expression of B-cell transcription factors
B-cell lymphoma, unclassifiable, with features intermediate between DLBCL and CHL	Intermediate cytomorphologic features with Hodgkin-like cells and variable expression of CD20, CD30 and CD15 as well as strong expression of B-cell transcription factors
Primary effusion lymphoma	Usually express CD45, CD138, CD30 and EBV EBER, but lack pan-B markers. May have associated T-cell marker expression. Rearranged Ig genes and also TCR is subset
Plasmablastic lymphoma	Express CD138, CD38 and partial CD79a and lack or show weak expression of CD45, CD20 and PAX5. Lack HHV8 and CD56. EBV EBER in 60–75%
	Clonal IgH rearrangements usually present
ALK + large B-cell lymphoma	Express ALK, CD138 and lack CD20, CD79a, CD3. CD45 and CD30 may be weak or negative. Usually express cytoplasmic Ig (IgA>IgG)
Large B-cell lymphoma arising in HHV8-associated multicentric Castleman disease	Variable expression of CD20 and CD38, and lack CD79a, CD138 and EBV EBER. Interfollicular plasma cells express cytoplasmic IgA and polytypic light chains (microlymphomas). Express HHV8

Table 2-4. Plasma cell proliferations.

Antibody panels	
1st tier antibodies	2nd tier antibodies
CD138	Pan B-cell: CD20
Kappa/lambda light chains (IHC or ISH)	Plasmacytoid differentiation: CD38, CD79a
	Viral: EBV EBER, HHV8
CD5	Germinal center (GC) B cells: CD10, BCL6
Specific applications and diagnostic entities	
Monoclonal gammopathy of undetermined significance (MGUS)	Less than 10% clonal plasma cells in bone marrow that express CD138
Plasma cell myeloma	At least 10% clonal plasma cells in the bone marrow that express CD138. Atypical morphology and coexpression of CD56 in subset
Extraosseous and solitary plasmacytoma of bone	Clonal CD138-positive plasma cells in extramedullary or bony sites; must be distinguished from lymphomas with prominent plasmacytoid differentiation such as marginal zone, plasmablastic and DLBCL
Monoclonal immunoglobulin deposition diseases (MIDD)	Visceral and soft tissue deposition of immunoglobulins compromising organ function.

from the list of second tier antibodies can be added as necessary. However, IHC cannot be the sole adjunct diagnostic tool, as correlation with cytogenetic and molecular genetic studies is required for some tumors.

Although many of the antibodies in basic panels have been used for years, some more recently characterized immunohistologic markers have shown clinical utility. For example, antibodies directed against two markers of germinal center (GC) B cells, HGAL [23] and LMO2, [24] are excellent adjuncts to CD10 and BCL6 in typing large B-cell lymphoma, and in demonstrating follicle center derivation (Figs. 2-4, 2-5, 2-6). Especially in cases with equivocal or absent CD10 and BCL6 expression, they are particularly useful in the separation of diffuse follicle center lymphomas, which express HGAL and LMO2, from marginal zone lymphomas, which do not. Unlike BCL6 whose expression in GC-associated T cells can complicate diagnosis of T-cell rich follicular proliferations, HGAL and LMO2 are not expressed in T cells [23,24]. Antibodies against two recently characterized markers of GC T cells, PD-1, [25,26] and CXCL13, [27] can identify angioimmunoblastic T-cell lymphoma as both markers stain the neoplastic cells (Fig. 2-7) whereas the other T-cell lymphomas do not. Another use of PD-1 is as a diagnostic marker of the nonneoplastic GC-type T cells that typically surround the neoplastic large B cells in nodular lymphocyte predominant Hodgkin lymphoma (NLPHL, Fig. 2-8).

Immunostaining for one or more of the B-cell transcription factors PAX5, OCT2, BOB1, and PU.1 [28,29] can be useful in the distinction between NLPHL and classical Hodgkin lymphoma (CHL) especially in those cases in which the latter expresses CD20 and/or lacks CD15. As documented by GEP studies, [30] Reed-Sternberg cells of classical Hodgkin lymphoma typically show absent or weak expression of the above four B-cell transcription factors (PAX5 shown in Fig. 2-9a), whereas they are expressed at higher levels in the tumor cells of NLPHL (OCT2 shown in Fig. 2-9b). Similarly, these markers can be used to support the diagnosis of large B-cell lymphoma over CHL in mediastinal tumors with limited sampling or unusual features and help to reduce the need to place cases in the borderline category

Table 2-5. Immunodiagnostic panels for diffuse large-cell and paracortical proliferations derived from T and NK cells.

Antibody panels	
1st tier antibodies	2nd tier antibodies
CD20	Additional pan-T-cell: CD3, CD2, CD7, CD4, CD8, CD43
CD5	Additional B/plasma cell: PAX5, CD79a, CD138, Kappa, lambda light
Ki-67	chains
CD21	Cytotoxic granule-associated proteins: Granzyme B, TIA1, perforin
	GC T cell: programmed death-1 (PD-1), CXCL13, CD10
	Histiocytic: CD163, CD68, Lysozyme
	NK and NK/T cell: CD56
	Hodgkin: CD30, CD15
	Viral: EBV EBER, HHV8
	Tyrosine kinase: ALK-1

Specific applications and diagnostic entities	
Peripheral T-cell lymphoma, NOS	T-cell proliferation with or without loss of pan-T-cell markers. Monoclonal TCR rearrangements are often present
	Secondary EBV-associated B-cell proliferations may be present and should be confirmed with B-cell clonality studies
Angioimmunoblastic T-cell lymphoma	Expanded CD21-positive FDC meshworks and expression of
	GC T-cell markers PD-1, CXCL13 and CD10
	Secondary EBV-associated B-cell proliferations may be present and should be confirmed with B-cell clonality studies
Anaplastic large cell lymphoma, ALK+	Typically sinusoidal infiltrate with pleomorphic horseshoe-shaped nuclei with expression of CD30 and ALK1
Anaplastic large cell lymphoma, ALK-	Identical to ALK+ lymphoma but without expression of ALK1
Extranodal NK/T-cell lymphoma, nasal type	Expression of CD56, CD2 and cytotoxic granule-associated proteins and absence of surface CD3 but positive for cytoplasmic CD3. None of these markers are specific (also in gamma/delta T cells); correlation with clinical features and sites of involvement is required
Enteropathy-associated T-cell lymphoma	Intraepithelial atypical lymphocytes express CD3, CD7, CD103, cytotoxic granule-associated proteins and TCR-gamma/delta with variable expression of CD30 and CD56, and lack of CD5 and CD8
Hepatosplenic T-cell lymphoma	Intrasinusoidal hepatosplenic and bone marrow infiltrates that express CD3, gamma-delta T cells, variably express CD56 and CD8, and usually lack CD5 and CD4. Express TIA1 but not granzyme B or perforin
Subcutaneous panniculitis-like T-cell lymphoma	Subcutaneous infiltrate involving fat lobules that express TCR-alpha/beta, CD8 and cytotoxic granule-associated proteins
EBV-positive T-cell lymphoproliferative disorders of childhood	Acute onset with systemic infiltrates of EBV-positive T cells of variably sized cells that express CD2, CD3, CD8, and TIA1 and lack CD56. Hydroa vacciniforme-like lymphoma with associated sensitivity to sun and insect bites
Mycosis fungoides	Epidermotropic primary cutaneous small-to-medium sized infiltrate that expresses CD2, CD3, CD4, CD5 and TCR-alpha/beta, and lacks CD7 and CD8
Primary cutaneous CD30+ T-cell lymphoproliferative disorders	Spectrum of overlap with reactive entities and nonepidermotropic infiltrates that express CD4, CD30, and cytotoxic granule-associated proteins with frequent loss of CD2, CD3 and CD5
Primary cutaneous peripheral T-cell lymphomas, rare subtypes	Includes gamma/delta T-cell lymphoma, aggressive epidermotropic CD8-positive T-cell lymphoma and CD4-positive small/medium pleomorphic T-cell lymphoma

Table 2-6. Panel for tumors with blastic morphology.

Antibody panels	
1st tier antibodies	2nd tier antibodies
CD79a	Progenitor: CD34, CD117
CD3	Additional B-cell: PAX5
TdT	Additional T-cell: CD3, CD2, CD7, CD4, CD8, CD43
MPO (myeloperoxidase)	Myelomonocytic: CD163, CD68, Lysozyme, CD43
	Megakaryocytic: CD61, CD31, Factor VIII, LAT
	Erythroid: glycophorin C, hemoglobin A
	Mast cell: Mast cell tryptase, CD117, CD25, CD2
	Plasmacytoid dendritic/NK: CD123, CD56
	If mantle cell lymphoma suspected: cyclin D1 (BCL1)
Specific applications and diagnostic entities	
B-lymphoblastic lymphoma/ leukemia	CD79a, TdT and CD10 with weak or absent CD20 and moderate to high Ki-67
	Correlation with cytogenetic studies is important for prognostic subclassification
T-lymphoblastic lymphoma/ leukemia	CD3, TdT and CD10 with moderate to high Ki-67
	Correlation with cytogenetic studies is important for prognostic subclassification
Acute myeloid leukemia	Presence of progenitor markers and myelomonocytic markers
	Coexpression of CD56 or CD7 may be present in a subset.
	Monocytic leukemias often lack CD34 and MPO
	Rarely, erythroid or megakaryocytic leukemias (also often CD34-negative) that present in extramedullary sites may require specialized lineage markers
	Correlation with cytogenetic studies is important for prognostic subclassification
Blastic mantle cell lymphoma	Expression of CD5 and BCL1
Mast cell proliferations/ leukemia	Expression of mast cell tryptase and CD117, CD2 and CD25; rule out concurrent involvement by associated myelomonocytic leukemia
Blastic plasmacytoid dendritic cell neoplasm	Expression of CD123, CD56 and CD4. Usually lacks EBV and other myelomonocytic and T-cell markers

of B-cell lymphoma, unclassifiable, with features intermediate between diffuse large B-cell lymphoma and classical Hodgkin lymphoma [7].

2.4. Immunoprofiling Uses Other Than for Lineage Assignment

Immunostaining can be used not only to define tumor lineage and assist in diagnosis but also to aid in tumor grading (e.g., quantification of the number of proliferating cells by Ki-67) and blast counts (e.g., CD34 or TdT stains), and to look for minimal residual disease. These applications are discussed in more detail in the other chapters. Here, we highlight the use of IHC in detecting expression of therapy targets (e.g., CD20 in lymphomas which might benefit from anti-CD20 immunotherapy), in detecting altered subcellular localization of proteins, and most especially in detecting biomarkers of outcome and therapy response.

Table 2-7. Panel for tumors with a sinusoidal to diffuse lymph node infiltration pattern.

Antibody panels

1st tier antibodies	2nd tier antibodies
Pankeratin	Additional histiocytic: CD68, lysozyme
CD45 (LCA)	Myeloid: myeloperoxidase
S100	Langerhans cell: CD1a, langerin
CD163	Follicular dendritic cell: CD21, CD23, CD35
	Plasmacytoid dendritic: CD123, CD56, CD4
	Additional neural, melanocytic and epithelial markers may be necessary depending on the clinical presentation

Specific applications and diagnostic entities

Histiocytic sarcoma	Diffuse, noncohesive, predominantly sinusoidal proliferation of mature histiocytes that express CD163 and CD68, and lack CD1a, langerin, CD21, CD35 and myeloid markers
Langerhans cell histiocytosis	Proliferation of spindled to ovoid Langerhans cells with minimal atypia, typically in a sinus distribution in lymph nodes, or diffusely in extranodal sites or bone with associated eosinophilia. Expression of CD1a, S100, CD68 and langerin. Birbeck granules on electron microscopy
Langerhans cell sarcoma	Langerhans cells with markedly atypical cytologic features that express the Langerhans cell immunophenotype above
Sinus histiocytosis with massive lymphadenopathy (Rosai–Dorfman disease)	Specialized macrophages exhibiting emperipolesis that express S100 and CD163, often associated with abundant reactive plasma cells and fibrosis
Interdigitating dendritic cell sarcoma	Spindled to ovoid cell proliferation arranged in fascicles in a paracortical distribution that expresses S100 but lacks specific markers of Langerhans and follicular dendritic cells
Follicular dendritic cell sarcoma	Spindled to ovoid cell proliferation arranged in fascicles or whorls with a sprinkling of small lymphoid cells sometimes surrounding blood vessels. Cells express CD21, CD23 and CD35, and variably positive for CD68, S100 and EMA
Disseminated juvenile xanthogranuloma	Proliferation of xanthomatous histiocytes with Touton-type giant cells that express CD68, CD163, Factor XIIIa with variable expression of S100

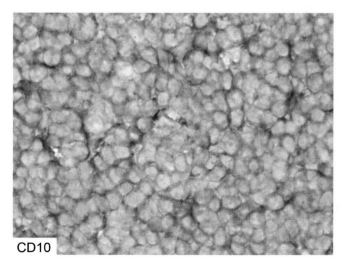

CD10

Fig. 2-4. *Immunohistochemistry for CD10.* Immunohistochemistry for CD10 protein shows staining localized primarily to the plasma membrane of the neoplastic cells in a case of diffuse large B-cell lymphoma

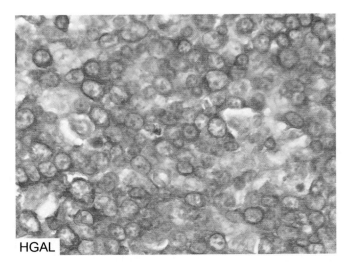

Fig. 2-5. *Immunohistochemistry for HGAL.* Immunohistochemistry for HGAL (human germinal center-associated lymphoma) protein shows staining within the cytoplasm of neoplastic cells in a case of diffuse large B-cell lymphoma

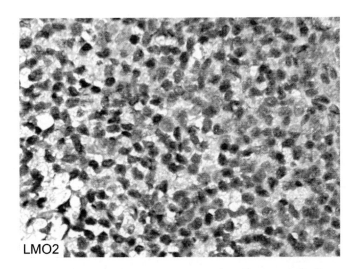

Fig. 2-6. *Immunohistochemistry for LMO2.* Immunohistochemistry for LMO2 protein shows staining localized primarily to the nucleus of neoplastic cells in a case of diffuse large B-cell lymphoma

Table 2-8 shows some examples of how immunohistologic markers may be used in each of these contexts (modified and expanded from Natkunam and Mason 2006) [9].

2.4.1. Use of Immunostaining to Detect Subcellular Localization of Proteins

Because it is performed in situ, IHC can be used to define the subcellular localization of proteins. Figs. 2-3–2-5 show the staining patterns of three GC B-cell-associated proteins that localize to the plasma membrane (CD10), cytoplasm (HGAL), [23] and nucleus (LMO2), respectively, [24] in a case of diffuse large B-cell lymphoma (DLBCL). Aberrant localiza-

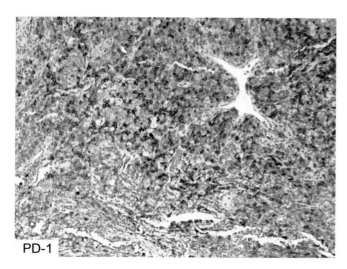

Fig. 2-7. *Immunohistochemistry for angioimmunoblastic T-cell lymphoma.* Immunohistochemistry for the germinal center T-cell-associated marker PD-1 shows labeling of a significant number of cells comprising the atypical lymphoid infiltrate

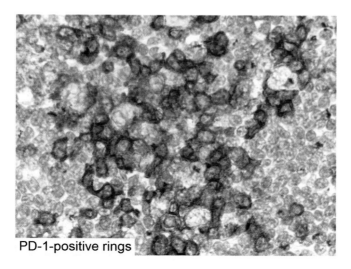

Fig. 2-8. *Immunohistochemistry for nodular lymphocyte predominant Hodgkin lymphoma.* Immunohistochemistry for PD-1 highlights T cells surrounding large atypical cells in a ring-like pattern in a case of nodular lymphocyte predominant Hodgkin lymphoma

tion of a protein can occasionally provide important clues to the underlying genetic event in a tumor. A well-known example is the abnormal accumulation of the NPM1-ALK fusion protein in the nuclei of anaplastic large cell lymphoma (ALCL) as a result of the t(2;5) translocation [31]. More recently in AML, cytoplasmic localization of the NPM1 protein (which normally shuttles between the cytoplasm and nucleus) has been shown to correlate with the

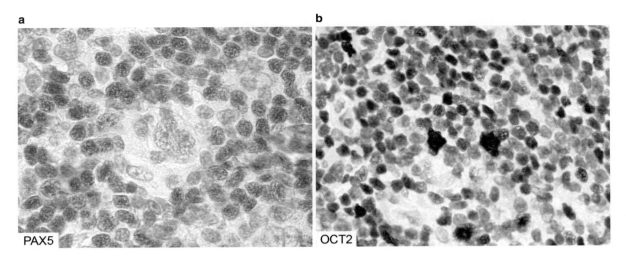

Fig. 2-9. *B-cell transcription factors in the subtyping of Hodgkin lymphoma.* (**a**) Diminished expression of the B-cell transcription factor PAX5 in Reed-Sternberg cells in a case of classical Hodgkin lymphoma in comparison to nonneoplastic small B cells in the background. (**b**) In contrast, intense expression of the B-cell transcription factor OCT2 in large atypical cells favors a diagnosis of lymphocyte predominant Hodgkin lymphoma in a case of Hodgkin lymphoma with expression of CD20 and CD30 but not CD15

Table 2-8. Examples of immunohistochemical markers used for tumor grading, prognostic prediction and as therapeutic targets.

Immunohistologic marker	Protein function, location	Association with genetic or prognostic feature
Ki-67 in B-cell lymphoma	S-phase marker of proliferating cells, nuclear	Increased expression (>50%) usually associated with aggressive lymphomas
BCL2 expression in follicular B cells	Anti-apototic protein, cytoplasmic	Overexpressed in follicular lymphoma due to t(14;18) (q32;q21)
BCL1 expression in small B-cell lymphoma	Cell cycle regulator, nuclear	Overexpressed in mantle cell lymphoma due to t(11;14) (q13;q32)
ALK expression in T-cell lymphoma	Dysregulated tyrosine kinase, nuclear if NPM1 is partner	Expressed due to t(2;5) (p23;q35) or variants
Cytoplasmic localization of NPM1 expression in AML	Transcriptional regulator, cytoplasmic localization suggests mutation	Mutated form confirms good prognosis in FLT3-unmutated AML
Lost or diminished expression of PAX5, OCT2, BOB1, or PU.1	Transcription factors that link BCR signaling to B-cell transcriptional program	Aids in the separation of CHL from NLPHL and other large B-cell lymphomas
CD20 expression in B-cell lymphomas	Pan-B-cell surface glycosylated phosphoprotein	Target of the therapeutic chimeric monoclonal antibody rituximab
CD33 expression in acute myeloid leukemia	Transmembrane receptor, expressed in myeloid cells and most AML	Target of anti-CD33 immunotherapy gemtuzumab ozogamicin (Mylotarg)

Abbreviations: *AML* acute myeloid leukemia, *CHL* classical Hodgkin lymphoma, *NLPHL* nodular lymphocyte predominant Hodgkin lymphoma

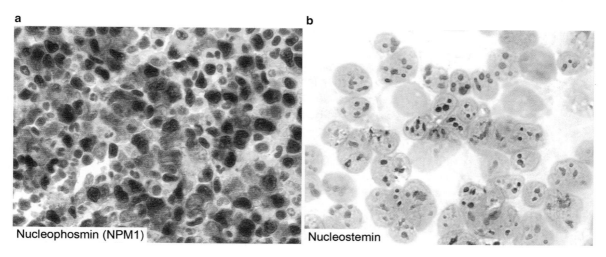

Fig. 2-10. *Nucleolar proteins in hematopoietic malignancy.* (**a**) Immunohistochemistry for nucleophosmin (NPM1) in a case of acute myeloid leukemia shows expression of the protein in the nucleus (normal pattern) as well as in the cytoplasm (aberrant pattern) resulting from a c-terminus mutation of the *NPM1* gene; (**b**) nucleostemin, a protein that localizes to the nucleolus is shown for comparison

presence of dominant-negative NPM1 truncation mutations, a finding that has prognostic implications (Fig. 2-10) [32–34].

2.4.2. Immunostaining to Detect Prognostic Markers: Successes and Failures

Translating GEP studies into IHC markers: The use of genome-wide discovery tools has vastly increased the number of new biomarkers whose detection may be relevant in tumor tissues. An important milestone in this regard was the use of GEP in DLBCL to link expression of genes indicative of B-cell differentiation state to clinical outcome. In the initial studies, two subsets of DLBCL were identified with expression profiles resembling either germinal center B cells (GCB) or activated peripheral blood B cells (ABC), with the ABC subtype having a worse outcome following standard chemotherapy (see Chaps. 17 and 33) [35,36]. Subsequent GEP studies in DLBCL identified expression signatures related to B-cell receptor signaling and the cell cycle, mitochondrial function and oxidative phosphorylation, and the background host inflammatory and immune response. These studies have shown that when the expression pattern of thousands of genes are simultaneously analyzed, different subsets of DLBCL are found that reflect many features of normal lymphocyte subsets and that these differences can have prognostic significance [37].

All of these GEP studies have identified a wealth of markers that require further testing and validation in IHC assays. Although immunohistologic methods can be used to assess many markers simultaneously, such high throughput screening is generally not practical or cost-effective [9]. Therefore, most IHC studies have selected a limited subset of markers for which high-quality IHC antibodies are available. Such confirmatory IHC studies using a limited number of markers have not always seen the clear-cut histogenetic differences produced by the RNA-based GEP profiles. For example, the GCB markers HGAL, [23] LMO2, [24] and JAW1/LRMP, [38] while expressed in the GCB-type of DLBCL, were also shown to be expressed in a significant number of cases with an apparent ABC GEP pattern. These results demonstrate that IHC detection of a small number of tumor-associated IHC markers may not provide the needed discriminatory power for meaningful clinical prognostication in a complex, biologically heterogeneous disease such as DLBCL.

The contribution of the tissue microenvironment to the genesis, prognosis, and progression of lymphomas has focused attention on the value of immunomarkers that stain nontumor elements instead. For example, tumor-infiltrating host inflammatory cells such as macrophages, and stromal molecules such as fibronectin and SPARC, have been shown to correlate with clinical behavior in DLBCL [37,39,40]. Signaling molecules such as the enzyme protein tyrosine phosphatase 1B (PTP1B) are differentially expressed in lymphoma subtypes, [41] and angiogenic parameters such as microvessel density (detected by CD34 IHC) and expression of vascular endothelial growth factor (VEGF) and/or its receptors may be useful, [42,43] especially if anti-VEGF agents are introduced for lymphoma therapy.

Problems with marker selection: Many IHC-based studies of prognostic significance have had inherent flaws in their selection of targets. Proteins are often chosen based solely on the availability of suitable antibodies and therefore may be irrelevant to disease pathogenesis, show expression which varies in different areas of the tumor, or have only modest differences in expression between subgroups that are difficult to separate using nonquantitative IHC [9]. Each year, the pathology literature contains hundreds of pilot studies on prognostic markers, however, only a small fraction of these markers are used clinically to aid in outcome prediction or in tailoring therapy. Some of these markers fail to advance because the reported differences between subgroups in expression level of the marker, while statistically significant, are slight and difficult to reproduce in subsequent studies. In this regard, studies of prognostic markers in DLBCL are particularly illustrative. Over 40 IHC markers have been described to date that predict prognosis in DLBCL, but the majority have never been confirmed in a second independent cohort of patients; other markers have yielded conflicting results in the subsequent studies [9].

One guide for selecting potential prognostic markers from GEP studies for IHC confirmation is to remember that most such successful markers have been directly related to the disease pathogenesis, namely those linked to a specific tumor-associated genetic abnormality or with therapeutic or experimental evidence for a central role in oncogenesis. For example, immunohistochemical detection of ALK as a clinical predictor of favorable outcome in ALCL was rapidly adopted precisely because it was the protein activated by a tumor-specific chromosomal translocation. Interestingly, such widespread use of ALK immunostaining in IHC panels then led to the identification of other lymphoma types that express this protein and these tumors (e.g., ALK + B-cell lymphoma) were then classified as distinct entities [44]. In this way, use of marker directly linked to disease pathogenesis can drive revisions in tumor classification due to its central transforming role.

The effect of shifts in therapy on IHC markers: Even if a useful biomarker is developed, advances in treatment may render its use obsolete. For example, the addition of the anti-CD20 monoclonal antibody rituximab to anthracycline-based chemotherapy (R-CHOP) was recently shown to improve the survival of DLBCL patients, which reduced the value of IHC-based algorithms for DLBCL subtyping [45–48]. Under certain circumstances, IHC may not be sensitive enough for the detection of subtle differences in the expression of receptors and signaling molecules that may predict response to targeted therapy. Emerging technologies such as phosphospecific flow cytometry, [49] proteomics [50] and automated imaging and quantitation [51] may increase a biomarker's diagnostic and prognostic utility and are discussed below.

2.5. Standardization Issues for IHC Studies

2.5.1. Establishing the Validity of a New Marker

To provide better translation of biomarkers into routine clinical practice, a standardized approach to marker development is needed. Once a new marker has been identified, well-defined antibody reagents to probe its expression in tumors should be developed. The specificity of an antibody for its target should be confirmed by the presence of an appropriately-sized band on Western immunoblot of protein lysates from a relevant cell type, and its subcellular localization pattern determined (usually by immunofluorescent confocal microscopy). Whenever possible, the antibody should also be tested for its ability to immunoprecipitate the target protein. Next, IHC should be performed on an appropriate control tissue with a variety of different dilutions of the primary antibody and several antigen retrieval conditions. Finally, the range of expression in normal tissues (tonsil, lymph node, thymus, spleen, bone marrow) and tumors should be analyzed, focusing on any expression seen in the host inflammatory cells and stroma that may complicate the scoring of tumor staining. Analysis of marker expression in nonhematopoietic tissues or in special niches (e.g., intraepithelial lymphocytes, tumor vasculature, etc.) may also identify unexpected uses for the marker. TMAs are extremely useful for these studies and a comprehensive system developed for the use of TMAs will be detailed below.

2.5.2. Scoring Criteria and Reproducibility of Stain Interpretation

Even with high quality reagents, the cumulative experience using IHC for prognostication suggests that differences in laboratory techniques, scoring definitions, and inter- and intra-observer variability in defining the positive results can lead to poor reproducibility of results. IHC is usually recorded on an ordinal scale (e.g., 0, 1+, 2+), but there are often widely variable cut-offs for the percentage of immunopositive cells regarded as significant and for the interpretation of varying staining intensities and differential subcellular localization. In clinical studies, there has been little effort to establish guidelines for the use of IHC markers in diagnostic studies, and this has resulted in a significantly low concordance rate across published studies for routinely used markers. These differences are magnified even more when scoring criteria used for one clinical trial are completely incongruent with thresholds used in a different trial.

The importance of uniform scoring criteria was demonstrated in studies on the use of IHC to replicate the GCB vs. ABC risk-model of DLBCL. The two large multi-institutional collaborative studies using CD5, CD10, CD20, BCL2, BCL6, and Ki-67 to distinguish DLBCL subtypes reported a high degree of variability in the laboratory methodology and scoring interpretation [10,11]. Across 24 participants in one study, concordance rates for IHC scoring varied from a dismal 35% for Ki-67 to an excellent 95% for CD20 staining; suggesting that some markers are more difficult to interpret than others [11]. When a uniform IHC methodology was used and the participants were trained using a predefined scoring criteria, concordance rates in a second round of scoring showed a vast improvement (up to 53–100%). These studies point to the importance of optimizing laboratory techniques and establishing and adhering to scoring definitions. As a result, centralized consensus review has now been adopted for many large multi-institutional clinical studies to minimize the impact of inter-institutional and inter-observer variability.

2.6. Tissue Microarrays and Databasing of Immunohistochemistry Results

TMA are a highly efficient method for studying protein and RNA expression, enabling a rapid survey of hundreds of patient samples in a single experiment [52]. TMAs are constructed from 0.6 to 2.0 mm tissue cores transferred from each individual tumor paraffin blocks to a recipient paraffin TMA block using a tissue arrayer and then sectioned by routine microtomy (Fig. 2-11). At least two to three different cores from each tumor block should be transferred to ensure the reproducibility of staining in different areas of the tumor. Selection of blocks with thicker sections of tumor tissue is recommended so that the TMA is not exhausted after a few sections.

Given the large numbers of tissue samples on each TMA, array design, scoring of staining and archiving of results can be problematic. Resources for TMA design and interpretation are listed in Table 2-9, and the Stanford Tissue Microarray Database (TMAD), which we

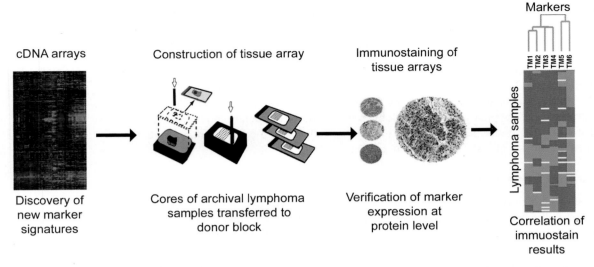

Fig. 2-11. *From gene expression profiling to tissue microarrays.* Schematic representation illustrating the discovery of novel gene targets from gene expression arrays that are subsequently validated at the protein level in human lymphoma biopsy samples with the aid of tissue microarrays. Hierarchical cluster and tree-view algorithms are used to database the high throughput information generated from multiple markers across multiple tumor samples

Table 2-9. Tissue microarray-based resources.

Resource	Description	References
The Stanford Tissue Microarray Database (TMAD) http://tma.stanford.edu	Information on standard probes as well as novel and emerging markers	53
	Includes 250,000 digitized images generated from approximately 1500 stained slides of TMAs	
The Human Protein Atlas Project http://www.proteinatlas.org/	Information on 48 normal human tissues and 20 cancers	54
	Includes over 400,000 images corresponding to over 700 antibodies	
The Nordic Immunohistochemical Quality Control Organization http://www.nordiqc.org	Stained images of thousands of clinically important protein targets	55
	Participation from > 100 laboratories	
	In-depth information on antibodies and protocols	

have built, is described in more detail below. Automated image acquisition and archiving software from TMAs is available from a number of sources. For example, the *BLISS* microscope-imaging system (Bacus Laboratories, Inc., Slide Scanner (*BLISS*), Lombard, IL) or the *Ariol* brightfield/fluorescence microscope (Applied Imaging, Hampshire, UK) can be used for digital image collection and storage. Both allow for easy access of images for comparisons to be made across multiple stains and TMAs.

TMAD is a free, web-based resource (http://tma.stanford.edu) that provides investigators with tools to design, annotate, score and archive TMA data [53]. Its main objective is to disseminate the annotated high resolution light and fluorescence microscopic images of tissue cores with associated protein and RNA expression data such that collaborators worldwide can retrieve, share, and analyze information of interest. To accommodate high throughput data from TMAs, TMAD offers a robust system for integrating commercially-available hardware and software together with custom-designed new software tools from gene micro-array analysis platforms [56,57]. The output from these programs is in a format that is ame-nable for statistical analysis. TMAD also incorporates the NCI thesaurus of oncology such that specific search parameters can be readily used to access the cancer tissues or diagnoses. This comprehensive system also allows for interpretative data to be accrued on an on-going basis such that staining results of novel markers can be analyzed and incorporated as they become available. Additional advantages include the ease of importing images and metadata such that the transport of samples and slides and the requisite permissions required for human tissue research is avoided [53]. We have also created a novel method to make TMAs from cells in suspension, such that low numbers of cells from bone marrow, fine needle aspirates, and cultured cells can be subjected to a large-scale protein expression studies [58,59].

2.7. Beyond Immunohistochemistry: New Methods to Measure Protein Expression

2.7.1. Limitations of the IHC Method

Although traditional IHC remains the primary method of detecting protein expression in tumors, it has a number of significant limitations. First, IHC analysis is typically limited to a single antibody–antigen target per slide. Staining patterns are also complex, and even if read by skilled pathologists, there is often poor intra- and inter-observer reproducibility. Also, ordinal scoring systems may oversimplify the clinically relevant gradations in protein expression. Lastly, tissue and subcellular localization of a protein is morphologically defined, rather than through colocalization with a molecular target so that it may not correlate with therapeutic response in a targeted therapy application. In recent years, a number of new methodologies have been developed to address these limitations. These new technologies fall into two broad categories: (1) more precise in situ analysis of multiple proteins; and (2) computer-assisted image acquisition and quantitation of protein expression on a continuous scale.

2.7.2. Confocal Microscopy on FFPE: Improved Resolution and Multiple Targets

Currently, the most commonly-used technique to analyze the expression of multiple proteins on a FFPE tissue slide is dual-label IHC, using two different chromogens, analyzed using light microscopy. To analyze three or more proteins, clinical laboratories have begun to use confocal microscopy on FFPE sections using the same fluorescence-tagged antibodies that are widely utilized for unfixed cytologic preparations in research laboratories [22,60]. This approach allows for the analysis of multiple proteins at higher resolution than possible using chromogenic substrates, with the added benefit of localizing protein expression in relation-ship to specific subcellular compartments.

Limitations of this approach include the need for (expensive) confocal microscope instru-ments to limit the effects of tissue autofluorescence, overlapping absorption/emission spectra of multiple fluorescent probes, photobleaching, and low stability of the fluorescent conju-gates over time. Many of these limitations have been overcome by the development of highly stable nanocrystal fluorophores (quantum dots) that exhibit a broad wavelength absorption, but sharply defined emission spectra [61,62]. Quantum dots have been conjugated to a variety of biologically useful macromolecules, including antibodies and streptavidin [63]. Demonstrating the usefulness of mulitplex immunofluoresence in detecting lymphocyte populations within the complex lymph node environment, Fountaine and colleagues reported results of staining for five distinct streptavidin-conjugated quantum dots on a single FFPE tonsil section [64]. With the development of new antibody-conjugated quantum dot reagents, the use of this technology is likely to increase in the near future.

2.7.3. In Situ Solubilization of FFPE Proteins for Multiplex Analysis

Several groups have adapted the Western blot technique to transfer partially enzymatically-digested FFPE tissue onto antibody-linked membranes (i.e., layered expression scanning) [65] or transfer of prebound antibodies to specific membranes containing peptides from the protein of interest (i.e., layered peptide arrays) [66]. Using these techniques, greater than twenty different proteins may theoretically be detected and quantified from a single specimen, far more than currently possible using conventional immunofluorescence techniques. After transfer to the membrane, much of the spatial orientation of protein expression from the original tissue is maintained. In addition, by blotting proteins bound to membranes, antibodies unsuitable for use on FFPE material may be used for the analysis. However, while these techniques increase the number of proteins that may be detected, they do so at the expense of morphologic detail.

2.7.4. Multispectral Data Analysis

With the complexity of the data generated by multiplex protein expression analysis, there is a concomitant need for computational strategies to enhance signal detection and integration. As the human eye is unable to reproducibly detect subtle variations in staining intensity, increasingly sophisticated algorithms are required to quantitate protein expression on a continuous scale. Perhaps most importantly, automated IHC detection systems have the potential to provide a more reliable and standardized interpretation of protein expression, which is especially critical with the advent of targeted drug therapy.

To fulfill this need, numerous companies have developed integrated digital imaging and analysis systems (recently reviewed by Cregger and colleagues) [67]. One of these technologies, termed AQUA (automated quantitative analysis) (HistoRx, New Haven, CT) utilizes an automated image capture system with the capability to detect up to five different fluorescent labels. The image data is then processed using a series of algorithms to reduce the background noise while simultaneously localizing pixels based on a user-defined molecular parameter, such as DAPI positivity for the nucleus [68]. The data is then expressed as a continuous measure of pixel intensity over unit area. In a demonstration of this technology, Gustavson and colleagues were able to detect subtle differences in thymidylate synthase expression in the nucleus and cytoplasm of colorectal carcinoma cells, and correlate the expression ratio to overall patient survival [69].

Other approaches include quantitative laser-scanning cytometry (CompuCyte, Westwood, MA), which adapts flow cytometry technology for multiplex immunofluorescence analysis in FFPE tissue [70]. Newer instruments can simultaneously detect chromogenic and fluorescent signals. While AQUA and laser-scanning cytometry provide a much greater degree of precision in measuring protein expression, the expense of the detection systems and reagents may largely limit the initial use of these technologies to the academic or industry setting.

2.8. Conclusions

Our ability to diagnose lymphoma has progressed rapidly from the characterization of the first antibodies against leukocyte surface markers to the ability to detect multiple proteins simultaneously in FFPE material. It is likely that advances in multiplex immunostaining technology will enable pathologists to further refine the diagnostic categories of lymphoma, and detect subtle alterations in the lymph node microenvironment that may be important for predicting patient prognosis. In the future, the use of TMA and multiplex immunofluorescence technology will certainly enhance our understanding of the biology of lymphoma and potentially lead to new therapeutic strategies based on a broader molecular understanding of hematolymphoid malignancy.

Selected References

1. Warnke RA, Gatter KC, Falini B, et al. Diagnosis of human lymphoma with monoclonal antileukocyte antibodies. N Engl J Med 1983;309:1275–81.
2. Natkunam Y, Mason DY. Prognostic immunohistologic markers in human tumors: why are so few used in clinical practice? Lab Invest 2006;86:742–7.
3. Cregger M, Berger AJ, Rimm DL. Immunohistochemistry and quantitative analysis of protein expression. Arch Pathol Lab Med 2006;130:1026–30.

References

1. Coons AH, Kaplan MH. Localization of antigen in tissue cells; improvements in a method for the detection of antigen by means of fluorescent antibody. J Exp Med 1950;91:1–13.
2. Schmalstieg FC Jr, Goldman AS, Ilya Ilich Metchnikoff (1845–1915) and Paul Ehrlich (1854–1915): the centennial of the 1908 Nobel Prize in Physiology or Medicine. J Med Biogr 2008;16:96–103.
3. Kohler G, Milstein C. Continuous cultures of fused cells secreting antibody of predefined specificity. Nature 1975;256:495–7.
4. Nakane PK, Pierce GB Jr. Enzyme-labeled antibodies for the light and electron microscopic localization of tissue antigens. J Cell Biol 1967;33:307–18.
5. Avrameas S. Enzyme markers: their linkage with proteins and use in immuno-histochemistry. Histochem J 1972;4:321–30.
6. Warnke RA, Gatter KC, Falini B, et al. Diagnosis of human lymphoma with monoclonal antileukocyte antibodies. N Engl J Med 1983;309:1275–81.
7. Swerdlow SH, Campo E, Harris NL, et al. WHO classification of tumours of haematopoietic and lymphoid tissues. Lyon: IARC, 2008.
8. Natkunam Y, van De Rijn M. The use of gene expression arrays and high density tissue microarrays in the study of hematolymphoid malignancies. Histopathology 2002;41:520–5.
9. Natkunam Y, Mason DY. Prognostic immunohistologic markers in human tumors: why are so few used in clinical practice? Lab Invest 2006;86:742–7.
10. Zu Y, Steinberg SM, Campo E, et al. Validation of tissue microarray immunohistochemistry staining and interpretation in diffuse large B-cell lymphoma. Leuk Lymphoma 2005;46:693–701.
11. de Jong D, Rosenwald A, Chhanabhai M, et al. Immunohistochemical prognostic markers in diffuse large B-cell lymphoma: validation of tissue microarray as a prerequisite for broad clinical applications–a study from the Lunenburg Lymphoma Biomarker Consortium. J Clin Oncol 2007;25:805–12.
12. Henry NL, Hayes DF. Uses and abuses of tumor markers in the diagnosis, monitoring, and treatment of primary and metastatic breast cancer. Oncologist 2006;11:541–52.
13. Taylor CR, Shi S, Barr NJ, Wu N. Techniques of immunohistochemistry: principals, pitfalls, and standardization. In: Dabbs DJ (eds.), Diagnostic Immunohistochemistry, Churchill Livingston, 2nd Edition, 2002; 3–43.
14. Popkov M, Mage RG, Alexander CB, Thundivalappil S, Barbas CF 3 rd, Rader C. Rabbit immune repertoires as sources for therapeutic monoclonal antibodies: the impact of kappa allotype-correlated variation in cysteine content on antibody libraries selected by phage display. J Mol Biol 2003;325:325–35.
15. Cheuk W, Wong KO, Wong CS, Chan JK. Consistent immunostaining for cyclin D1 can be achieved on a routine basis using a newly available rabbit monoclonal antibody. Am J Surg Pathol 2004;28:801–7.
16. Cordell JL, Falini B, Erber WN, et al. Immunoenzymatic labeling of monoclonal antibodies using immune complexes of alkaline phosphatase and monoclonal anti-alkaline phosphatase (APAAP complexes). J Histochem Cytochem 1984;32:219–29.
17. Hsu SM, Raine L, Fanger H. A comparative study of the peroxidase–antiperoxidase method and an avidin–biotin complex method for studying polypeptide hormones with radioimmunoassay antibodies. Am J Clin Pathol 1981;75:734–8.
18. Adams JC. Biotin amplification of biotin and horseradish peroxidase signals in histochemical stains. J Histochem Cytochem 1992;40:1457–63.

19. Sabattini E, Bisgaard K, Ascani S, et al. The EnVision++ system: a new immunohistochemical method for diagnostics and research. Critical comparison with the APAAP, ChemMate, CSA, LABC, and SABC techniques. J Clin Pathol 1998;51:506–11.

20. Vyberg M, Nielsen S. Dextran polymer conjugate two-step visualization system for immunohisto-chemistry. Appl Immunohistochem 1998;6:3.

21. Marafioti T, Jones M, Facchetti F, et al. Phenotype and genotype of interfollicular large B cells, a subpopulation of lymphocytes often with dendritic morphology. Blood 2003;102:2868–76.

22. Mason DY, Micklem K, Jones M. Double immunofluorescence labelling of routinely processed paraffin sections. J Pathol 2000;191:452–61.

23. Natkunam Y, Lossos IS, Taidi B, et al. Expression of the human germinal center-associated lymphoma (HGAL) protein, a new marker of germinal center B-cell derivation. Blood 2005;105:3979–86.

24. Natkunam Y, Zhao S, Mason DY, et al. The oncoprotein LMO2 is expressed in normal germinal-center B cells and in human B-cell lymphomas. Blood 2007;109:1636–42.

25. Roncador G, Garcia Verdes-Montenegro JF, Tedoldi S, et al. Expression of two markers of germinal center T cells (SAP and PD-1) in angioimmunoblastic T-cell lymphoma. Haematologica 2007;92:1059–66.

26. Dorfman DM, Brown JA, Shahsafaei A, Freeman GJ. Programmed death-1 (PD-1) is a marker of germinal center-associated T cells and angioimmunoblastic T-cell lymphoma. Am J Surg Pathol 2006;30:802–10.

27. Grogg KL, Attygalle AD, Macon WR, Remstein ED, Kurtin PJ, Dogan A. Expression of CXCL13, a chemokine highly upregulated in germinal center T-helper cells, distinguishes angio-immunoblastic T-cell lymphoma from peripheral T-cell lymphoma, unspecified. Mod Pathol 2006;19:1101–7.

28. McCune RC, Syrbu SI, Vasef MA. Expression profiling of transcription factors Pax-5, Oct-1, Oct-2, BOB.1, and PU.1 in Hodgkin's and non-Hodgkin's lymphomas: a comparative study using high throughput tissue microarrays. Mod Pathol 2006;19:1010–8.

29. Loddenkemper C, Anagnostopoulos I, Hummel M, et al. Differential Emu enhancer activity and expression of BOB.1/OBF.1, Oct2, PU.1, and immunoglobulin in reactive B-cell populations, B-cell non-Hodgkin lymphomas, and Hodgkin lymphomas. J Pathol 2004;202:60–9.

30. Schwering I, Brauninger A, Klein U, et al. Loss of the B-lineage-specific gene expression program in Hodgkin and Reed–Sternberg cells of Hodgkin lymphoma. Blood 2003;101:1505–12.

31. Pulford K, Lamant L, Morris SW, et al. Detection of anaplastic lymphoma kinase (ALK) and nucleolar protein nucleophosmin (NPM)-ALK proteins in normal and neoplastic cells with the monoclonal antibody ALK1. Blood 1997;89:1394–404.

32. Schnittger S, Schoch C, Kern W, et al. Nucleophosmin gene mutations are predictors of favorable prognosis in acute myelogenous leukemia with a normal karyotype. Blood 2005;106:3733–9.

33. Noguera NI, Ammatuna E, Zangrilli D, et al. Simultaneous detection of NPM1 and FLT3-ITD mutations by capillary electrophoresis in acute myeloid leukemia. Leukemia 2005;19:1479–82.

34. Cazzaniga G, Dell'Oro MG, Mecucci C, et al. Nucleophosmin mutations in childhood acute myel-ogenous leukemia with normal karyotype. Blood 2005;106:1419–22.

35. Alizadeh AA, Eisen MB, Davis RE, et al. Distinct types of diffuse large B-cell lymphoma identi-fied by gene expression profiling. Nature 2000;403:503–11.

36. Rosenwald A, Wright G, Chan WC, et al. The use of molecular profiling to predict survival after chemotherapy for diffuse large-B-cell lymphoma. N Engl J Med 2002;346:1937–47.

37. Monti S, Savage KJ, Kutok JL, et al. Molecular profiling of diffuse large B-cell lymphoma identifies robust subtypes including one characterized by host inflammatory response. Blood 2005;105:1851–61.

38. Tedoldi S, Paterson J, Cordell J, et al. Jaw1/LRMP, a germinal centre-associated marker for the immunohistological study of B-cell lymphomas. J Pathol 2006;209:454–63.

39. Lenz G, Wright G, Dave SS, et al. Stromal gene signatures in large-B-cell lymphomas. N Engl J Med 2008;359:2313–23.

40. Lossos IS, Czerwinski DK, Alizadeh AA, et al. Prediction of survival in diffuse large-B-cell lym-phoma based on the expression of six genes. N Engl J Med 2004;350:1828–37.

41. Lu X, Malumbres R, Shields B, et al. PTP1B is a negative regulator of interleukin 4-induced STAT6 signaling. Blood 2008;112:4098–108.

42. Gratzinger D, Zhao S, Tibshirani RJ, et al. Prognostic significance of VEGF, VEGF receptors, and microvessel density in diffuse large B cell lymphoma treated with anthracycline-based chemo-therapy. Lab Invest 2008;88:38–47.

43. Gratzinger D, Zhao S, Marinelli RJ, et al. Microvessel density and expression of vascular endothelial growth factor and its receptors in diffuse large B-cell lymphoma subtypes. Am J Pathol 2007; 170:1362–9.

44. Gascoyne RD, Lamant L, Martin-Subero JI, et al. ALK-positive diffuse large B-cell lymphoma is associated with Clathrin-ALK rearrangements: report of 6 cases. Blood 2003;102:2568–73.

45. Coiffier B, Lepage E, Briere J, et al. CHOP chemotherapy plus rituximab compared with CHOP alone in elderly patients with diffuse large-B-cell lymphoma. N Engl J Med 2002;346:235–42.

46. Habermann TM, Weller EA, Morrison VA, et al. Rituximab-CHOP versus CHOP alone or with maintenance rituximab in older patients with diffuse large B-cell lymphoma. J Clin Oncol 2006;24:3121–7.

47. Pfreundschuh M, Trumper L, Osterborg A, et al. CHOP-like chemotherapy plus rituximab versus CHOP-like chemotherapy alone in young patients with good-prognosis diffuse large-B-cell lymphoma: a randomised controlled trial by the MabThera International Trial (MInT) Group. Lancet Oncol 2006;7:379–91.

48. Sehn LH, Donaldson J, Chhanabhai M, et al. Introduction of combined CHOP plus rituximab therapy dramatically improved outcome of diffuse large B-cell lymphoma in British Columbia. J Clin Oncol 2005;23:5027–33.

49. Irish JM, Czerwinski DK, Nolan GP, Levy R. Kinetics of B cell receptor signaling in human B-cell subsets mapped by phosphospecific flow cytometry. J Immunol 2006;177:1581–9.

50. Elenitoba-Johnson KS, Crockett DK, Schumacher JA, et al. Proteomic identification of oncogenic chromosomal translocation partners encoding chimeric anaplastic lymphoma kinase fusion proteins. Proc Natl Acad Sci U S A 2006;103:7402–7.

51. Kohrt HE, Nouri N, Nowels K, Johnson D, Holmes S, Lee PP. Profile of immune cells in axillary lymph nodes predicts disease-free survival in breast cancer. PLoS Med 2005;2:e284.

52. Kononen J, Bubendorf L, Kallioniemi A, et al. Tissue microarrays for high-throughput molecular profiling of tumor specimens. Nat Med 1998;4:844–7.

53. Marinelli RJ, Montgomery K, Liu CL, et al. The Stanford tissue microarray database. Nucleic Acids Res 2008;36:D871–7.

54. Uhlen M, Bjorling E, Agaton C, et al. A human protein atlas for normal and cancer tissues based on antibody proteomics. Mol Cell Proteomics 2005;4:1920–32.

55. Vyberg M, Torlakovic E, Seidal T, Risberg B, Helin H, Nielsen S. Nordic immunohistochemical quality control. Croat Med J 2005;46:368–71.

56. Liu CL, Montgomery KD, Natkunam Y, et al. TMA-Combiner, a simple software tool to permit analysis of replicate cores on tissue microarrays. Mod Pathol 2005;18:1641–1648.

57. Liu CL, Prapong W, Natkunam Y, et al. Software tools for high-throughput analysis and archiving of immunohistochemistry staining data obtained with tissue microarrays. Am J Pathol 2002;161:1557–65.

58. Hazard F, Zhao S, Schiffman J, Lacayo N, Dahl G, Natkunam Y. Tissue microarrays from bone marrow aspirates for high throughput assessment of immunohistologic markers in pediatric acute leukemia. Pediatr Dev Pathol 2007;1.

59. Montgomery K, Zhao S, van de Rijn M, Natkunam Y. A novel method for making "tissue" microarrays from small numbers of suspension cells. Appl Immunohistochem Mol Morphol 2005;13:80–4.

60. Robertson D, Savage K, Reis-Filho JS, Isacke CM. Multiple immunofluorescence labelling of formalin-fixed paraffin-embedded (FFPE) tissue. BMC Cell Biol 2008;9:13.

61. Bruchez M Jr, Moronne M, Gin P, Weiss S, Alivisatos AP. Semiconductor nanocrystals as fluorescent biological labels. Science 1998;281:2013–6.

62. Chan WC, Nie S. Quantum dot bioconjugates for ultrasensitive nonisotopic detection. Science 1998;281:2016–8.

63. Tholouli E, Sweeney E, Barrow E, Clay V, Hoyland JA, Byers RJ. Quantum dots light up pathology. J Pathol 2008;216:275–85.

64. Fountaine TJ, Wincovitch SM, Geho DH, Garfield SH, Pittaluga S. Multispectral imaging of clinically relevant cellular targets in tonsil and lymphoid tissue using semiconductor quantum dots. Mod Pathol 2006;19:1181–91.

65. Englert CR, Baibakov GV, Emmert-Buck MR. Layered expression scanning: rapid molecular profiling of tumor samples. Cancer Res 2000;60:1526–30.

66. Gannot G, Tangrea MA, Erickson HS, et al. Layered peptide array for multiplex immunohistochemistry. J Mol Diagn 2007;9:297–304.

67. Cregger M, Berger AJ, Rimm DL. Immunohistochemistry and quantitative analysis of protein expression. Arch Pathol Lab Med 2006;130:1026–30.

68. Camp RL, Chung GG, Rimm DL. Automated subcellular localization and quantification of protein expression in tissue microarrays. Nat Med 2002;8:1323–7.

69. Gustavson MD, Molinaro AM, Tedeschi G, Camp RL, Rimm DL. AQUA analysis of thymidylate synthase reveals localization to be a key prognostic biomarker in 2 large cohorts of colorectal carcinoma. Arch Pathol Lab Med 2008;132:1746–52.

70. Harnett MM. Laser scanning cytometry: understanding the immune system in situ. Nat Rev Immunol 2007;7:897–904.

Chapter 3

Flow Cytometry in the Evaluation of Hematologic Malignancies

Jeffrey L. Jorgensen

Abstract/Scope of Chapter The chapter reviews the procedures and analysis techniques used in flow cytometry studies for the diagnosis and follow-up of residual disease in lymphomas and leukemias. The particular antibodies used are summarized, and the basics of staining, gating, and reporting are outlined. Pitfalls that can be encountered are discussed. Also covered is the use of flow cytometry in T-cell subset analysis, blast enumeration, cell cycle/DNA ploidy determination, as well as in quantitative assessment of marker expression.

Keywords Flow cytometry, procedure • Flow cytometry, gating strategies • Flow cytometry, quality control • Cell cycle analysis, flow cytometry • Flow cytometry, T-cell subset analysis • Flow cytometry, quantitative marker assessment

3.1. Use of Flow Cytometry in the Diagnosis of Lymphomas and Leukemias

Flow cytometry (FC) is a method for analysis of the expression patterns of molecules on single cells in a fluid. In most applications, protein levels are analyzed using monoclonal antibodies conjugated to fluorochromes (fluorescent tags, ranging from small organic molecules to large protein complexes). Other applications include enumeration of DNA and RNA levels using nucleic acid binding dyes, and functional cell biology assays (e.g., apoptosis) using fluorescent indicators. The technology was first developed by Herzenberg and colleagues in the early 1970s [1] and soon synergized with the development of a method for routinely making large quantities of purified mouse monoclonal antibodies by Milstein and Kohler [2]. In its basic configuration, a flow cytometer consists of a laser, a detector, and a fluidics system which creates a single-file stream of cells along a precise pathway (Fig. 3-1a). The laser excites the fluorochromes bound to or within each cell, and an optical system of mirrors, filters, and detectors captures the emitted fluorescence over a range of wavelengths appropriate for each fluorochrome; electronic components convert the measured fluorescent signals to a digital output (Fig. 3-1b).

The development of a large number of highly specific monoclonal antibodies (Table 3-1) and a range of different fluorochromes with largely nonoverlapping absorption/emission spectra has permitted the development of multicolor FC using multiple lasers for excitation and multiple mirrors and filters for detection. Four-color FC is now performed routinely in most diagnostic laboratories, allowing incorporation of routine antibody panels for the detection of acute myeloid leukemia (AML), acute/precursor lymphoblastic leukemia (ALL), chronic

From: *Neoplastic Hematopathology*: Contemporary Hematology,
Edited by: D. Jones, DOI 10.1007/978-1-60761-384-8_3,
© Humana Press, a part of Springer Science+Business Media, LLC 2010

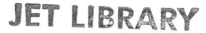

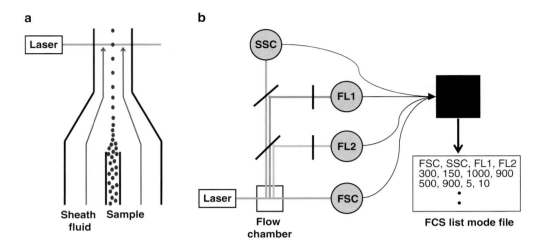

Fig. 3-1. *Schematic structure of a flow cytometer.* (**a**) Flow chamber: Continuous flow of sheath fluid creates laminar flow, enabling precise control of the stream of cells through the laser beam. (**b**) Optics and electronics: Total emitted light from the stained cells is separated by mirrors and filters (*black bars*) and directed to detectors (*gray circles*) for forward scatter (FSC), side scatter (SSC), and fluorescence channels (FL1 and FL2) corresponding to each fluorochrome in this two-color example. Voltage signals from the detectors are converted by electronics in the cytometer (*black box*) into digital output to an attached computer, resulting in a list mode file with one line of data per cell

lymphocytic leukemia (CLL), and lymphomas (Table 3-2). In the last few years, five-color to eight-color FC panels have been implemented in a growing number of laboratories. Analyzing samples with more antibodies in a single tube leads to more efficient sample processing, particularly for scant specimens, such as fine needle aspirates, and it can lead to much more efficient antibody panels for complex applications such as minimal residual disease (MRD) assessment. However, establishing the panels is more technically challenging than for standard four-color staining.

Fluorescent-activated cell sorting (FACS) utilizing FC methodology can also be used to produce purified populations of cells with a particular surface immunophenotype, though this technique currently has more research than clinical applications.

3.2. Performing a Flow Cytometry Assay

3.2.1. Steps in the Process

Figure 3-2 outlines the steps involved in a typical clinical FC study, including staining, RBC lysis, washing, fixation, data acquisition, and analysis. FC can be performed on a variety of clinical specimen types, including peripheral blood, bone marrow (BM) aspirates (usually collected in EDTA), dissociated tissue biopsies, fine needle aspirates, and body fluids. In clinical practice, most antibodies are directly conjugated to fluorochromes, whereas in some research applications, incubation with an unlabeled primary antibody generated in one species (often mouse) is followed by a washing step and then incubation with a fluoro-chrome-conjugated secondary antibody from a second species (e.g., goat), directed against immunoglobulins from the first species. For peripheral blood and BM aspirates, leukocytes must be separated at some stage of processing from the much more numerous red blood cells (RBCs). Historically, this was often performed by density gradient centrifugation, but this technique risks the loss of the cells of interest [3]. RBC lysis requires much less sample

Table 3-1. Antigens used in diagnostic panels for leukemia and lymphoma.

Antigen	Normal expression	Function	May be aberrantly expressed in:	Panel (see Table 3-2)
CD1	Pre-T, DC	Antigen presentation	T-ALL	ALL-extended
CD2	T, NK	T-cell regulation	AML, MCD	T, MCD, AL
CD3 (surface)	T, NK	Components of the TCR	TCL (dec)	All panels
CD3 (cytoplasmic)	T, NK	signaling complex	TCL (dec)	AL
CD4	T, mono	TCR complex	TCL (dec), PCM	TCL, ID
CD5	T, B subset	T-cell costimulatory regulator	CLL, MCL, TCL (dec), AML	Lymphoma, CLL, AL
CD7	T	T-cell costimulatory	AML, TCL (dec)	TCL, AL
CD8	T, NK	TCR complex	TCL (dec)	TCL, ID
CD10	Pre-B, follicular B & T, mature My, nonheme	Peptidase	ALL (inc or dec), AITL	Lymphoma, AL
CD13	My, mono	Zinc metalloproteinase	ALL, AML (dec), MDS (inc on myelocytes)	AL, MDS
CD14	Mono, my (dim)	Endotoxin receptor		AL
CD15	My, mono	Adhesion molecule	ALL, AML (inc)	AL
CD16	NK, my, mono, T subset	IgG Fc receptor	MDS, TCL	MDS, TCL
CD19	B, PC	B-cell signal transduction	ALL (inc), AML [t(8;21)], PCM (dec)	Lymphoma, CLL, AL, PCM
CD20	B, T subset	B-cell activation	ALL (inc)	Lymphoma, CLL, AL
CD22	B, baso	B-cell adhesion, stimulation	ALL (inc or dec)	Lymphoma, AL
CD23	B, DC	IgE Fc receptor	CLL (inc)	Lymphoma, CLL
CD25	B activated, T activated, mono	IL-2 receptor chain	ATLL (bright), MCD	TCL, MCD
CD26	T activated	Dipetidyl peptidase	TCL (dec)	TCL
CD30	B activated, T activated	TNF-associated factor receptor	ALCL	Lymphoma-extend
CD33	My, mono (bright)	Adhesion molecule	ALL, AML (dec)	AL
CD34	Blasts (Pre-B, Pre-T, My)	Adhesion molecule	ALL (inc or dec), APL usually neg	AL
CD38	PC, Pre-B, NK, my blasts, B, T	Adhesion molecule	ALL (dec), CLL (inc in some cases)	AL, PCM, CLL
CD41	MK, Plts	GpIIb	AMKL	AL
CD43	All heme except mature B	Adhesion molecule	CLL, MCL, some MZL (not FL, splenic MZL)	Lymphoma, CLL
CD45	All heme, dim in Ery, Plts	Phosphatase	ALL (dec)	All panels
CD56	NK, T subset, nonheme	Adhesion molecule (NCAM)	TCL, PCM, AML	Lymphoma, AL, PC
CD64	Mono, activated my	IgG Fc receptor		AL
CD79a	B, late Pre-B, PC	B-cell receptor signaling	T-ALL	ALL-extend
CD103	T subset, mono, MC	Adhesion molecule β7 integrin	HCL	HCL
CD117	Blasts, MC	Stem cell factor receptor kinase	T-ALL, PCM	AL
CD123	PDC, baso bright; my, mono moderate	Interleukin-3 receptor	BPDCN (bright)	AL
CD138	PC, nonheme	Adhesion molecule	PCM (dec)	PCM
HLA-DR	Most heme	Antigen presentation (class II)	APL usually neg	AL
TdT	Pre-B, pre-T	TCR, Ig gene rearrangement	AML	AL
Myeloperoxidase	My, mono	Lysosomal protein	Mixed phenotype AL	AL

Abbreviations: Normal cell types (column 1): B, B cells; DC, dendritic cells; Ery, erythroid cells; heme, hematopoietic cells; MC, mast cells; MK, megakaryocytes; mono, monocytes; my, myeloid cells; NK, NK cells; nonheme, nonhematopoietic cell types; PC, plasma cells; PDC, plasmacytoid dendritic cells; Plts, platelets; Pre-B, precursor B cells ("hematogones"); Pre-T, precursor T cells (thymocytes). Neoplastic cell types and panels (columns 3 and 4): inc, increased; dec, decreased; neg, negative; AITL, angioimmunoblastic T-cell lymphoma; AL, acute leukemia screening panel; ALCL, anaplastic large cell lymphoma; ALL, acute lymphoblastic leukemia; AMKL, acute megakaryocytic leukemia; AML, acute myeloid leukemia; APL, acute promyelocytic leukemia; ATLL, adult T-cell leukemia/lymphoma; BPDCN, blastic plasmacytoid dendritic cell neoplasm; CLL, chronic lymphocytic leukemia; FL, follicular lymphoma; HCL, hairy cell leukemia; ID, immunodeficiency; MCD, mast cell disease; MCL, mantle cell lymphoma; MDS, myelodysplastic syndrome; MZL, marginal zone lymphoma; PCM, plasma cell myeloma; T-ALL, precursor T-cell acute lymphoblastic leukemia; TCL, T-cell lymphoma

Table 3-2. Basic four-color flow cytometric panel for acute leukemia diagnosis.

FITC	PE	PerCPCy5.5	APC
IgG2ac	IgG1	CD45	IgG1
CD10	CD19	CD45	CD20
CD41	CD64	CD45	CD14
HLA-DR	CD13	CD45	CD5
CD7	CD33	CD45	CD2
CD34	CD117	CD45	CD38
CD15		CD45	CD34
cyto IgG1 + IgG2	IgG1	CD45	IgG1
cyto TdT	CD34	CD45	CD19
IgG1	cyto IgG1	CD45	IgG1
CD56	cyto CD3	CD45	CD3
cyto IgG1	cyto IgG1	CD45	
cyto MPO	cyto LF	CD45	

Panels are those used at MD Anderson Cancer Center. In most cases, blasts are identified by gating on CD34+/CD117+ cells. These are displayed on CD45 vs. SSC plots ("back-gated") in order to establish a blast gate, which is used to analyze the remaining tubes. For lymphoma panels with a pan B-cell marker (such as CD19) or a pan T-cell marker (usually CD3) in each tube, uniform gating may be performed on CD19 or CD3 vs. SSC plots. *Abbreviations*: cyto, cytoplasmic and/or nuclear stain; LF, lactoferrin (secondary granule protein, used to exclude mature granulocytes); MPO, myeloperoxidase; TdT, terminal deoxynucleotidyl transferase

Fig. 3-2. Steps in a typical clinical flow cytometry study

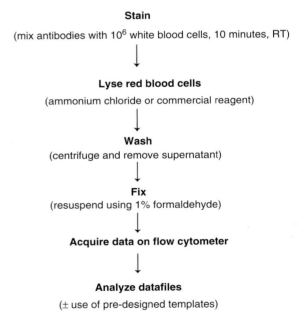

Stain

(mix antibodies with 10^6 white blood cells, 10 minutes, RT)

↓

Lyse red blood cells

(ammonium chloride or commercial reagent)

↓

Wash

(centrifuge and remove supernatant)

↓

Fix

(resuspend using 1% formaldehyde)

↓

Acquire data on flow cytometer

↓

Analyze datafiles

(± use of pre-designed templates)

manipulation and can easily be performed with a hypotonic ammonium chloride solution or other commercial lysis buffer. Antibody staining may be performed either before or after RBC lysis. However, in most cases, staining before lysis is recommended, [3] as this avoids potential effects of the lysis buffer on cell viability and on antigenicity of the target molecule. In most protocols, excess antibody is finally removed by one or more washing steps, by centrifugation of the sample and removal of the supernatant. Some protocols, predominantly for CD34 and T-cell subset enumeration, may be performed with no washing step, in order to minimize potential cell loss. Sample viability can be assessed on the cytometer by the light scatter properties of the cells or by using intravital dyes.

Prior to running the samples on the cytometer, the instrument must be properly calibrated, commonly by using standardized fluorescent beads and automated software. The gain on each detector is set so as to optimize the signal-to-noise ratio. Compensation settings are made by determining the amount of spectral overlap into all detectors from beads or cells stained with each separate fluorochrome [4]. Data are then acquired by running the stained cells one by one through the cytometer and recording the intensity of fluorescence and light scatter properties. Forward scatter (FSC) is proportional to cell size, while side scatter (SSC) is increased by subcellular complexity, particularly cytoplasmic granules (as in granulocytes) or cytoplasmic projections (as in hairy cell leukemia). The cytometer generates a line of data for each cell, with one data element for each light scatter and fluorescent parameter, organized into a list-mode data file. The number of cells collected for each analysis tube ranges from a few hundred in a scant CSF specimen, to 10,000 in a standard leukemia analysis, to several hundred thousand or more in a test for minimal residual disease. The resulting data files may be analyzed using the same software on the same computer workstation used for data acquisition on the flow cytometer, or by any of a number of independent software packages on another workstation ("off-line" analysis).

There are two approaches to analyzing and reporting FC data. The first is to catalog the percentages of subsets of leukocytes that have a particular antibody staining pattern (e.g., percentage of CD19+CD10+ lymphocytes, or %CD34+ cells in the blast gate). This simple method can lead to misleading results in evaluation of leukemias and lymphomas for a number of reasons, particularly if a specimen includes a high proportion of nonneoplastic background cells, and/or a subset of nonneoplastic cells shows a partial overlap with the neoplastic phenotype (see Sect. 3.2.3 for specific examples). As a result, most clinical reporting is now done using the second approach, "cluster analysis," where the distinctive antigen density/fluorescence intensity and scatter properties of an abnormal cell population are used for enumeration. The data collected on a single cell may be regarded as coordinates for a point in multidimensional space, one dimension for each fluorochrome and two for light scatter. Similar cells form clusters of data points in this space, and a well-designed antibody panel should result in neoplastic cells forming a distinct cluster from normal background cells. For convenience of analysis, clinical FC data are usually displayed on two-dimensional dotplots, with each cell represented by one point. Particularly useful plots include FSC vs. SSC, which provides reasonable separation of lymphocytes, monocytes, and granulocytes (Fig. 3-3a), and CD45 vs. SSC, [5,6] which leads to better separation of lymphocytes, immature precursors ("blasts," including myeloid and B-cell precursors), and erythrocytes (Fig. 3-3b).

3.2.2. Detecting Abnormal Cell Populations: Cluster Analysis

FC data analysis usually involves a process of *gating*, which is selection of cell subsets of interest, based on their levels of fluorescence using one or more antibodies, and/or light scatter properties. In most cases, clusters of cells are gated for further characterization. Common gates for initial analysis of lymphomas or leukemias include a lymphocyte gate (on cells with low FSC and low SSC, or CD45 bright cells with low SSC) and a blast gate (on CD45 dim cells with low SSC). However, it is also important to examine total ungated data. This is because, in some cases, neoplastic lymphocytes may lie outside of the standard lymphocyte gate, as in hairy cell leukemia (Fig. 3-4), large B-cell lymphoma, and anaplastic large cell lymphoma, all of which show increased side scatter. Similarly, the neoplastic cells in some AMLs lie outside the standard blast gate, as in acute promyelocytic leukemia with moderate to high SSC, and acute monoblastic leukemia, with moderate SSC and brighter CD45 expression. Viewing ungated data on a set of plots displaying each fluorochrome vs. SSC is one convenient way to help ensure that no unusual neoplastic populations are missed (see Fig. 3-4c).

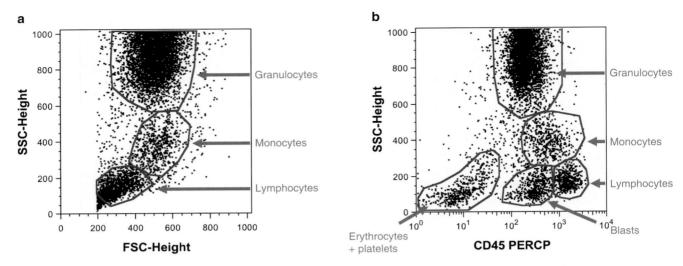

Fig. 3-3. *Typical gating strategies* for clinical flow cytometry studies on bone marrow (*shown*) or peripheral blood (**a**) FSC vs. SSC plot. Lymphocytes are commonly gated. (**b**) Side scatter vs. CD45 plot. Lymphocytes and/or blasts are commonly gated. Note that blasts are increased in this bone marrow from a patient recovering after chemotherapy

Once a cell gate is established, the staining levels of these selected cells for the other antibodies in the same analysis tube are evaluated for patterns of expression indicative of the disease state. Phenotypic aberrancies include: expression of antigens not usually present in that lineage (e.g., expression of myeloid antigens such as CD13 or CD33 on precursor B-lymphoblastic leukemia); altered levels of expression of antigens normally expressed in that lineage (e.g., dim CD20 expression in CLL); and/or temporal aberrancies, with coexpression of immature and mature antigens that would not normally be seen on the same cells (e.g., coexpression of TdT and surface CD3 in T-cell ALL). Various controls are employed to assess for specificity of staining (see Table 3-3 and below). However, when testing highly expressed antigens, such as those for T-cell subset analysis, the positive and negative cell clusters are sufficiently well separated that controls may not be necessary.

The FC report for a specimen positive for a neoplastic population should describe the neoplastic phenotype and enumerate the aberrant cells, usually either as a percentage of total analyzed cells, CD45+ cells (excluding erythroid cells and platelets), or total lymphocytes. In some cases, primarily for peripheral blood, enumeration of the absolute number of aberrant cells may be useful for staging or for monitoring disease levels after therapy. Current recommendations are to report the level of staining for each antigen as positive, negative, or partially positive [7]. It is often highly informative to further specify the intensity of staining as bright, dim, or normal, with reference to the closest normal counterpart. Thus, antigen expression on CLL cells should be compared to normal mature B lymphocytes, B-ALL cells to normal precursor B lymphocytes, etc. This approach should help to keep results consistent from laboratory to laboratory, despite the numerous possible technical differences in antibody panels, cell preparation, instrumentation, and analysis technique. This reporting approach also emphasizes the aberrancies in antigen expression by the neoplastic cells.

A sample FC report for a CLL case would include:
Interpretation: Positive for chronic lymphocytic leukemia.
Aberrant cells are 77% of lymphocytes and 65% of total analyzed cells.
POSITIVE: CD5 bright, CD19, CD20 dim, CD22 dim, CD23 bright, and dim monoclonal immunoglobulin kappa light chain.
NEGATIVE: CD10 and FMC-7.

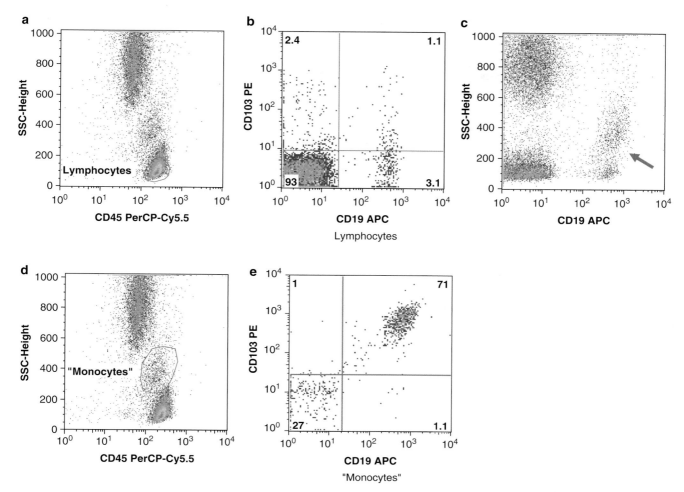

Fig. 3-4. *Neoplastic cells lying outside of the usual lymphocyte gate*, in hairy cell leukemia. Gating on CD45 bright lymphocytes with low SSC (**a**) yields mostly CD103-negative B cells. (**b**). Displaying CD19 vs. SSC on ungated cells (**c**) reveals an atypical B-cell population with increased SSC (*red arrow*). The neoplastic cells lie within the "monocyte" gate on a CD45 vs. SSC plot (**d**), and are CD103+ (**e**)

Table 3-3. Control tubes for quantitative flow cytometry analysis.

Control	Composition	Assesses
Autofluorescence	Only antibodies used for gating (e.g., CD45)	Degree of fluorescence contributed by cells themselves (higher in myeloid forms with increased granules)
Isotype control	Antibody against antigen not seen on human cells, labeled with the same fluorochrome and of the same isotype as the antibody being tested (e.g., mouse IgG1-FITC)	Nonspecific and Fc binding of antibodies
Fluorescence-minus-one (FMO) or leave-one-out	All antibodies except one that is to be measured quantitatively	Autofluorescence specific to target population, plus spectral overlap contributed from other fluorochromes
Negative control cells	Normal tissue stained with same antibody panel	Off-target binding of primary or secondary antibodies

3.2.3. Detecting Abnormal Cell Populations: Quantitative Analysis

It is also possible to summarize the FC data as the percentage of cells positive for each antigen or for selected antigen combinations. This presentation of data is particularly important for markers which are therapeutic targets (e.g., CD52 levels used to select patients for alemtuzumab immunotherapy) or for biomarkers which are heterogeneously expressed and have clinically relevant expression cut-offs (e.g., CD38 expression in ≥30% of CLL cells).

In quantitative reporting of an FC marker, the level of background signal in the corresponding fluorescence channel must be determined to set appropriate threshold levels (Fig. 3-5). The analysis software then superimposes the background thresholds, set based on the controls, on the datasets from each tube. Background signal is the sum of four components: autofluorescence, often from cytoplasmic granules and thus higher in myeloid lineage cells than in lymphocytes; nonspecific or off-target binding of the primary and/or secondary antibody, due to nonspecific protein binding or binding to FC receptors; nonspecific adherence of free fluorochrome in the labeled antibody preparation; and signal contributed from other antibody–fluorochrome pairs with overlapping emission spectra present in the same analysis tube. For some bright fluorochromes with very high antibody binding, this false signal cannot be completely eliminated even with proper compensation.

To assess the relative contribution of each of these components to background staining, several controls, such as autofluorescence, isotype, and fluorescence-minus-one (FMO)/leave-one-out types, [4] can be used (Table 3-3). Isotype controls have limitations as a control for assessment of specificity of antibody binding, as every antibody has a charge and hydrophobicity profile that will influence nonspecific binding affinity [8]. Also, each preparation of antibody may have a different efficiency of fluorochrome conjugation or varying amounts of free fluorochrome. Thus, many laboratories avoid isotype controls for surface antibody stains, and instead use autofluorescence or FMO controls. However, an isotype control is usually necessary for intracytoplasmic or nuclear antigens, since cell permeation exposes cytoplasmic components that have a higher potential for nonspecific antibody binding.

Even with careful background assessment, use of numerical threshold reporting can be misleading. For example, if a normal B-cell population is stained with CD5 conjugated to a bright fluorochrome, such as PE, a substantial number of B cells may be CD5+, but with dim to moderate levels of staining. In contrast, a CLL population usually shows brighter,

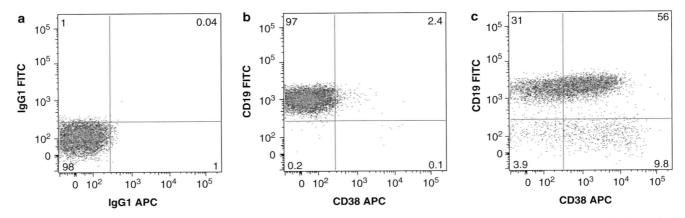

Fig. 3-5. *Threshold gating to determine quantitative levels of protein expression.* (**a**) CLL cells stained with isotype-matched negative control antibodies, with thresholds set so that 99% of cells are negative. (**b**) Same CLL cells with CD38 staining quantitated using the same threshold; the case is scored as negative (<30% of cells positive). (**c**) Another CLL case, positive for CD38

more uniform expression of CD5, but the percentage of CD5+/CD19+ cells could be the same in both cases. T-cell neoplasms may show partial loss of pan-T-cell antigens, such as CD3, resulting in an aberrant cell cluster on dot-plots (Fig. 3-6); however, by threshold reporting, the aberrant cells would still be enumerated as "positive" compared with isotype controls. Another situation which may lead to highly misleading numerical results arises when the gated population includes cells from multiple lineages. For example, in bone marrow from an AML patient after treatment, the CD45-dim mononuclear "blast gate" may contain an admixture of regenerating benign myeloid precursors and B-cell precursors – giving a false impression of mixed-lineage blasts. However, using careful cluster analysis, myeloid and B-lineage markers may be demonstrable on distinct subsets of the blasts, with no aberrancies in comparison with normal bone marrow.

FC may be used for absolute quantitation of antigen expression, using carefully prepared staining reagents with a 1:1 ratio of fluorochrome to antibody. Calibration beads, with known numbers of fluorochrome molecules per bead, are used to establish a standard curve [9]. Specialized analysis software is then used to plot FC data based on the number of antigen molecules per cell, and to calculate the mean level of antigen expression in a population of interest (Fig. 3-7).

3.2.4. Troubleshooting and Panel Design Considerations

Cell viability may be decreased in specimens more than 24–48 hours old or in neoplasms with increased apoptosis or necrosis. Nonviable cells tend to show decreased FSC and increased SSC, as well as increased nonspecific binding to multiple antibodies (often detectable as events along the diagonal on 2D dotplots). Viability can be assessed using a DNA-binding dye which does not cross an intact cell membrane, with positive events indicating nonviable cells. In specimens with extremely poor preservation, diagnostic information can sometimes still be obtained by including a viability dye in every tube, and excluding all positive events representing nonviable cells from the analysis. For four-color antibody panels, the dye 7-AAD in the PerCP channel may be used to exclude dead cells. Given the critical time-dependent nature of many diagnoses, clinical specimens submitted for workup of a possible new lymphoma or leukemia should not be rejected solely on the basis of low viability.

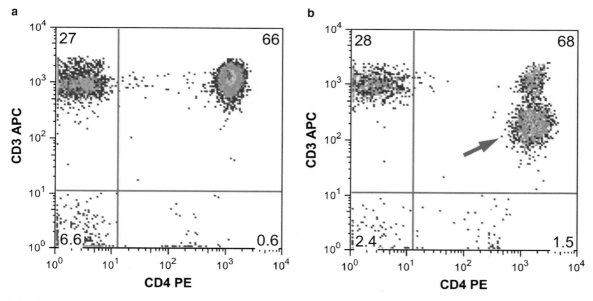

Fig. 3-6. *Potentially misleading results from numerical threshold reporting.* Similar numbers of CD3+CD4+ cells are seen among (**a**) normal peripheral blood lymphocytes, and (**b**) peripheral blood involved by T-cell lymphoma. However, the lymphoma cells in (**b**) form a distinct aberrant cell cluster (*red arrow*)

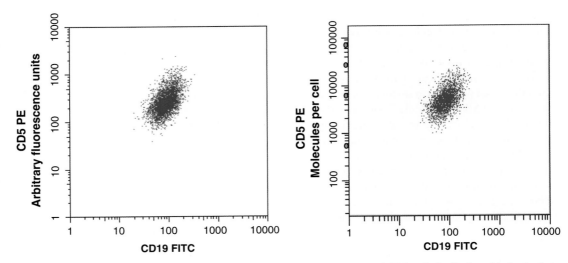

Fig. 3-7. *Quantitation of antigen expression levels.* The same population of CLL cells is displayed in both plots, with the *Y*-axis showing CD5 PE expression in terms of (**a**) arbitrary fluorescence units (i.e., the usual plot), or (**b**) antigen molecules per cell. The green dots on the *Y*-axis indicate the positions of calibration beads, with known numbers of PE molecules per bead

Even in viable specimens, some cell types are often significantly under-represented in FC analysis, presumably due to cell fragility and disruption during analysis. These disrupted cells, if they are not washed out during processing, may show such low forward scatter that they are excluded from analysis. Cell types which are particularly susceptible to this problem include plasma cells, mast cells, and large lymphoma cells. In addition, tumor cells in neoplasms associated with bone marrow fibrosis, such as mast cell disease and follicular lymphoma, may be under-represented or absent in bone marrow aspirates.

When choosing combinations of antibody for a panel, it is important to be aware of the differential brightness of different fluorochromes and to try to match low-expressing antigens with brighter fluorochromes for ease of detection. In general, PE and its conjugates and APC and its conjugates are relatively bright, while FITC and some of the dyes excited by violet lasers are somewhat dimmer. Compensation issues should also be taken into account in order to avoid staining an abundant antigen with a fluorochrome which shows high spillover into a detection channel used for a dim, heterogeneously-expressed antigen. One important step in establishing a new antibody panel is to stain a control sample with each antibody–fluorochrome combination individually to determine the degree of spillover into other channels. The performance of the antibody panel should be established on normal control specimens (peripheral blood, bone marrow, or reactive lymphoid tissue such as tonsil). The resulting dotplots may be valuable as a baseline, for comparison to results from clinical samples.

3.3. MRD Assessment by FC

Minimal residual disease (MRD) after therapy is defined as disease that is not detectable by morphologic examination, conventionally regarded as 5% of the total cellularity (usually in bone marrow). MRD detection requires the ability to distinguish a small population of neoplastic cells from a complex background which may contain the normal counterparts of a given tumor type. MRD assays require extensive knowledge of benign populations, including the spectrum of changes which normal cells may undergo following chemotherapy [10–13]. In some cases, "aberrant" phenotypes such as dim myeloid antigen expression on immature B-lineage cells may be seen at low frequencies in normal recovering bone marrow.

The sensitivity of MRD detection by FC is dependent in large part on the number of cells acquired for analysis in each tube. Enough data must be acquired to identify a cluster of at least 10–20 aberrant cells to distinguish MRD from nonspecific low-level background events. At least 100 aberrant cells must be present for accurate quantitation. Thus, for a level of detection of 1 in 10^4 (0.01%), 100,000–200,000 cells must be analyzed. For MRD analysis of bone marrow aspirates for mast cell disease, even more cells must be analyzed (500,000 or more), since the mast cells are usually under-represented, as discussed in Sect. 3.2.4.

MRD panels contain antibodies against one or more antigens for gating to track the same population of interest in each tube, and one or more antigens which may show aberrant expression patterns. While neoplastic cells may entirely gain or lose various antigens, they also frequently express aberrantly increased or decreased levels of antigens compared to the levels seen on their normal counterparts (Fig. 3-8). Common gating antigens and possible aberrant antigens are shown in Table 3-4, for several different diseases (B-ALL, T-ALL, PCM, MCD, and AML). The newest generation of clinical flow cytometers, with capabilities to examine 5–10 antibodies simultaneously in one tube, allow more efficient panels to

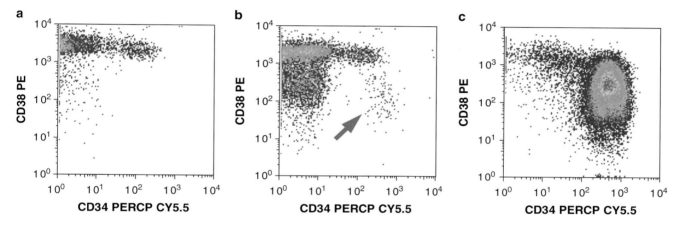

Fig. 3-8. *Minimal residual disease detection.* Shown are total CD19+ mononuclear cells in each specimen. (**a**) Normal bone marrow, with all CD34+ cells showing bright CD38 expression. (**b**) Minimal residual B-ALL, with aberrantly decreased CD38 expression (*red arrow*), in a background of normal B-cell precursors. Leukemic blasts comprise 0.1% of total cells. (**c**) Same patient during subsequent relapse, with 81% leukemic blasts

Table 3-4. Approaches to MRD detection.

Tumor type	Antigens for gating[a]	Possible aberrant antigens[b]
Precursor B-ALL	CD19, CD34, CD10	CD13, CD20, CD22, CD25, CD33, CD38, CD45, CD58, CD81
Precursor T-ALL	Cytoplasmic CD3, CD7	CD1, CD2, surface CD3, CD4, CD5, CD7, CD8, CD10, CD13, CD33, CD34, CD56, TdT
AML	CD45, CD34, CD117	CD2, CD5, CD7, CD13, CD15, CD19, CD33, CD56, CD65
CLL	CD19, CD5	Kappa/lambda, CD20, CD22, CD38, CD43, CD79b, CD81
B-cell lymphoma	CD19	Kappa/lambda, CD5, CD10, CD20, CD22
T-cell lymphoma	CD3	CD2, CD4, CD7, CD8, CD10, CD26
Mast cell disease	CD117	CD2, CD25, CD35, CD59, CD63, CD69

[a] Possible antigens to include in each staining reaction, depending on the number of colors available for analysis. Note that the gating antigens may also show aberrantly increased or decreased expression

[b] These lists are intended to be relatively comprehensive but not exhaustive

be constructed. In the extreme case, a panel using three antigens for gating and testing five antigens for aberrancy would require five staining tubes on a four-color cytometer, but could instead be performed in a single tube on an eight-color cytometer. Knowledge of the original phenotype is often helpful, but not essential in order to perform MRD testing. Phenotypes may change following chemotherapy, [14–16] due to direct effects of chemotherapy or radiation therapy, or clonal evolution possibly induced by therapy, or selection by therapy of minor subclones that were only present at low levels in the original neoplastic population.

3.4. Other FC Applications

3.4.1. CD4/CD8 Ratios and Immunophenotyping for Immunodeficiency

Lymphocyte subset analysis is one of the mainstays of therapeutic monitoring in human immunodeficiency virus (HIV) infection, and in the workup of patients with presumed genetic or iatrogenic immunodeficiency. A typical four-color panel for HIV is CD3, CD4, and CD8, and CD45 to assist in gating. Some centers also perform lymphocyte subset typing routinely in tumor types, such as CLL, that produce immune suppression. Finally, monitoring of immune function following stem cell transplantation may identify those patients with graft failure earlier than molecular assays. The use of FC to detect loss of GPI-linked proteins in paroxysmal nocturnal hemoglobinuria is discussed in Chap. 6.

3.4.2. Stem Cell Enumeration in Transplant Harvests

Stem cell transplantation requires the infusion of pluripotent stem cells which show CD34 expression with variable density of expression of CD38 and CD117. FC is used to quantitate the numbers of putative stem cells present in a harvest (e.g., blood following stem cell mobilization, donor BM harvests, or in vivo expanded cell populations). A standardized protocol has been established for stem cell enumeration, [17,18] using sequential gating to identify the rare cells with the expected levels of CD34 and CD45 expression and expected forward and side light scatter properties (Fig. 3-9). These gates should exclude events with nonspecific staining.

3.4.3. Staining for Phosphoproteins and Intracellular Proteins

Most of the routine FC antigens used for diagnostic and MRD applications are cell surface proteins. This obviates the need for cell permeabilization. However, several nuclear and cytoplasmic markers are routinely evaluated, such as terminal deoxynucleotidyl transferase (TdT), positive primarily in lymphoblastic cells, and myeloperoxidase (MPO) in myeloid and monocytic cells. Some surface antigens on mature cells are expressed in the cytoplasm at immature stages, and can be important for lineage assignment. These include cytoplasmic CD3 in T-lineage cells, and cytoplasmic CD22 in B-lineage cells.

The activation state of proteins can also be assessed using antisera (usually polyclonal) directed against phosphotyrosine (p-Tyr) residues that become phosphorylated upon activation of particular signaling pathways. These assays allow direct interrogation of the actions of inhibitors directed against particular signaling molecules. For example, intracellular levels of phosphorylated CRKL can be used as a marker or the activity of the BCR-ABL kinase in CML, and its level of inhibition by the kinase inhibitor imatinib (Gleevec) [19]. A similar strategy uses stimulators of signaling pathways, along with FC analysis of the p-Tyr status of downstream targets, to determine which pathways remain intact in neoplastic cell populations [20].

3.4.4. Maturation Abnormalities in MDS and MPN

Myelodysplastic syndromes and myeloproliferative neoplasms affect multipotent hematopoietic stem cells, which often lead to aberrant antigen expression in multiple cell lineages [21,22].

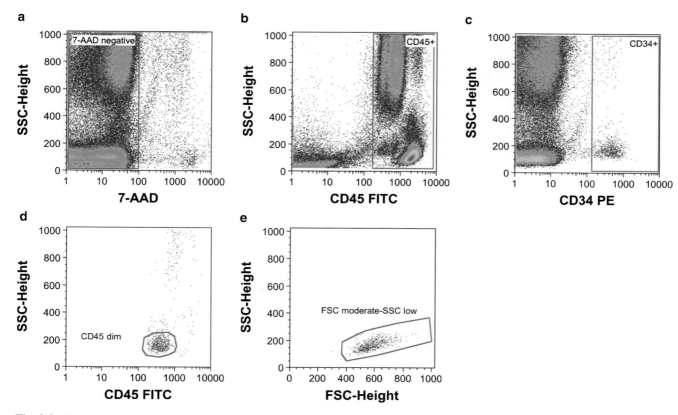

Fig. 3-9. *Stem cell enumeration by the ISHAGE sequential gating protocol, with assessment of viability.* The gated cells from each plot are displayed on the subsequent plot. (**a**) Total peripheral blood leukocytes, with gating on viable 7-AAD-negative cells (93%); (**b**) Gating on CD45 positive cells (81%); (**c**) Gating on CD34 positive cells (0.5%); (**d**) Gating on CD45 dim mononuclear cells in the blast gate (0.4%); (**e**) Gating on cells with low SSC and moderate FSC (0.4%)

Within the myeloid lineage, blasts may show aberrant phenotypes including lymphoid antigen expression. Later stages of granulocyte maturation may also be affected, with altered expression of developmentally-regulated antigens like CD13, CD11b, CD16 and CD10. For example, in normal maturation, CD13 is brightly expressed on promyelocytes, shows decreased expression on myelocytes, and then is again brightly expressed on metamyelocytes and later cells. In MDS, often the myelocytes fail to appropriately downregulate CD13 expression, altering the pattern of maturation seen on plots of CD13 vs. CD11b or CD13 vs. CD16 [23]. Other common abnormalities in MDS and MPN are aberrant increases of expression of CD56 on granulocytes and/or monocytes, and decreased side scatter of granulocytes, reflecting their aberrant cytoplasmic hypogranularity. Similar findings may be seen in both entities, so FC may not be helpful in the differential diagnosis between MDS and MPN.

3.4.5. DNA Content Analysis

FC assays using DNA-binding dyes may be used to detect altered DNA content (aneuploidy) in neoplastic cells, as well as to estimate the proliferating S-phase cell fraction [24]. Propidium iodide (PI), the most commonly used dye in clinical assays, shows increased fluorescence when it intercalates between bases in double-helical nucleic acid. Assays may be performed on clinical specimens, such as blood or bone marrow, or on nuclei isolated from paraffin-embedded tissue. PI does not cross the cell membrane, so assays on viable specimens require cell permeabilization. Data on cell aggregates must be removed during analysis by gating on the basis of their altered signal pulse characteristics (e.g., on signal height vs. area plots) compared with single cells. Control cells, such as peripheral blood lymphocytes, are used to establish the degree of fluorescence corresponding to diploid cells in G0/G1 phase. Aneuploid cells will show a brighter or dimmer G0/G1 peak. G2/M phase cells will show twice the fluorescent intensity of G0/G1 phase cells, and cells in S-phase show intermediate intensity.

3.4.6. Functional Assays

A number of specialized dyes are available for flow cytometric analysis of various functional cellular parameters, which are currently used predominantly in research studies. Changes in calcium concentration during cellular activation can be measured using calcium-sensitive dyes such as indo-1 [25]. Cell proliferation in vitro can be quantitated using dyes which covalently attach to cellular proteins, such as carboxyfluorescein diacetate succinimidyl ester (CFSE) [26]. During each subsequent cell division, the amount of bound dye decreases by one-half. After a time interval, the entire population can be analyzed to determine the number of cells with decreased labeling corresponding to one, two, three, or more cell divisions, and the doubling time can be thus calculated. Apoptosis can be assessed by several methods, including surface staining with annexin V, which binds phosphatidyl serine [27]. In viable cells, this phospholipid is sequestered in the inner layer of the plasma membrane, but in apoptotic cells it flips to the outer layer. Mitochondrial polarization may also be lost during apoptosis, and this function can be measured by FC using dyes which accumulate and fluoresce within normal mitochondria, such as JC-1 [28].

Suggested Readings

Wood B. Multicolor immunophenotyping: human immune system hematopoiesis. Methods Cell Biol 2004;75:559–76

Wood B. Nine-color and ten-color flow cytometry in the clinical laboratory. Arch Pathol Lab Med 2006;130:680–90.

McCoy JP Jr. Basic principles in clinical flow cytometry. In: Carey JL, McCoy JP Jr, Keren DF, eds. Flow cytometry in clinical diagnosis. 4th ed. Chicago, IL: American Society for Clinical Pathology Press, 2007:15–34.

Craig FE, Foon KA. Flow cytometric immunophenotyping for hematologic neoplasms. Blood 2008; 111:3941–67.

Campana D. Status of minimal residual disease testing in childhood hematological malignancies. Br J Haematol 2008;143:481–9.

References

1. Bonner WA, Hulett HR, Sweet RG, Herzenberg LA. Fluorescence activated cell sorting. Rev Sci Instrum 1972;43:404–9.
2. Kohler G, Milstein C. Continuous cultures of fused cells secreting antibody of predefined specificity. Nature 1975;256:495–7.
3. Stelzer GT, Marti G, Hurley A, McCoy P Jr, Lovett EJ, Schwartz A. U.S.–Canadian Consensus recommendations on the immunophenotypic analysis of hematologic neoplasia by flow cytometry: standardization and validation of laboratory procedures. Cytometry 1997;30:214–30.
4. Roederer M. Spectral compensation for flow cytometry: visualization artifacts, limitations, and caveats. Cytometry 2001;45:194–205.
5. Loken MR, Brosnan JM, Bach BA, Ault KA. Establishing optimal lymphocyte gates for immunophenotyping by flow cytometry. Cytometry 1990;11:453–9.
6. Stelzer GT, Shults KE, Loken MR. CD45 gating for routine flow cytometric analysis of human bone marrow specimens. Ann N Y Acad Sci 1993;677:265–80.
7. Wood BL, Arroz M, Barnett D, et al. 2006 Bethesda International Consensus recommendations on the immunophenotypic analysis of hematolymphoid neoplasia by flow cytometry: optimal reagents and reporting for the flow cytometric diagnosis of hematopoietic neoplasia. Cytometry B Clin Cytom 2007;72(Suppl 1):S14–22.

8. Keeney M, Gratama JW, Chin-Yee IH, Sutherland DR. Isotype controls in the analysis of lymphocytes and CD34+ stem and progenitor cells by flow cytometry–time to let go!. Cytometry 1998;34:280–3.

9. Schwartz A, Fernandez-Repollet E. Quantitative flow cytometry. Clin Lab Med 2001;21:743–61.

10. Weir EG, Cowan K, LeBeau P, Borowitz MJ. A limited antibody panel can distinguish B-precursor acute lymphoblastic leukemia from normal B precursors with four color flow cytometry: implications for residual disease detection. Leukemia 1999;13:558–67.

11. van Lochem EG, Wiegers YM, van den Beemd R, Hahlen K, van Dongen JJ, Hooijkaas H. Regeneration pattern of precursor-B-cells in bone marrow of acute lymphoblastic leukemia patients depends on the type of preceding chemotherapy. Leukemia 2000;14:688–95.

12. van Wering ER, van der Linden-Schrever BE, Szczepanski T, et al. Regenerating normal B-cell precursors during and after treatment of acute lymphoblastic leukaemia: implications for monitoring of minimal residual disease. Br J Haematol 2000;110:139–46.

13. McKenna RW, Washington LT, Aquino DB, Picker LJ, Kroft SH. Immunophenotypic analysis of hematogones (B-lymphocyte precursors) in 662 consecutive bone marrow specimens by 4-color flow cytometry. Blood 2001;98:2498–507.

14. van Wering ER, Beishuizen A, Roeffen ET, et al. Immunophenotypic changes between diagnosis and relapse in childhood acute lymphoblastic leukemia. Leukemia 1995;9:1523–33.

15. Borowitz MJ, Pullen DJ, Winick N, Martin PL, Bowman WP, Camitta B. Comparison of diagnostic and relapse flow cytometry phenotypes in childhood acute lymphoblastic leukemia: implications for residual disease detection: a report from the children's oncology group. Cytometry B Clin Cytom 2005;68:18–24.

16. Chen JS, Coustan-Smith E, Suzuki T, et al. Identification of novel markers for monitoring minimal residual disease in acute lymphoblastic leukemia. Blood 2001;97:2115–20.

17. Sutherland DR, Anderson L, Keeney M, Nayar R, Chin-Yee I. The ISHAGE guidelines for CD34+ cell determination by flow cytometry. International Society of Hematotherapy and Graft Engineering. J Hematother 1996;5:213–26.

18. Gratama JW, Orfao A, Barnett D, et al. Flow cytometric enumeration of CD34+ hematopoietic stem and progenitor cells. European Working Group on Clinical Cell Analysis. Cytometry 1998;34:128–42.

19. Hamilton A, Elrick L, Myssina S, et al. BCR-ABL activity and its response to drugs can be determined in CD34+ CML stem cells by CrkL phosphorylation status using flow cytometry. Leukemia 2006;20:1035–9.

20. Irish JM, Hovland R, Krutzik PO, et al. Single cell profiling of potentiated phospho-protein networks in cancer cells. Cell 2004;118:217–28.

21. Kussick SJ, Wood BL. Using 4-color flow cytometry to identify abnormal myeloid populations. Arch Pathol Lab Med 2003;127:1140–7.

22. Loken MR, van de Loosdrecht A, Ogata K, Orfao A, Wells DA. Flow cytometry in myelodysplastic syndromes: report from a working conference. Leuk Res 2008;32:5–17.

23. Stetler-Stevenson M, Arthur DC, Jabbour N, et al. Diagnostic utility of flow cytometric immunophenotyping in myelodysplastic syndrome. Blood 2001;98:979–87.

24. Darzynkiewicz Z, Huang X. Analysis of cellular DNA content by flow cytometry. Curr Protoc Immunol 2004;Chapter 5:Unit 5.7.

25. Rabinovitch PS, June CH, Grossmann A, Ledbetter JA. Heterogeneity among T cells in intracellular free calcium responses after mitogen stimulation with PHA or anti-CD3. Simultaneous use of indo-1 and immunofluorescence with flow cytometry. J Immunol 1986;137:952–61.

26. Lyons AB. Divided we stand: tracking cell proliferation with carboxyfluorescein diacetate succinimidyl ester. Immunol Cell Biol 1999;77:509–15.

27. Koopman G, Reutelingsperger CP, Kuijten GA, Keehnen RM, Pals ST, van Oers MH. Annexin V for flow cytometric detection of phosphatidylserine expression on B cells undergoing apoptosis. Blood 1994;84:1415–20.

28. Cossarizza A, Baccarani-Contri M, Kalashnikova G, Franceschi C. A new method for the cytofluorimetric analysis of mitochondrial membrane potential using the J-aggregate forming lipophilic cation 5, 5', 6, 6'-tetrachloro-1, 1', 3, 3'-tetraethylbenzimidazolcarbocyanine iodide (JC-1). Biochem Biophys Res Commun 1993;197:40–5.

Chapter 4

Molecular Diagnostics and Cytogenetic Testing

Su Chen, Zhuang Zuo, and Dan Jones

Abstract/Scope of Chapter This chapter covers the basic molecular diagnostic techniques of polymerase chain reaction (PCR), quantitative PCR, reverse transcription PCR and DNA sequencing. Advantages and pitfalls in the use of these different techniques for clonality assays and chromosomal translocation detection in lymphomas and leukemias are discussed. The types of high-throughput genomic and expression array technologies are also discussed with a review of the common data analysis techniques employed to handle these techniques.

Keywords Central dogma • MicroRNA • Epigenetics • Polymerase chain reaction (PCR) • PCR, reverse transcription • PCR, quantitative • PCR, real-time • Fluorescence in situ hybridization (FISH) • Karyotype, G-banded • Microarray, gene expression • Micoarray, genomic • Microarray, heat-map • Microarray • Analysis methods • High-throughput sequencing • PCR methylation • Comparative genomic hybridization

4.1. A Short History of Molecular Biology: The Central Dogma

The discovery of DNA as the heritable material by Avery and McLeod (1944) and Hershey and Chase (1950) followed by the elucidation of its structure as a double-stranded helix by Watson and Crick in 1953 opened the molecular era [1]. The first human chromosome studies (cytogenetics) were occurring at the same time. The recognition of discrete chromosomes as the structures responsible for Mendelian segregation of genes (by Barbara McClintock and others) focused attention on the role of chromosomes in human cancers. Beginning in 1952 with the correct enumeration of the human chromosome complement by T.C. Hsu, tumors have been routinely cultured and their chromosomes visualized (*karyotyping*). The recognition of the translocation of a portion of chromosome 9 to chromosome 22 (i.e., the Philadelphia chromosome) as the defining genetic event in chronic myelogenous leukemia by Nowell and Hungerford in 1962 was the first of many cancer-associated genetic changes identified.

Understanding of the structure of the chromosome, as a single continuous strand of DNA with A (adenine), C (cytosine), G (guanine), and T (thymine) nucleotides attached to a complementary strand (A with T, and G with C) by hydrogen bonds, led to methods to sequence and replicate DNA in vitro using purified DNA polymerases. Techniques to study specific segments of DNA (genes) followed soon thereafter, including the discovery and purification of a range of different restriction endonucleases from bacteria that cut DNA at specific base pair sequences (e.g., GGATCC), and the parallel development of bacterial and yeast vectors

From: *Neoplastic Hematopathology*: Contemporary Hematology,
Edited by: D. Jones, DOI 10.1007/978-1-60761-384-8_4,
© Humana Press, a part of Springer Science+Business Media, LLC 2010

to clone and express such cleaved human DNA fragments in model organisms. These methods allowed the construction of genomic libraries containing the full range of human DNA sequences whose base pair composition could then be determined by the enzymatic DNA sequencing methods described below.

In parallel, studies identified messenger (m)RNA as the substrate which is transcribed from the DNA sequence of a gene and then moves into the cytoplasm to the ribosomes to translate the genetic code into a protein (Fig. 4-1). The process of RNA transcription is initiated by the recruitment of RNA polymerases and transcription factors. *Promoter* DNA sequences upstream of the start site of the gene and additional regulatory *enhancer* sequences help control gene expression so that mRNA is transcribed in cell-specific patterns. Many of the oncogenes in leukemias and lymphomas are altered transcription factors that bind to promoter and enhancer sequences upstream of different genes than their normal counterparts, or block binding of the normal factors. This dominant-negative action of these cancer-causing altered transcriptional factors leads to a block in cell maturation that produces increased blasts.

Since RNA is labile and easily degrades, its use in molecular biology was limited until the discovery of the retrovirus-encoded reverse transcriptase (RT) enzymes that allow RNA to be converted into more stable *complementary (c)DNA*. mRNA, which initially is transcribed as an intact copy of the DNA sequence of a gene, is then processed by *RNA splicing* to remove the noncoding *introns* from a gene and link the coding *exons* together. This greatly shortens the length of a gene and makes RNA (or its cDNA copy) an ideal substrate for amplification and cloning of the coding sequence of a gene, or to detect DNA mutations that arise in cancer. However, RNA splicing is not exact and sometimes different mRNA sequences from the same gene are created by *alternative splicing*.

The cloning of cDNA of human genes into bacterial, yeast, and eventually into retroviral and eukaryotic expression vectors (that allowed expression in mammalian cells) was greatly facilitated by the development of the polymerase chain reaction (PCR) technique. First reported by Cory Mullis in 1983, PCR uses repetitive cyclic binding and extension of bidirectional primers that flank a target DNA sequence to greatly expand a limited number of DNA molecules to allow their easy cloning and sequencing.

A recent important development in molecular biology was the elucidation of the function of small nonprotein-coding RNAs (*micro RNAs or miRs*) as mediating the simultaneous degradation of multiple mRNAs through the RISC (RNA inhibitory silencing complex) mechanisms. This type of posttranscriptional method of gene regulation represents an *epigenetic* change, and coexists with other epigenetic processes such as methylation and acetylation of the histones that compact the chromosomes and methylation of DNA around promoter sites. Methylation

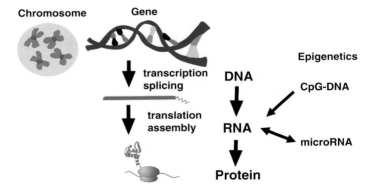

Fig. 4-1. *The central dogma: DNA to RNA transcription to protein translation.* Illustrated is a flowchart of DNA replication, DNA transcription to RNA, and RNA translation to protein. Epigenetic mechanisms including microRNA regulation of RNA transcript levels and reversible silencing of gene expression due to methylation of DNA at CpG islands around gene promoters represent recently understood shifts in the central dogma model

of DNA at cytosine-guanine sequences that are often found near the transcription start sites in genes (so-called "CpG" islands) has profound effects on the level of transcription. This process, termed *promoter silencing by CpG methylation*, has been shown to be important in both gene-specific and global gene regulation and underlies many of the gene expression changes seen in cancer cells.

4.2. Sample Preparation and Nucleic Acid Isolation

4.2.1. Sample Preparation

Specimens obtained for molecular studies in hematopathology commonly include peripheral blood (PB), bone marrow (BM) aspirate, fresh surgical biopsies, needle aspirates (FNA), body fluids, and formalin-fixed, paraffin-embedded (FFPE) tissues. Each of these sample types presents different challenges for processing, storage, and extraction of DNA, RNA, and protein for analysis. The decline in the use of open surgical biopsies for obtaining diagnostic material and the resulting disappearance of fresh-frozen biopsy material for testing has led to the increased use of FFPE and fixed material from cytology cell blocks for molecular testing. With the exception of G-banded karyotype and Southern blot, all of these methods discussed here, including FISH, arrays, and quantitative PCR, are now routinely performed on fixed materials in the clinical setting. Whole genomic DNA amplification methods are also now available to expand limited material [2].

The handling times and storage requirements for different tissue sources are summarized in Table 4-1, and generally reflect the regulatory guidelines of the College of American Pathology

Table 4-1. Specimen handling according to type.

Processing step	Peripheral blood and bone marrow aspirates	Fresh solid tissues	Formalin-fixed, paraffin-embedded (FFPE) tissue
Sample collection	EDTA (lavender-topped) tubes, not heparin (green-topped) tubes since heparin inhibits PCR amplification	Sterile container with a saline-dampened gauze to prevent drying, or frozen in OCT or liquid nitrogen	Prolonged formalin fixation increases degradation of nucleic acid with excessive cross-linking of proteins
Sample storage	2–8°C: ~2–3 days 22–25°C (room temp.): 2–3 days[a] −20°C: ~1 year −80°C: indefinitely	Some tissues (e.g., bowel, brain) degrade extremely rapidly so should be processed immediately or snap frozen, LN is stable for several hours to 2 days in media	Room temperature, avoid excess heating; adequate dehydration of tissues during paraffin embedding will limit degradation
Sample preparation	Remove red blood cells by lysis, pelleting, or Ficoll separation; wash leukocytes with PBS since contaminating hemoglobin inhibits PCR amplification	LN: create cell suspension in media DNA: lyse directly RNA: homogenize tissue immediately in Trizol, or flash freeze in liquid nitrogen and powder with pestle, or place in RNA stabilization solutions (e.g., RNA*later*)	Deparaffinize (using xylene or other oganics) and rehydrate through an alcohol series to a dilute salt buffer before scraping or microdissection, samples may be lysed directly into protein-containing buffer for DNA extraction

Abbreviations: *EDTA* ethylene-diamine-tetra-acetic acid, *LN* lymph node, *PBS* phosphate buffered saline
[a]Blood is more stable at room temperatures than BM aspirates which degrade rapidly and should be refrigerated

(CAP) [3]. More rigorous recommendations have been proposed by the National Institutes of Health and some of the cooperative oncology groups (e.g., NCCN, COG, etc) [4].

4.2.2. DNA Isolation

After initial processing of specimens, DNA isolation begins with cell lysis using proteases (typically proteinase K) and a detergent solution to break down cellular membranes. Various methods are available to purify the DNA contained in these cell lysates (Table 4-2). In organic solubilization, proteins and other cellular debris are fractionated into either the phenol or chloroform phases, and the DNA remaining in the aqueous phase is precipitated using ethanol, washed to remove salts, and resuspended in a low-salt buffer. In column chromatography methods, DNA is separated from protein and RNA, based on differential charge and size through a series of wash steps. In solid-phase (bead) methods, DNA is adsorbed onto a solid support while proteins and other cellular contents are washed away.

Solid-phase extraction methods are commercially available in fully-validated manual, semiautomated, and fully-automated formats. Automated nucleic acid isolation can minimize handling time significantly, provide consistent yields, minimize sample mix-ups, and be integrated with downstream applications like PCR. However, when minimal sample is present manual extraction methods are preferred.

After DNA is isolated, it is assessed for quantity and quality, most commonly using ultraviolet (UV) spectrophotometry by measuring the absorbance of a nucleic acid solution at several UV wavelengths. The quantity of nucleic acids is determined by absorbance at 260 nm wavelength (A_{260}) and the purity of the sample is indicated by A_{260}/A_{280} ratio which should range from 1.65 to 1.85 (Table 4-3). Nucleic acid quality can also be assessed using gel electrophoresis followed by staining with a DNA-binding dye, such as SYBR green or ethidium bromide. High-quality genomic DNA forms a sharp band near the well of the gel, whereas degraded samples produce a smear representing nucleic acids of varying sizes (Fig. 4-2a). Newer microfluidic separation methods (e.g., the Agilent Bioanalyzer) can provide more sensitive assessment of DNA quantity and quality. Purified genomic DNA can be stored at 2–8°C for weeks to months, and at −20°C or −80°C for years without significant degradation.

4.2.3 RNA Isolation and Reverse Transcription

Cellular RNA species include messenger (m)RNAs comprising transcripts from the protein-encoding genes (representing 1–5% of total RNA in most cells), the much more abundant ribosomal RNA (including the 28S, 18S, and 5S subunits), and the small micro RNAs (miRs), snRNPs, and transfer RNAs which carry amino acids to the elongating proteins at the ribosome.

The general techniques for isolation of RNA are similar to those for DNA (Table 4-2), however, RNase inhibitors are added, and RNase-free reagents are used to minimize degradation. The most common RNA extraction method uses a chaotropic salt (guanidinium thiocyanate) to aid in RNA:DNA phase separation during density centrifugation, and to help inhibit RNases (an example is the TRIzol reagent). Column and bead-based methods of RNA extraction are becoming more popular and generally result in RNA of higher purity. Additionally, when removal of all DNA is required, digestion using the DNase I enzyme can be added. RNA quantity and purity are assessed using UV spectrophotometry (Table 4-3). RNA quality can be assessed by ethidium bromide staining following slab gel electrophoresis since intact total RNA produces two distinct bands corresponding to the 18S and 28S rRNA. A 28S to 18S intensity ratio of 2.0 or more is consistent with minimal degradation whereas degraded samples will show indistinct 18S and 28S rRNA bands and a shift of staining to lower molecular weights (Fig. 4-2b). Purified RNA can be stored at −20°C for several weeks, but should be shifted to −80°C or liquid nitrogen for longer-term storage.

Table 4-2. Techniques for isolation of DNA and RNA.

Technique	Method	Advantages	Disadvantages
DNA extraction			
Organic solvent-based	Separation of DNA into soluble phase by phenol: chloroform extraction with subsequent ethanol precipitation	High recovery; scalability of sample size using batch method	Uses volatile hazardous solvents, labor-intensive, low throughput of sample volume
Column-based	DNA is adsorbed to silica-coated membrane, while proteins and other cell lysate components flow-through; membrane is then washed and the purified DNA eluted	Simple, fast, consistent, automation available	Membrane clogging problem, poor sample-size scalability, low throughput of sample volume
Bead-based	DNA is adsorbed to silica-coated beads, which are then pelleted or aggregated using a magnet, and washed, followed by elution of purified DNA	Scalable, high throughput of sample volume using multiwell plates, automation available	Lower recovery
RNA extraction			
Guanidinium-based cell lysis (e.g., TRIzol)	Organic separation with addition of chaotropic salt guanidium isothiocyanate to inactivate RNase and aid density separation	Scalable: 50×10^6 cells/ml of reagent	Volatile organics require special disposal
Column-based	Chromatography with addition of RNase inhibitors, with/without DNase I to remove residual DNA	Higher purity than TRIzol methods, can be used in tandem with other methods	Limited volumes unless multiple columns run per sample
Bead-based	Solid phase separation with RNase inhibitors to prevent degradation	Automatable and potentially scalable	Lower recovery than column methods, often

Table 4-3. Spectrophotometric quantification and purity assessment of DNA, RNA, and protein.

Substrate	Maximal absorption	Conversion factor	Purity assessment Quality assessment	Fixes for problems
DNA	260 nm	dsDNA = $A_{260} \times 50$ μg/mL ssDNA = $A_{260} \times 35$ μg/mL	$A_{260}/A_{280} = 1.65$–1.85 Electrophoresis	Repurify over sizing columns or extract with phenol
RNA	260 nm	$A_{260} \times 40$ μg/mL	$A_{260}/A_{280} = 1.8$–2.0 Electrophoresis	Repurify over columns Add RNase inhibitors
Protein	Several maxima, including at 280 nm	Absorbance with Bradford reagent at 595 nm, mapped against a standard curve (albumin dilutions)	Electrophoresis	Dialyze to concentrate. Add protease and phosphatase inhibitors for degradation problems

Abbreviations: *dsDNA* double-stranded DNA, *ssDNA*: single-stranded DNA

For use in PCR applications, RNA must be converted to cDNA using *reverse transcriptase* (RT) as the polymerase and either random hexamers or poly(T)-oligonucleotide (that bind to the mRNA poly(A)-tail) as primers to amplify the entire mRNA pool. Gene-specific primers can also be used to more selectively convert particular mRNAs to cDNA. Variability in the activity of different RT enzyme preparations makes conversion of RNA to cDNA the most variable step in PCR quantification of gene transcripts [5]. Since miRs and occasional noncoding RNA species cannot be amplified by conventional cDNA synthesis, it is recommended to preserve some sample within the laboratory as total RNA for any subsequent miR profiling needed.

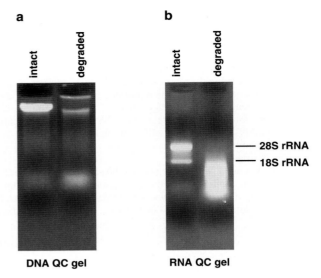

Fig. 4-2. *Quality assessment of DNA and RNA.* (**a**) Quality control (QC) assessment of DNA on an ethidium bromide-stained agarose gel shows fragmented low-molecular weight material in a degraded sample (*right lane*). (**b**) RNA QC gels show strong ribosomal (r)RNA bands in intact RNA, which are lost in a degraded sample (*right lane*)

4.3. Core Techniques of Molecular Diagnostics

4.3.1. Solid-Phase Hybridization (Southern and Northern Blot and Reverse Hybridization)

In classical hybridization methods, DNA, RNA, or specific PCR products are size-separated using slab gel electrophoresis and then the products are transferred in place from the agarose or polyacrylamide gel to a nylon or nitrocellulose membrane. This membrane is then hybridized with a labeled DNA probe that detects a gene or sequence target of interest. The binding of that probe is then visualized using autoradiography. Probes may be labeled with radioactive, colorimetric, or fluorescent markers (Fig. 4-3).

The first such probe hybridization technique to be developed, *Southern blot*, is illustrated in Fig. 4-3a. In this application, genomic DNA is digested with one or more restriction endonucleases that cut within the gene(s) of interest so that any disruption of the gene (whether by insertion, deletion, or rearrangement) is detected by an alternately-sized banding pattern following electrophoresis and probing. Radioactively-labeled DNA probes are typically more sensitive in detecting signal than colorimetric tags. The size difference between DNA molecules that can be unambiguously resolved using standard agarose gel electrophoresis is approximately 50 base pairs, although the use of gradient polyacrylamide gels especially with running buffers of different pHs can improve detection of smaller base pair changes. Nonetheless, Southern blot cannot be used to detect many clinically-significant alterations in genes such as point mutations, small insertions or deletions, or changes in DNA methylation status.

Southern blot is a labor-intensive technique which typically requires 3 days to complete. Currently, the principal uses of Southern blot in hematopathology include detection of rearrangements in the immunoglobulin (Ig) and T-cell receptor (TCR) genes for clonality assessment in lymphoid tumors, and for probing deletions or amplifications in large genes that are too long to be conveniently spanned by PCR and PCR-based DNA sequencing.

a

Hybridization against a sample

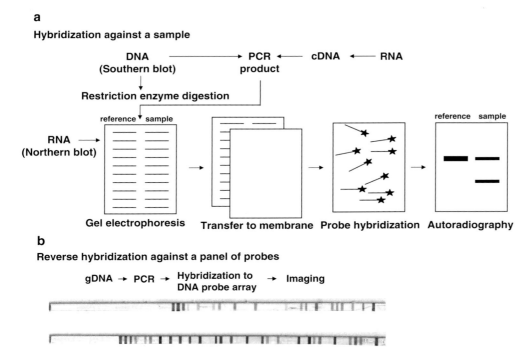

b

Reverse hybridization against a panel of probes

Fig. 4-3. *Solid phase hybridization.* (**a**) Steps in the Southern blot are illustrated for a reference and a patient sample. (**b**) Example of reverse hybridization using a sequence-specific oligonucleotide (SSO) array for HLA typing. Illustrated are HLA-A and HLA-Cw typing, showing A*02010101, 250101 type and Cw*0102, 150201 type, respectively

Other common applications of direct hybridization include Northern blot, where the range of transcripts expressed by a particular gene are assessed, and post-PCR hybridization, where the specificity of a particular band observed on a gel following PCR is confirmed by hybridizing against a probe for that gene.

A related blotting application is *reverse hybridization* in which DNA sequences from a tumor or body fluid are PCR-amplified and then labeled and hybridized against an array of probes that have been spotted onto a membrane or other matrix. These applications are widely used to detect the specific haplotype of the HLA loci (Fig. 4-3b and Chap. 29) or type the specific strain of a particular virus present in a sample. This technique also serves as the basis of most high-throughput array-based genomic and RNA expression methods that will be discussed in subsequent sections.

4.3.2. Polymerase Chain Reaction

Because of the inherent lack of sensitivity and nonquantitative nature of solid-phase hybridization techniques, PCR-based assays with fluorescent-label detection have gradually replaced membrane blotting in most clinical applications. The principal advantage of PCR is its ability to massively amplify the number of target nuclei acid sequences using a pair of oligonucleotide primers that flank the target DNA segment. PCR is a simple, iterative process consisting of: (1) denaturation of DNA double-strands at high temperature (94°C); (2) annealing of one copy of each primer to the opposite strands of the template at a lower temperature; and (3) extension of primers to create a new copy using a DNA polymerase (Fig. 4-4). PCR reactions contain, in addition to the sample DNA template, the four deoxynucleotide triphosphates (dNTPs) needed to extend the DNA, a thermostable polymerase capable of surviving heat denaturation (usually *Taq* polymerase), and the DNA primers at sufficient concentrations to allow amplification for at least 30 PCR cycles. In a well-designed

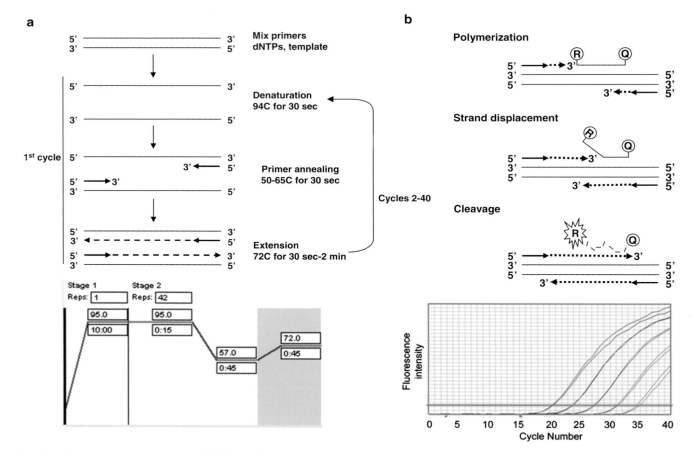

Fig. 4-4. *Polymerase chain reaction (PCR).* (**a**) Three-stage conventional PCR, with denaturation, annealing, and extension steps. (**b**) Quantitative PCR using the TaqMan method; the output for tenfold dilutions of a reference sample is shown below

PCR reaction, the amount of template DNA doubles with every cycle during the exponential phase. During the plateau phase, amplification gradually ceases as the progressively higher concentrations of template (relative to primers) leads to reannealing of double-stranded templates rather than further primer binding and extension.

Variants of PCR include, *multiplex PCR* in which several sets of primers for different genes (or different parts of the same gene) are combined together in the same tube, and *asymmetric PCR* in which only one primer is included so that only the opposite strand is amplified (utilized in Sanger sequencing described below). *Allele-specific (ASO) PCR* refers to the design of one primer, so it recognizes only one specific allelic DNA sequence (or mutated sequence) that usually only differs by a single base pair from the other allele or the unmutated sequence. Such single base pair mismatches in the primers require careful titration of the PCR annealing temperature so that the primer binds only to the desired sequence.

Reverse transcriptase PCR (RT-PCR) of RNA is done following cDNA conversion, either in two steps (RT followed by PCR) or in one step. The list of methodologic variations and applications for PCR and RT-PCR in the clinical laboratories is vast (Table 4-4), and has been greatly expanded with the introduction of capillary electrophoresis (CE) which can readily separate PCR products that differ from each other by as little as one or two base pairs (Fig. 4-5). In PCR with CE detection, one of the primers is labeled with a fluorochrome which is incorporated into the PCR products during amplification. A laser then detects the migration though the capillary matrix of the labeled PCR product(s) and compares its mobility to

Table 4-4. General categories of molecular techniques.

Categories	Methods	Applications
Size and charge separation of DNA fragments	Slab gel electrophoresis, capillary gel electrophoresis, microfluidic separation (e.g., Agilent Bioanalyzer), HPLC, mass spectrophotometry	DNA fragment size analysis (insertion/ deletion mutation detection), restriction fragment length analysis, SSCP and heteroduplex analysis, DNA sequencing methods
Use of fluorescent labels of DNA with/without amplification	*DNA binding dyes*: SYBR green, ethidium bromide *Fluorescent tags*: FITC, Cy3, Cy5 (arrays, FISH) *PCR probes*: TaqMan; dual hybridization probe; molecular beacons, scorpions, Lux, Uniprimer *Signal amplification probes*: bDNA, Invader cleavase, rolling circle, ramification	Detection of sequencing and PCR products by capillary electrophoresis, quantitative PCR methods, FISH, arrays
Nucleic acid hybridization	Southern blot (genomic DNA), Northern blot (total RNA), post-PCR detection with radioactive, colorimetric or fluorescent probes	B-cell and T-cell clonality assays (Southern), genetic deletion syndromes (Southern), chromosomal translocations, alternative splicing (Northern)
Nucleic acid amplification	*PCR variants*: RT-PCR, qPCR/RQ-PCR, ASO-PCR; multiplex PCR, nested PCR, DNA methylation-specific PCR *Isothermal amplification*: ligase chain reaction; TMA; strand displacement amplification; NASBA	Gene expression, fusion transcript detection and quantification, viral load assays, mutation detection T-cell and B-cell clonality assays, DNA methylation analysis
Reverse nucleic acid hybridization (arrays)	Strand-specific oligonucleotide probe arrays (SSOP), line probe assay (LiPA), array comparative genomic hybridization (CGH), oligonucleotide arrays, liquid bead arrays	HLA haplotyping, viral typing (HPV, HCV, etc.), genome-wide expression analysis
DNA sequencing	Sanger/chain-terminator method Pyrosequencing Nano- or high-throughput methods such as single molecule synthesis or hybridization, or high-scale pyrosequencing or hybridization methods	DNA mutation or SNP detection, fusion transcript verification Multigene mutation detection, genome-wise DNA methylation analysis
Conventional and probe-based visual chromosomal inspection	G-banded karyotype, FISH, SKY	Routine genomic profiles, translocation, target detection (e.g., HER2 amplification in breast cancer)

Abbreviations: *HPLC* high performance liquid chromatography, *SSCP* single-strand conformation polymorphism, *FITC* fluorescein isothiocyanate, *Cy3* cyanine 3, *Cy5* cyanine 5, *bDNA* branched-DNA, *FISH* fluorescence in situ hybridization, *RT-PCR* reverse-transcription PCR, *qPCR* quantitative real-time PCR, *RQ-PCR* real-time quantitative RT-PCR, *ASO-PCR* allele-specific oligonucleotide PCR, *TMA* transcription mediated amplification, *NASBA* nucleic acid sequence-based amplification, *SNP* single nucleotide polymorphism

that of reference size standards. The ability of CE to detect small size differences in PCR products has permitted assays that detect microsatellite polymorphisms between individuals that differ by as little as one to five base pairs which are the basis of tissue identity/forensics and donor/recipient chimerism determinations in transplant (see Chap. 29). CE-PCR also enables assays that detect small insertions and deletions that occur in cancer-causing genes in lymphomas and leukemias (Fig. 4-5).

Variables that can influence the efficiency of PCR include the quality of the DNA template, the length and specific sequence of the primers (particularly avoiding primer self-annealing, primer dimers, and binding of primers to other nontarget sites in the genome), the temperature of annealing, the time of PCR extension, and the amount of magnesium in the reaction buffer. Online freeware computer applications are available to assist in primer design and selection of thermocycling conditions. However, empirical optimization is often required for a new assay. PCR efficiency is highest when primers are located no more than 200–600 base pairs apart, but longer extension times and more stable DNA polymerases can be used to easily amplify up to 10 kb of DNA. However, for such long-range PCR protocols, the fragmented DNA isolated from formalin-fixed tissue specimens is frequently not usable.

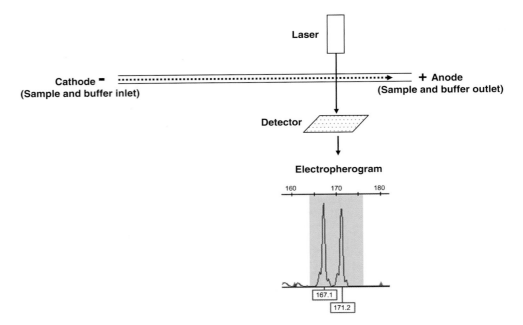

Fig. 4-5. *Capillary electrophoresis.* The sample electropherogram illustrated is from a case of leukemia with a 167 base pair (bp) PCR amplicon from an unmutated NPM1 allele and a 171 bp amplicon from the other allele with a 4 bp insertion

Common inhibitors of PCR present in extracted DNA include heme and heparin (from blood samples), melanin (from skin and hair samples), excess salt (from poor extraction techniques), and heavy metals present in some fixatives. DNA fragmentation, as occurs with acid treatment (of bone biopsies) or prolonged fixative exposure, can limit the number of amplifiable targets. The most effective measures for overcoming each of these problems are summarized in Table 4-5.

Given the high sensitivity of PCR, which can detect even a single DNA target, contamination of the initial starting material with stray DNA sequences is a common problem. This usually results from amplicons from previous PCR reactions which contaminate the reagents, tubes, or pipettes used for the setup of new reactions. Among the steps to prevent such contamination are: physical separation of preamplification/PCR setup and post-PCR areas, prealiquoted reagents, positive-displacement pipettes to minimize aerosolization, and the inclusion of a "reagent control" containing all components of the reaction except template to detect process-related contamination. PCR can also be done using the base pair dUTP which will be incorporated instead of dTTP so any prior amplicons present in a new reaction will be degraded by uracil-*N*-glycosylase (UNG). The use of real-time PCR, where amplicon detection and characterization can be done in a closed-tube system, has also helped greatly in controlling amplicon contamination.

4.3.3. Quantitative PCR and RQ-PCR

Real-time or quantitative (q)PCR is the technique by which amplicons are detected and quantified during their exponential expansion phase rather than at the end of cycling (plateau phase) when logarithmic doubling has ceased. Using genomic DNA as starting material, such qPCR can be used to calculate the copy numbers of amplified or deleted genes, or detect the percentage of mutated DNA sequences in a mixed population. When cDNA is used as the starting material, such RQ-PCR can be used to sensitively detect the level of gene expression over a 6-log range. Such closed-system qPCR systems also have advantages, in that a single

Table 4-5. Inhibitors of PCR and their fixes.

Type	Reason	Possible fixes
Contaminates in DNA template		
Heparin (from blood collection)	Binds to template and inhibits polymerase	Dilute sample, heparinase can be used
High salt, heavy metals (from alternative fixatives)	Inhibit DNA polymerase	Repurify DNA using column chromatography, dilute sample
Melanin	Inhibits DNA polymerase	Addition of albumin or alcohol extraction [33,34]
Heme from lysed blood cells		Repurify DNA using column chromatography, dilute sample
Reduced efficiency of PCR amplification		
Damaged DNA template	Effects of tissue drying, decalcification or fixation	Increase input template, shorten amplicon
Primer self-annealing	Hairpin formation in primers	Redesign primers
Unpredictable amplification results	Lack of adequate DNA polymerase processivity	Titrate magnesium concentration Switch to high fidelity polymerase
DNA sequence changes (errors) introduced during PCR		Switch to high fidelity polymerase

reaction tube is used for amplification and fluorescence monitoring so chances of contamination due to aerosolization or carryover is practically eliminated.

Common to all qPCR techniques is the detection of a fluorescent signal whose intensity is proportional to the amount of PCR amplicon generated during the reaction. The fluorochrome tag present in each reaction well is repeatedly excited (by a laser or other light source) and its emission measured at least once during every cycle of PCR. For example, the SYBR green dye fluoresces when it binds to double-stranded DNA, so increases in the copy number of DNA amplicons during PCR will result in an exponential rise in SYBR fluorescence corresponding to a two-fold rise during each PCR cycle (or a tenfold rise approximately every 3.3 cycles).

The more specific TaqMan probe chemistry relies on the design of a short, gene-specific probe that has a reporter fluorophore at its 5' end and a quencher molecule at the 3' end. The probe hybridizes to its target amplicon during the annealing step of each PCR cycle and is then hydrolyzed by the 5' exonuclease activity of *Taq* polymerase during DNA extension. When the TaqMan probe is hydrolyzed, the reporter fluorophore is detached from the adjacent quencher molecule and fluoresces in an amount proportional to the degree of PCR product amplification. Thus, as more and more probe is bound, hydrolyzed, and its reporter released, the detected fluorescence rises exponentially (Fig. 4-4b). Fluorescence detected above a set background (threshold) is interpreted as authentic, with the threshold cycle (Ct) determined by the inflection point of the rising curve used to calculate the quantity of target DNA. The Ct is converted to absolute target copy number in the initial sample by plotting it on a standard curve (log Ct vs. starting copy number) constructed from samples with a known target copy number. Target quantities can also be expressed relative to a coamplified normalizer control (e.g., expression levels of a housekeeping gene such as GUSB in RQ-PCR applications). This delta-Ct method for relative quantitation $[2^{-(Ct\ of\ gene\ target - Ct\ of\ reference\ gene)}]$ is used commonly when reference standards are not available.

In order for quantitative results to be comparable among different laboratories, assays must be calibrated to standards of known quantity. Unfortunately, commercially-available calibrators are not available for most molecular hematopathology assays, so standards must be made by individual laboratories in most cases. If multiple TaqMan probes are labeled with different fluorochromes, expression from several genes can be assessed simultaneously in the same reaction. However, such multiplex PCR can be technically challenging since the emission spectra of different fluorochromes overlap and will complicate accurate quantitation, analogous to the compensation problem in multicolor flow cytometry (see Chap. 3).

4.3.4. DNA Sequencing and the Interpretation of Base Pair Changes

The most common method for sequencing of DNA is the dideoxy chain-termination method, first reported by Fred Sanger in 1977, [6] which uses DNA polymerase to expand a single-stranded DNA template from a primer in the presence of chain-extending dNTPs and chain-terminating ddNTPs. PCR amplification of the extension reaction generates a complex population of different-sized DNA molecules which are terminated at every position following the primer (+1-T, +2-A, +3-C, +4-C, etc.). In the fluorescent-tag version of this technique, each of the four dideoxynucleotide chain-terminating base analogs (dGTP, dCTP, dATP and dTTP) are each labeled with a differently-colored fluorochrome. Incorporation of a colored terminator ddNTP into a growing chain stops the extension, and allows the terminal nucleotide of a DNA fragment of that size to be identified by capillary electrophoresis (Fig. 4-6). Software converts the fluorescent pattern from CE into an automated sequence base call, and compares the results from the samples to the reference sequence known for that gene.

The Sanger method can accurately sequence up to 500–1,000 base pairs of DNA from the template but is complex, taking 2–3 days to perform and is subject to many artifacts. The cycle-sequencing PCR reaction (step 3 in Fig. 4-6) is asymmetric so that a sequence is only obtained from one strand. To confirm changes seen, cycle sequencing is usually performed using a primer from the other strand (going in the reverse direction) prior to clinical reporting.

After confirming the presence of a sequence variation, the significance of the variation needs to be interpreted, differentiating between tumor-associated mutations, inherited single nucleotide polymorphisms (SNPs), and passenger mutations that make no functional difference to tumor growth (Table 4-6). Extensive public databases of known SNPs are now available that also include data on the population frequency. If an unexpected base pair change is encountered (i.e., one that is not an established SNP or has never or only rarely been previously associated with disease) including a caveat in the report on its unknown significance is critical.

Step 1:   PCR to create enough product
Step 2:   Remove unincorporated primers
Step 3:   Cycle-sequence by PCR with
           chain terminator fluorescent dNTPs

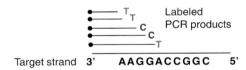

Step 4:   Clean up products
Step 5:   Detect products with capillary electrophoresis

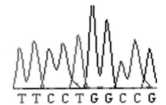

Step 6:   Compare base sequence to template in software

Fig. 4-6. *DNA sequencing.* The dideoxy chain-termination (Sanger) method is illustrated

Table 4-6. Types of DNA base pair changes encountered in tumors, and how to evaluate their significance.

Type	Feature(s)	Sample type	How to determine significance	Consequence	Database resources[a]
Germline mutation, disease-causing, inherited or sporadic	Inherited disease syndrome, usually manifest in childhood	Compare tumor with blood, or buccal swab	Occurrence in prior families with disease; Pedigree analysis to determine disease association	Pre- and posttest genetic counseling may be required Testing of family members Lifetime affect on disease monitoring Homozygous or heterozygous inheritance patterns	OMIN HGMD HGVS
Germline genetic polymorphisms (SNPs), population-based	Inherited monoallelic or biallelic base pair change without clear disease-causing role Often synonymous (noncoding change)	Compare tumor with blood or buccal swab	Population-based association studies comparing specific SNPs with disease risk;	Major contributor to individual differences in susceptibility to polygenic disease, immune response, and drug metabolism	dbSNP HapMap GeneSNP
Somatic mutation, disease-associated (driver mutation)	Seen in diagnostic samples or acquired with progression	Only seen in tumor sample	Previously reported in same tumor type; disease causing in in vitro or animal models	May indicate prognosis or suggest target for treatment	COSMIC
Somatic mutation, passenger	Acquired, but no discernable effect on the fitness of the neoplasm	Only seen in tumor sample	Not previously reported Absence of effect in vitro or in animal models	A byproduct of somatic evolution of tumor; may indicate an acquired defect in DNA repair with tumor progression	
PCR artifact	Due to mistake in early cycles of PCR by low-fidelity Taq polymerase	Any specimen	Repeat PCR with high-fidelity polymerase; Use non-PCR-based method to detect	No significance once confirmed	

[a]*Location of databases*: OMIN: http://www.ncbi.nlm.nih.gov/omim; HGMD: http://www.hgmd.cf.ac.uk/ac/index.php; HGVS: http://www.hgvs.org/dblist/dblist.html; COSMIC: www.sanger.ac.uk/genetics/CGP/cosmic; dbSNP: www.ncbi.nlm.nih.gov/SNP; HapMap: http://www.hapmap.org; GeneSNP: http://www.niehs.nih.gov/research/supported/programs/egp/genesnps/index.cfm

It is also important to use standard nomenclature in reporting the genes and the mutation to avoid confusion (Fig. 4-7) [7]. The American College of Medical Genetics (ACMG) [8] has published recommendations on interpreting sequence variation, with standardized nomenclature for reporting formalized by the Human Genome Variation Society (HGVS) [9]. The HUGO Gene Nomenclature Committee (HGNC) [10] now serves as the repository of official gene names, all of which must be composed of upper-case letters (with or without Arabic numerals) with no intervening punctuation allowed (i.e., lower-case letters are no longer used) Italics are often used but can be omitted (as in this textbook).

4.3.5. Other Methods of Sequencing and Mutation Detection

There are several other methods for interrogating the DNA sequence, including pyrosequencing, in which nucleotides are added one-by-one sequentially to a template and incorporation detected by the release of pyrophosphate (PPi) whenever a trinucleotide is added to a growing DNA strand. In contrast to the 20% sensitivity of mutation detection by Sanger sequencing, pyrosequencing can detect mutations present at levels as low as 1–5% of the template. For highly-sensitive detection of known single base pair mutations, allele-specific qPCR is often used, comparing the amplification levels of PCR probes or primers that differentially recognize the wild-type/unmutated and mutated sequences [11]. This method can routinely detect the presence of a mutation down to 0.01% of the template in the sample.

4.3.6. DNA CpG Methylation Analysis

Epigenetic changes such as DNA methylation and acetylation and histone acetylation can alter the ability of transcription factors and polymerases to attach to DNA and mediate transcription. Methylation of DNA occurs predominantly at cytosine residues within the CpG islands often present in the promoter regions of genes. When these CpG sequences located near a promoter are hypermethylated, the expression of the associated gene is suppressed.

Various qualitative and quantitative techniques are available to detect methylated CpG DNA. In most methods, the nonmethylated cytosines are converted to uracil (and then to thymidine during PCR replication) using sodium bisulfite treatment, whereas the methylated cytosines remain unchanged. Methylation-specific PCR (MSP) or qPCR can then be performed using different primers (or TaqMan probes) for the converted/unmethylated sequences (all "Cs" now converted to "Ts") vs. the unchanged sequence in methylated DNA. MSP protocols have now been adapted to the oligonucleotide-based microarray format for

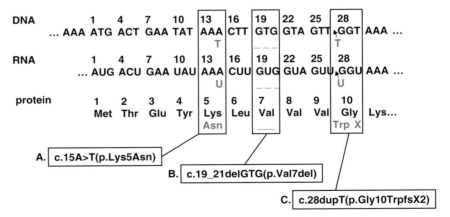

Fig. 4-7. *Nomenclature for DNA changes.* (**a**) Point mutation at position 15, corresponding to position 15 in the RNA transcript, and codon 5 of the protein resulting in a change from lysine (Lys) to asparagine (Asp). (**b**) Deletion of the whole codon GTG at DNA position 19–21. (**c**) Duplication of T at DNA position 28 causing frameshift resulting in glycine (Gly) to tryptophan (Trp) changes, and a stop codon ("X") at position 2

simultaneously interrogating a larger number of genes. The level of unmethylated vs. methylated DNA at any particular residue can also be directly assessed using PCR-based DNA sequencing or pyrosequencing on bisulfite-converted DNA.

4.4. Genomic Analysis

4.4.1. The Standard G-Banded Karyotype

Cytogenetic analysis is used to detect gross abnormalities of the chromosomes that can be seen by light or fluorescent microscopy. In conventional karyotyping, cells are trapped in metaphase and their chromosomes spread on a glass slide and stained with Giemsa (G) or another DNA-binding dye (Fig. 4-8a). Each stained chromosome has a different length and characteristic pattern of light and dark bands (cytobands). To assemble the karyotype, the full metaphase chromosomal complement from a cell is photographed and arranged in a linear array from chromosome 1–22 in order of length, with the X and Y chromosomes shown at the end. Each chromosome is arranged along its long axis with the short arm (p) facing up and the long arm (q) facing down (Fig. 4-8b) [12].

In traditional tumor cytogenetics, the metaphase chromosomes from 20 cells are examined and reported, giving a maximal sensitivity of 5% (1 in 20) for detection of any aberration. The same aberration must be seen in at least two cells (or in three cells for some aberrations)

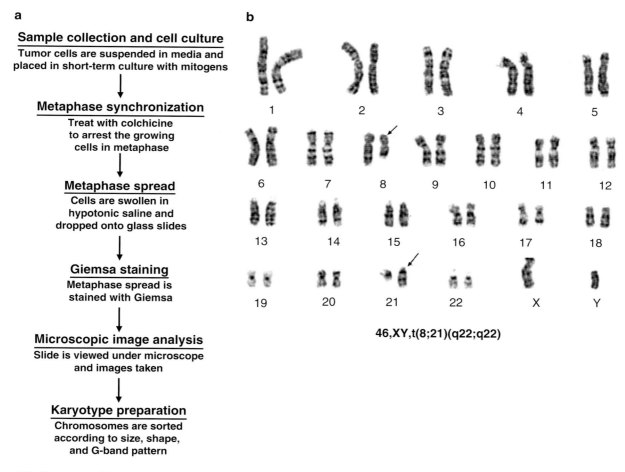

a

Sample collection and cell culture
Tumor cells are suspended in media and placed in short-term culture with mitogens

↓

Metaphase synchronization
Treat with colchicine to arrest the growing cells in metaphase

↓

Metaphase spread
Cells are swollen in hypotonic saline and dropped onto glass slides

↓

Giemsa staining
Metaphase spread is stained with Giemsa

↓

Microscopic image analysis
Slide is viewed under microscope and images taken

↓

Karyotype preparation
Chromosomes are sorted according to size, shape, and G-band pattern

b

1   2   3   4   5

6   7   8   9   10   11   12

13   14   15   16   17   18

19   20   21   22   X   Y

46,XY,t(8;21)(q22;q22)

Fig. 4-8. *Conventional karyotyping.* (**a**) Steps in the preparation of a G-banded metaphase preparation from short-term cultures. (**b**) Example of a karyotype showing 46,XX,t(8;21)(q22;q22)

to be regarded as a "clonal" change since short-term culture with mitogens occasionally produces artifactual chromosomal changes. An informative karyotype requires obtaining dividing tumor cells in culture so metaphases can be obtained. This is most difficult to achieve in low-grade lymphomas and easiest in aggressive lymphoma and myeloid leukemias. Therefore, the finding of a diploid karyotype (i.e., 46,XX or 46,XY) may be due to lack of any gross cytogenetic aberrations in the tumor or to a false-negative result because of the failure of the tumor cells to divide and generate metaphases in culture.

Alterations in chromosome copy numbers (aneuploidy) are common in cancer and are represented according to standard nomenclature in the karyotype (Table 4-7). Reciprocal chromosomal translocations represent an identifiable swap of chromosomal material between two (or more) chromosomes and some are common cancer-initiating events in lymphoma and leukemia. Other structural aberrations of chromosomes (e.g., deletion, amplifications, and inversions) are detected by abnormal banding patterns and ascribed as best as possible to specific cytoband intervals. However, the detection frequency and accuracy of describing such structural changes will be affected by the quality of the metaphase preparation, the quality of the staining, and the complexity of the changes. Chromosomes that are not morphologically identifiable are listed as markers ("mar" in the karyotype) and may be further clarified using chromosome or gene-specific FISH probes.

4.4.2. Fluorescence in Situ Hybridization (FISH)

FISH is performed by hybridizing a fluorescently-labeled DNA probe to chromosomal material to detect copy number or chromosomal alterations of the region covered by the probe. FISH can be performed on previously prepared metaphase spreads or on cells not in mitosis ("interphase FISH") from fresh samples or formalin-fixed tissues preparations. The procedure involves cell lysis (if needed), denaturation of the chromosomal DNA, hybridization of the labeled DNA probe, washing off of unbound probe, and then visualization under a fluorescence microscope. Multiple probes labeled with different colored fluorochromes

Table 4-7. Cytogenetic nomenclature for karyotype.

Type of aberrations	Definition	Nomenclature
Chromosome copy number terminology		
Diploid	Two copies of chr 1–22, and the XY or XX	46, XY [20}
Trisomy	Extra copy of a particular chromosome (in this case, trisomy 8 in 6 of 20 cells)	47,XY,+8 [6]/ 46,XY [14]
Monosomy	Loss of one copy of a chromosome	45,XY,−7
Tetraploid	Two extra copies of all chromosomes	92,XXXX
Unstable karyotype	Different numbers of chromosomes in different cell examined	45–47,XY,−3,+8,+21
Structural chromosomal abnormalities		
Reciprocal translocation	Swap of parts of two chromosomes with no loss of material	46,XX,t(9;22)(q34;q11)
Interstitial deletion	Loss of material between two cytobands	46,XX,del(5)(q13.3q33.1)
Terminal deletion	All material lost after indicated cytoband	46,XX,del(16)(q22)
Additional chromosomal material	Insertions of material after a cytoband	46,XX,add(14)(q32)
Pericentric inversion	Reversal in orientation of cytobands in same chromosome across the centromere	46,XY,inv(16)(p13q22)
Paracentric inversion	Reversal in orientation of certain cytobands in same arm of a chromosome	46,XX,inv(14)(q11q32.1)
Isochromosome	Duplication of one arm of the chromosome and loss of the other arm	46,XX,i(17q)

Additional guidance on nomenclature is provided in references [35,36]

can be combined together to assess multiple chromosomal aberrations simultaneously in the same cells. Because fluorescent signals are easy to count, many cells can be analyzed and most applications examine between 200 and 400 cells giving a sensitivity of FISH detection of between 1–3% for most alterations. Detection of aberrations is best in metaphase spreads where cells are separated from each other, and is worst in thick, fixed tissue sections where signals from multiple overlapping cells may give false-positive signals. Automated counting of FISH signals with image-processing algorithms, not yet in wide use, may increase sensitivity and reduce false calls due to cell overlap.

There are many clinical applications for FISH in hematopathology, including detecting chromosomal aberrations in tissues and in tumor types where culture is suboptimal (e.g., CLL and low-grade lymphomas) and in fixed material where metaphase karyotyping cannot be performed. The routine use of gene-specific FISH panels in CLL genomic profiling has been invaluable in identifying genomic losses or amplifications that are too small to be seen with conventional karyotyping. FISH can also quantify copy number changes in particular chromosomes using "painting probes" which are directed against chromosome-specific repeat sequences. FISH also has a large role in confirmatory testing to resolve complex changes seen in karyotypes or array-based genomic profiles (see Sect. 4.4.3). Finally, FISH is the best method to definitively detect the common reciprocal chromosomal translocations in lymphoma and leukemias.

Dual-color fusion FISH is the method used when both partner genes in a translocation are known (e.g., PML-RARA in AML), with each gene probe labeled with a different color fluorochrome. Whenever the translocation producing the fusion is present in a cell, a fusion signal merging the two fluorescent colors will be detected, along with the unfused signals from the nonrearranged alleles (Fig. 4-9a). When assessing a gene that can have multiple translocation partners (e.g., MLL in AML, or ALK in ALCL), break-apart probes are used with probes

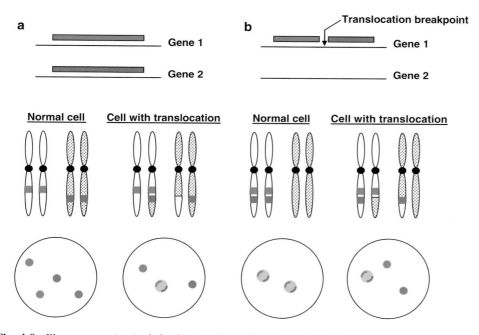

Fig. 4-9. *Fluorescence in situ hybridization.* (**a**) FISH illustrating a fusion probe approach to detect reciprocal chromosomal translocations. In a normal cell that lacks translocation, two green and two red signals are observed, reflecting two intact copies of each gene. In an abnormal cell with a translocation, one green, one red, and one yellow (fusion of green and red) signals are seen. (**b**) FISH illustrating a breakapart probe approach to detect translocation or disruption of a chromosomal locus. In a normal cell with two intact copies of a gene, due to the close proximity of the green and red probes, two yellow (fusion of green and red) signals are observed. In an abnormal cell with translocation occurring at the breakpoint between the green and red probes in one allele, one red, one green, and one yellow (normal allele) signals are observed

mapping to the 5' and the 3' regions of the target, each labeled with a different fluorochrome. In this case, the unrearranged allele will show a fusion signal, and presence of a translocation will be detected by splitting of the other signal due to separation of the probes (Fig. 4-9b). In metaphase spreads, the likely identity of the partner gene in the translocation can then be determined by which chromosome acquired the split signal.

4.4.3. Comparative Genomic Hybridization

Given the laborious nature of conventional karyotyping and the ability of FISH to only detect limited, previously defined genomic changes, high-throughput microarray techniques have begun to play a larger role in genomics. Array comparative genomic hybridization (CGH) is a powerful technique that derives the *consensus karyotype* (or average) of all of the DNA copy number changes in a sample by competitively hybridizing the fluorescently-tagged extracted DNA from a tumor against a normal reference sample that has been labeled with a different fluorescent tag (Fig. 4-10). Differences with conventional karyotyping include no need for short-term culture but the inability to detect chromosomal inversions or translocations where there is no net loss or gain of chromosomal material. SNP arrays represent another method of typing the genomic changes in a tumor. Unexpected finding of a small genomic gain or loss in a tumor by either technique must be interpreted with caution, since copy number variations (CNVs) are now known to be extensively present throughout the genome [13]. Comparison of a tumor sample with a nonneoplastic sample (e.g., buccal swab)

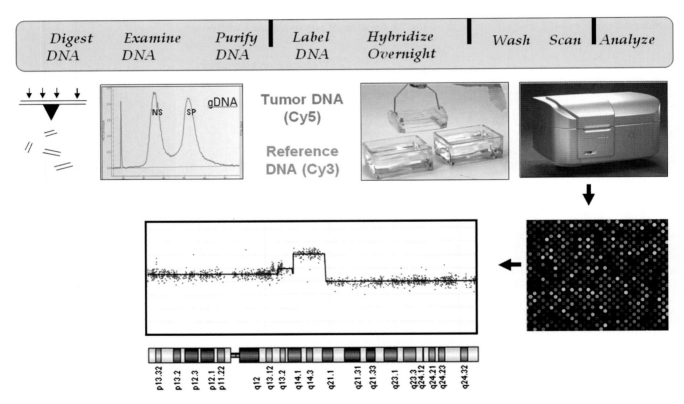

Fig. 4-10. *Array comparative genomic hybridization.* Illustration of the step in the process of DNA digestion, labeling with a red fluorescent probe, and competitive hybridization to a glass slide along with a test sample against reference (normal) DNA labeled with a green fluorescent probe. The glass slide is spotted with thousands of oligonucleotide probes from areas across the whole genome at an average resolution of one probe every several thousand base pairs. Hybridization signals are quantified and then normalized against the background following scanning of the relative red (sample) vs. green (reference) fluorescence for each spot. The values for each probe are then reconstructed into a karyotype of the sample

Table 4-8. Applications of molecular tests in hematopathology.

Categories	Clinical utility	Assay examples	Methods
Lymphoid clonality assays	Detection of clones	IGH rearrangement	Southern
	MRD monitoring	TCR rearrangement	PCR
Chromosomal translocation testing	Diagnosis	t(11;14)/CCND1-IGH	G-banded karyotype
	Prognosis	inv(16)/CBFB-MYH11	FISH
	MRD monitoring	t(14;18)/IGH-BCL2	PCR, RT-PCR
	Therapy response prediction	t(9;22)/BCR-ABL1	qPCR, RQ-PCR
Gene mutation testing	Diagnosis	KIT D816V	DNA sequencing ASO-PCR
	Prognosis	FLT3 ITD, NPM1	Electrophoresis
	MRD monitoring	JAK2 V617F	DNA sequencing
	Therapy response prediction	BCR-ABL kinase domain (acquired)	
Somatic hypermutation assessment (IGH)	Prognosis	CLL subtyping	ZAP70 IHC as surrogate marker

Abbreviations as in text

from the same patient is the best way to exclude a CNV, but public databases on known human variations are also widely available [14,15].

4.5. The Uses of Molecular Testing in Hematopathology

Molecular diagnostic techniques now have a wide range of uses in hematopathology. A core function is to help in diagnosis by detection of specific chromosomal translocations or mutations that define specific subtypes of lymphoma and leukemia (Chap. 1). A critical use of molecular testing is in the monitoring of patients under treatment with the detection of minimal residual disease (MRD) by molecular methods which may lead to continuation of therapy or change to a different drug. This application is most well-developed in CML (Chap. 9) but is also widely used in acute lymphoid leukemias (ALL) and acute myeloid leukemias that have specific defining chromosomal translocations (Table 4-8).

A more recent use of molecular studies has been their role in developing prognostic models for risk stratification. These commonly include transcript panels with RQ-PCR of a small number of genes that have been identified as prognostically important from retrospective whole genome gene expression microarray studies. An example of such an approach for diffuse large B-cell lymphoma is discussed in Chap. 33. Finally, the use of molecular testing to assist in therapy selection has begun to emerge as an important application. This is most developed for CML where the location of specific secondary resistance point mutations detected in the BCR-ABL kinase (following imatinib therapy) can be used to help select a new inhibitor (see Chaps. 10 and 11).

4.6. Lymphoid Clonality Assays

4.6.1. The Structure of the BCR and TCR Antigen Receptors

The process of DNA recombination of the variable (V), diversity (D), and joining (J) segments of the Ig and the TCR genes in B cells and T cells, respectively, provides the molecular basis of clonality testing. The surface B-cell receptor (BCR) is composed of one Ig light chain (either kappa or lambda produced from the IGK and IGL loci) and one heavy chain from the IGH locus (Fig. 4-11). B cells express only one clonotypic type of Ig (i.e., only one heavy and light chain protein per cell), and T cells similarly express only one TCR-α/β or TCR-γ/δ receptor.

During maturation of each precursor B cell in the bone marrow, one of the many possible V, D, and J segments in the IGH allele are recombined to create an intact V–D–J segment,

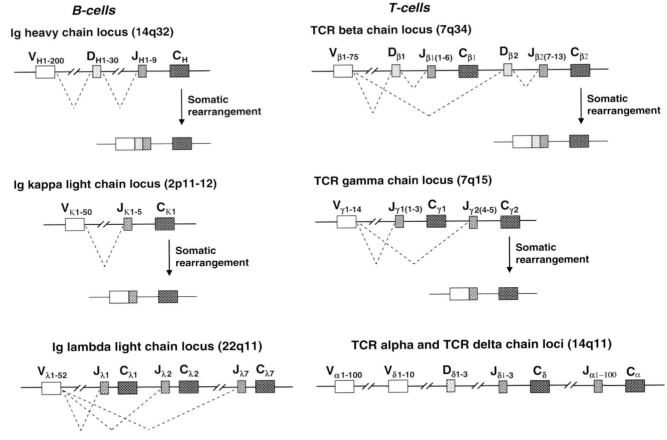

Fig. 4-11. *Structure of the antigen receptor genes used for lymphoid clonality assessment.* The IGH, IGK, IGL loci are rearranged in B cells, and the TCRB, TCRG, and TCRA/TCRD loci are rearranged in T cells. Acute lymphoblastic lymphoma/leukemia can rearrange any of these loci (promiscuous recombination) due to their frequent expression of the proteins in the recombination machinery (TdT and the Rag recombinases)

which is then spliced together with one of the five constant (C) regions during transcription to create a single transcript encoding IgM/IgD or (after class-switch) IgA, IgG, or IgE. Additional size and sequence variation of the V–D–J segment is created during this recombination by the addition or deletion of base pairs at the V–D and D–J junctions. If the VDJ rearrangement is "in-frame", meaning it is translated into a functional IGH protein, recombination of the light chain IGK locus proceeds by VJ recombination. If the VDJ recombination from the first IGH allele is out-of-frame, resulting in a nonfunctional IGH, the second IGH allele is recombined prior to IGK rearrangement. This process of *allelic exclusion* also occurs with the light chain genes so that a nonfunctional IGK allele leads to rearrangement of the second allele, and then sequentially at the two IGL loci until a functional Ig light chain protein is produced. As a result, every mature B cell has one or both of its IGH alleles rearranged and one or both of its IGK alleles rearranged, as well as one or both of its IGL loci rearranged if it expresses lambda light chain.

Similarly, in precursor T-cell development in the thymus, the TCRG loci undergoes V–J rearrangement until a functional gamma chain is made, followed by V–D–J rearrangement of TCRD until a functional TCR-γ/δ protein is expressed. If either of these recombination events fails to produce an intact receptor, the TCRB loci undergoes V–D–J rearrangement followed by VJ rearrangement of the TCRA loci. Thus, mature γ/δ-T cells have TCRG and TCRD rearrangements and α/β-T cells have rearrangements of TCRG, TCRB, and TCRA

(TCRD is usually deleted during the process of TCRA recombination, see Fig. 4-11). When examining the entire lymphocyte population, marked overrepresentation of one particular size V–(D)–J rearrangement in the Ig or TCR genes is thus indicative of an expanded population of lymphocytes derived from a common progenitor (i.e., a clonal proliferation). A comparison of the different IGH and TCR clonality detection techniques is presented in Table 4-9.

4.6.2. B-cell Clonality by IGH Southern Blot Analysis

In IGH Southern blot, restriction enzyme-digested genomic DNA fragments are separated by agarose gel electrophoresis, transferred to a nylon membrane, and hybridized with a DNA probe specific to the IGH J or C region. Since only B cells undergo IGH rearrangement, all non-B cells in the sample have an identical pattern of bands detected (i.e., the unrearranged germline pattern) whereas polyclonal B cells show a range of different-sized bands due to variable VDJ recombination which appears as a smear on the autoradiogram. In contrast, monoclonal B-cell proliferations show discrete bands different in size from the germline

Table 4-9. Comparison of lymphocyte clonality assays.

Test	Uses	Diagnostic sensitivity	Analytical Sensitivity	Limitations
IGH, Southern blot	Gold-standard for B-cell clonality in diagnostic fresh/frozen samples	>95% of B-cell tumors, if tumor cells ≥ 10% of cells in sample	5–10%	• Laborious technique with lower analytical sensitivity than PCR • Requires 5–10 μg of genomic DNA from fresh or frozen samples • Negative in some primitive B-ALL • Up to 40% positivity in T-ALL (promiscuous rearrangement)
IGH PCR (Biomed-2)	B-cell clonality in any sample type MRD monitoring	79–100%[37]	1–5%[a]	• Up to 30% false-negative rates in GC/post-GC B-cell tumors due to somatic hypermutation changing primer binding sites (improved with use of FR1 and FR2 primers sets in addition to FR3) • Up to 20% positivity in T-ALL[38] • Occasional false-positive signals using Biomed-2 FR2 primer sets[39]
Clone-specific IGH PCR	MRD monitoring	Varies in different tumor types	1:1,000–100,000	• IGH rearrangement in diagnostic clone must be sequenced, and a clone-specific CDR3 primer made • Sensitivity will depend on the levels of amplification seen in polyclonal B cells
IGK PCR	2nd-tier assay for B-cell clonality	80–100%[37]	1–10%	• Up to 20% positivity in T-ALL[38]
TCRB, Southern blot	Gold-standard for T-cell clonality in diagnostic fresh/frozen samples	80–95%,[40] if tumor cells ≥ 10% of cells in sample	5–10%[40]	• Negative in γ/δ-T-cell tumors and primitive T-ALL • Up to 50% positivity in B-ALL (promiscuous rearrangement)
TCRB PCR (Biomed-2)	T-cell clonality in any sample type MRD monitoring	74–100%[38]	0.1–10%[a]	• Limited sensitivity in mixed polyclonal/monoclonal T-cell samples • 3–14% positivity in B-cell tumors (mostly B-ALL)[37]
TCRG PCR (Biomed-2)	Same as TCRB PCR	74–96%[38]	1–10%	• Many false-positive calls due to overinterpretation of canonical or pseudoclonal peaks (see text) • 2–18% positivity in B-cell tumors (mostly B-ALL)[37]

[a]Average sensitivity, although greatly dependent on the level of polyclonal lymphocytes in sample

bands (Fig. 4-3). To be seen above the smear background of polyclonal B cells, monoclonal populations must comprise 10% or more of the total B cells in the sample, greatly limiting the sensitivity of Southern blot. Inclusion of a digestion control (nonlymphoid) tissue is recommended for each assay. To ensure specificity, separate digests of the sample DNA with three different enzymes are usually done with detection of rearranged bands in at least two digests necessary for unequivocal determination of clonality. Southern blot of the IGK locus can also be done by similar methodology.

4.6.3. B-cell Clonality by IGH and IGK PCR Analysis

PCR clonality assays for IGH and IGK rely on detecting size differences in the length of V–(D)–J segment due to additions/deletions introduced at random during the recombination of the progenitor B cells. The design and assay conditions for assessing B-cell clonality using PCR for the IGH and IGK loci have now been standardized [16]. The IGH-VJ assay, which is the most commonly-used test, employs a single consensus J primer that recognizes all IGH J regions, combined with forward primers directed against the conserved framework region (FR)1, FR2, and FR3 regions in three separate tubes. An illustration of the results for monoclonal, oligoclonal, and polyclonal B-cell populations is shown in Fig. 4-12. Polyclonal lymphocyte populations demonstrate a Gaussian/normal distribution pattern due to the presence of multiple PCR amplicons of different sizes which represent the diverse V(D)J recombination and the random nucleotide insertion/deletion at the ends of rearranging V, (D), and J segments. In contrast, monoclonal lymphoid cells produce amplicons of identical size which will manifest as a single peak or two different peaks if biallelic IGH rearrangements are present in the tumor clone. The IGK or IGH D–J PCR assays [16] may be useful in detecting clonality in lymphoblastic leukemias since these tumors often have incomplete recombination of the antigen receptor genes.

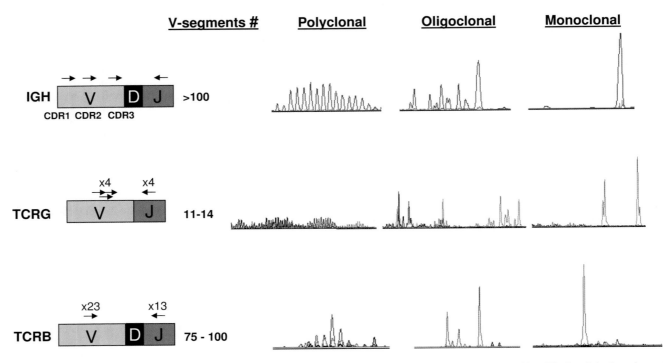

Fig. 4-12. *Lymphoid clonality PCR assays for the IGH, TCRG, and TCRB loci.* Structure of the rearranged V–(D)–J and the locations of the primers are shown on the left. Examples of polyclonal, oligoclonal, and monoclonal amplification patterns detected using multicolor capillary electrophoresis detection

A specialized use of quantitative (q)PCR in B-cell clonality determination is *clone-specific qPCR,* where the expressed IGH variable region in a B-cell tumor is sequenced and a specific primer is made that binds to the unique V–D–J junction (CDR3) and then used as the forward primer in qPCR with a reverse universal J primer (similar to conventional IGH PCR) and a family-specific J TaqMan probe. If the probe is designed well, only the B-cell tumor cells will amplify (and not the polyclonal background B cells which lack the unique CDR3 sequences), and quantification of tumor levels can be obtained down to 1 in 100,000–1,000,000 sensitivity levels [17].

4.6.4. T-cell Clonality by TCRB and TCRD Southern Blot Analysis

T-cell clonality can be determined using Southern blot of the TCRB, TCRG, TCRA, and TCRD loci (Fig. 4-11). TCRB is most commonly used for Southern blot since the large size of the locus means that V–D–J rearrangement usually results in large differences between the germline and rearranged bands that are easy to detect by routine agarose gel electrophoresis. As with IGH, separate digestion with three different restriction enzymes is recommended, with size changes seen in at least two digests used as the criteria for clonality. Southern blot of the TCRD locus can also be used for clonality assessment since it resides within the TCRA locus and the generation of a functional TCR-α/β will result in deletion of the intervening TCRD locus. Southern blot assays for T-cell clonality determination have been increasingly replaced by PCR due to the former's lower intrinsic sensitivity which is especially a problem in mixed tumor/inflammatory conditions where the polyclonal smear from nonneoplastic T cells may obscure clonal TCRB or TCRD rearrangements.

4.6.5. T-cell Clonality by TCRG and TCRB PCR Analysis

Consensus PCR primers, developed by the BIOMED-2 group, [16] are highly sensitive with false-negative rates in T-cell malignancies of only 5-10% with either the TCRG or TCRB assay (Table 4-9). However, TCR clonality by PCR is difficult to interpret given the propensity for false-positive results and distinguishing oligoclonal from monoclonal patterns of amplification, particularly in the TCRG assay (Fig. 4-12). These false-positive results have two main causes: pseudoclonality, which gives PCR spikes whenever only a small number of T cells are present in the sample, and amplification of nonclonal T cells with canonical TCRG rearrangements giving a false-positive clonal pattern.

Canonical rearrangements occurring in γ/δ-T cells are a function of the limited V-region diversity of the TCRG and TCRD loci. Many γ/δ-T cells have TCRG V-J rearrangements that utilize the same V and J segments and lack deletion or insertion compared to the germline sequence. This results in single spike PCR amplification patterns from polyclonal γ/δ-T cells that appear monoclonal. Spurious clonality due to canonical rearrangements is particularly a problem in clinical settings (e.g., postchemotherapy or stem cell transplant) and at sites where gamma/delta T cells are prominent (i.e., spleen, blood, and bone marrow), and is not seen in lymph node samples. Finally, it should be remembered that ~40% of all precursor B leukemias will display clonal TCRG or TCRB rearrangements due to lineage infidelity. As a result, whenever possible, the results of TCRG and TCRB assays should be correlated with the histologic findings before assuming T-cell clonality. The term "oligoclonal rearrangement" should be used liberally whenever discordances are noted.

4.7. Detection of Fusion Transcripts in Leukemia by RQ-PCR

Chromosomal translocations in CML, AML, ALL, and some lymphomas (e.g., NPM1-ALK in anaplastic large cell lymphoma) lead to the creation of an aberrant chimeric gene with a fusion transcript containing parts of two genes from each of the partner chromosomes. These translocations can be detected by karyotype or by fusion FISH (Fig. 4-9), but these techniques lack the sensitivity and ease of automation of PCR. Since each translocation creates

Table 4-10. RQ-PCR assays for detecting and quantifying fusion transcripts in leukemia and lymphoma.

Translocation	Genes	Transcript pattern Reference for method	Alternative methods	Comments
Myeloid neoplasms				
t(9;22)(q34;q11)	BCR-ABL1	Separate primer-probes for: e13a2 in CML e14a2 in CML e1a2 in Ph+ALL [41]	Dual-fusion FISH G-banded karyotype	Rare alternate fusions not detected by RQ-PCR (see Chap. 9)
t(15;17)(q22;q21)	PML-RARA	10–15% of AML in younger pts; separate primer-probes for long and short forms (PML breakpoint variation) [41]	Dual-fusion FISH G-banded karyotype	Rare variants require other primers
inv(16)(p13q22)	CBFB-MYH11	8–10% of AML in younger pts; isoform A is the only common breakpoint in AML [41]	Dual-fusion FISH	Karyotype has high false-negative rate
t(8;21)(q22;q22)	RUNX1/RUNX1T1 (AML1-ETO)	8% of AML in younger pts; single common fusion [41]	Dual-fusion FISH G-banded karyotype	
Lymphoid malignances				
t(4;11)(q21;q23)	MLL-AFF1 (MLL-AF4)	5% of B-ALL, some biphenotypic AL; several alternate fusions requiring two or more primer sets [41]	Dual-fusion FISH	
t(1;19)(q23;p13)	TCF3-PBX1 (E2A-PBX1)	3–5% of B-ALL, single common fusion [41]	Dual-fusion FISH	
t(12;21)(p13;q22)	ETV6-RUNX1 (TEL-AML1)	25% of childhood B-ALL; two recurrent breakpoints [41]	Dual-fusion FISH	
t(11;18)(q21;q21) and other MALT lymphoma fusions	API2-MALT1	RQ-PCR methods preferred due to variations in levels of fusion transcript [42]	Dual-fusion FISH Nuclear BCL10 IHC Long-range DNA PCR	Hybrid approach with IGH and MALT1 break-apart FISH probes may be best for MALT lymphomas [43]
t(2;5)(p23q35)	NPM1-ALK	RQ-PCR assay allows use in blood, BM for staging/ prognosis [44]	Dual-fusion FISH ALK IHC	Alternate fusion partners make break-apart FISH a better choice

a unique mRNA that is not present at all in normal cells, highly-sensitive RT-PCR assays can be designed by selecting a forward primer from one gene and a reverse primer from the other and then using cDNA to look for PCR products that reflect the abnormal fusion genes. When designing such assays, it is important to consider the types of fusion transcripts that can occur so that PCR will amplify all of the common variants. Table 4-10 summarizes the most commonly employed RQ-PCR assays for fusion transcripts in hematologic diseases, for which most have had extensively validated primer and probe sequences published.

Qualitative testing of cDNA for such fusion transcripts with probe-based detection following gel electrophoresis is gradually giving way to RQ-PCR, which has the ability to precisely quantify the disease levels.

4.8. Detecting Chromosomal Translocations in Lymphoma by DNA PCR

Characteristic chromosomal translocations in lymphoma such as t(14;18)/IGH-BCL2 in follicular lymphoma, t(11;14)/IGH-CCND1 in mantle cell lymphoma (MCL), and the t(8;14)/IGH-MYC in Burkitt lymphoma lead to increased expression of a structurally normal oncogene by bringing it under the transcriptional regulation of *cis*-acting elements (promoters and enhancers) of the IGH gene which are highly active in mature B cells. These translocations are typically detected by break-apart or fusion FISH probes or by Southern blot looking for rearrangement of the target gene loci (Table 4-11).

Because these IGH translocations do not generate a unique fusion transcript, PCR must be done across the chromosomal breakpoint using genomic DNA and cannot utilize the highly sensitive RQ-PCR strategies described above. This presents difficulties since many of the breakpoints in these translocations can occur across a wide region, including up to 100,000–1,000,000 base pairs in some cases. Detection strategies by PCR rely on designing multiple IGH-target gene PCR primer sets and focusing on the most common areas of translocation within the partner genes. For follicular lymphoma, this is the major breakpoint region (MBR), which is a ~150 base pair region in the 3' noncoding region of BCL2, which is the site of the chromosome 18 breakpoint in 65–70% of follicular lymphoma cases. For mantle cell lymphoma, the most commonly tested area involves a 100–1000 base pair major translocation cluster (MTC) upstream of the CCND1 (cyclin D1) gene which will detect 35% of cases. For those lymphomas with PCR-detectable breakpoints, MRD analysis can be done on followup samples with highly-sensitive qPCR to monitor for residual lymphoma (Fig. 4-13).

Table 4-11. Detection of lymphoma-associated translocations involving immunoglobulin gene enhancers.

Translocation	Gene involved	PCR strategy	Alternate methods
t(14;18)(q32;q21)	BCL2	Mbr breakpoint primers detect 60–70% of cases	Dual-fusion FISH G-banded karyotype
t(11;14)(q13;q32)	CCND1	MTC breakpoint primer detect 30–35% of cases	Dual-fusion FISH G-banded karyotype
t(8;14)(q24;q32) t(2;8)(p12;q24) t(8;22)(q24;q11)	MYC	None, given large size of breakpoint area at MYC	Breakapart FISH to detect any MYC partner
t(3;14)(q27;q32)	BCL6	None, given large size of breakpoint area at BCL6	Breakapart FISH to detect any BCL6 partner

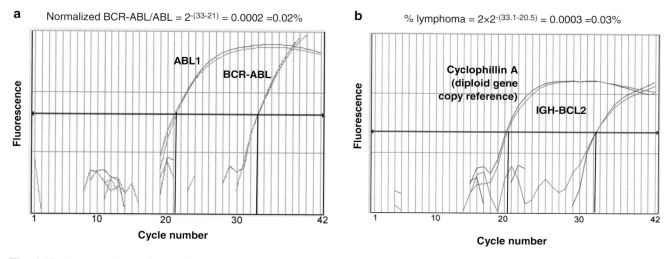

Fig. 4-13. *Quantitation of disease levels in followup samples.* (**a**) TaqMan RQ-PCR assay illustrated for detection of the BCR-ABL fusion transcript with normalization to total ABL1 levels. The level of disease calculated by the ΔCt method is shown above. (**b**) Detection of MRD in follicular lymphoma by qPCR using genomic DNA shows residual disease detected by Mbr-IGH primer sets normalized to the cyclophilin A (PP1A gene at chr 7p13) corresponding to 0.03% of lymphoma cells in this blood sample

4.9. Mutation Analysis in Acute Leukemias

One increasing use of molecular testing in hematopathology has been the detection of point mutations and gene deletions that have prognostic importance in AML. These include small duplications in the NPM1 gene that occur in normal karyotype AML, and internal tandem duplications (ITDs) in the FLT3 tyrosine kinase that occur in 25–30% of AML and are correlated with poor outcome. Since both mutations produce size changes, they can be detected using PCR-CE assays (Fig. 4-5). Other alterations, such as NRAS and KRAS point mutations and more complex deletions and mutations in the CEBPA and RUNX1 genes, require DNA sequencing.

Another indication for gene mutation testing is for predicting therapy response. This is best exemplified by assays to detect BCR-ABL point mutations mediating imatinib resistance in CML which can not only demonstrate the cause of such therapy resistance but, based on which particular mutation is detected, help in selecting an alternate therapy [18]. The use of JAK2 and MPL gene mutation profiling to assist in classification of myeloproliferative neoplasms (MPNs) is another application (see Chap. 9).

4.10. IGH Somatic Hypermutation Analysis of B-cell Tumors

Somatic hypermutation (SH) of the IGH locus is present in B cells that have undergone germinal center (GC) affinity maturation (see Chap. 12) and thus mark GC or post-GC derivation in B-cell tumors. This result is most relevant clinically for CLL where the post-GC subset has been shown to have a better prognosis and a different pathogenesis than the pre-GC subset (see Chap. 14) [19–21]. The mutation status of the IGH locus is typically assessed using multiplex RT-PCR of total cellular RNA followed by DNA sequencing. The sequence of the expressed IGH transcript is then compared to the germline sequence from a public database, with a homology of less than 98% (i.e., > 2% sequence variation) considered to be evidence for somatic hypermutation. This cutoff is established since some few germline changes in the IGH locus can occur between different individuals due to inherited IGH gene polymorphism. SH mutation testing is a complex assay to perform, so use of surrogate markers that partially predict SH status, such as detection in CLL of the expression of the ZAP70 kinase or surface CD38 (both associated with unmutated/pre-GC status), is favored by many centers.

4.11. Expression Microarray Techniques

4.11.1. History of Microarray Development and Applications

Microarrays were first reported in 1995 as a research tool to simultaneously detect transcriptional levels of many different genes [22]. All current microarray platforms for DNA and RNA are based on the complementary hybridization between nucleic acid sequences. Using photolithography (i.e. Affymetrix chips), "inkjet" technology, or precise spotting with small pins, tens of thousands gene-specific probes (longer cDNAs or shorter oligonucleotides) can be applied to a glass slide or silicon chip. Appropriate target nucleic acid extracted from a specimen is then labeled with a fluorescent dye and hybridized to the array. Hybridization is then assayed by measuring the fluorescence for each probe using a confocal laser scanner. Other medium to high-scale "array" platforms for multiparameter DNA and RNA assessment have also been developed including liquid bead arrays, or solid-phase "bar-coded" substrates to distinguish individual sequences (Table 4-12).

Global gene expression profiling in cancer began in 1999 with the discovery that the expression pattern of a set of genes could distinguish acute lymphoblastic leukemia (ALL) and acute myeloid leukemia (AML) [23]. The use of expression microarrays to provide prognostic and predictive gene signatures in hematopoietic neoplasms was first demonstrated in studies of diffuse large B-cell lymphoma [24] and are discussed in greater detail in Chap. 33. The range of analytes that can be measured by microarray now includes DNA mutations and

Table 4-12. Types of microarrays.

Technology type	Principle	Uses	Example of platforms	Range of events
Single-color system	Test and reference samples hybridized to different chips/slides, data compared computationally	Expression (including microRNA) SNP, CGH, ChIP-on-chip, methylation resequencing, exon arrays, tiling arrays	Affymetrix GeneChip, NimbleGen	Millions
Competitive hybridization (dual-color)	Test and reference samples labeled with different colors, and competitively hybridized	Expression (including microRNA) SNP, CGH, ChIP-on-chip analysis Methylation	Agilent oligonucleotide microarrays; conventional spotted cDNA microarrays; BAC arrays; Roche NimbleGen	Tens to millions
Liquid bead microarray	Oligonucleotides linked to uniquely colored micro-sphere beads and then hybridized to labeled samples	Expression on focused sets of genes/microRNA; genotyping on focused sets of DNA polymorphisms	Luminex xMAP technology	Tens to hundreds
Tagged methods	Fixing nebulized and adapter-ligated DNA fragments to small DNA-capture beads in a water-in-oil emulsion, emulsion PCR to generate "bead clones"	Sequencing	454 Life Sciences (Roche); ABI SOLiD	Millions to hundreds of millions
Bead array	Oligonucleotides attached to decoded silica beads (barcoding) or beads randomly deposited into wells on substrate (glass slide)	Expression, SNP, CGH, ChIP-on-chip analysis, methylation sequencing, exon arrays	Illumina	Tens of thousands to >one million

SNPs, chromosomal gains and losses, micro RNA (miRs), epigenetic changes on DNA (e.g., methylation arrays), proteins, and antibodies. The goals of microarray applications now extend from mechanistic studies to disease classification, and to biomarker and therapeutic target identification.

4.11.2. Microarray Analysis Techniques

Regardless of the analyte measured or the hybridization techniques used, analysis of micro-array data uses similar analysis algorithms. Microarray data analysis begins with collecting the raw data which is an image file acquired from the microarray scanner. This image must first be converted into a numerical format that quantifies the fluorescence signals from each measurement. This is usually accomplished by the image-processing algorithms built into the microarray vendor's software package. Following collection, the data are normalized to minimize the variations attributable to measurement, i.e., differences in the efficacy of probe labeling, hybridization, or signal detection. The locally-weighted scatter-plot smoothing algorithm is commonly used for this purpose. The data are then generally filtered for minimal variance genes to reduce the number of data elements requiring analysis. These normalization and filtering transformations must be carefully applied as they can have a profound effect on the analysis results.

A large variety of statistical and data-mining techniques can be applied to the next stage of data analysis, depending on the study design and goals. Table 4-13 summarizes the commonly-used methods and algorithms. One common purpose of a microarray study is to identify the differentially-expressed genes among study groups to establish potential cor-relations between genes and specific phenotypes. Simply evaluating the significance of the fold-changes in expression levels using the t-test or ANOVA is applicable. However, when

Table 4-13. Algorithms and analysis methods used in genome-wide analysis.

Type of analysis	Use/strength	Limitations
Analysis of differentially expressed genes		
Fold change methods: • k-fold change or unusual ratios Parametric test: • Paired and unpaired t-tests • Nearest neighbor analysis • Fisher's discriminant criterion • ANOVA (> two groups)	• Straightforward and intuitive • Suitable for data sets without replicates • Two-way ANOVA ideal for normalization of microarray data	• Arbitrary threshold • Low-level expression subject to noise • Assume normal distribution of data, • Design studies for two-way ANOVA can be expensive
Nonparametric tests: • Mann–Whitney test • Kruskal–Wallis Test (> two groups)	• Makes no assumptions about the distribution pattern of the data • Less sensitive to outliers and noise	• Less powerful than parametric tests, especially when sample size is small
Model-fitting techniques	• Best for large gene sets • Suitable for data sets without replicates	• Assumes normality of the data • Not applicable for smaller gene sets
Corrections for multiple variable effects: • Family wise error rate (FWER) • False discovery rate (FDR) • Permutation correction • SAM • Bootstrap analysis	• Estimates error rate (false positives) • Independent of statistical method used • FWER and FDR control global rate • Resampling methods (SAM, permutation and bootstrapping) correct among data objects • Bootstrapping is more sensitive and accurate for microarray data	• FWER and FDR can be too stringent • Assumes genes are independent • SAM, permutation and bootstrapping are computation intensive
Pattern/class discovery (unsupervised methods for identification of distinct gene expression patterns among sample groups)		
Hierarchical clustering	• Most widely used in microarray analysis • Dendrogram and heatmaps allow thorough inspection of entire data set	• High computational complexity • May lack robustness • Difficult to assess strength of cluster • No guide to choose number of clusters
Principal component analysis (PCA)	• Reduces dimensionality of data while still captures the salient variations • Visualization of sample clusters by signature	• Components are not biologically selected • May not be an ideal initial approach to identify significant genes
k-means clustering	• Partition-based clustering method • Simple and fast for smaller gene sets	• Require initial stipulation of some global parameters, e.g., number of clusters • Assumes genes are independent and normally distributed • Empirical, black box approach, may not be practical for lager gene sets • Sensitive to noise
Self-organizing map	• Single layered neural network • Partition-based, efficient and robust • Hierarchical structure can be built	• Require initial stipulation of some global parameters, e.g., number of clusters • Sensitive to noise
Class prediction (supervised methods that impose known groups on datasets, assign unknown sample to a defined group)		
Linear discriminant analysis	• Classic statistical classification method	• Linear discriminant functions need to be prespecified
k-nearest neighbor classification	• Instance-based classification • Simple, flexible and effective	• Can be slow with larger data set • No explicit generalization is done
Decision tree	• Easy to build and understand • No prior assumptions about data required • Able to model complex functions	• Requires discretized expression levels into categorical values • Prone to overfitting • Unstable and can be quite complex
Support vector machine	• More powerful, handles nonlinear separability	• Prone to overfitting • Posterior probability not provided • Extension to multiple classes is difficult
Artificial neural network	• Ideal for finding relationships among large complex data set	• Black box approach, lack of explanation • Can be difficult to build • Can be slow with larger data set

analyzing tens of thousands of genes, the false discovery rate (FDR) associated with multiple testing has to be considered. The significance analysis of microarrays (SAM) method has been developed to specifically address this issue [25]. SAM uses permutation of measurements to estimate the FDR, and assigns a score to each gene according to its change in gene expression. Genes with scores greater than a threshold are considered as "potentially" significant. SAM is widely applied in gene expression profiling studies (Fig. 4-14).

While SAM is a supervised algorithm that requires prior knowledge of the classification type of sample groups, unsupervised approaches are used to discover new distinct groups of phenotypes defined by gene expression patterns (class discovery). Hierarchical clustering is the most commonly-used technique in this category and it generates a tree graph (dendrogram) to represent the hierarchical series of nested clusters of the phenotype groups. The associated gene expression patterns are visualized by a heatmap (Fig. 4-15). Self-organizing maps (SOM), *k*-nearest neighbor, and principal component analysis [26] are examples of other techniques that can be used to identify subclasses in the data by determining relationships of groups that share similar patterns of gene expression.

The most attractive and promising application of microarrays in clinical practice is for predicting outcome and therapy response. This process generally includes: (1) identification of the informative genes (gene signature) using training set samples; (2) establishing a model system that reflects the relationship between phenotypes and the gene expression patterns; and (3) validation of the model system by a different set of testing samples. Several such applications have recently been cleared by the Food and Drug Administration (FDA) using guidelines for in vitro diagnostic multivariate index assays (IVDMIA) tests.

One potential challenge in gene expression profiling studies is that, very often, the identified signatures are not easily interpreted causally or mechanistically with respect to the

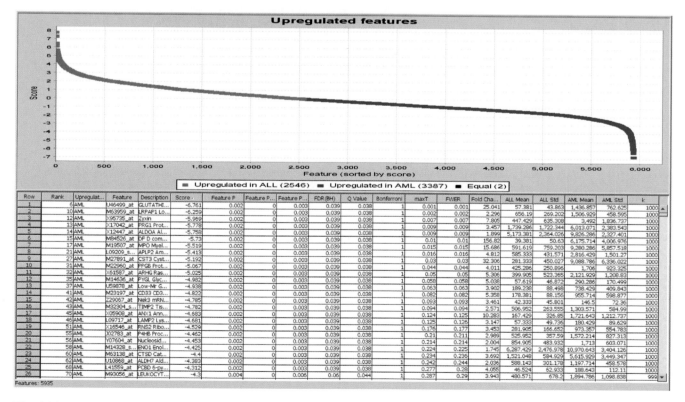

Fig. 4-14. *An example of comparative gene marker selection by SAM score.* Plot of genes (*x* axis) and their SAM scores (*y* axis) using data from Golub et al. (1999) [23]. Statistical significance of each gene is determined by the *p* value as shown in the table

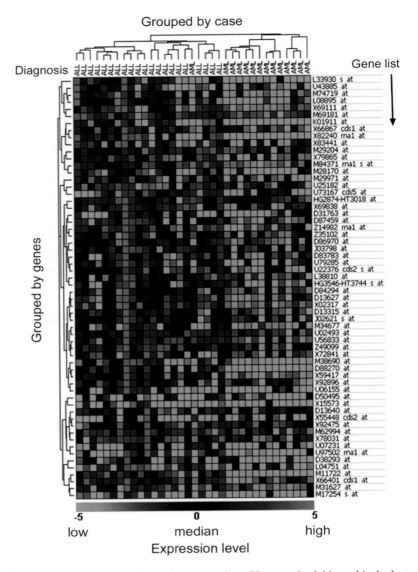

Fig. 4-15. *A heat map of expression microarray data.* Unsupervised hierarchical clustering was performed using a subset of genes are expressed in DLBCL from the dataset of Golub et al. (1999). Pearson correlation coefficient was used to compute gene and case similarity. The cluster-to-cluster distance was computed using the average linkage. The relative gene expression scale is depicted at the bottom with the normalized scores ranging from −5 to 5. Gene cluster and case cluster dendrograms are plotted to the top and left sides of the heatmap, respectively. The Affymetrix probeset identifiers are shown to the right side

underlying diseases. It is therefore an active area of bioinformatics research to develop tools that enable the association of genes with particular biological pathways and networks. The most authoritative content currently in this area is the Gene Ontology coding, which is a controlled vocabulary produced by the Gene Ontology Consortium to describe the function of gene products, their location in the cell, and the biological process that they are involved in. However, a large number of other techniques and algorithms have been developed to enrich the gene expression data with biological function information, and incorporate pathway analysis into microarray studies [27].

4.12. Assay Validation and Quality Control in Molecular Testing

4.12.1. Regulations in the United States Governing Molecular Assays

Clinical diagnostic laboratories in the United States are regulated through the Clinical Laboratory Improvement Amendments (CLIA), with routine compliance inspections and certification performed through one of its "deemed status" authorities such as the College of American Pathologists (CAP). As such, testing laboratories must abide by the regulations of the FDA regarding validation of diagnostic and predictive molecular assays. In vitro diagnostic (IVD) kits marketed for diagnostic use require formal FDA approval of their claims and performance characteristics, and as a result do not need extensive validation if used as intended in the testing laboratory [28]. However, as of 2009, there were limited numbers of IVD kits in hematopathology applications so most testing is still done through "home-brew" or laboratory-developed assays (LDA) that require full validation studies [29]. Such LDAs typically combine in-house developed reagents (e.g., controls and buffers) with commercially-available and validated analyte-specific reagents (ASR) such as enzymes, primers, and probes.

4.12.2. The Components of an Appropriate Assay Validation

For an FDA-approved IVD kit, the testing laboratory need only periodically verify the already established performance characteristics of the test, whereas the performance characteristics of LDAs must be first established and then periodically validated. All test results from a LDA must include a disclaimer that the performance characteristics of the assay have been determined by a validation study within the laboratory. Analytical validation of the assay performance characteristics involves demonstration of the accuracy, reproducibility/precision, sensitivity, and specificity on an adequate number of samples with a range of expected values (Table 4-14). For quantitative assays, the linear dynamic range of the assay must also be demonstrated using external calibrators. The CAP assay validation requirements are publicly available in CAP's Molecular Pathology Checklist and are periodically updated to be in compliance with practice standards and the CLIA guidelines. Clinical validation of

Table 4-14. Analytic validation of assay performance characteristics.

Terms	Definitions	How to establish
Analytic sensitivity	Lowest level of an analyte that can be reliably detected	Test on serial dilution of a sample of known quantity and ascertain the limit of detection
Diagnostic sensitivity	Ability to detect all samples containing the analyte [=TP/(TP+FN)]	Assess for false negatives (FN) by analyzing all variants of a disease condition diagnosed by a combination of other methods
Specificity	Ability to detect only the analyte and not other interfering analytes or substances [=TN/(TN+FP)]	Assess for false positive (FP) results by testing a range of different relevant substances besides the analyte
Accuracy	Extent to which results are close to the true values	Compare to a gold standard method
Precision	Reproducibility of results when tests are run repeatedly	Calculate standard deviation and coefficient-of-variation
Linear dynamic range	The concentration range of the analyte that can be reliably quantitated	Find the linear segment of a calibration curve by testing a serial dilution of the analyte; the lower and the upper end of the linear segment represents the lower and the upper limit of quantitation

the significance of an assay is often beyond the means of an individual laboratory and draws heavily on published studies and cooperative and consensus group efforts.

4.12.3. Run Controls and Sample Calibrators

Once an assay has been validated, quality control (QC) procedures have to be established to monitor every step in the analytical testing process from sample receipt to results reporting. Critical for such QC is inclusion of appropriate controls on every test run with the control samples processed in the same manner as the routine patient samples (Table 4-15). For quantitative assays in which standard curves are not generated for each run, controls with low, mid, and high positive levels should be included to ensure the expected dynamic range. Performance can be monitored over a period of time using tools such as the Levey–Jennings chart, which plots the mean and the standard deviation (SD) of the controls (vertical-axis) against time (horizontal-axis) to assess for assay drift (Fig. 4-16). When the controls fall within the ± 2 SD limit the test run is in control and the test results are considered acceptable. When the controls fall outside the ± 2 SD limit the test run is considered out-of-control, and a decision about accepting or rejecting the test results needs to be made. Westgard proposed six rules (Table 4-16) to determine acceptance or rejection of test runs based on QC results on a Levey–Jennings chart [30].

Strict QC criteria are most important for those assays in which quantitative results are used to guide therapy, such as viral load for hepatitis C or BCR-ABL quantitation in CML [31]. Translocation-bearing cell lines available from commercial sources or public cell banks are the most useful for creating assay controls that are stable over time [32]. Some quantitative assays are designed to have calibrators that are spiked into the sample before nucleic acid extraction for normalization of loss of target molecule during extraction, and for detection and normalization of any inhibitory factors.

4.12.4. Competency and Proficiency Testing

Molecular diagnostic testing is regarded as high-complexity according to CLIA regulations and thus calls for stringent quality assessment (QA) standards, including participation in an external proficiency testing (PT) program, such as the Laboratory Accreditation Program offered by CAP, for all tests at least once a year. PT exchanges with another laboratory performing

Table 4-15. Types of controls used in PCR assays.

Control types	Examples	Comments
Positive control	A known positive sample	Test result should be positive to assure the sensitivity of the test
Sensitivity control	A known positive sample with concentration close to the limit of detection	Test result should be positive to assure the sensitivity of the test
Negative control	A known negative sample	Test result should be negative to assure the specificity of the test
No template/reagent control	Only reagents without any DNA	Test result should be negative to assess for DNA contamination
Internal/inhibitor control	Endogenous housekeeping gene or an exogenous spiked-in artificial DNA	Test result should be positive to assess for inhibition of PCR amplification
Quantitative control	A positive sample with known quantity (low-, mid-, high-positive controls)	Needed for quantitative assays Test result should fall within acceptable range, usually within ± 2 standard deviation, to assure accuracy of quantitation

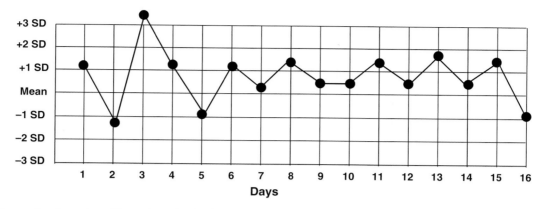

Fig. 4-16. *Levey–Jennings chart.* Illustration of a plot for monitoring quantitative controls over 16 days. A Westgard rule 1:3s violation on day 3 and rule 10: mean violation from day 6 to 15 are shown

Table 4-16. Westgard's rules for quantitative molecular assays.

Rules	Explanation
1:2s	Warning when one control observation exceeds the mean ±2 SD limit
1:3s	Reject when one control observation exceeds the mean ±3 SD limit
2:2s	Reject when two consecutive observations exceed the same mean ±2 SD limit
R:4s	Reject when one control observation exceeds +2 SD limit, and another exceeds −2 SD limit
4:1s	Reject when four consecutive control observations exceed the same mean ±1 SD limit
10:mean	Reject when ten consecutive control observations fall on one side of the mean

the same test are acceptable if no external program is available. Personnel performing the test must have appropriate qualifications, training, and demonstrable competence in technical skills, as well as adequate knowledge of the procedure, equipment operation, and laboratory safety. Competency training must also include a continuing education program and an annual assessment. For participating sites, CAP inspection of the entire laboratory is done every 2 years by an external team using the CAP General Laboratory and Molecular Pathology Checklists as guidelines. Failure to comply is documented as a deficiency which requires a plan for corrective action plan. If deficiencies are not fixed in a timely manner, loss of certification may result.

Suggested Readings

Finan JE, Zhao RY. From molecular diagnostics to personalized testing. Pharmacogenomics 2007; 8:85–99.
- An excellent review of PCR detection methods.

Roberts PC. Gene expression microarray data analysis demystified. Biotechnol Annu Rev. 2008; 14:29-61.
Wang J. Computational biology of genome expression and regulation--a review of microarray bioinformatics. J Environ Pathol Toxicol Oncol. 2008;27:157-79.
- Introductions to analysis of microarray data.

References

1. Wilkins MH, Strokes AR, Wilson HR. Molecular structure of deoxypentose nucleic acids 1953. Nature 2003;421:398–400; discussion 396.
2. Luthra R, Medeiros LJ. Isothermal multiple displacement amplification: a highly reliable approach for generating unlimited high molecular weight genomic DNA from clinical specimens. J Mol Diagn 2004;6:236–42.

3. Molecular Pathology Checklist. Commission on Laboratory Accreditation, College of American Pathologist. 2007 (Accessed 2009, at www.cap.org)

4. Compton C. The cancer and leukemia group B pathology committee at 50. Clin Cancer Res 2006;12:3617s–21.

5. Hughes T, Deininger M, Hochhaus A, et al. Monitoring CML patients responding to treatment with tyrosine kinase inhibitors: review and recommendations for harmonizing current methodology for detecting BCR-ABL transcripts and kinase domain mutations and for expressing results. Blood 2006;108:28–37.

6. Sanger F, Nicklen S, Coulson AR. DNA sequencing with chain-terminating inhibitors. Proc Natl Acad Sci U S A 1977;74:5463–7.

7. Ogino S, Gulley ML, den Dunnen JT, Wilson RB. Standard mutation nomenclature in molecular diagnostics: practical and educational challenges. J Mol Diagn 2007;9:1–6.

8. Richards CS, Bale S, Bellissimo DB, et al. ACMG recommendations for standards for interpretation and reporting of sequence variations: Revisions 2007. Genet Med 2008;10:294–300.

9. Horaitis O, Cotton RG. The challenge of documenting mutation across the genome: the human genome variation society approach. Hum Mutat 2004;23:447–52.

10. Wain HM, Bruford EA, Lovering RC, Lush MJ, Wright MW, Povey S. Guidelines for human gene nomenclature. Genomics 2002;79:464–70.

11. Gibson NJ. The use of real-time PCR methods in DNA sequence variation analysis. Clin Chim Acta 2006;363:32–47.

12. Schreck RR, Disteche CM, Adler D. ISCN standard idiograms. Current Protocols in Human Genetics, Appendix 1998;18:4B.1-A.4B.21.

13. Redon R, Ishikawa S, Fitch KR, et al. Global variation in copy number in the human genome. Nature 2006;444:444–54.

14. McCarroll SA, Kuruvilla FG, Korn JM, et al. Integrated detection and population-genetic analysis of SNPs and copy number variation. Nat Genet 2008;40:1166–74.

15. Won HH, Kim HJ, Lee KA, Kim JW. Cataloging coding sequence variations in human genome databases. PLoS ONE 2008;3:e3575.

16. van Dongen JJ, Langerak AW, Bruggemann M, et al. Design and standardization of PCR primers and protocols for detection of clonal immunoglobulin and T-cell receptor gene recombinations in suspect lymphoproliferations: report of the BIOMED-2 Concerted Action BMH4-CT98–3936. Leukemia 2003;17:2257–317.

17. Cazzaniga G, Biondi A. Molecular monitoring of childhood acute lymphoblastic leukemia using antigen receptor gene rearrangements and quantitative polymerase chain reaction technology. Haematologica 2005;90:382–90.

18. Jones D, Kamel-Reid S, Bahler D, et al. Laboratory practice guidelines for detecting and reporting BCR-ABL drug resistance mutations in chronic myelogenous leukemia and acute lymphoblastic leukemia: a report of the Association for Molecular Pathology. J Mol Diagn 2009;11:4–11.

19. Tobin G, Rosenquist R. Prognostic usage of V(H) gene mutation status and its surrogate markers and the role of antigen selection in chronic lymphocytic leukemia. Med Oncol 2005;22:217–28.

20. Damle RN, Wasil T, Fais F, et al. Ig V gene mutation status and CD38 expression as novel prognostic indicators in chronic lymphocytic leukemia. Blood 1999;94:1840–7.

21. Hamblin TJ, Davis Z, Gardiner A, Oscier DG, Stevenson FK. Unmutated Ig V(H) genes are associated with a more aggressive form of chronic lymphocytic leukemia. Blood 1999;94:1848–54.

22. Schena M, Shalon D, Davis RW, Brown PO. Quantitative monitoring of gene expression patterns with a complementary DNA microarray. Science 1995;270:467–70.

23. Golub TR, Slonim DK, Tamayo P, et al. Molecular classification of cancer: class discovery and class prediction by gene expression monitoring. Science 1999;286:531–7.

24. Alizadeh AA, Eisen MB, Davis RE, et al. Distinct types of diffuse large B-cell lymphoma identified by gene expression profiling. Nature 2000;403:503–11.

25. Tusher VG, Tibshirani R, Chu G. Significance analysis of microarrays applied to the ionizing radiation response. Proc Natl Acad Sci U S A 2001;98:5116–21.

26. Wilson CS, Davidson GS, Martin SB, et al. Gene expression profiling of adult acute myeloid leukemia identifies novel biologic clusters for risk classification and outcome prediction. Blood 2006;108:685–96.

27. Subramanian A, Tamayo P, Mootha VK, et al. Gene set enrichment analysis: a knowledge-based approach for interpreting genome-wide expression profiles. Proc Natl Acad Sci U S A 2005;102:15545–50.

28. Kaul KL, Leonard DG, Gonzalez A, Garrett CT. Oversight of genetic testing: an update. J Mol Diagn 2001;3:85–91.

29. Amos J, Patnaik M. Commercial molecular diagnostics in the U.S.: The Human Genome Project to the clinical laboratory. Hum Mutat 2002;19:324–33.

30. Westgard JO, Barry PL, Hunt MR, Groth T. A multi-rule Shewhart chart for quality control in clinical chemistry. Clin Chem 1981;27:493–501.

31. van der Velden VH, Hochhaus A, Cazzaniga G, Szczepanski T, Gabert J, van Dongen JJ. Detection of minimal residual disease in hematologic malignancies by real-time quantitative PCR: principles, approaches, and laboratory aspects. Leukemia 2003;17:1013–34.

32. Yao R, Rich SA, Schneider E. Validation of sixteen leukemia and lymphoma cell lines as controls for molecular gene rearrangement assays. Clin Chem 2002;48:1344–51.

33. Eckhart L, Bach J, Ban J, Tschachler E. Melanin binds reversibly to thermostable DNA polymerase and inhibits its activity. Biochem Biophys Res Commun 2000;271:726–30.

34. Giambernardi TA, Rodeck U, Klebe RJ. Bovine serum albumin reverses inhibition of RT-PCR by melanin. Biotechniques 1998;25:564–6.

35. ISCN rules for listing chromosomal rearrangements. Current Protocols in Human Genetics, Appendix 1998;17;A.4C.1-A.4C.55.

36. Schreck RR, Disteche C. Karyotyping. Current Protocols in Human Genetics, Appendix 1998;18:A4A.1-A.4A.3.

37. Evans PA, Pott C, Groenen PJ, et al. Significantly improved PCR-based clonality testing in B-cell malignancies by use of multiple immunoglobulin gene targets. Report of the BIOMED-2 concerted action BHM4-CT98–3936. Leukemia 2007;21:207–14.

38. Bruggemann M, White H, Gaulard P, et al. Powerful strategy for polymerase chain reaction-based clonality assessment in T-cell malignancies. Report of the BIOMED-2 concerted action BHM4 CT98–3936. Leukemia 2007;21:215–21.

39. Donisi PM, Di Lorenzo N, Paparella A, Riccardi M, Stracca-Pansa V. Molecular diagnosis of non-Hodgkin B lymphomas by capillary electrophoresis and Genescan analysis: a molecular pathology laboratory experience. Pathologica 2006;98:139–46.

40. Langerak AW, Wolvers-Tettero IL, van Dongen JJ. Detection of T cell receptor beta (TCRB) gene rearrangement patterns in T cell malignancies by Southern blot analysis. Leukemia 1999;13:965–74.

41. Gabert J, Beillard E, van der Velden VH, et al. Standardization and quality control studies of 'real-time' quantitative reverse transcriptase polymerase chain reaction of fusion gene transcripts for residual disease detection in leukemia – a Europe Against Cancer program. Leukemia 2003; 17:2318–57.

42. Suguro-Katayama M, Suzuki R, Kasugai Y, et al. Heterogeneous copy numbers of API2-MALT1 chimeric transcripts in mucosa-associated lymphoid tissue lymphoma. Leukemia 2003;17:2508–12.

43. Vinatzer U, Gollinger M, Mullauer L, Raderer M, Chott A, Streubel B. Mucosa-associated lymphoid tissue lymphoma: novel translocations including rearrangements of ODZ2, JMJD2C, and CNN3. Clin Cancer Res 2008;14:6426–31.

44. Damm-Welk C, Busch K, Burkhardt B, et al. Prognostic significance of circulating tumor cells in bone marrow or peripheral blood as detected by qualitative and quantitative PCR in pediatric NPM-ALK-positive anaplastic large-cell lymphoma. Blood 2007;110:670–7.

Section 2

Neoplasms of the Bone Marrow

Chapter 5

The Bone Marrow in Normal and Disease States

Dan Jones and Roberto N. Miranda

Abstract/Scope of Chapter This chapter presents an overview to the morphologic findings in normal and disease states in the bone marrow (BM). We begin with a discussion of the maturation and function of the normal marrow elements. The effects of microanatomical localization of hematopoietic elements in relation to specialized stromal cell types on promoting growth and maturation are considered.

Keywords Bone marrow, aspiration • Bone marrow, touch preparation • Bone marrow, trephine biopsy • Bone marrow, differential count • Platelet, function: platelet, granules • Neutropenia • Granulocytosis • Eosinophilia • Basophilia • Monocytosis • Monocytopenia • Megaloblastic anemia • Megaloblastoid erythroid maturation • Parvovirus B19 • Bone marrow, dysplastic changes • Bone marrow, lymphoma patterns • Bone marrow, lymphoid aggregates • Bone marrow, anaplastic large cell lymphoma • Bone marrow, fibrosis grading • Bone marrow, iron stain • Bone marrow, microanatomy • Adventitial reticular cell, bone marrow • Growth factor effect, bone marrow • T-cell lymphoma, bone marrow • B-cell lymphoma, bone marrow • Lysosomal storage disease • Gaucher disease • Bone marrow, carcinoma

5.1. Performing the Bone Marrow Biopsy and Aspirate

For the diagnosis of most bone marrow (BM) conditions, examination of both a cytologic preparation (i.e., BM aspirate) and a tissue sample (i.e., BM core biopsy) is preferred. The large bones in the hip, particularly the posterior superior iliac crest, are the usual site sampled. Following infiltration of the skin and periosteum with a local anesthetic, a small skin incision is made and the BM aspiration needle inserted with aspirate collected into a syringe. The first pull from the aspirate needle usually contains the most bone marrow elements (spicules) and should be used for making smears for morphological examination. Subsequent aspirate pulls can be allocated for flow cytometric [collected in purple top (EDTA) tubes], cytogenetic [collected in green top (heparin) tubes], or molecular (purple top tubes) studies. Trephine BM biopsy is done in a separate site adjacent to the aspirate using a tapered needle with a bevelled sharp edge (e.g., Jamshidi needle) to avoid crush artifact. Core biopsy length of at least 1.5 cm is required for adequate assessment and should be ≥2 cm for lymphoma evaluation [1].

To make smears, aspirate material is typically dispensed into a saucer, where the spicules/particles rise to the surface and are then transferred to glass slides by pipette. The particles are then drawn across the slides by capillary action using the edge of another slide, before air drying, fixing, and staining them with Wright-Giemsa. After making slides, unused aspirate

From: *Neoplastic Hematopathology*: Contemporary Hematology,
Edited by: D. Jones, DOI 10.1007/978-1-60761-384-8_5,
© Humana Press, a part of Springer Science+Business Media, LLC 2010

material is used to generate a clot specimen and submerged into formalin or B5 fixative, embedded in paraffin and cut by microtomy. Most centers also prepare a squash prep from unused particles, or a touch imprint from the marrow biopsy by gently touching the surface of the biopsy 3–4 times to a glass slide. This preparation is especially useful for conditions in which the aspirate is suboptimal or in which marrow fibrosis precludes extraction of cells through the aspirate needle. Before paraffin-embedding and sectioning, the BM biopsy requires decalcification to soften the bone which can be done by brief treatment in dilute acid, or by use of acidified formalin preparations. Prolonged decalcification results in poor morphology and degradation of nucleic acids precluding molecular studies.

For acute leukemia workups, unstained aspirate smears are subjected to cytochemical stains to detect myeloperoxidase and nonspecific (butyrate) esterase, which are indicative of myeloid and monocytic differentiation, respectively. Periodic acid Schiff (PAS) stain can highlight cytoplasmic inclusions in dysplastic erythroid elements. Unstained fixed aspirate smears may be kept for several weeks to months with acceptable morphology maintained, although enzyme activity degrades rapidly unless slides are kept frozen. A common difficulty encountered in aspirate preparation is clotting of aspirate material due to delays in drawing the sample. For preparation of the clot section, thrombin can be added to hasten coagulation.

For some purposes, such as monitoring of acute myeloid leukemia (AML), chronic myelogenous leukemia (CML), or chronic lymphocytic leukemia (CLL), marrow aspiration without biopsy may be adequate given that flow cytometry and molecular studies provide the needed information on residual disease levels. However, routine biopsy is recommended for all diagnostic workups, as metastatic tumors, plasma cell disorders, and many lymphoma types may be poorly sampled by aspirate only because of their focal infiltration and associated reticulin fibrosis. BM biopsy is also needed for evaluation of most myeloproliferative neoplasms (MPNs), such as primary myelofibrosis, since marrow fibrosis often results in a "dry tap". Tumor necrosis will also make the morphology of marrow elements on aspirate smears largely uninterpretable.

5.2. Overview of Hematopoiesis and the Bone Marrow Cell Differential

Hematopoietic elements, including lymphocytes and dendritic cells, emerge from the bone marrow following a programmed development sequence involving several morphologically recognizable maturation stages, with simultaneous expansion of cell number at each stage (Table 5-1). The earliest progenitors for each lineage are referred to as stem cells, and are likely all derived from a single population of pluripotent stem cells with essentially unlimited replicative potential. The exact interrelationships between each hematopoietic lineage are still being investigated, but lymphoid lineages diverge from the other marrow elements at an early stage of development (see Chap 31 for a discussion of molecular aspects of hematopoiesis).

Table 5-1. Maturation characteristics of hematopoietic elements.

Lineage	Mature form	Maturation time in bone marrow	Normal lifespan in circulation
Myeloid	Neutrophil	10–14 days	10–24 h
	Eosinophil	8–18 days	Variable
	Basophil	?	?
Monocyte/ dendritic cell	Monocyte	6–8 days	1–3 days
	Dendritic cell	days	Variable
Erythroid	Erythrocyte	4–6 days	120 days
Megakaryocytic	Platelet	5–6 days	10 days

5.2.1. Maturation and Function of Neutrophils, Eosinophils and Basophils

The term "myeloid" is often used to refer broadly to the nonlymphoid, nonerythroid components of the BM, including granulocytic and monocytic lineages. The progressive maturation of granulocytes or polymorphonuclear leukocytes (PMNs) occurs over a 10–14 day period in the BM. Morphologically recognizable stages of myeloid maturation include the myeloblast, promyelocyte (progranulocyte), myelocyte, metamyelocyte, nonsegmented (band or stab) form, and the mature segmented (or polymorphonuclear) form. Mature granulocytes are distinguished based on the immune functions imparted by their different cytoplasmic granules. Granulopoiesis can occur more quickly in emergency states such as overwhelming infection which results in an increase of immature forms in the marrow and in the circulation (i.e., "left-shifted" myelopoiesis with increased immature neutrophils or "band" forms).

Neutrophils, the predominant granulocyte cell type representing 50%–60% of all peripheral blood white blood cells (leukocytes), contain granules rich in proteases (e.g., elastase), acid hydrolases (e.g., cathepsins), and anti-microbial compounds (e.g., myeloperoxidase and defensins). They produce free radicals through catalase activity that aid in tissue cleanup and bacterial clearance from sites of active inflammation. Neutrophils have a limited life span in blood of 1–2 days, and mediate their effects by migrating to sites of inflammation by binding to blood vessel endothelium and transmigrating into tissues. Overproduction of granulocytes is seen in infection, reactive stress conditions, and in myeloid leukemias (Table 5-2).

Eosinophils function in microbial immunity and by altering vascular permeability at sites of inflammation through release of products in their granules, including highly cationic polypeptides such as major basic protein that alter membrane permeability. Eosinophils are increased in response to parasitic infection, some metabolic and autoimmune diseases, and have a pathogenetic role in allergic reactions due to immunoglobulin-triggered degranulation and release of inflammatory mediators such as leukotrienes. A range of myeloid neoplasms, including CML, CMML, and rare primary eosinophilic leukemias, can produce marked eosinophilia (Chap. 9). Some lymphoid neoplasms, particularly Hodgkin's lymphoma and T-cell lymphomas, produce abundant cytokines including interleukin (IL)-4 and eotaxin which induce eosinophil proliferation and tissue infiltration (Table 5-2). Any cause of eosinophilia is often accompanied by edema and intense itching (pruritis).

Basophils, which contain coarse basophilic granules rich in histamine, proteoglycans such as heparin and chondroitin sulfate, and proteases, participate in IgE-mediated immune responses and are present in low numbers in the marrow and blood, but can be increased in certain pathologic states (Table 5-2). Mast cells are a similar tissue-based cell type, which have a distinct phenotype and maturation pathway, but share with basophils an Fc receptor for IgE [2]. Mast cells in bone marrow are located adjacent to the blood vessels and bony trabeculae and thus are usually trapped in the spicules when marrow aspirates are prepared. Distinction of mast cells from basophils can be difficult but usually basophils have multilobate nuclei and a clearing of granules over their nucleus, whereas mast cells have oval, monolobate nuclei and abundant, uniformly distributed, minute cytoplasmic granules.

5.2.2. Monocyte and Dendritic Cell Maturation and Function

Monocytic precursors diverge from the myeloid lineage at the granulocyte-macrophage colony forming unit (CFU) stage, progressing through committed monoblast and promonocyte stages. Mature monocytes circulate in the blood and enter blood vessel walls to further differentiate before entering tissues as terminally differentiated macrophages or histiocytes. Subsets of macrophages function in phagocytosis, and processing of pathogens, with presentation of such digested microbial protein antigens to lymphocytes. Another subset of macrophages resemble the specialized sinus lining cells in the reticuloendothelial system (RES) of the spleen and act in the BM to recycle iron obtained by breaking down and processing hemoglobin from engulfed erythrocytes.

Table 5-2. Peripheral blood counts, abnormal processes and disease states.

Cell type	Normal PB ranges in adults (x 10^9/L)[a]	Overproduction	Causes	Underproduction or loss	Causes
Myeloid					
Neutrophil	1.4–6.5	Granulocytosis (neutrophilia)	Infection, leukemoid reaction, CML, CNL, paraneoplastic	Neutropenia	MDS, drug reaction, CVD, infection, congenital genetic syndromes
Eosinophil	0–0.5	Eosinophilia	Allergy/asthma, parasites, TLPD, HL, HES/MPN	Eosinopenia	Corticosteroid therapy
Basophil	0–0.2	Basophilia	CML, MDS	nd	nd
Monocyte	0.11–0.59	Monocytosis	CMML, sarcoidosis, infections	Monocytopenia	MDS, Hairy cell leukemia
Erythroid (erythrocyte)	Hemoglobin (g/dL) Men: 14–18 Women: 12–16	Erythrocytosis (polycythemia)	PV, volume depletion, smoking, kidney failure, paraneoplastic EPO	Anemia[b] Macrocytic Microcytic Normocytic	B12/folate deficiency, MDS Iron deficiency AIHA, drug/toxins, blood loss
Megakaryocyte (platelet)	150–400	Thrombocytosis	ET, volume depletion, paraneoplastic, iatrogenic TPO	Thrombocytopenia	MDS, ITP, TTP, drug/toxin
Lymphocyte	1.0–4.8	Lymphocytosis	LPD, viral and some bacterial infections	Lymphopenia	HL, immunosuppressive drugs, HIV, congenital

[a]Normal ranges vary somewhat with age, and laboratory methodology. Absolute count rather than percentage is favored

[b]Determined by mean corpuscular volume (MCV) derived from RBC histogram. For males, normal range is 80–94 fl; for females, normal range is 81–99 fl

CML: chronic myelogenous leukemia; *CNL*: chronic neutrophilic leukemia; *MDS*: myelodysplastic syndrome; *CVD*: collagen vascular diseases such as lupus; *TLPD*: T-cell lymphoma/leukemia; *HL*: Hodgkin lymphoma; *HES*: hypereosinophilic syndrome (myeloid leukemia); *MPN*: myeloproliferative neoplasm; *nd*: not defined; *CMML*: chronic myelomonocytic leukemia; *PV*: polycythemia vera; *EPO*: erythropoietin; *AIHA*: autoimmune hemolytic anemia; *ET*: essential thrombocythemia; *TPO*: thrombopoietin; *ITP*: idiopathic thrombocytopenic purpura; *TTP*: thrombotic thrombocytopenic purpura; *LPD*: lymphoproliferative disorder; *HIV*: human immunodeficiency virus

Other terminally differentiated cells of the monocyte series that are specialized for antigen presentation (APCs) include the Langerhans cells (LCs), which function in mucosal immunity, and the classical (or myeloid-derived) dendritic cells (DCs). In addition to presenting processed microbial antigens to CD4+ and CD8+ T cells, DCs can also present intact foreign antigens to T cells expressing gamma-delta T-cell receptor in association with nonclassical MHC-like glycoproteins, including CD1 isoforms. A second subset of antigen-presenting cells, the plasmacytoid dendritic cells (pDCs), which are round lymphoid-appearing cells, function primarily in viral and mucosal immunity by secreting large amounts of the antiviral cytokine interferon. The progenitor cell origins of pDCs remains unresolved.

DCs of all types participate in a system of self-/nonself- recognition in the innate immune system through a series of polymorphic killer inhibitory receptors (KIRs) which shift with antigenic activation to either growth-promoting or lysis-inducing KIRs on the surface of cytotoxic lymphocytes. Subsets of DC, other APCs and gamma-delta T cells also express different toll-like receptors (TLRs) that recognize foreign molecules associated with pathogens or cell stress, such as lipopolysaccharide (LPS), lipoproteins, unmethylated CpG DNA, and double-stranded RNA. Signaling through TLRs promotes cytokine production that attracts additional inflammatory cells, activates cytotoxic lymphocytes, and promotes pathogen clearance.

5.2.3. Erythroid Maturation

Erythropoiesis occurs continuously particularly in the marrow of the long bones, producing up to two million erythrocytes or red blood cells (RBCs) per second. The morphologically distinct maturation stages are the pronormoblast (proerythroblast), basophilic normoblast, polychromatophilic and orthochromatic normoblasts, reticulocyte, and the circulating erythrocyte which lacks a nucleus.

RBCs function in oxygen exchange between lung and tissues through their iron-containing hemoglobin. The average life span of an erythrocyte is approximately 90–120 days. RBCs obtain their hemoglobin iron through a complex cycle, whereby senescent or abnormally shaped RBCs are phagocytized by cells of the RES with the recycled iron loaded onto transferrin and released into the blood, recaptured by resident marrow macrophages, and then reloaded into developing RBCs. The cytokine erythropoietin (EPO), which binds a transmembrane JAK-STAT-linked receptor (EPOR), drives both erythrocyte differentiation and production. Recombinant EPO can be used to boost RBC production in patients with anemia or following chemotherapy. Anemia can result from RBC underproduction due to iron or vitamin deficiencies, bone marrow failure states due to toxic or immune injury (i.e., aplastic anemia), and genetic defects in maturation (i.e., myelodysplastic syndromes, MDS). Anemia can also result from RBC loss such as bleeding, or RBC destruction associated with infections (e.g., malaria) or hemolytic (immune-mediated) causes. Erythrocytosis can be due to ectopic or paraneoplastic EPO production or due to polycythemia vera, which has an acquired activating JAK2 mutation which leads to hyper-responsive EPO signaling (Table 5-3).

5.2.4. Megakaryocytic Maturation

Platelets are produced from megakaryocytes and function in blood clotting and wound healing. Clear morphologic stages of the multinucleated megakaryocytes (produced by endomitotic reduplication) are difficult to define [3], as are the subtle dysplastic features that occur with megakaryocyte disease processes [4]. Mature platelets bud off from the megakaryocyte cytoplasm in stages and contain alpha-granules, with abundant growth factors and mediators of platelet aggregation, and dense bodies, rich in vasoactive amines and calcium, involved in clot retraction and vasoconstriction. Prior to their release into the circulation, platelets are held within secondary membranes within the cytoplasm of megakaryocytes. The cytokine thrombopoietin (TPO) which binds to a JAK-STAT-linked receptor (TPOR or MPL) helps mediate platelet release, and is used to treat thrombocytopenia. The drug anagrelide inhibits TPO-mediated platelet release so it is used to control thrombocytosis in MPNs (Table 5-3).

Table 5-3. Selected soluble factors involved in maturation, release, and chemotaxis of hematopoietic elements.

Lineage	Growth factor (recombinant form)	Receptor	Signaling pathway	Function	Therapeutic use
Myelomonocytic Early myeloid	SCF (ancestim)	KIT	Receptor tyrosine kinase	Proliferation and survival of HSC Differentiation effects on myeloid and erythroid lineages	Graft failure[38]
All myeloid	GM-CSF (sargramostim)	CD116	JAK-STAT	Stimulates CFU-GM growth and differentiation to increase neutrophils and monocytes	GF to combat neutropenia
Granulocytic	G-CSF (filgrastim)	CD114	JAK-STAT	Growth and differentiation of mature neutrophils	GF to combat neutropenia
Neutrophilic	CXCL13/SDF-1	CXCR4	Chemokine	Chemotactic/adhesion factor that blocks release of neutrophils from BM	Anti-CXCR4 antibodies for stem cell mobilization
Eosinophilic	IL-5	CD125	JAK-STAT	BFU-E growth, differentiation of eosinophils	Anti-IL-5 antibodies to block allergy
Eosinophilic	Eotaxin /CCL11	CCR3	Chemokine	Selective chemotaxis agent for eosinophils	
Erythroid	Erythropoietin (EPO)	EPOR	JAK-STAT	Growth and differentiation of erythroid elements	GF to combat anemia
Megakaryocyte	Thrombopoietin (TPO)	MPL	JAK-STAT	Growth of megakaryocytes and platelet release	GF to combat thrombocytopenia

5.2.5. Lymphoid Maturation and Localization in the Marrow

The stages of lymphoid maturation and the molecular pathways involved are discussed in Chap. 31. Only the earliest stages of T cell maturation occur in the marrow before precursor T cells migrate to the thymus. In contrast, B cells mature in the marrow and then are released into the circulation and enter secondary lymphoid tissues where they encounter antigen. Since B-cell maturation peaks in the perinatal period, immature B cells can be quite numerous in pediatric bone marrows; such precursor B cells have a hyperchromatic appearance and are termed *hematogones*. The majority of lymphocytes in the normal adult bone marrow are mature T cells, ranging from 5 to 15% of the cells in an aspirate differential.

5.2.6. The Bone Marrow Differential Cell Count and Interpretation of the BM Aspirate

Approach to the interpretation of the aspirate includes a general assessment of marrow cellularity, quantification of the relative levels of each marrow element by differential count, and examination of the morphologic features of maturation for each lineage.

5.2.6.1. Assessment of Cellularity
Although it will be influenced by the degree of dilution introduced during smear preparation, the overall degree of marrow cellularity can usually be accurately assessed by the number of cells observed around the spicules on smears (Fig. 5-1). The presence of "bare spicules", i.e., stroma, plasma cells, small lymphocytes, or mast cells with few hematopoietic elements, is indicative of adequate sampling of a hypocellular marrow.

5.2.6.2. Assessment of Proportions of Marrow Elements
It is recommended that a 400-cell differential count be performed on all patients (Fig. 5-2). The normal ranges of hematopoietic elements that should be observed in the bone marrow differential at various ages are summarized in Table 5-4. Megakaryocytes are not usually enumerated on the marrow aspirate, but their numbers are assessed on the trephine biopsy.

5.2.6.3. Assessment of Morphologic Maturation
Normal morphologic findings include orderly maturation of all lineages with no expansions of cell number. Morphologic changes in hematopoietic maturation can be induced by genetic changes such as myelodysplastic syndromes (MDS), nutritional deficiency (such as megaloblastic changes in Vitamin B12 or folate deficiency), or infection (such as erythroid maturation arrest seen in Parvovirus B19 infection). The dysplastic changes in MDS can be limited to one lineage or affect all hematopoietic lines (Fig. 5-3). Changes in the nuclei of maturing hematopoietic forms are the easiest dysplastic features to appreciate and include abnormal shape of the nuclear membrane, such as budding in erythroid precursors or increased numbers of or widely spaced nuclear lobes, hypolobation, and bridging between nuclei of cells which have divided in megakaryocytes. Cytoplasmic changes also occur with dysplasia, but are more difficult to quantify and include hypo- or hypergranulation in myeloid elements

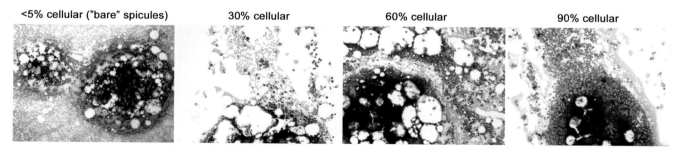

| <5% cellular ("bare" spicules) | 30% cellular | 60% cellular | 90% cellular |

Fig. 5-1. *Bone marrow aspirate, assessment of cellularity.* Left panel illustrates an adequate aspirate with numerous spicules but essentially no marrow elements. Representative aspirate cellularity in more cellular marrows are illustrated in other panels

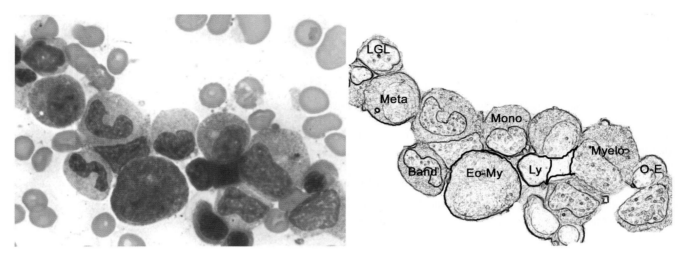

Fig. 5-2. *Bone marrow aspirate, normal morphology.* Giemsa stain on left, with a shadow diagram on right, with a large granular lymphocyte (LGL), myelocyte/metamyelocyte transitional form (meta), neutrophil band form (band), monocyte (mono), eosinophilic myelocyte (Eo-My), small lymphocyte (Ly), neutrophilic myelocyte (Myelo), and orthochromatic normoblast (O-E) highlighted

Table 5-4. Normal ranges of cell types in bone marrow aspirates from patients of various ages.

Cell types	Adult	Early childhood	Newborn
Marrow cellularity (%)	40–60	60–80	80–100
Myeloid (%)			
Myeloblast	<2	2–4	2–5
Promyelocyte	1–4	2–5	2–4
Myelocyte	6–8	4–6	4–6
Metamyelocyte	8–10	6–8	6–8
Band/mature neutrophil	15–20	20–25	25–30
Eosinophil	1–3	3	2
Basophil	<1	<1	<1
Monocyte (%)	1–3	2	1
Erythroid (%)			
Pronormoblast	0–1.5	0–2	0–2
Orthochromatic normoblast	5–30	5–11	6–20
Polychromatophilic normoblast	5–10	0–8	0–5
Lymphocyte (%)	5–15	20–45	15–45
Plasma cell (%)	0–2	<1	<1
Myeloid: erythroid ratio	3:1	3:1	≥ 4:1

Values derived from references 22,39

and abnormal coloration on Giemsa stain. Finally, maturation defects in MDS or nutritional deficiencies are reflected by abnormally large or small cell size for appropriate maturation stage and dyssynchrony between the cytoplasmic and nuclear features (i.e., megaloblastoid and megaloblastic maturation, respectively).

5.2.6.4. Criteria for Inadequate Sample

Causes of inadequate marrow aspirate smears are mostly due to suboptimal sampling, or poor staining technique. It is important to distinguish hypocellular marrow (with bare spicules) from inadequate samples (spicules absent). If only rare marrow elements are sampled, BM

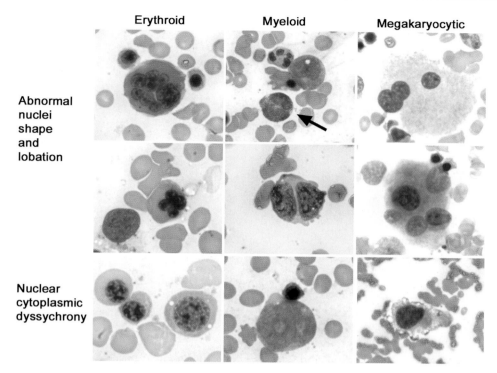

Erythroid   Myeloid   Megakaryocytic

Abnormal nuclei shape and lobation

Nuclear cytoplasmic dyssychrony

Fig. 5-3. Categories of hematopoietic dysplastic changes, on bone marrow aspirates

differential should not be done, as the numbers will be misleading, but a qualitative comment should still be made if blasts, tumor, or other abnormal findings are detected.

5.2.7. Stains on the Marrow Aspirate

Although no longer required for AML classification in the WHO schema, cytochemical staining for myeloperoxidase (expressed in the myeloid lineage) and butyrate esterase (expressed in the monocytic lineage) is an extremely useful and rapid method to type blasts and choose additional subsequent studies for workup. Counterstaining of cytochemical stains with Giemsa helps to identify blast morphology, but can obscure minimal enzyme positivity (Fig. 5-4). Promyelocytes and blasts in promyelocytic leukemia are uniformly (100%) positive for MPO, which aids in distinguishing hypogranular variants from other AML types. Globular cytoplasmic inclusions noted in early erythroid precursors on PAS stain are supportive of erythroleukemia.

5.2.8. Interpretation of the Bone Marrow Biopsy and Clot Section

A stepwise approach to evaluating a BM biopsy includes assessment of sample adequacy, structure and appearance of trabecular bone, BM cellularity, maturation, identification of any abnormal infiltrates, and a semi-quantitative assessment of megakaryocyte number. The overall cellularity of the BM has wide variation but normally declines with age, with a rough approximation of the appropriate level represented by 100% – minus the patient's age. As discussed below, marrow elements mature in different locations within the interstitial space and abnormal localization of one or more lineages can hint at an abnormality.

5.2.9. Stains to Assess Iron Stores and Erythroid Maturation

The Perl stain is commonly performed on marrow aspirate (or on clot or biopsy sections) to assess total iron stores, and scored on a 4- or 5- tier scale (0-absent to 4-markedly increased).

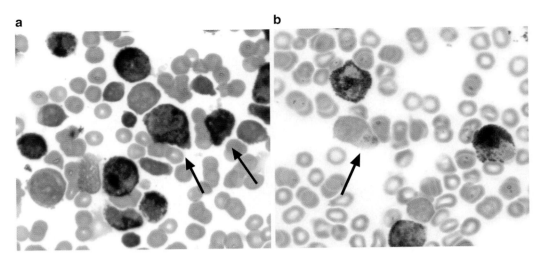

Fig. 5-4. *Myeloperoxidase (MPO) cytochemical staining of marrow aspirates.* (**a**) MPO positivity in blasts and maturing myeloid forms in AML, with nuclear morphology highlighted by Giemsa counterstain. (**b**) Focal positivity in a blast (*arrow*) revealed in MPO stain without counterstain

Iron staining should be done in all new cases of anemia, and in all suspected cases of MDS, as iron stores are usually increased in MDS and decreased or absent in MPNs. The degree of hemosiderin deposition, reflecting the increased RBC turnover often seen in autoimmune or MDS states, can be assessed as well as the amount of iron present in the cytoplasm of erythroid precursors. In sideroblastic anemias, including MDS, alcohol toxicity and genetic causes, abnormally increased erythrocyte iron is seen, including nonheme iron deposited in mitochondria producing the ring sideroblast (Fig. 5-5a) or abnormal globular deposition in the cytoplasm of RBCs or other marrow elements (Fig. 5-5b). The ineffective hematopoiesis associated with MDS can be highlighted by abundant iron deposition around abnormal erythroid CFUs (Fig. 5-5c).

5.2.10. Stains to Assess Marrow Fibrosis

Marrow fibrosis can be seen in a wide variety of conditions, including MPNs, metastatic infiltration by solid tumors, or marrow injury. The degree of extracellular matrix deposition in the marrow can be more precisely assessed using silver impregnation techniques (e.g. Snook's reticulin stain) and histochemical methods for collagen detection (e.g., Masson's trichrome stain). In MPNs, marrow fibrosis is typically graded on a 4-tier score using the European criteria (Table 5-5) [5]. The presence of dense bundles of collagen highlighted by the trichrome stain is a sign of disease progression in myelofibrosis.

5.3. Bone Marrow Anatomy and Microenvironment

5.3.1. Microanatomy of the Marrow Space

During childhood, bone marrow elements are present in the hollow interior (intertrabecular) space of most bones. However, in adults, the marrow in the large bones of extremities and pelvis produce most blood cells. The marrow is organized into an interstitial compartment where hematopoiesis occurs in a space bounded by the bone lining cells (BLC, osteoblasts) which anchor a radial network of fibroblastic adventitial reticular cells (ARC) (Fig. 5-6a). The ARC network surrounds a parallel vascular network that is dominated by venous sinuses

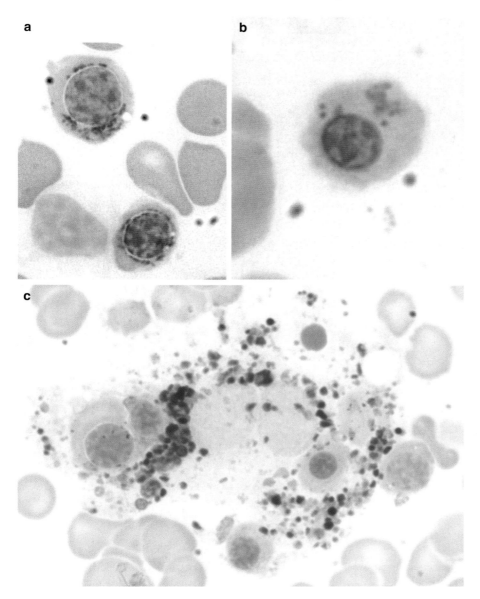

Fig. 5-5. *Findings on iron stain in MDS.* (**a**) A ring sideroblast showing perinuclear cytoplasmic iron-containing granules representing nonheme deposition of iron in mitochondria. (**b**) Erythroid elements with globular cytoplasmic iron deposit. (**c**) Erythroid CFU shows marked increases in iron deposition associated with ineffective erythropoiesis (all panels are Perl stain)

lined by specialized endothelial cells (EC). The sinus ECs, which possess only rudimentary basal laminae, allow hematopoietic cells to pass into the circulation after being released from their attachments within the interstitial compartment [6–8]. This three-dimensional sinus-EC-ARC structure is easiest to visualize in fibrotic marrow processes where there is increased reticulin deposition by ARC leading to distended sinuses (Fig. 5-6b) [9].

Hematopoiesis is highly compartmentalized within the interstitial space, with erythroid maturation occurring in association with supportive macrophages around larger blood vessels in the interior of the marrow space (Fig. 5-7). The more immature myeloid elements typically abut the BLC adjacent to the bone trabeculae, with maturation occurring toward the interior. Due to the complex marrow topography, these localization patterns can be difficult to appre-

Table 5-5. Semiquantitative grading system for bone marrow fibrosis.

Grade	Quantity of reticulin	Type of fibrotic change
MF-0	Scattered linear reticulin fibers with no intersections	No bundles of collagen
MF-1	Loose network of reticulin fibers with many intersections, especially in perivascular areas	No bundles of collagen
MF-2	Diffuse and dense increase in reticulin fibers with extensive intersections	Focal bundles of collagen and/or focal osteosclerosis
MF-3	Diffuse and dense increase in reticulin fibers with extensive intersections	Frequent bundles of collagen and/or osteosclerosis

Fiber density should be assessed in hematopoietic (cellular) areas. Criteria according to the European consensus group [5]

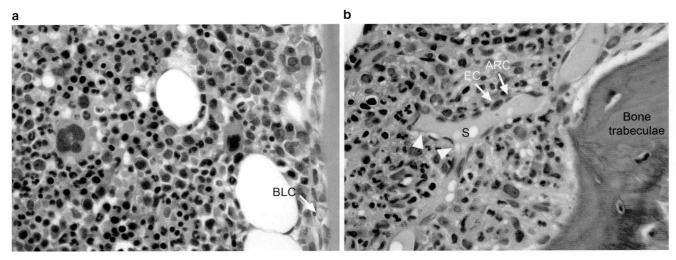

Fig. 5-6. *Bone marrow, microanatomy.* (**a**) Normal bone marrow with bone lining cells (BLC) and adjacent maturing myeloid elements, with erythroid elements and megakaryocytes in more central areas. (**b**) The relationship between the sinus endothelium (EC) with discontinuous basal lamina (*arrowheads*) and the closely apposed adventitial reticular cells (ARC) lining the interstitial space is illustrated in a case of essential thrombocythemia

ciate in normal marrow but can be easily observed in marrow expanded by CML (Fig. 5-8) or in post-therapy marrow with sparse recovering marrow. Megakaryocytes mature in close association with cytoplasmic extensions of ARC (Fig. 5-9) and extend cytoplasmic projections across the EC barrier into the sinuses [3]. In fibrotic marrow states, such as in MPNs, megakaryocytes may translocate across the EC and mature in the sinuses (Fig. 5-10).

5.3.2. Role of Bone Marrow Stromal Cells in Hematopoietic Maturation

In addition to the sinus EC and the fibroblastic ARC, the intertrabecular space also contains a range of stromal elements including adipocytes and stromal macrophages. These are not passive cell types, but actively participate in providing trophic signals for hematopoiesis and expand and contract in number in response to marrow injury (Fig. 5-11), neoplasms, and deposition conditions. Stromal progenitor cells ("mesenchymal stem cells") isolated from aspirate specimens and propagated in culture initially have an ARC phenotype, [10] but can differentiate into other stromal cell types (e.g., adipocytes) with addition of growth factors, raising the promise of their use in organ regeneration [11]. Differentiation in situ occurs in part through expression of neurotrophin growth factors and their receptors [12]. The degree of stromal marrow injury can influence engraftment following stem cell transplant [12].

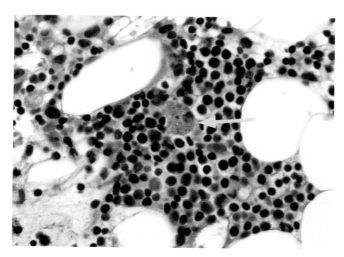

Fig. 5-7. *Bone marrow, microanatomy.* Localization of maturing erythroid elements in the interior of the marrow space. The E-CFU is centered around a hemosiderin-laden macrophage (*yellow arrow*)

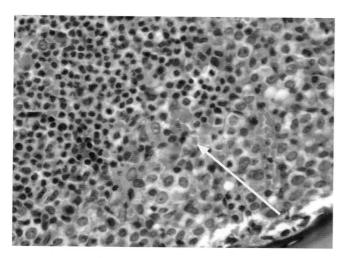

Fig. 5-8. *Bone marrow, microanatomy.* Paratrabecular localization of immature myeloid elements is noted with maturation toward the interior of the marrow space (direction of *white arrow*)

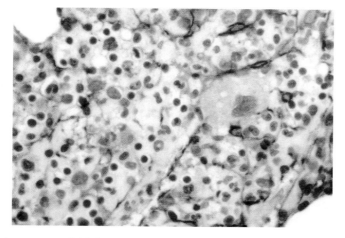

Fig. 5-9. *Megakaryocyte and ARC interaction.* Low-affinity nerve growth factor receptor (LNGFR) immunostaining highlights the cytoplasmic extensions of an adventitial reticular cell wrapping around a megakaryocyte

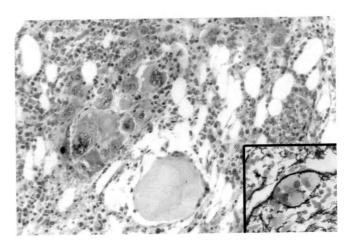

Fig. 5-10. *Megakaryocyte displacement in myeloproliferative neoplasm.* Marrow fibrosis in MPNs leads to a shift of maturing megakaryocytes into intrasinusoidal locations. This abnormal localization is highlighted by reticulin stain (inset)

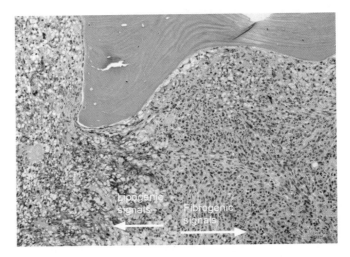

Fig. 5-11. *Adipocyte proliferation in the spent phase of a myeloproliferative neoplasm* (left side). An adjacent area of fibrosis is present (right side of picture)

5.3.3. Release of Hematopoietic Elements

As hematopoiesis proceeds, marrow elements move across the fenestrated endothelium of the sinus and enter the circulation. The factors mediating release of hematopoietic elements from the marrow into the periphery include cytokines and chemotactic chemokines secreted by marrow stromal elements, and are influenced by dynamic changes in the activation state of adhesion molecules expressed on both stromal and hematopoietic elements. For example, chemokine receptor CXCR4 expressed on myeloid elements and lymphocytes retains hematopoietic elements in the BM through interactions with its ligand CXCL13 produced by BM stroma [13]. CXCL13 production is downregulated by G-CSF facilitating neutrophil release [13]. Thus, the use of cytokines with myeloid maturation effects can speed the release of granulocytes into the circulation.

5.4. Bone Marrow Regeneration and Growth Factor Effects

A number of recombinant versions of hematopoietic growth factors are in clinical use to support blood production in BM failure states and following chemotherapy and stem cell transplantation [14]. The most commonly-used growth factors (GFs) are G-CSF, GM-CSF, EPO, and TPO   (Table 5-2). The response of any patient's BM to exogenous growth factors is highly idiosyncratic, and are superimposed on any underlying bone marrow dyspoiesis. Left-shifted granulopoiesis with coarse cytoplasmic granulations is characteristic of patients treated with G-CSF/filgastrim (Fig. 5-12a). EPO can reverse the effects of erythroid maturation defects [15] and also has stimulatory effects on stromal proliferation [17]. The degree and kinetics of platelet rebound observed with TPO treatment is difficult to predict, [14] with age-related [16] and probable genetic differences [17].

A number of chemotherapeutic agents also produce dysplastic changes that may mimic MDS. For example, arsenic trioxide treatment for AML-M3 results in marked erythroid dysplasia in the immediate post-treatment setting (Fig. 5-12b).

5.5. Evaluation of the Bone Marrow in Lymphoma

BM examination in patients with lymphomas assists in outcome prediction and choice of therapy [18]. Examination of multiple tissue sections cut from a unilateral BM core biopsy that is at least 2 cm is now considered the standard of care for staging of lymphoma [1,19]. Bilateral sampling may be useful when there is a high suspicion of marrow involvement based on radiologic findings or evidence of cytopenias [20]. The percentage of the total cellularity involved by lymphoma should be estimated, as well as the total area of the biopsy involved. Flow cytometry immunophenotyping performed on the BM aspirate is extremely helpful in detecting low-level disease, especially in those lymphoproliferative disorders with a subtle interstitial pattern of BM infiltration [21]. However, flow cytometry may miss completely or underestimate the amount of lymphomatous involvement due to poor aspirate sampling in cases with focal involvement or tumor-associated fibrosis. Use of immunohistochemical stains are highly useful in resolving discrepancies when an atypical infiltrate is seen by morphology but no immunophenotypically abnormal population is detected by flow cytometry (Table 5-6).

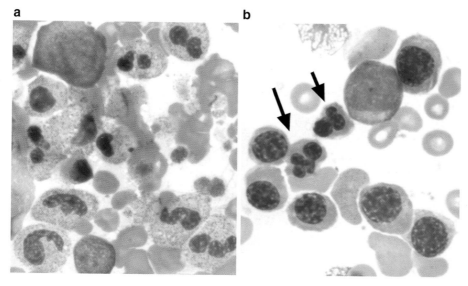

Fig. 5-12. *Effects of treatment on bone marrow morphology.* (**a**) Left-shifted granulopoiesis with coarse granulations in a patient treated with G-CSF (filgastrim). (**b**) Marked erythroid dysplasia in follow-up marrow from a patient with promyelocytic leukemia treated with arsenic trioxide

Table 5-6. Patterns of lymphoma infiltration in bone marrow.

Type	Primary and secondary patterns	Incidence	Helpful IHC stains	Associated morphologic features
SLL/CLL	Interstitial, random nodules or diffuse	~70% (SLL)	CD5+, CD23+, cyclin D1−	Proliferation centers
Mantle cell lymphoma	Interstitial or random nodules	~60%	CD5+, CD23−, cyclin D1+	Monomorphous cellularity; pink histiocytes
Follicular lymphoma	Paratrabecular nodules to diffuse	20–70% (by grade)	CD10+, BCL2+, BCL6+	Cleaved cells and/or centroblasts
Splenic marginal zone lymphoma	Nodules surrounding GC and intrasinusoidal	~80%	CD5−, CD10−, CD21+ germinal center stroma	Lymphocytosis, polar cytoplasmic projections
Nodal and extranodal MZL	Random nodules	<10%	CD5−, CD10−	No lymphocytosis
Lymphoplasmacytic lymphoma	Diffuse or random nodules	>90%	Restricted cytoplasmic light chain immunoglobulins	Plasmacytic or plasmacytoid differentiation
Diffuse large B-cell lymphoma	Diffuse or single cells	10–30%	BCL6+, large CD20+ cells	Tumor necrosis
Burkitt lymphoma	Diffuse	40–60%	CD10+, BCL2−, Ki-67: ~100%	Starry-sky appearance, tumor necrosis
Peripheral T-cell lymphoma	Loose aggregates, lymphohistiocytic	40–80% (by type)	BCL6, CD10, and CXCL13 in AILT	Polymorphic T cell infiltrate
Hepatosplenic T-cell lymphoma	Sinusoidal and interstitial	>90% (focal)	CD56+, γ/δ-TCR+	
Anaplastic large cell lymphoma	Single cells/clusters to diffuse	10–30% (focal)	CD30+ and ALK+ in subset	Blastoid morphology
NK-cell lymphoma	Single cells/clusters	by type	EBER+, CD56+	Hemophagocytosis, necrosis
LGL leukemia	Interstitial, with benign B-cell aggregates	>90%	CD8+, TIA-1+, α/β-TCR+	Granular cytoplasm

AILT: Angioimmunoblastic T-cell lymphoma; *ALK*: anaplastic lymphoma kinase-1; *CLL/SLL*: Chronic lymphocytic leukemia/small lymphocytic lymphoma; *GC*: reactive germinal center; *EBER*: *EBV-encoded RNA*; *IHC*: Immunohistochemistry; *MZL*: marginal zone lymphoma; *NK*: Natural killer

Molecular testing for T-cell and B-cell clonality using PCR is not recommended for routine BM staging, given its high sensitivity and frequent false-positive rates (See Chap. 4) [24].

Small lymphocytes normally comprise up to 15% of BM cellularity, of which 60–85% are usually T cells. Although most lymphocytes are randomly distributed in the BM, [22] small, intertrabecular, T-cell rich lymphoid aggregates are a normal finding, particularly in older individuals (Fig. 5-13). Lymphoma should be suspected whenever lymphoid aggregates are large (greater than 50% of a high-power field), paratrabecular in location, are predominantly B cells, or have atypical morphology [23,24]. Distinct patterns of infiltration are characteristic of particular lymphoma types, and in combination with immunophenotyping, can often allow classification of lymphomas on BM material alone (Table 5-6) [25]. Paratrabecular lymphoid aggregates are most characteristic of follicular lymphoma (FL), but can occur in other lymphoproliferative disorders, although not as the predominant pattern (Fig. 5-14) [25]. Intertrabecular aggregates are common in mantle cell lymphoma (MCL), CLL/SLL, and marginal zone lymphoma (MZL), with B cells cuffing around reactive germinal centers seen in some MZLs. However, reactive germinal centers can also occur in the BM in autoimmune diseases and systemic infections.

Interstitial to diffuse BM lymphoid infiltrates are seen in diffuse large B-cell lymphoma (DLBCL), Burkitt lymphoma (BL), MCL, CLL/SLL, hairy cell leukemia, acute lymphoblastic leukemia (ALL), lymphoplasmacytic lymphoma, and plasma cell neoplasms (PCN). An intrasinusoidal growth pattern may occur in marginal zone lymphoma, intravascular large cell lymphoma, large granular lymphocyte leukemia, and hepatosplenic T-cell lymphoma.

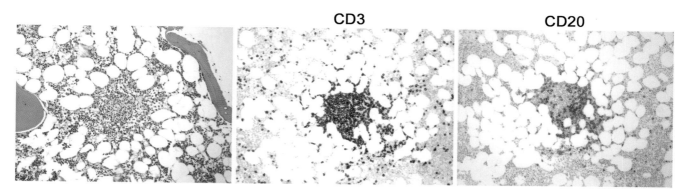

Fig. 5-13. *Benign lymphoid infiltrates, bone marrow.* A single small, interstitial lymphoid aggregate shows mixed population of CD3+ T cells and CD20+ B cells. Interstitial lymphocytes outside of the aggregate are randomly distributed

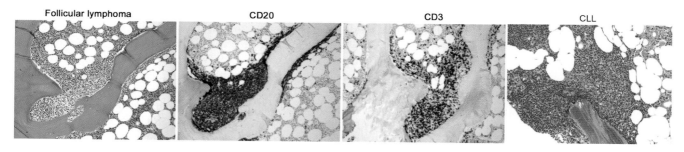

Fig. 5-14. *Paratrabecular lymphoid aggregates.* Follicular lymphoma cells are closely apposed to the bone trabeculae (paratrabecular pattern). Most of lymphocytes within the aggregates are CD20+ B cells but numerous CD3+ T cells are also present. The right panel shows a case of CLL with interstitial and paratrabecular lymphoid aggregates that are not as closely opposed to the bone trabeculae as in follicular lymphoma

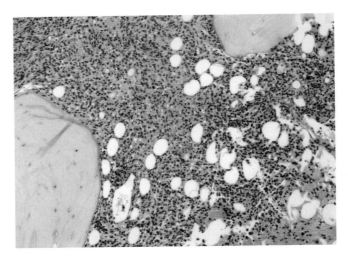

Fig. 5-15. *Peripheral T-cell lymphoma, bone marrow biopsy.* Ill-defined fibrotic lymphohistiocytic aggregates are present

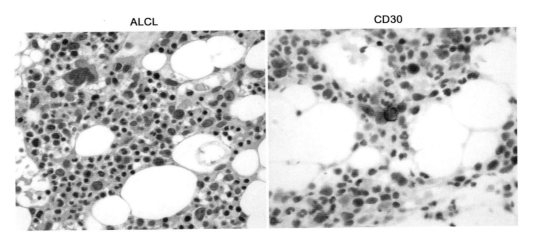

Fig. 5-16. *Anaplastic large cell lymphoma (ALCL), focal marrow involvement.* ALCL often shows subtle interstitial infiltrate that is best highlighted with CD30 immunostain

T-cell lymphomas frequently involve the marrow as poorly defined lymphohistiocytic aggregates, sometimes with admixed plasma cells and eosinophils (Fig. 5-15) [26]. Focal patterns of marrow infiltration can be seen in ALL, PCN, DLBCL, CD30+ anaplastic large cell lymphoma (Fig. 5-16), and NK-cell lymphomas, so immunophenotyping for these tumors is recommended whenever the BM appearance is abnormal to any degree. Finally, aggressive B-cell lymphomas including DLBCL, BL, lymphoblastic lymphoma/leukemia, and some FL may produce coagulative necrosis which can obscure involvement (Fig. 5-17). CD20 immunostain will highlight the necrotic cells in B-cell lymphomas.

The percentage of BM lymphomatous infiltration has established prognostic significance in CLL/SLL, [29,30] MCL, [27] FL, [28] DLBCL, [29,30] and NK-cell lymphomas [32]. However, conflicts arise when the lymphoma shows a lower or higher histologic grade in the BM than in the tissue biopsy. This is a particularly common issue in patients

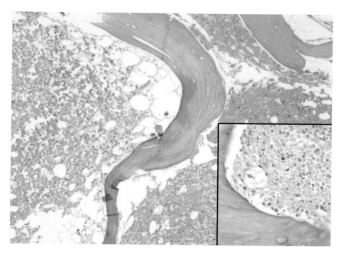

Fig. 5-17. Necrotic lymphoblastic lymphoma, bone marrow

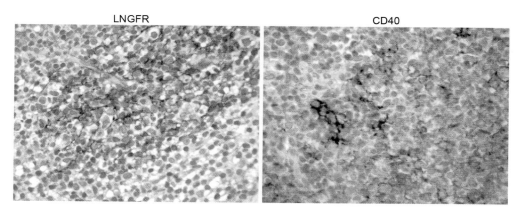

Fig. 5-18. *Bidirectional immunophenotypic shifts in BM stroma and lymphoma cells.* The FDC marker low-affinity nerve growth factor receptor (LNGFR) is upregulated in BM ARC stroma in the center of a FL aggregate. FL tumor cells upregulate the growth receptor CD40 in the same areas with FDC differentiation in the stroma

with DLBCL at other sites who are found to have low-grade paratrabecular lymphoma infiltrates in the BM (indicative of an underlying undetected low-grade FL), as these do not carry the same poor prognostic implication as large cell infiltrates found in the BM [29,31]. Detection of lymphoid infiltrates in the BM can also have different meanings in allogeneic stem cell transplant (SCT), where it may be a sign of helpful graft-versus-tumor effects, whereas it would reflect relapse in autologous SCT.

Microenvironmental influences in the growth of lymphoma in the BM include differential expression of adhesion molecules, [32,33] differential expression of chemokine receptors, [34]. and the effects of growth factors produced by the lymphoma cells on adjacent marrow stroma and bone [35]. For example, the paratrabecular localization of lymphoid aggregates in FL is associated with conversion of the existing BM stroma to an immunophenoype more similar to lymph node follicular dendritic cells (Fig. 5-18) [36].

5.6. Non-Hematopoietic Elements in the Marrow

Lysosomal storage diseases often manifest in the BM, most commonly Gaucher disease which is due to a deficiency of the enzyme glucocerebrosidase (Fig. 5-19). The nonhematopoietic tumors that most frequently involve the BM include neuroblastoma and rhabdomyosarcoma in children, and carcinomas of the breast (Fig. 5-20), prostate, and kidney in adults. Keratin immunostains are recommended for detecting lobular breast carcinoma, and neuron-specific enolase (NSE) or beta-catenin for detecting neuroblastoma [37]. Finally, bone pathology can be detected on routine BM biopsy. This is most commonly the thinned bone trabeculae of osteoporosis which can be noted, but whose diagnosis is best done with more sensitive bone density radiologic studies. The changes of Paget's disease are more distinctive (scalloping of the trabecular bone and irregular cement cells) and, if observed, should always be noted in the report (Fig. 5-21).

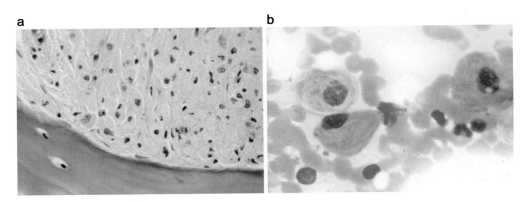

Fig. 5-19. *Gaucher disease.* (**a**) Bone marrow biopsy shows sheets of histiocytes with cytoplasm distended by striated tubular inclusions. (**b**) Bone marrow aspirate shows characteristic wrinkled tissue paper-like appearance of storage histiocytes

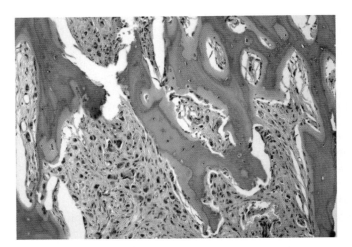

Fig. 5-20. *Metastatic carcinoma, bone marrow.* Infiltration by poorly differentiated breast cancer is accompanied by osteosclerosis and fibrosis resembling myelofibrosis

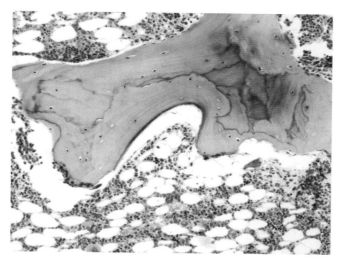

Fig. 5-21. *Paget's disease.* Bone biopsy shows thickened bone trabeculae with irregular scalloping and haphazard cement lines that imparts the radiologic jigsaw puzzle appearance

References

1. Cheson BD, Pfistner B, Juweid ME, et al. Revised response criteria for malignant lymphoma. J Clin Oncol 2007;25:579–86.
2. Metcalfe DD. Mast cells and mastocytosis. Blood 2008;112:946–56.
3. Tavassoli M, Aoki M. Localization of megakaryocytes in the bone marrow. Blood Cells 1989;15:3–14.
4. Tefferi A, Thiele J, Orazi A, et al. Proposals and rationale for revision of the World Health Organization diagnostic criteria for polycythemia vera, essential thrombocythemia, and primary myelofibrosis: recommendations from an ad hoc international expert panel. Blood 2007;110: 1092–7.
5. Thiele J, Kvasnicka HM, Facchetti F, Franco V, van der Walt J, Orazi A. European consensus on grading bone marrow fibrosis and assessment of cellularity. Haematologica 2005;90:1128–32.
6. Tavassoli M. Structural alterations of marrow during inflammation. Blood Cells 1987;13:251–61.
7. Lichtman MA, Chamberlain JK, Weed RI, Pincus A, Santillo PA. The regulation of the release of granulocytes from normal marrow. Prog Clin Biol Res 1977;13:53–75.
8. Inoue S, Osmond DG. Basement membrane of mouse bone marrow sinusoids shows distinctive structure and proteoglycan composition: a high resolution ultrastructural study. Anat Rec 2001;264:294–304.
9. Wickramasinghe SN. Observations on the ultrastructure of sinusoids and reticular cells in human bone marrow. Clin Lab Haematol 1991;13:263–78.
10. Jones E, McGonagle D. Human bone marrow mesenchymal stem cells in vivo. Rheumatology (Oxford) 2008;47:126–31.
11. Zhang N, Mustin D, Reardon W, et al. Blood-borne stem cells differentiate into vascular and cardiac lineages during normal development. Stem Cells Dev 2006;15:17–28.
12. Cattoretti G, Schiro R, Orazi A, Soligo D, Colombo MP. Bone marrow stroma in humans: antinerve growth factor receptor antibodies selectively stain reticular cells in vivo and in vitro. Blood 1993;81:1726–38.
13. Petit I, Szyper-Kravitz M, Nagler A, et al. G-CSF induces stem cell mobilization by decreasing bone marrow SDF-1 and up-regulating CXCR4. Nat Immunol 2002;3:687–94.
14. Vadhan-Raj S, Cohen V, Bueso-Ramos C. Thrombopoietic growth factors and cytokines. Curr Hematol Rep 2005;4:137–44.
15. Cortelezzi A, Colombo G, Pellegrini C, et al. Bone marrow glycophorin-positive erythroid cells of myelodysplastic patients responding to high-dose rHuEPO therapy have a different gene expression pattern from those of nonresponders. Am J Hematol 2008;83:531–9.

16. Pastos KM, Slayton WB, Rimsza LM, Young L, Sola-Visner MC. Differential effects of recombinant thrombopoietin and bone marrow stromal-conditioned media on neonatal versus adult megakaryocytes. Blood 2006;108:3360–2.

17. Zeng SM, Murray JC, Widness JA, Strauss RG, Yankowitz J. Association of single nucleotide polymorphisms in the thrombopoietin-receptor gene, but not the thrombopoietin gene, with differences in platelet count. Am J Hematol 2004;77:12–21.

18. Igarashi T, Kobayashi Y, Ogura M, et al. Factors affecting toxicity, response and progression-free survival in relapsed patients with indolent B-cell lymphoma and mantle cell lymphoma treated with rituximab: a Japanese phase II study. Ann Oncol 2002;13:928–43.

19. Campbell JK, Matthews JP, Seymour JF, Wolf MM, Juneja SK. Optimum trephine length in the assessment of bone marrow involvement in patients with diffuse large cell lymphoma. Ann Oncol 2003;14:273–6.

20. Franco V, Tripodo C, Rizzo A, Stella M, Florena AM. Bone marrow biopsy in Hodgkin's lymphoma. Eur J Haematol 2004;73:149–55.

21. DiGiuseppe JA, Borowitz MJ. Clinical utility of flow cytometry in the chronic lymphoid leukemias. Semin Oncol 1998;25:6–10.

22. Harmening DM. In: Clinical hematology and fundamentals of hemostasis. 5th ed. Philadelphia, PA: F. A. Davis, 2009.

23. Thiele J, Zirbes TK, Kvasnicka HM, Fischer R. Focal lymphoid aggregates (nodules) in bone marrow biopsies: differentiation between benign hyperplasia and malignant lymphoma–a practical guideline. J Clin Pathol 1999;52:294–300.

24. Horny HP, Wehrmann M, Griesser H, Tiemann M, Bultmann B, Kaiserling E. Investigation of bone marrow lymphocyte subsets in normal, reactive, and neoplastic states using paraffin-embedded biopsy specimens. Am J Clin Pathol 1993;99:142–9.

25. Arber DA, George TI. Bone marrow biopsy involvement by non-Hodgkin's lymphoma: frequency of lymphoma types, patterns, blood involvement, and discordance with other sites in 450 specimens. Am J Surg Pathol 2005;29:1549–57.

26. Grogg KL, Morice WG, Macon WR. Spectrum of bone marrow findings in patients with angioimmunoblastic T-cell lymphoma. Br J Haematol 2007;137:416–22.

27. Todorovic M, Pavlovic M, Balint B, et al. Immunophenotypic profile and clinical characteristics in patients with advanced stage mantle cell lymphoma. Med Oncol 2007;24:413–8.

28. Canioni D, Brice P, Lepage E, et al. Bone marrow histological patterns can predict survival of patients with grade 1 or 2 follicular lymphoma: a study from the Groupe d'Etude des Lymphomes Folliculaires. Br J Haematol 2004;126:364–71.

29. Chung R, Lai R, Wei P, et al. Concordant but not discordant bone marrow involvement in diffuse large B-cell lymphoma predicts a poor clinical outcome independent of the International Prognostic Index. Blood 2007;110:1278–82.

30. Campbell J, Seymour JF, Matthews J, Wolf M, Stone J, Juneja S. The prognostic impact of bone marrow involvement in patients with diffuse large cell lymphoma varies according to the degree of infiltration and presence of discordant marrow involvement. Eur J Haematol 2006;76:473–80.

31. Hodges GF, Lenhardt TM, Cotelingam JD. Bone marrow involvement in large-cell lymphoma. Prognostic implications of discordant disease. Am J Clin Pathol 1994;101:305–11.

32. Domingo A, Gonzalez-Barca E, Castellsague X, et al. Expression of adhesion molecules in 113 patients with B-cell chronic lymphocytic leukemia: relationship with clinico-prognostic features. Leuk Res 1997;21:67–73.

33. Angelopoulou MK, Kontopidou FN, Pangalis GA. Adhesion molecules in B-chronic lymphoproliferative disorders. Semin Hematol 1999;36:178–97.

34. Jones D, Benjamin RJ, Shahsafaei A, Dorfman DM. The chemokine receptor CXCR3 is expressed in a subset of B-cell lymphomas and is a marker of B-cell chronic lymphocytic leukemia. Blood 2000;95:627–32.

35. Marcelli C, Chappard D, Rossi JF, et al. Histologic evidence of an abnormal bone remodeling in B-cell malignancies other than multiple myeloma. Cancer 1988;62:1163–70.

36. Vega F, Medeiros LJ, Lang WH, Mansoor A, Bueso-Ramos C, Jones D. The stromal composition of malignant lymphoid aggregates in bone marrow: variations in architecture and phenotype in different B-cell tumours. Br J Haematol 2002;117:569–76.

37. Krishnan C, Twist CJ, Fu T, Arber DA. Detection of isolated tumor cells in neuroblastoma by immunohistochemical analysis in bone marrow biopsy specimens: improved detection with use of beta-catenin. Am J Clin Pathol 2009;131:49–57.

38. Korper S, Hutter G, Blau W, et al. Successful treatment of partial graft failure after matched unrelated donor stem cell transplantation by a combination of ancestim (stem cell factor) and granulocyte colony stimulating factor in a patient with heavily pre-treated chronic lymphocytic leukemia. Leuk Lymphoma 2008;49:2015–7.

39. Foucar K, Viswanatha DS, Wilson CS. In: Atlas of nontumor pathology: Non-neoplastic disorders of bone marrow. ARP Press, 2008:397–8.

Chapter 6

Myelodysplastic Syndromes and Myelodysplastic/Myeloproliferative Neoplasms

Sa A. Wang

Abstract/Scope of Chapter This chapter provides updated information on the myelodysplastic syndromes (MDS) and the myelodysplastic/myeloproliferative neoplasms (MDS/MPN). The different biological features are illustrated in their variable clinical presentation, morphologic characteristics, molecular genetic findings, and flow cytometric anomalies. The diagnostic criteria recommended by the International Working Group (IWG) and disease classification by World Health Organization (WHO) are incorporated into the discussion of diagnostic approaches to MDS and MDS/MPD. Specifically, the significance and diagnostic challenges of some unusual forms of MDS and MDS/MPD are discussed, including MDS with fibrosis, hypoplastic MDS, MDS with a PNH clone, MDS with minimal dysplasia, MDS with erythroid predominance or aplasia, and morphological assessment following treatment.

Keywords Myelodysplastic syndrome (MDS), minimal diagnostic criteria • Myelodysplastic syndrome, international working group • Abnormal localization of immature precursors (ALIP) • Bone marrow, dysplastic features • Ringed sideroblasts, definition • Myelodysplastic syndrome, cytogenetic findings • Myelodysplastic syndrome, flow cytometry • Myelodysplastic syndrome, international prognostic scoring system (IPSS) • Myelodysplastic syndrome, immune-mediated • Myelodysplastic/myeloproliferative neoplasms (MDS/MPN) • Idiopathic cytopenia with uncertain (undetermined) significance (ICUS) • Paroxysmal nocturnal hemoglobinuria (PNH) • Aplastic anemia • Myelodysplastic syndrome, hypocellular • Myelodysplastic syndrome, fibrotic • Chronic myelomonocytic leukemia (CMML) • Chronic myeloid leukemia, atypical (aCML) • Refractory anemia with ring sideroblasts and marked thrombocytosis (RARS-T)

6.1. Overview of the Myelodysplastic Syndromes

6.1.1. Definitions

The myelodysplastic syndromes (MDS) are a group of heterogeneous clonal hematopoietic stem cell diseases characterized by ineffective hematopoiesis with peripheral cytopenia(s), morphological dysplasia, and increased risk of development of acute myeloid leukemia (AML) [1]. MDS are classified according to their etiology as primary (de novo) or as therapy-related, if preceded by exposure to DNA-damaging chemotherapy or radiation. This chapter will focus on primary adult MDS, and therapy-related MDS will be discussed under therapy-related MDS/AML in Chap. 7.

From: *Neoplastic Hematopathology*: Contemporary Hematology,
Edited by: D. Jones, DOI 10.1007/978-1-60761-384-8_6,
© Humana Press, a part of Springer Science+Business Media, LLC 2010

6.1.2. Diagnostic Criteria

Cytopenia(s), as defined by the International Prognostic Scoring System (IPSS) for MDS, are hemoglobin (Hb) <10 g/dL, absolute neutrophil count (ANC) <1.8×10^9/L, and platelets <100×10^9/L [[2]. Cytopenia(s) are often unremitting and, at minimum, last for more than 6 months. However, in some patients, cytopenia(s) can be less severe at presentation, and a diagnosis of MDS can still be rendered if definitive morphologic and/or cytogenetic findings are present [3,4]. Myeloblasts in the peripheral blood (PB) and bone marrow (BM) may be increased, but if they comprise 20% or more of the cellularity, the diagnosis of AML is rendered. Abnormal cytogenetic findings can be helpful in confirming a clonal stem cell disease, with del(20q),+8, −7, del(7q), and del(5q) (particularly bands q13-33) being the most frequent cytogenetic alterations in MDS.

In many patients, the diagnosis of MDS using the 2008 WHO criteria [1] is straightforward but can be challenging when: (1) there is no detectable cytogenetic abnormality and only mild cytopenia; (2) there is both a karyotypic abnormality and cytopenia but only minimal morphologic dysplasia; or (3) there is isolated persistent thrombocytopenia, neutropenia, or transfusion-dependent macrocytic anemia without either a karyotype abnormality or overt morphologic dysplasia. Therefore, the international working conference composed of representatives from the US National Comprehensive Cancer Network (NCCN), the International Working Group (IWG), and the European Leukemia Net proposed consensus guidelines for the minimal diagnostic criteria for MDS (Table 6-1). The diagnosis of MDS can be established when *both* prerequisite criteria and at least one decisive criterion are fulfilled. If no decisive criterion is fulfilled, co-criteria should be applied. It is noteworthy that some patients may have MDS coexisting with another hematological or nonhematological disease; therefore, detection of another disease potentially causing cytopenia does not exclude a diagnosis of MDS.

Table 6-1. Minimal diagnostic criteria in myelodysplastic syndromes recommended by the International Working Conference (IWP) (2007).

Minimal diagnostic criteria for MDS
(A) Prerequisite criteria
1. Constant cytopenia in one or more of the following cell types:
• Erythrocyte (hemoglobin <11 g/dL), and/or
• Neutrophil (ANC < 1.5×10^9/L), and/or
• Megakaryocyte (platelets <100×10^9/L)
2. Exclusion of all other hematopoietic or nonhematopoietic disorders as primary reason for cytopenia/dysplasia
(B) MDS-related decisive criteria
• Dysplasia in at least 10% of all cells in one of the following lineages in the bone marrow smear: erythroid; myeloid; or megakaryocytic, or >15% ringed sideroblasts (iron stain)
• 5–19% blasts in bone marrow or peripheral blood
• Typical chromosomal abnormality (by conventional karyotyping or FISH)
(C) Co-criteria (for patients fulfilling "A" but not "B", and otherwise show typical clinical features, e.g., macrocytic transfusion-dependent anemia)
• Abnormal phenotype of bone marrow cells clearly indicative of a monoclonal population of erythroid or/and myeloid cells, determined by flow cytometry.
• Clear molecular signs of a monoclonal cell population by HUMARA assay, gene chip profiling, or mutational analysis (e.g., somatic point mutation in ras genes)
• Markedly and persistently reduced colony formation (±cluster formation) in bone marrow or/and circulating progenitor cells (CFU-assay)

ANC absolute neutrophil count, *FISH* fluorescence in situ hybridization, *CFU* colony-forming units

6.1.3. Epidemiology

MDS occur principally in older adults with a median age of 70 years at presentation. Data from 2001 through 2003 in the Surveillance, Epidemiology & End Reports (SEER) registry at the National Cancer Institute indicates an abrupt rise in incidence (> five-fold) for patients over 60 years, with 86% of MDS cases arising in that age group. Men have a significantly higher incidence than women (4.5 vs. 2.7 per 100,000) [5]. The prevalence of MDS is currently estimated at 3.3 per 100 000 cases in the United States and is highest among whites and non-Hispanics [6]. An apparent increase in incidence is likely related to the aging of the population, although recent changes in diagnostic criteria are also relevant.

6.1.4. Historical Overview of MDS Classifications

Several classification systems have been developed to predict survival and risk for transformation to AML following the diagnosis of MDS. The French-America-British (FAB) classification system was introduced in 1976 and is primarily based on the percentage of blasts classifying MDS into refractory anemia (RA); refractory anemia with ring sideroblasts (RARS); MDS-unspecified (MDS-U), refractory anemia with excess blasts (RAEB) (5–19% myeloblasts), and refractory anemia with excess blasts in transformation (RAEB-t) (20–29% myeloblasts) [7]. Chronic myelomonocytic leukemia (CMML) was also included as one of the MDS subcategories. The FAB system served as the standard for MDS classification for two decades and provided considerable prognostic information. However, the clinical outcomes of patients assigned to the same MDS subgroup was variable.

In 2001, the WHO proposed a revision of the FAB morphologic approach that included lowering the threshold for the percentage of blasts required to make the diagnosis of AML from 30 to 20%, thus eliminating the MDS subcategory of RAEB-t. In addition, CMML was removed from MDS and reclassified under myelodysplastic/myeloproliferative neoplasm (MDS/MPD). Morphologic dysplasia was further divided into unilineage and multilineage types, and as a result, two new subcategories, refractory anemia with multilineage (RCMD) and RCMD with ring sideroblasts (RCMD-RS), were created. RAEB was further divided into RAEB-1 (5–9% blasts) and RAEB-2 (10–19% blasts), acknowledging the importance of increasing blasts in predicting patients' survival and risk for transformation to AML. Most importantly, the WHO classification incorporated cytogenetic data into subcategorization of MDS. For example, MDS with isolated del(5)(q13-33) and <5% BM blasts was separately delineated as the 5q- syndrome because of its favorable prognosis and excellent response to the drug lenalidomide [8]. Several studies conducted retrospectively and prospectively using the 2001 WHO classification criteria have confirmed its value in risk stratification and prediction of clinical outcomes [9,10].

In 2008, in order to further stratify the risk in cases with fewer than 5% BM blasts, the WHO group added a subcategory of refractory cytopenia with unilineage dysplasia (RCUD) to include refractory anemia (RA), refractory neutropenia (RN), and refractory thrombocytopenia (RT) [1]. The type of cytopenia in MDS generally corresponds with the lineage showing the most obvious morphologic dysplasia, although discordance may be observed [4]. This followed recognition that RCUD is relatively indolent clinically with a favorable prognosis. The subcategories of MDS in the 2008 revised WHO classification and their respective PB and BM features are summarized in Table 6-2. Since many clinical studies and trials are based on different classification systems, Table 6-3 lists the corresponding subcategories in the three most common classification schemes.

6.1.5. Clinical Features and Etiologic Associations

The majority of patients with MDS present with symptoms related to cytopenia. Symptoms related to anemia, such as fatigue, malaise, tiredness, and transfusion-dependence are most common. Patients can also present with petechiae, ecchymoses, and nose and gum bleeding due to thrombocytopenia. Fever, cough, dysuria, or shock may be manifestations of serious

Table 6-2. 2008 World Health Organization classification of myelodysplastic syndromes.

MDS subcategories	Blood findings	Bone marrow features
Refractory cytopenias with unilineage dysplasia (RCUD) • Refractory anemia (RA); • Refractory neutropenia (RN); • Refractory thrombocytopenia (RT)	Unicytopenia or bicytopenias Blasts <1%	1. Unilineage dysplasia 2. <5% blasts 3. <15% of erythroid precursors are ringed sideroblasts
Refractory anemia with ring sideroblasts (RARS)	Anemia Blasts <1%	1. dyserythropoiesis 2. <5% blasts 3. ≥15% of erythroid precursors are ringed sideroblasts
Refractory cytopenia with multilineage dysplasia (RCMD) Cytopenia(s) with or without Ringed-sideroblasts (RCMD-RS)	Blasts <1% Monocytes <1 × 10⁹/L	1. Dysplasia in ≥ two myeloid lineages 2. <5% blasts 3. No Auer rods 4. < or ≥15% ringed sideroblasts
Refractory anemia with excess blasts-1 (RAEB-1)	<5% blasts No Auer rods <1 × 10⁹/L monocytes	1. Unilineage or multilineage dysplasia 2. 5-9% blasts 3. No Auer rods
Refractory anemia with excess blasts-2 (RAEB-2) Cytopenia(s)	5–19% blasts Auer rods <1 × 10⁹/L monocytes	1. Unilineage or multilineage dysplasia 2. 10–19% blasts 3. Auer rods (if present)
*Myelodysplastic syndrome – unclassified (MDS-U)		1. RCUD, RARS, RCMD with 1% blasts in blood 2. Dysplasia in <10% of cells of each lineage but with a cytogenetic abnormality presumptive for a diagnosis of MDS 3. Unilineage dysplasia with bicytopenias
MDS associated with isolated del(5q)	Anemia Platelet usually normal or increased Blasts <1%	1. Normal to increased megakaryocytes with hypolobated nuclei 2. <5% blasts, no Auer rods 3. Isolated del(5q) cytogenetic abnormality

*Any case meeting any of the 3 features listed here are classified as MDS-U

bacterial or fungal infections associated with neutropenia. Organomegaly is infrequently observed.

Primary or de novo MDS occurs without a known history of chemotherapy or radiation exposure. Environmental agents possibly related to MDS include cigarette smoking, occupational exposure to benzene, other solvents or agricultural chemicals, and viral infection [11]. Genetic risk factors, as revealed by epidemiologic studies and genomic arrays, are beginning to emerge. Some inherited hematological disorders, such as Fanconi anemia, dyskeratosis congenita, Schwachmann-Diamond syndrome, and Diamond-Blackfan syndrome are also associated with an increased risk of MDS, especially in the pediatric population, which will not be discussed further here.

Table 6-3. Translation across different myelodysplastic classification schemes.

FAB classification	2001 WHO classification	2008 WHO classification
RA	RA	RCUD-RA
	RCMD	RCMD
	5q- syndrome	5q- syndrome
RARS	RARS	RARS
	RCMD-RS	RCMD
	5q- syndrome	5q- syndrome
MDS-unspecified	MDS-unclassifiable	RCUD-RN
		RCUD-RT
		RCMD-U
	RCMD	RCMD
RAEB	RAEB-1	RAEB-1
	RAEB-2	RAEB-2
RAEB-t	AML	AML with MDS-related
CMMoL	MDS/MPD	MDS/MPD
	CMML-1	CMML-1
	CMML-2	CMML-2

RA refractory anemia, *RARS* refractory anemia with ring sideroblasts, *RAEB* refractory anemia with excess blasts, *RAEB-T* refractory anemia with excess blasts in transformation, *CMML or CMMoL* chronic myelomonocytic leukemia, *RCMD* refractory cytopenia with multilineage dysplasia, *RCUD* refractory cytopenia with unilineage dysplasia, *RN* refractory neutropenia, *RT* refractory thrombocytopenia

6.1.6. Morphologic Features

6.1.6.1. Bone Marrow Biopsy Evaluation

BM biopsy is important for assessment of cellularity, relative cell proportions, fibrosis, stromal alterations, and degree of dysplasia in the megakaryocytic lineage. The normal BM usually shows a cellularity appropriate for age (calculated as 100 minus the patient's age), with orderly maturation and cell distribution. As described in Chap. 5, the myeloid precursors are normally found along the bone trabeculae, whereas the erythroid and megakaryocytic precursors are located more centrally. In MDS, the BM is usually hypercellular, and the BM topography is disrupted. Altered stroma is common, including shifts in the distribution of adipocytes, increased histiocytes, proliferations of small blood vessels, and fibrosis (Fig. 6-1a). Abnormal localization of immature precursors (ALIP) describes the findings of clusters or aggregates of centrally localized myeloblasts and promyelocytes (Fig. 6-1b). Although ALIP is not unique to MDS and can be seen in active BM regeneration or growth factor treatment, the presence of ALIP in MDS is often associated with a poor outcome and increased risk for AML progression [12].

6.1.6.2. Bone Marrow Aspirate Interpretation

Good quality BM aspirate smears are critical for diagnosis and classification of MDS. BM aspirate evaluation includes recording the percentage of blasts, and the degree of (unilineage or multilineage) dysplasia. Dysplasia has to present in at least 10% cells of any lineage described as dysplastic, and the particular dysplastic changes seen may be relevant in predicting biology and the relationship to specific cytogenetic abnormalities.

6.1.6.3. Dyserythropoiesis and Ring Sideroblasts

Dyserythropietic features include nuclear budding, internuclear bridging, karyorrhexis, multinuclearity, nuclear hyperlobation, megaloblastoid change (i.e., nuclear-cytoplasmic dyssynchrony), and cytoplasmic basophilic stippling. Cytoplasmic vacuoles which may be positive with the periodic acid-Schiff (PAS) cytochemical stain in some cases (Fig. 6-2a–e). Ring sideroblasts are an erythroid abnormality detected on iron stain when nucleated erythrocytes have at least five perinuclear siderotic granules present, or the granules cover at least one-third of the circumference of the nucleus (IWG and WHO criteria). Erythroblasts with less than five granules or more than five granules, but not in a perinuclear location, should not be counted as ring sideroblasts (RS) [1,13]. The presence of 15% or more RS in a BM with <5% blasts would be classified as either RARS, if dysplasia is confined to the erythroid lineage, or RCMD with RS if dysgranulopoiesis and/or dysmegakaryopoiesis is present. However, the presence of increased RS cells in other MDS types such as RAEB or the 5q-syndrome does not change subclassification.

6.1.6.4. Dysgranulopoiesis

Dysgranulpoiesis includes nuclear hypolobation such as the pseudo-Pelger-Huet anomaly (Fig. 6-3a and b), hypersegmentation of the nuclei with abnormal condensed chromentin, and agranularity, hypogranularity, or hypergranularity of the cytoplasm, such as the large irregularly shaped eosinophilic pseudo-Chediak-Higashi granules. Abnormally large or small granulocytes are also evidence of dysplasia, but giant bands can also be seen in Vitamin 12 or folate deficiency (i.e., *megaloblastic anemia*). Dysplasia in earlier stages of myeloid lineage is often underappreciated. Those features include hypogranulation, abnormal granulation (such as coarse chunky granules), abnormal nuclear lobation and nuclear/cytoplasmic dyssynchrony.

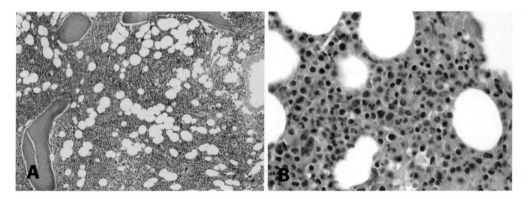

Fig. 6-1. Myelodysplastic syndromes: refractory cytopenia with multilineage dysplasia (RCMD). (**a**) Bone marrow (BM) biopsy shows hypercellularity, altered fat and cellular distribution, dysplastic megakaryocytes. (**b**) Abnormal localization of immature precursors (ALIPS)(clusters or aggregates of centrally localized myeloblasts and promyelocytes)

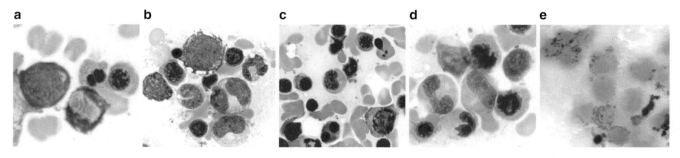

Fig. 6-2. Dysplastic erythropoiesis in MDS. (a) Megaloblastoid changes and basophilic stippling; (**b**) nuclear vacuolization; (**c**) nuclear budding and binucleated forms; (**d**) karyorrhexis; (**e**) ring sideroblasts

6.1.6.5. Dysmegakaryopoiesis

Megakaryocyte dysplasia in MDS is characterized by micromegakaryocytes with hypolobated nuclei, megakaryocytes of all sizes with nonlobated nuclei (Fig. 6-3c), or megakaryocytes with multiple, widely separated nuclei ("pawn-ball" appearance, Fig. 6-3d). Megakaryocytes can be increased, decreased, or normal in number. Some changes are characteristic, including megakaryocytes with nonlobated and hypolobated nuclei in the 5q- syndrome. When a limited number of megakaryocytes are present on the aspirate smears, megakaryocytic dysplasia is more reliably evaluated in the BM biopsy. In evaluating megakaryocyte dysplasia, the best approach is to make initial evaluation based on the biopsy (Fig. 6-1a), and then verify that impression on the BM aspirate smears. At least 30 megakaryocytes should be evaluated.

6.1.6.6. Evaluating blasts

The recognition and enumeration of blasts is of critical importance in diagnosis, risk stratification and assessment of treatment response in MDS. Blast cutoffs are <5%, 5–9%, and 10–19% for different diagnostic categories and <5%, 5–10%, and 11–19% for IPSS risk assessment respectively (Table 6-4) [2]. A 500-cell differential count is required for accurate blast enumeration. The presence of Auer rods shifts the classification to RAEB-2 regardless

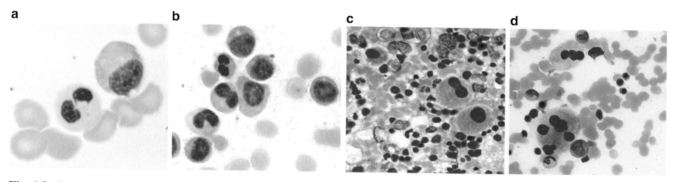

Fig. 6-3. Dysplastic myelopoiesis in MDS. (**a**) Pseudo-Pelger-Huet anomaly and hypogranulation; (**b**) nuclear hypolobation; (**c**) hypolobated/monolobated megakaryocytes; (**d**) dysplastic megakaryocytes with nuclear hypersegmentation and widely separated nuclei

Table 6-4. The international prognostic scoring system (IPSS) for myelodysplastic syndromes.

Score					
Variables	**0**	**0.5**	**1.0**	**1.5**	**2.0**
Bone marrow blasts (%)	<5	5–10	–	11–20	21–30
Cytogenetics	Good	Intermediate	Poor	–	–
Cytopenia (s)	0 or 1	2 or 3	–	–	–

Risk category	Overall score	Median overall survival (years)*	25% AML progression (years)*
Low	0	5.7	9.4
INT-1	0.5	3.5	3.3
INT-2	1.5-2.0	1.1	1.1
High	≥2.5	0.4	0.2

*Absence of therapy. Adapted from Greenberg et al [28·84].

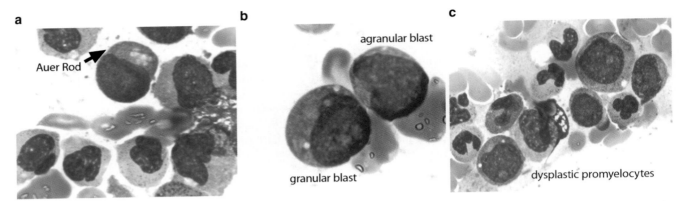

Fig. 6-4. Blast morphology in MDS. (**a**) Agranular blast containing no visible granules and a high nuclear/cytoplasmic ratio and a granular blast containing visible granules (³20 granules/cell). (**b**) In contrast, dysplastic promyelocytes have a lower nuclear/cytoplasmic ratio, less prominent nucleoli, and a Golgi zone. (**c**) If a blast contains Auer rods, the case is always classified as RAEB-2

of the blast percentage (Fig. 6-4a) according to the WHO classification. Cases of MDS with <5% blasts in the BM and <1% in the PB rarely contain Auer rods but such cases have been reported to be associated with an adverse prognosis [14]. However, the prognostic significance of finding Auer rods in MDS remains controversial, and requires further clarification [15,16].

Myeloblasts in MDS often show marked heterogeneity in size and can be classified into three morphologic types. Type I and II blasts have high nuclear/cytoplasmic ratios, and blastic chromatin but show conspicuous nucleoli with agranular cytoplasm in type I, and scant granules in type II (Fig. 6-4b). Type III blasts have at least 20 fine azurophilic granules and were originally designated as promyelocytes in the FAB classification [7], but their inclusion in the blast count gives a better separation of survival curves [17]. In 2008, the IWG proposed a revised definition to cover both agranular and granular types effectively merging the three morphologic types [13]. Promyelocytes, especially in MDS, can be misinterpreted as granular blasts; therefore, it is important to recognize dysplastic changes that can occur in promyelocytes (Fig. 6-4c). Normal promyelocytes have a visible Golgi zone, uniformly dispersed azurophilic granules, and, in most instances, basophilic cytoplasm. Dysplastic promyelocytes may have reduced or irregular cytoplasmic basophilia, a poorly developed Golgi zone, hyper or hypogranularity, or irregular distribution (clumps) of granules, but still contain a round, oval, or indented nucleus that is often eccentric, a Golgi zone (at least faintly visible), and a nucleus with fine or coarse chromatin and an easily visible nucleolus [13].

6.1.6.7. Peripheral Blood Evaluation

The peripheral blood in MDS always shows some evidence of cytopenia. Anemia is often macrocytic and the red cell distribution width (RDW) is often increased. Patients with significant RS in the marrow will show a dimorphic red cell appearance due to a combination of macrocytic anemia and hypochromatic microcytic anemia. Granulocytic dysplasia may be more visible in PB in comparing to BM. It is important to recognize and report circulating blasts, since it can change classification and predict outcome. It is noteworthy that circulating immature cells including blasts can also be seen in patients who have received growth factor treatment, have an actively regenerating BM, or following stem cell transplant.

6.1.7. Application of Immunohistochemistry

Immunohistochemistry (IHC) can be very useful in assessing MDS, especially in fibrotic or hypocellular BM. CD34, a stem cell/early progenitor marker, is positive in the majority of blasts, regardless of MDS subtype [18]. The presence of increased and/or clustered CD34+ blasts not only helps confirm a diagnosis of MDS (Fig. 6-5a), but also assists in identifying ALIP and reliably predicts risk of transformation to AML and adverse outcome [19,20].

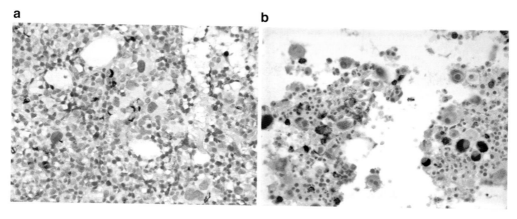

Fig. 6-5. Value of immunostaining in MDS. (**a**) Immunostains for CD34 (clone: QBEND-10) shows focal CD34+ myeloblast clustering in a case of refractory cytopenia with multilineage dysplasia (RCMD) (**b**) strong megakaryocyte reactivity CD34 seen in case of refractory anemia with excess blasts-1 (RAEB-1)

CD34 also stains endothelium and sinus lining cells, so highlighting the increased angiogenesis characteristic of MDS. We have also observed that strong CD34 positivity in megakaryocytes characterizes some cases of RAEB with a high IPSS score (Fig. 6-5b). However, focal and weak CD34 positivity in megakaryocytes can be seen in normal regenerating BM and should not be considered as an abnormal feature. In rare cases, blasts in MDS are negative for CD34. In these instances, CD117/KIT can be used as an alternative blast marker; however, CD117 will also stain early erythroid precursors (pronormoblasts), some promyelocytes, and mast cells. This last pattern of reactivity is helpful since detection of aggregates of more than 15 mast cells may be a sign of MDS-associated systemic mastocytosis.

Paraffin section markers of megakaryocytes, including CD61, CD42b, von Willebrand factor (VWF)-associated protein and LAT (linker of activation of T-cells), are useful in highlighting micromegakaryocytes and abnormal grouping or clustering of megakaryocytes, especially in fibrotic BM. These markers are also helpful in differentiating MDS from acute megakaryocytic leukemia where the megakaryoblasts have an abnormal phenotype, commonly CD61+ but negative for CD42 and the VWF-associated protein.

6.1.8. Flow Cytometry Immunophenotyping

Immunophenotyping by flow cytometry (FC) represents a highly sensitive and reproducible method for quantitative and qualitative evaluation of hematopoietic cell maturation. Although no abnormal marker is entirely specific for MDS, differentiation block is reflected in patterns of altered antigen expression, as indicated by either altered fluorescence intensity or in the percentage of blasts, maturing myeloid cells, and monocytes (Table 6-5).

FC immunophenotypic abnormalities in MDS have been shown to be highly correlated with morphologic dysplasia and cytogenetic abnormalities [18,21,22]. Compared to normal myeloblasts, blasts in MDS can show increased fluorescence intensity for CD117, CD13 or CD33, decreased CD45 and CD38, or aberrant expression of lymphoid antigens such as CD2, CD5, CD7, and CD56, and paradoxical expression of mature myeloid antigens, such as CD65, CD15, CD10, CD11b. Maturing myeloid cells can show decreased side scatter (SS) as indicative of hypogranulation (Fig. 6-6), altered maturation patterns of CD13/CD16 and CD11b/CD16, or decreased fluorescence intensity of mature myeloid antigens such as CD10, CD15, and CD33. Monocytes can show increased numbers, decreased CD14, CD64, CD33, CD11b, CD13, or aberrant CD56 and CD2 expression. The normal precursor B cells (hematogones) are usually decreased in MDS. Recently, the European Leukemia Network has published standardized protocols for the use of FC in the diagnosis of MDS, thus providing a model for panel design and data interpretation [85].

Table 6-5. Frequency of antigenic abnormalities detected by flow cytometry in patients with myelodysplastic syndrome.

Blasts

- Increased ≥3%
- A discrete population
- Aberrant expression of CD2, CD5, CD7, CD56
- Increased CD117, CD123, and/or CD33 expression intensity
- Decreased CD45 and/or CD38
- Paradoxical expression of mature myeloid antigens, CD15, CD65, CD11b, CD
- Decreased hematogones

Myeloid

- Hypogranulation
- Increased CD14
- Decreased CD64
- Decreased or absence of CD10 on granulocytes
- Decreased CD33
- Decreased CD15 and/or CD65
- Aberrant expression of CD2, CD5, CD7
- Partial CD117
- Partial CD34
- CD11b/CD13/CD16 abnormalities
- CD56 expression (>15%)

Monocytes

- CD34 and/or CD117 partial expression
- Decreased CD14
- Decreased CD64
- Decreased HLA-DR
- Decreased CD13, CD33
- Decreased CD11b
- Increased CD15
- CD56 (>25%)
- Aberrant CD2, CD5, and/or CD7 expression

The use of FC as an ancillary test in diagnosing MDS has been gradually accepted, but thus far is only recommended for experienced laboratories given the wide range of findings observed in MDS and in reactive and recovering hematopoiesis. Substitution of the percentage of CD34+ cells determined by FC for a visual blast count is discouraged. Not all myeloblasts express CD34, and not all CD34 positive cells are myeloblasts (e.g., stage I hematogones are CD34+). Furthermore, the number of blasts enumerated by FC is affected by hemodilution, incomplete red blood cell lysis or lysis of late stage nucleated red blood cells, suboptimal cell viability due to sample aging, or cell loss due to sample processing.

Some studies suggest that FC may also assist in outcome prediction in MDS as a supplement to current prognostic scoring systems [23,26]. Such use of FC in risk stratification will require standardized reporting and consensus on standard reagent panels and protocols, the method for enumerating abnormal blasts, and the most diagnostically useful abnormal antigen pattern to separate MDS findings from those seen in BM recovery and stress. Larger prospective clinical studies must be completed to better define the importance of each

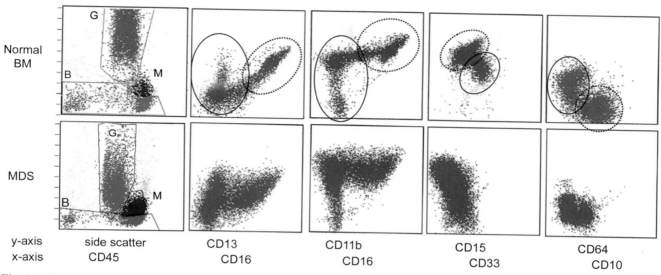

Fig. 6-6. Flow cytometric findings in MDS. *Upper panel*: A case of normal lymphoma staging bone marrow. The myeloid cells encircled by the solid lines are relatively immature cells; the ones encircled by the dashed lines are mature myeloid cells. *Lower panel*: A case of refractory anemia with multilineage dysplasia demonstrates hypogranularity on in the CD45/side-scatter gate (**left**) with the myeloid marker sets showing abnormal maturation patterns

abnormality to eventually generate a scoring system that is easy to interpret, reproducible within and between laboratories, and encodes the maximal information for assisting diagnosis and improving on the IPSS outcome predictors.

6.1.9. Cytogenetic Analysis

Cytogenetic studies have a long-established role in diagnosis and outcome prediction in MDS, but have recently emerged as important factors in treatment selection and in monitoring response.

Conventional karyotyping remains an essential component of the diagnostic work-up of any patient with suspected MDS (see Chap. 8), but needs to be interpreted with caution. Isolated (nonclonal) cytogenetic abnormalities are commonly observed in BM samples and may represent an artifact of short-term culture prior to harvesting. Use of a standardized definition for clonality, such as finding the same chromosomal gain or structural aberration in at least two BM cells and the same chromosome loss in at least three cells, is essential to avoid false-positive results. In borderline cases or in the posttreatment setting where low numbers of metaphases are obtained, confirmation of the suspected chromosome changes by fluorescence in situ hybridization (FISH) on interphase (noncultured) cells is recommended.

Clonal cytogenetic abnormalities are observed in approximately 50% of MDS cases and include a large number of different alterations. For example, a recent multicenter analysis showed 684 different types of chromosome abnormalities among the 1,080 MDS patients who had abnormal karyotypes [27]. The IPSS uses cytogenetic abnormalities to define three risk categories: "good", which includes a normal karyotype, isolated del(5q), isolated del(20q), and −Y; "poor", which includes a complex karyotype with more than three abnormalities, as well as del(7q) and −7 either present as alone or in combination with other anomalies; and "intermediate", which includes all other abnormalities (Table 6-4) [2,28]. More recent series have shown that some of the less common cytogenetic abnormalities seen in MDS may have very significant roles in clinical outcome suggesting a more sophisticated classification scheme is needed [27,29,30]. Such attempts at improving the IPSS scoring identified additional favorable cytogenetic findings such as del(12p), del(9p), +21, −21, del(11p), del(15p), and del(11q), reclassified sole del(7q) as intermediate risk, and added i(17q) and other forms of 17p loss as poor risk changes [31]. As therapy shifts, additional reconsideration of these associations will be required.

6.1.10. The Role of Molecular Testing

Molecular clonality assays (such as G6PD isoenzymes, restriction-linked polymorphisms, and X-linked DNA polymorphisms of the androgen receptor) have helped to define MDS as a clonal disorder but are rarely used in clinical practice. In contrast, molecular genetic analyses looking for mutations and copy number changes in oncogenes and tumor suppressor genes are now common in MDS. Following the model in AML (Chap. 7), such mutations have been grouped as class I when the target genes are involved in signal transduction (commonly FLT3, RAS genes, and KIT), or as class II if they involve transcription factors involved in differentiation block (e.g., RUNX1/AML1, EVI1, and WT1) [32]. In early stages of MDS, class I mutations are usually absent except in specialized subgroups (e.g., RAS gene mutations in CMML), but a variety of class II mutations may be observed in MDS.

Tumor suppressors are regulatory genes whose loss promotes growth and cell cycle progression in nearly all neoplasms. These genes can be lost by mutation, deletion, promoter methylation silencing, transcriptional regulation or posttranscriptional mechanisms such as microRNA targeting. Since large chromosomal deletions and numerical chromosomal defects are the most common feature of de novo MDS, loss of tumor suppressors by gene deletion was proposed as an extremely important mechanism of progression. However, to date, with the exception of the 17p deletion, which causes the loss of one TP53 allele, followed by either the mutation or the submicroscopic deletion of the other allele on the apparently normal chromosome 17 in 70% of del(17p) patients, [33], other tumor suppressor gene loss has not been clearly implicated in most common MDS-associated chromosomal losses. Instead, recent data has implicated copy number loss of genes involved in cell metabolism such as ribosome biogenesis, protease function and cytoskeleton regulation [34]. Microarray-based gene expression profiling (GEP) may help to define which gene levels are most critical and establish prognostically relevant gene signatures that correlate with FAB, WHO, or IPSS subtypes [35,36]. However, these studies have shown a considerable overlap in gene expression profiles between high risk MDS and AML, as well as low risk MDS and nonneoplastic bone marrow samples.

6.2. Specialized Presentations of MDS and Bone Marrow Failure States

A number of patients will present with changes that do not meet current criteria for diagnosis of MDS (Table 6-1) or with features overlapping with other hematologic conditions. Diagnostic difficulties also result when MDS acquires secondary genetic changes that lead to a proliferative phenotype mimicking myeloproliferative neoplasms (MPNs) which is described in the next section. Here, we describe the most commonly encountered problems in variant and unusual MDS presentations.

6.2.1. Cytopenias Without Other Diagnostic Criteria of MDS

Idiopathic cytopenia of uncertain significance (ICUS)[3,37] is a newly coined term for conditions where there are persistent cytopenias (lasting ≥ 6 months) that cannot be explained by any other disease and where the full diagnostic criteria for MDS are lacking. ICUS usually encompasses hematologic changes such as transfusion-dependent macrocytic anemia that are suggestive of MDS. As such, ICUS is a diagnosis of exclusion requiring careful BM examination (with use of IHC and FC), chromosome analysis, and a search for infectious or other identifiable causes. An approach to the diagnosis of these borderline ICUS cases is presented in Fig. 6-7. Careful follow-up is advised as ICUS may progress quickly to full-blown MDS [85].

6.2.2. Clonal Cytogenetic Abnormalities in the Absence of Morphologic Dysplasia

Some MDS cases show the presence of cytopenias and a clonal karyotypic abnormality but minimal morphologic dysplasia. The 2008 WHO classification suggests handling these cases based on the type of cytogenetic change identified [1,3]. When the sole aberration is −Y, +8 or del(20q), the recommendation is to diagnose as "suspicious for MDS" because such changes can occasionally be encountered in metaphases analysis of "normal" BM. The finding of any other cytogenetic abnormality would be regarded as presumptive evidence for MDS (Fig. 6-7).

6.2.3. Hypocellular MDS Versus Aplastic Anemia

Hypocellular MDS, where the marrow cellularity at diagnosis is less than 30% in patients under 70 years of age and less than 20% in patients over 70, comprises 10–20% of MDS and can be diagnostically problematic [38]. The low cellularity and cell-poor aspirates makes appreciation of morphologic dysplasia difficult, leading to problems distinguishing these cases from aplastic anemia. Patterns of apoptotic cell death and genetic changes different from those normally seen in hypercelluar MDS may underlie the hypocellularity [39,40]. Similar to aplastic anemia, hypocellular MDS may respond to anti-thymocyte globulin (ATG) suggesting a similar immune-mediated attack on stem cells [41]. In recent studies, hypo-cellularity in MDS has shown to be an independent predictor of favorable outcome, compared to hyper-or normal cellularity MDS [40,42] indicating that hypocellular MDS is worth recognizing as a separate MDS subgroup.

6.2.4. MDS with Bone Marrow Fibrosis

Moderate to severe degrees of marrow fibrosis are observed in approximately 10–20% of MDS, [43,44] either at diagnosis or over the course of disease. The presence of moderate to severe marrow fibrosis is an adverse prognostic factor independent of IPSS score or MDS subtype [44,45]. and needs to be highlighted and scored in diagnostic and follow-up mate-

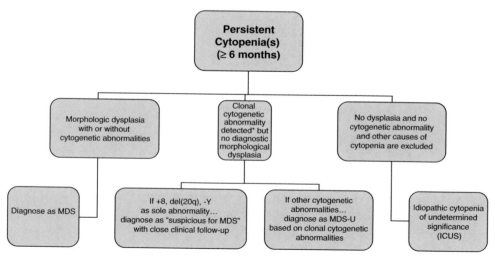

Fig. 6-7. Algorithm for diagnosis of cytopenias when full criteria for MDS are lacking. Common MDS-type clonal cytogenetic abnormalities include -7, -5, del(7q), del(5q), del(11q), i(17q) or t(17p), -13 or del(13q), del(11q), del(12p), and del(9q). Common balanced translocations involve chromosome locations 3(q26.2) [EVI1] and 11(q23) [MLL] and t(6;9)(p23;q34)[DEK-CAN fusion]

rial using trichrome and reticulin stains. MDS with moderate and severe BM fibrosis usually have high transfusion requirement and show multilineage dysplasia and high-risk cytogenetic changes, with a faster progression to fatal BM failure. Because of the dry tap, aspirate smears are generally of poor quality and IHC for CD34 and CD117 are recommended to estimate blast percentages. Unlike MDS/MPN with fibrosis, *JAK2 V617F* mutation is infrequent in MDS with BM fibrosis [43,45,46].

6.2.5. MDS Associated with a Minor PNH Clone

Classic paroxysmal nocturnal hemoglobinuria (PNH) is an acquired hemolytic anemia characterized by an increased number of cells with loss of glycosyl phosphatidylinositol-anchored membrane proteins (GPI-AP) as a result of a phosphatidlyinositol glycan complementation group A (PIGA) gene mutation in hematopoietic stem cells. A small population of GPI-AP-deficient blood cells can be present in patients with BM failure who show no clinical or laboratory signs of hemolysis or PNH signs and symptoms. The presence of such small populations of GPI-AP–deficient cells in the setting of aplastic anemia or MDS has been shown to have important prognostic and therapeutic implications [47]. and has been defined as PNH-subclinical (sc) [48]. In PNH-sc, the PIGA-mutated cells appear to be an independent clonal expansion that arises because of a selective growth advantage over the ineffective MDS clone or the immune-mediated destruction of the normal marrow in aplastic anemia (Fig. 6-8a). PNH-sc in MDS is usually seen in low-grade MDS subtypes with a low cellularity, infrequent cytogenetic abnormalities, and minimal granulocytic or megakaryocytic dysplasia (i.e., RA type). The frequency is 10–20% [47,49,50] in low grade MDS.

Diagnosis of PNH-sc is performed by FC looking for loss of expression on a subpopulation of granulocytes of a number of GPI-APs, including CD55, CD59, CD16, CD66b, CD24, CD14, and CD58. Application of a stringent gating strategy with at least 100,000 total events acquired is important to ensure detection sensitivity (Fig. 6-8b). Since alterations of GPI-

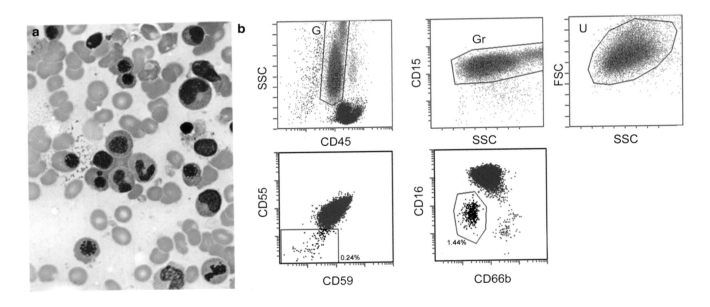

Fig. 6-8. Refractory anemia with a small paroxysmal nocturnal hemoglobinuria (PNH) clone. (**a**) Dyserythropoiesis is present, no dysgranulopoiesis; (**b**) flow cytometric findings: *Upper panel*: Gating strategy: granulocytes are followed through the following sequential gates: CD45/SSC, further defined by CD15/SSC followed by FSC/SSC. *Lower panel*: The granulocytes from the three combined analysis regions (G, Gr and U) show a small PNH clone (CD55/CD59 and CD16/CD66b)

APs can be associated with granulocytic/monocytic dysplasia and immaturity. Definitive diagnostic criteria should include identification of loss of at least two GPI-AP proteins on the same cell population or the GPI-AP protein loss in two different cell populations [48].

6.2.6. Erythroid-Predominant MDS

In approximately 10–20% of MDS, there is overwhelming erythroid hyperplasia with erythroblasts comprising at least 50% of total BM nucleated cell, in the absence of erythropoietin treatment [51,52]. Although erythroid-predominant MDS includes a group of true low-grade de novo MDS, such as RARS, many such cases are therapy-related MDS or primary MDS with a similar aggressive clinical course. In the FAB and WHO classifications, BM blasts in erythroleukemia (AML-M6a) are enumerated by counting only the nonerythroid rather than all nucleated cells (See Chap. 7). However, in erythroid-predominant MDS, there is no clear guidance from the FAB, 2001 WHO or IWG on whether to enumerate blast percentages from nonerythroid elements (as in AML-M6a) or from all nucleated cells (as for all other MDS) [53]. Several studies have shown that in erythroid-predominant MDS, blast calculation as a proportion of marrow nonerythroid rather than total nucleated cells can better stratify patients into prognostically relevant groups [51,52]. In 2008 WHO, in erythroid-predominent MDS, if blast calculation does not meet the diagnosis of M6a, the blast number is enumerated as the percentage of total nucleated cells.

6.2.7. MDS with Erythroid Aplasia

MDS with pure red cell aplasia (PRCA) is rare, representing much less than 5% of MDS and can present at the time of diagnosis or during the course of MDS. Patients with PRCA have strong male predominance, are almost always red cell transfusion-dependant, and have markedly increased serum erythropoietin. There is no association with the presence of anti-erythropoietin autoantibodies or with Parvovirus B19 infection [54]. In the past, PRCA in MDS has been assumed to be a result of defective erythroid stem cell differentiation or due to erythroid precursors that undergo excessive apoptosis. However, several recent studies have demonstrated monoclonal or oligoclonal T-cell expansion in a large proportion of cases [54,55]. indicating that immune-mediated destruction or dysregulation of erythroid precursors, as in aplastic anemia, might be more important in the pathogenesis. Correspondingly, some cases of MDS-associated PRCA have shown an excellent response to cyclosporine treatment [54,56].

6.3. Evaluation of PostTreatment Samples

Since MDS comprise a heterogeneous group of diseases, the therapeutic goals and endpoints are similarly broad including achieving objective disease responses (e.g., cytogenetic remission), hematologic improvement (reduction of transfusion needs), altering the natural history of the disease (decreasing leukemia progression) or improving quality of life (See Chap. 8) [53].

Standardized criteria for assessing response are crucial. When evaluating posttreatment BM in MDS, blast percentage is the most important parameter in assessing a patient's response and for indicating persistent disease. Dysplastic changes in posttreatment samples are more difficult to interpret, since common therapeutic agents such as hydroxyurea, cytarabine, azacitidine, and decitabine can all alter normal hematopoiesis to some degree. In particular, megaloblastic changes, mild dyserythropoiesis and mild dysgranulopoiesis are commonly seen with DNA-damaging therapies and their presence should be mentioned and documented but not used to indicate residual disease in a patient who otherwise meets the criteria for complete response.[53] However, severe dysplastic changes, particularly the presence of micromegakaryocytes, always favor residual MDS.

6.4. Prognosis of MDS and Transformation to Acute Leukemia

The most significant causes of mortality in patients with MDS are BM failure and transformation to acute leukemia, which is almost always AML, with rare cases of acute precursor B-lymphoblastic leukemia (ALL) reported [57,58]. The overall incidence of transformation to AML in MDS is approximately 30% but varies significantly by subtype, being 25–35% for patients with RAEB and 2% for RA [59]. The IPSS 4-tier score (Table 6-4), combining the percent marrow blasts, specific cytogenetic abnormalities, and number of cytopenias, effectively predicts overall survival and evolution to AML [2]. Multiple other factors [59,61]. have been shown to add significant prognostic information to that provided by the IPSS, such as patient age, performance status, transfusion dependence, WHO disease subtype, presence of marrow fibrosis, and presence of molecular alterations including in the FLT3, TP53 and RAS genes [62,63]. Although 20% blasts in PB or BM now distinguishes AML from MDS (RAEB), it is not a requirement to treat as AML, and therapy algorithms are currently based on a complex matrix of patient age, performance status, risk and benefit assessment (See Chap. 8).

6.5. Overview of the Myelodysplastic/Myeloproliferative Neoplasms

Myelodysplastic/myeloproliferative neoplasms (MDS/MPN) represent a group of clonal myeloid neoplasms characterized, at the time of their initial presentation, by the simultaneous presence of myelodysplastic and myeloproliferative features. In addition to MDS-like features such as cytopenia(s) and dysplastic changes, MDS/MPD patients often present with elevated white blood cell (WBC) counts, thrombocytosis and organomegaly, features more commonly associated with MPN. The three best-defined entities within the MDS/MPN group are chronic myelomonocytic leukemia (CMML), atypical chronic myeloid leukemia (aCML) and juvenile myelomonocytic leukemia (JMML). The latter is a leukemic condition seen in young children that is usually considered within the group of pediatric myeloid neoplasms; it will not be discussed any further in this chapter. Less well-defined is a group of MDS/MPN unclassifiable disorders that are different from both CMML and aCML. Among these, the most well-characterized is the rare refractory anemia with ring sideroblasts and thrombocytosis (RARS-T).

6.6. Chronic Myelomonocytic Leukemia

6.6.1. General Features

Chronic Myelomonocytic Leukemia (CMML) is defined by persistent monocytosis (3 months or more of at least 1×10^9/L in PB) with fewer than 20% blasts in the PB and BM and dysplasia involving one or more myeloid lineages. CMML cases lack the Philadelphia (Ph) chromosome/BCR-ABL1 fusion gene seen in CML and lack the PDGFRA or PDGFRB translocations seen in MPNs with monocytosis (See Chap. 9). The 2008 WHO classification subdivides the entity into CMML-1, when blasts are less <5% in PB or <10% BM, and CMML-2 when there are 5–19% in PB or 10–19% in BM, or when Auer rods are seen. CMML-1 patients have shown a better survival than CMML-2 patients [64]. Most cases of CMML are de novo but can evolve from a preexisting MDS [65]. The incidence of CMML is aproximately three cases per 100,000 individuals older than 60 years [7]. CMML patients show a male predominance with a male to female ratio of 1.5-3:1.

6.6.2. Morphologic and Flow Cytometric Features

The BM findings in CMML resemble MDS but with increased number of monocytes to varying degrees. In cases with significant granulocytic dysplasia, it can be difficult to distinguish monocytes from myeloid cells, and nonspecific esterase cytochemical studies on smears are helpful in confirming their monocytic origin [66]. Myeloblasts, monoblasts, and promono-cytes should all be combined in the final blast count. If this number is 20% or greater, AML should be diagnosed instead. If morphological dysplasia is minimal, CMML may still diag-nosed when persistent idiopathic monocytosis is present for at least 3 months or an acquired clonal cytogenetic or molecular genetic abnormality can be demonstrated.

Flow cytometry immunophenotyping with CD64, CD14, HLA-DR, CD13, CD36, CD11b, CD2, and CD56 are useful in assessing monocytic maturation or aberrant expres-sion to distinguish CMML from reactive monocytosis, even in the absence of morphologic dysplasia. The most common aberrant immunophenotypic characteristics are overexpres-sion of CD56 (often more than 25% of total monocytes), aberrant expression of CD2, decreased expression of CD14 and decreased expression of HLA-DR, CD13, CD64 and/or CD36 [22,67]. FC is also effective in distinguishing CMML from AML-M5a [68]. However, distinguishing CMML from AML-M5b can be challenging immunophenotypi-cally, since CD34 and CD117 are often negative in both M5b and CMML and monocytic antigen expression patterns are very similar. Morphological examination, especially a BM biopsy, is more informative.

6.6.3. Molecular Genetic Findings

Although clonal cytogenetic abnormalities are found in 20–40% [64,69]. of patients with CMML, this frequency is lower than MDS with multilineage dysplasia (RCMD) or RAEB. The cytogenetic alterations are very similar to that seen in MDS (described above). Abnormalities of chromosome 11q23 are uncommon in CMML and should suggest a diag-nosis of AML. PDGFRA or PDGRB gene alterations which occur de novo in other MPNs have been rarely reported to occur as a secondary genetic event rarely in CMML [70]. Point mutations in either NRAS or KRAS occur in 40–50% of CMML, [71,72]. and RUNX1 alterations occur with a frequency of 40% [71]. JAK2 V617F mutation is infrequent (less than 5%), and if discovered, should raise the differential with variants of MPNs [65,73].

6.6.4. The Significance of Myelodysplastic Versus Myeloproliferative Types of CMML

Historically, CMML was grouped under MDS in FAB. The 2001 WHO classification included it under MDS/MPD, acknowledging its proliferative features in addition to dysplasia [74]. Regardless of its classification, CMML can be grouped into myelodysplastic (MD) and myeloproliferative (MP) subtypes on the basis of a WBC count of greater or less than $13 \times 10^9/L$. Patients with MP-CMML have a higher incidence of splenomegaly, high serum lactate dehydrogenase (LDH) levels, high frequency of point mutation in RAS genes and shorter survival [71,75,76]. However, it remains to be clarified whether the MD and MP forms of CMML represent distinct clinical-biological entities rather than different stages of the same disease [64·65]. It also has yet to be decided if it would be appropriate to shift MD-CMML, i.e., WBC $<12 \times 10^9/L$, back into the MDS group, since these patients clearly have no prolifer-ative features and only differ by the presence of more than 1,000 monocytes/μL. Although the WHO classification does not distinguish MP-CMML from MD-CMML,[1,74]. the IPSS[2]. group excludes CMML with a WBC of more than 12,000/μL from its calculations.

6.7. Atypical Chronic Myeloid Leukemia (aCML)

Atypical chronic myeloid leukemia (aCML) is a rare and poorly characterized MDS/MPD presenting with high WBC count (at least $13 \times 10^9/L$), hypercellular myeloid-predominant bone marrow, and dysgranulopoiesis. There is no evidence of BCR-ABL1 or PDGFRA or PDGFRB gene alterations. Compared to CML, the percentage of mature neutrophils is higher, with less-prominent myeloid left-shift maturation and virtual absence of basophilia.

An absence of monocytosis excludes CMML. A variety of different karyotypic abnormalities have been reported in aCML in up to 80% of cases, as have mutations in RAS genes in up to 30% [77]. Some cases of t(8;9)(p22;p24) with the *PCM1-JAK2* fusion gene have been reported as "aCML" but data currently available suggest they have eosinophilia and lack dysplasia and may be better regarded as chronic eosinophilic leukemia [78]. aCML is a more aggressive disease than CML, with an overall median survival being 11–25 months [77,79].

6.8. Refractory Anemia with Ring Sideroblasts Associated with Marked Thrombocytosis

Refractory anemia with ring sideroblasts associated with marked thrombocytosis (RARS-T) is a recognized MDS/MPN variant that combines the features of RARS with thrombocytosis ($\geq 450 \times 10^9$/L) and abnormal marrow megakaryopoiesis. Megakaryocyte morphology can range from MDS-like to MPD-like (Fig. 6-9a), and there is a high frequency of JAK2 V617F mutation (50–75%) [80,83]. Median overall survival is inferior to RARS, essential thrombocythemia, or 5q- syndrome with thrombocytosis [81]. Whether RARS-T represents progression of RARS with an acquired (JAK2) genetic abnormality, or MPN with ring sideroblasts (Fig. 6-9b), is still unresolved signifying its provisional status in the 2008 WHO classification.

6.9.   MDS/MPN-Unclassifiable

MDS/MPN-U is a residual diagnostic category reserved for those de novo myeloid neoplasms with mixed dysplastic and proliferative features that do not meet the criteria for CMML, JMML or aCML and lack BCR-ABL1, PDGFRA, PDGFRB or FGFR1 gene alterations. Cases showing isolated del(5q) or t(3;3)(q21;q26), or inv(3)(q21q26) where thrombocytosis is frequently present, should be diagnosed as MDS, as should cases which show leukocytosis only following treatment with growth factors. Nonetheless, such disorders with mixed features are not rare, and may include cases of MDS that went undiagnosed in the hypoproliferative phase and were diagnosed after acquiring a secondary (growth-promoting) genetic change. Similarly, undiagnosed MPN may develop dysplastic features and cytopenia with disease progression. The most common presentation of MDS/MPN-U is anemia of varying severity combined with marrow hypercellularity and thrombocytosis (platelet count $\geq 450 \times 10^9$/L) and/or leukocytosis (WBC $>13 \times 10^9$/L). Cytogenetic findings are variable, as would be expected.

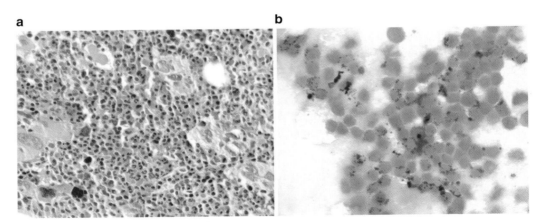

Fig. 6-9. Refractory anemia with ring sideroblasts associated with marked thrombocytosis (RARS-T) (a case positive for JAK2 V617F mutation). (**a**) Megakaryocytes show a mixed myeloproliferative neoplasm-like and myelodysplastic syndromes-like morphology. (**b**) Numerous ring sideroblasts are present.

Suggested Readings

Valent P, Horny HP, et al. Definitions and standards in the diagnosis and treatment of the myelodysplastic syndromes: Consensus statements and report from a working conference. Leuk Res 2007;31(6):727–36.

Haase D. Cytogenetic features in myelodysplastic syndromes. Ann Hematol 2008;87(7):515–26.

Orazi A, Germing U. The myelodysplastic/myeloproliferative neoplasms: Myeloproliferative diseases with dysplastic features. Leukemia 2008;22(7):1308–19.

References

1. Swerdlow SH, Campo E, Harris NL, et al. eds. WHO classification of tumours of haematopoietic and lymphoid tissues, 4th ed. Lyon, IARC, 2008.

2. Greenberg P, Cox C, LeBeau MM, et al. International scoring system for evaluating prognosis in myelodysplastic syndromes. Blood 1997;89:2079–88

3. Valent P, Horny HP, Bennett JM, et al. Definitions and standards in the diagnosis and treatment of the myelodysplastic syndromes: Consensus statements and report from a working conference. Leuk Res 2007;31:727–36

4. Verburgh E, Achten R, Louw VJ, et al. A new disease categorization of low-grade myelodysplastic syndromes based on the expression of cytopenia and dysplasia in one versus more than one lineage improves on the WHO classification. Leukemia 2007;21:668–77

5. Ma X, Does M, Raza A, Mayne ST. Myelodysplastic syndromes: incidence and survival in the United States. Cancer 2007;109:1536–42

6. Rollison DE, Howlader N, Smith MT, et al. Epidemiology of myelodysplastic syndromes and chronic myeloproliferative disorders in the United States, 2001–2004, using data from the NAACCR and SEER programs. Blood 2008;112:45–52

7. Bennett JM, Catovsky D, Daniel MT, et al. Proposals for the classification of the myelodysplastic syndromes. Br J Haematol 1982;51:189–99

8. Giagounidis AA, Germing U, Haase S, et al. Clinical, morphological, cytogenetic, and prognostic features of patients with myelodysplastic syndromes and del(5q) including band q31. Leukemia 2004;18:113–9

9. Malcovati L, Porta MG, Pascutto C, et al. Prognostic factors and life expectancy in myelodysplastic syndromes classified according to WHO criteria: a basis for clinical decision making. J Clin Oncol 2005;23:7594–603

10. Germing U, Strupp C, Kuendgen A, et al. Prospective validation of the WHO proposals for the classification of myelodysplastic syndromes. Haematologica 2006;91:1596–604

11. Strom SS, Gu Y, Gruschkus SK, Pierce SA, Estey EH. Risk factors of myelodysplastic syndromes: a case-control study. Leukemia 2005;19:1912–8

12. Verburgh E, Achten R, Maes B, et al. Additional prognostic value of bone marrow histology in patients subclassified according to the International Prognostic Scoring System for myelodysplastic syndromes. J Clin Oncol 2003;21:273–82

13. Mufti GJ, Bennett JM, Goasguen J, et al. Diagnosis and classification of myelodysplastic syndrome: International Working Group on Morphology of myelodysplastic syndrome (IWGM-MDS) consensus proposals for the definition and enumeration of myeloblasts and ring sideroblasts. Haematologica 2008;93:1712–7

14. Willis MS, McKenna RW, Peterson LC, Coad JE, Kroft SH. Low blast count myeloid disorders with Auer rods: a clinicopathologic analysis of 9 cases. Am J Clin Pathol 2005;124:191–8

15. Seymour JF, Estey EH. The prognostic significance of auer rods in myelodysplasia. Br J Haematol 1993;85:67–76

16. Yoshida Y, Oguma S, Ohno H. John Auer and Auer rods; controversies revisited. Leuk Res 2009;33(5):614–6

17. Goasguen JE, Bennett JM, Cox C, Hambley H, Mufti G, Flandrin G. Prognostic implication and characterization of the blast cell population in the myelodysplastic syndrome. Leuk Res 1991;15:1159–65

18. Ogata K, Nakamura K, Yokose N, et al. Clinical significance of phenotypic features of blasts in patients with myelodysplastic syndrome. Blood 2002;100:3887–96

19. Oriani A, Annaloro C, Soligo D, Pozzoli E, Cortelezzi A, Lambertenghi Deliliers G. Bone marrow histology and CD34 immunostaining in the prognostic evaluation of primary myelodysplastic syndromes. Br J Haematol 1996;92:360–4

20. Baur AS, Meuge-Moraw C, Schmidt PM, Parlier V, Jotterand M, Delacretaz F. CD34/QBEND10 immunostaining in bone marrow biopsies: an additional parameter for the diagnosis and classification of myelodysplastic syndromes. Eur J Haematol 2000;64:71–9

21. Kussick SJ, Fromm JR, Rossini A, et al. Four-color flow cytometry shows strong concordance with bone marrow morphology and cytogenetics in the evaluation for myelodysplasia. Am J Clin Pathol 2005;124:170–81

22. Stachurski D, Smith BR, Pozdnyakova O, et al. Flow cytometric analysis of myelomonocytic cells by a pattern recognition approach is sensitive and specific in diagnosing myelodysplastic syndrome and related marrow diseases: emphasis on a global evaluation and recognition of diagnostic pitfalls. Leuk Res 2008;32:215–24

23. Wells DA, Benesch M, Loken MR, et al. Myeloid and monocytic dyspoiesis as determined by flow cytometric scoring in myelodysplastic syndrome correlates with the IPSS and with outcome after hematopoietic stem cell transplantation. Blood 2003;102:394–403

24. Ogata K, Kishikawa Y, Satoh C, Tamura H, Dan K, Hayashi A. Diagnostic application of flow cytometric characteristics of CD34+ cells in low-grade myelodysplastic syndromes. Blood 2006;108:1037–44

25. Scott BL, Wells DA, Loken MR, Myerson D, Leisenring WM, Deeg HJ. Validation of a flow cytometric scoring system as a prognostic indicator for posttransplantation outcome in patients with myelodysplastic syndrome. Blood 2008;112:2681–6

26. van de Loosdrecht AA, Westers TM, Westra AH, Drager AM, van der Velden VH, Ossenkoppele GJ. Identification of distinct prognostic subgroups in low- and intermediate-1-risk myelodysplastic syndromes by flow cytometry. Blood 2008;111:1067–77

27. Haase D, Germing U, Schanz J, et al. New insights into the prognostic impact of the karyotype in MDS and correlation with subtypes: evidence from a core dataset of 2124 patients. Blood 2007;110:4385–95

28. Greenberg P, Cox C, LeBeau MM, et al. International scoring system for evaluating prognosis in myelodysplastic syndromes. Blood 1997;89:2079–88, [see comment][erratum appears in Blood 1998 Feb 1;91(3):1100]

29. Pozdnyakova O, Miron PM, Tang G, et al. Cytogenetic abnormalities in a series of 1029 patients with primary myelodysplastic syndromes: a report from the US with a focus on some undefined single chromosomal abnormalities. Cancer 2008;113:3331–40

30. Sole F, Luno E, Sanzo C, et al. Identification of novel cytogenetic markers with prognostic significance in a series of 968 patients with primary myelodysplastic syndromes. Haematologica 2005;90:1168–78

31. Haase D. Cytogenetic features in myelodysplastic syndromes. Ann Hematol 2008;87:515–26

32. Deguchi K, Gilliland DG. Cooperativity between mutations in tyrosine kinases and in hematopoietic transcription factors in AML. Leukemia 2002;16:740–4

33. Sankar M, Tanaka K, Kumaravel TS, et al. Identification of a commonly deleted region at 17p13.3 in leukemia and lymphoma associated with 17p abnormality. Leukemia 1998;12:510–6

34. Bernasconi P. Molecular pathways in myelodysplastic syndromes and acute myeloid leukemia: relationships and distinctions-a review. Br J Haematol 2008;142:695–708

35. Pellagatti A, Esoof N, Watkins F, et al. Gene expression profiling in the myelodysplastic syndromes using cDNA microarray technology. Br J Haematol 2004;125:576–83

36. Hofmann WK, de Vos S, Komor M, Hoelzer D, Wachsman W, Koeffler HP. Characterization of gene expression of CD34+ cells from normal and myelodysplastic bone marrow. Blood 2002;100:3553–60

37. Wimazal F, Fonatsch C, Thalhammer R, et al. Idiopathic cytopenia of undetermined significance (ICUS) versus low risk MDS: the diagnostic interface. Leuk Res 2007;31:1461–8

38. Tuzuner N, Cox C, Rowe JM, Watrous D, Bennett JM. Hypocellular myelodysplastic syndromes (MDS): new proposals. Br J Haematol 1995;91:612–7

39. Raza A, Gezer S, Mundle S, et al. Apoptosis in bone marrow biopsy samples involving stromal and hematopoietic cells in 50 patients with myelodysplastic syndromes. Blood 1995;86:268–76

40. Huang TC, Ko BS, Tang JL, et al. Comparison of hypoplastic myelodysplastic syndrome (MDS) with normo-/hypercellular MDS by International Prognostic Scoring System, cytogenetic and genetic studies. Leukemia 2008;22:544–50

41. Killick SB, Mufti G, Cavenagh JD, et al. A pilot study of antithymocyte globulin (ATG) in the treatment of patients with 'low-risk' myelodysplasia. Br J Haematol 2003;120:679–84

42. Yue G, Hao S, Fadare O, et al. Hypocellularity in myelodysplastic syndrome is an independent factor which predicts a favorable outcome. Leuk Res 2008;32:553–8

43. Lambertenghi-Deliliers G, Orazi A, Luksch R, Annaloro C, Soligo D. Myelodysplastic syndrome with increased marrow fibrosis: a distinct clinico-pathological entity. Br J Haematol 1991;78:161–6

44. Della Porta MG, Malcovati L, Boveri E, et al. Clinical relevance of bone marrow fibrosis and CD34-positive cell clusters in primary myelodysplastic syndromes. J Clin Oncol 2008;27(5):754–62

45. Buesche G, Teoman H, Wilczak W, et al. Marrow fibrosis predicts early fatal marrow failure in patients with myelodysplastic syndromes. Leukemia 2008;22:313–22

46. Kremer M, Horn T, Dechow T, Tzankov A, Quintanilla-Martinez L, Fend F. The JAK2 V617F mutation occurs frequently in myelodysplastic/myeloproliferative diseases, but is absent in true myelodysplastic syndromes with fibrosis. Leukemia 2006;20:1315–6

47. Dunn DE, Tanawattanacharoen P, Boccuni P, et al. Paroxysmal nocturnal hemoglobinuria cells in patients with bone marrow failure syndromes. Ann Intern Med 1999;131:401–8

48. Parker C, Omine M, Richards S, et al. Diagnosis and management of paroxysmal nocturnal hemoglobinuria. Blood 2005;106:3699–709

49. Wang SA, Pozdnyakova O, Jorgensen JL, et al. Detection of paroxysmal nocturnal hemoglobinuria clones in patients with myelodysplastic syndromes and related bone marrow diseases, with emphasis on diagnostic pitfalls and caveats. Haematologica 2009;94:29–37

50. Wang H, Chuhjo T, Yasue S, Omine M, Nakao S. Clinical significance of a minor population of paroxysmal nocturnal hemoglobinuria-type cells in bone marrow failure syndrome. Blood 2002;100:3897–902

51. Wang SA, Tang G, Fadare O, et al. Erythroid-predominant myelodysplastic syndromes: enumeration of blasts from nonerythroid rather than total marrow cells provides superior risk stratification. Mod Pathol 2008;21:1394–402

52. Mazzella FM, Smith D, Horn P, et al. Prognostic significance of pronormoblasts in erythrocyte predominant myelodysplastic patients. Am J Hematol 2006;81:484–91

53. Cheson BD, Greenberg PL, Bennett JM, et al. Clinical application and proposal for modification of the International Working Group (IWG) response criteria in myelodysplasia. Blood 2006;108:419–25

54. Wang SA, Yue G, Hutchinson L, et al. Myelodysplastic syndrome with pure red cell aplasia shows characteristic clinicopathological features and clonal T-cell expansion. Br J Haematol 2007;138:271–5

55. Shimamoto T, Iguchi T, Ando K, et al. Successful treatment with cyclosporin A for myelodysplastic syndrome with erythroid hypoplasia associated with T-cell receptor gene rearrangements. Br J Haematol 2001;114:358–61

56. Takata S, Kojima K, Fujii N, et al. Successful treatment with cyclosporin A of myelodysplastic syndrome with erythroid hypoplasia associated with t(6;8)(q15;q22). Cancer Genet Cytogenet 2003;140:167–9

57. Disperati P, Ichim CV, Tkachuk D, Chun K, Schuh AC, Wells RA. Progression of myelodysplasia to acute lymphoblastic leukaemia: implications for disease biology. Leuk Res 2006;30:233–9

58. Zainina S, Cheong SK. Myelodysplastic syndrome transformed into acute lymphoblastic leukaemia (FAB:L3). Clin Lab Haematol 2006;28:282–3

59. Malcovati L, Germing U, Kuendgen A, et al. Time-dependent prognostic scoring system for predicting survival and leukemic evolution in myelodysplastic syndromes. J Clin Oncol 2007;25:3503–10

60. Kantarjian H, O'Brien S, Ravandi F, et al. Proposal for a new risk model in myelodysplastic syndrome that accounts for events not considered in the original International Prognostic Scoring System. Cancer 2008;113:1351–61

61. Balducci L. Transfusion independence in patients with myelodysplastic syndromes: impact on outcomes and quality of life. Cancer 2006;106:2087–94

62. Shih LY, Lin TL, Wang PN, et al. Internal tandem duplication of fms-like tyrosine kinase 3 is associated with poor outcome in patients with myelodysplastic syndrome. Cancer 2004;101:989–98

63. Kita-Sasai Y, Horiike S, Misawa S, et al. International prognostic scoring system and TP53 mutations are independent prognostic indicators for patients with myelodysplastic syndrome. Br J Haematol 2001;115:309–12

64. Germing U, Strupp C, Knipp S, et al. Chronic myelomonocytic leukemia in the light of the WHO proposals. Haematologica 2007;92:974–7

65. Wang SA, Galili N, Cerny J, et al. Chronic myelomonocytic leukemia evolving from preexisting myelodysplasia shares many features with de novo disease. Am J Clin Pathol 2006;126:789–97

66. Orazi A, Germing U. The myelodysplastic/myeloproliferative neoplasms: myeloproliferative diseases with dysplastic features. Leukemia 2008;22:1308–19

67. Xu Y, McKenna RW, Karandikar NJ, Pildain AJ, Kroft SH. Flow cytometric analysis of monocytes as a tool for distinguishing chronic myelomonocytic leukemia from reactive monocytosis. Am J Clin Pathol 2005;124:799–806

68. Dunphy CH, Orton SO, Mantell J. Relative contributions of enzyme cytochemistry and flow cytometric immunophenotyping to the evaluation of acute myeloid leukemias with a monocytic component and of flow cytometric immunophenotyping to the evaluation of absolute monocytoses. Am J Clin Pathol 2004;122:865–74

69. Fenaux P, Beuscart R, Lai JL, Jouet JP, Bauters F. Prognostic factors in adult chronic myelomonocytic leukemia: an analysis of 107 cases. J Clin Oncol 1988;6:1417–24

70. Zota V, Miron PM, Woda BA, Raza A, Wang SA. Eosinophilia with FIP1L1-PDGFRA fusion in a patient with chronic myelomonocytic leukemia. J Clin Oncol 2008;26:2040–1

71. Gelsi-Boyer V, Trouplin V, Adelaide J, et al. Genome profiling of chronic myelomonocytic leukemia: frequent alterations of RAS and RUNX1 genes. BMC Cancer 2008;8:299

72. Hirsch-Ginsberg C, LeMaistre AC, Kantarjian H, et al. RAS mutations are rare events in Philadelphia chromosome-negative/bcr gene rearrangement-negative chronic myelogenous leukemia, but are prevalent in chronic myelomonocytic leukemia. Blood 1990;76:1214–9

73. Jones AV, Kreil S, Zoi K, et al. Widespread occurrence of the JAK2 V617F mutation in chronic myeloproliferative disorders. Blood 2005;106:2162–8

74. Jaffe ES, Harris N, Stein H, Vardiman JW, ed. Pathology and genetics: tumors of haematolopoietic and lymphoid tissues. Lyon: IARC Press, 2001

75. Breccia M, Latagliata R, Mengarelli A, Biondo F, Mandelli F, Alimena G. Prognostic factors in myelodysplastic and myeloproliferative types of chronic myelomonocytic leukemia: a retrospective analysis of 83 patients from a single institution. Haematologica 2004;89:866–8

76. Voglova J, Chrobak L, Neuwirtova R, Malaskova V, Straka L. Myelodysplastic and myeloproliferative type of chronic myelomonocytic leukemia – distinct subgroups or two stages of the same disease? Leuk Res 2001;25:493–9

77. Breccia M, Biondo F, Latagliata R, Carmosino I, Mandelli F, Alimena G. Identification of risk factors in atypical chronic myeloid leukemia. Haematologica 2006;91:1566–8

78. Bousquet M, Quelen C, De Mas V, et al. The t(8;9)(p22;p24) translocation in atypical chronic myeloid leukaemia yields a new PCM1-JAK2 fusion gene. Oncogene 2005;24:7248–52

79. Oscier D. Atypical chronic myeloid leukemias. Pathol Biol (Paris) 1997;45:587–93

80. Ceesay MM, Lea NC, Ingram W, et al. The JAK2 V617F mutation is rare in RARS but common in RARS-T. Leukemia 2006;20:2060–1

81. Wang SA, Hasserjian RP, Loew JM, et al. Refractory anemia with ringed sideroblasts associated with marked thrombocytosis harbors JAK2 mutation and shows overlapping myeloproliferative and myelodysplastic features. Leukemia 2006;20:1641–4

82. Gattermann N, Billiet J, Kronenwett R, et al. High frequency of the JAK2 V617F mutation in patients with thrombocytosis (platelet count>600×10⁹/L) and ringed sideroblasts more than 15% considered as MDS/MPD, unclassifiable. Blood 2007;109:1334–5

83. Remacha AF, Nomdedeu JF, Puget G, et al. Occurrence of the JAK2 V617F mutation in the WHO provisional entity: myelodysplastic/myeloproliferative disease, unclassifiable-refractory anemia with ringed sideroblasts associated with marked thrombocytosis. Haematologica 2006;91:719–20

84. Greenberg PL. Risk factors and their relationship to prognosis in myelodysplastic syndromes. Leuk Res 1998;22(Suppl 1):S3–6

85. van de Loosdrecht AA, Alhan C, Béné MC, Della Porta MG, Dräger AM, Feuillard J, Font P, Germing U, Haase D, Homburg CH, Ireland R, Jansen JH, Kern W, Malcovati L, Te Marvelde JG, Mufti GJ, Ogata K, Orfao A, Ossenkoppele GJ, Porwit A, Preijers FW, Richards SJ, Schuurhuis GJ, Subirá D, Valent P, van der Velden VH, Vyas P, Westra AH, de Witte TM, Wells DA, Loken MR, Westers TM. Standardization of flow cytometry in myelodysplastic syndromes: report from the first European LeukemiaNet working conference on flow cytometry in myelodysplastic syndromes. Haematologica. 2009;94(8):1124–34

86. Truong F, Smith BR, Stachurski D, Cerny J, Medeiros LJ, Woda BA, Wang SA. The utility of flow cytometric immunophenotyping in cytopenic patients with a non-diagnostic bone marrow: a prospective study. Leuk Res. 2009;33(8):1039–46

Chapter 7

Acute Myeloid Leukemia

Carlos E. Bueso-Ramos

Abstract/Scope of Chapter This chapter focuses on the diagnosis of acute myeloid leukemia (AML) according to the current standard of practice and discusses some of recent changes in the field of AML. Many phenotypic defects of AML can be mapped to specific molecular abnormalities. It is now recognized that not only genetic but also epigenetic alterations are similarly important in this process. The expectation is that the understanding of such alterations will allow implementation of genotype-specific therapies and patients will be entered into different treatment protocols based of their individual genetic profiles.

Keywords Acute myeloid leukemia (AML), diagnosis • Acute myeloid leukemia, cytogenetics • Acute myeloid leukemia, mutation analysis • NPM1 mutation • Acute myeloid leukemia, secondary • Topoisomerase inhibitors, risk of AML • Alkylating agents, risk of AML • AML, personalized risk assessment • Leukemia stem cells • Acute myeloid leukemia, epigenetic changes • MicroRNA (miR), AML subtyping

7.1. Classification Approaches to AML Reflect Its Plasticity and Stem/Progenitor Cell Origin

Acute myeloid leukemia (AML) comprises a heterogeneous group of clonal neoplasms arising from hematopoietic stem/progenitor cells [1]. As discussed in Chap. 31, stem/progenitor cells give rise to the full range of bone marrow (BM) hematopoietic elements through largely irreversible sequential maturation steps. A common finding in all AML subtypes is the acquisition, early in tumor development, of genetic alterations, which limit the full differentiation of hematopoietic precursors into erythrocytes, granulocytes, and platelets [2,3]. These changes result in an accumulation of less-mature "blast" forms whose different morphologic appearances were the basis of the first AML classification schemes. The basis of current AML subclassification (Table 7-1) is more complex combining clinical features with the stage of maturation arrest in the blasts and the dominant initiating genetic event(s). This move away from basing the diagnosis of AML on the morphological or immunophenotypic features of the blasts toward a genetic classification is a reflection of our understanding of its morphologic heterogeneity and plasticity.

In this regard, AML represents the prototypic example of neoplasia arising from cancer stem cells that have multilineage potential [1]. As with non-neoplastic hematopoietic stem/progenitor cells, leukemia stem cells (LSC) are not functionally homogeneous, but appear to comprise distinct hierarchically-arranged classes [4]. This heterogeneity is apparent in human AML samples and has been simulated in animal models. For example, investigators

From: *Neoplastic Hematopathology*: Contemporary Hematology,
Edited by: D. Jones, DOI 10.1007/978-1-60761-384-8_7,
© Humana Press, a part of Springer Science+Business Media, LLC 2010

Table 7-1. The 2008 WHO classification of acute myeloid leukemias.

Acute myeloid leukemia (AML) with recurrent genetic abnormalities
AML with t(8;21)(q22;q22), *RUNX1-RUNX1T1*
AML with inv(16)(p13.1q22) or t(16;16)(p13.1;q22), *CBFB-MYH11*
Acute promyelocytic leukemia (APL) with t(15;17)(q22;q12), *PML-RARA*
AML with t(9;11)(p22;q23); *MLLT3-MLL*
AML with t(6;9)(p23;q34); *DEK-NUP214*
AML with inv(3)(q21q26.2) or t(3;3)(q21;q26.2): *RPN1-EVI1*
AML (megakaryoblastic) with t(1;22)(p13;q13); *RBM15-MKL1*
Provisional entity: AML with mutated *NPM1*
Provisional entity: AML with mutated *CEBPA*
Acute myeloid leukemia with myelodysplasia-related changes
Therapy-related myeloid neoplasms
Acute myeloid leukemia, not otherwise specified
AML with minimal differentiation
AML without maturation
AML with maturation
Acute myelomonocytic leukemia
Acute monoblastic/monocytic leukemia
Acute erythroid leukemias
Pure erythroid leukemia
Erythroleukemia, erythroid/myeloid
Acute megakaryoblastic leukemia
Acute basophilic leukemia
Acute panmyelosis with myelofibrosis
Myeloid sarcoma
Myeloid proliferations related to Down syndrome
Transient abnormal myelopoiesis
Myeloid leukemia associated with Down syndrome
Blastic plasmacytoid dendritic cell neoplasms

Source: Derived from Vardiman et al. [11].

have provided direct evidence for plasticity and a variety of different cooperating events in leukemic transformation in a mouse transplant model [5]. This experiment stimulates AML development by blocking differentiation and promoting self-renewal through expression of the TLS-ERG oncogene and telomerase. The transduced cells can then undergo stepwise transformation to AML through spontaneous acquisition of a variety of different additional changes replicating the heterogeneity of human AML [5]. This chapter will discuss how such heterogeneity in molecular pathogenesis provides challenges for how best to identify and represent the most important genetic changes for classification, risk stratification, and therapy response prediction in AML.

7.2. Incidence and Demographics

The incidence of AML varies with gender, age, and race. Approximately 11,000 cases of AML are diagnosed annually in the United States, with a male predominance (1.5:1 male to female-ratio) and a median age of 68 years at presentation [6,7]. In the United States, during

2002 to 2003, the incidence of AML was lower for blacks than for whites [8]. The overall annual incidence of AML in adults below 65 years of age is 3.4 cases per 100,000, rising to 17.9 cases per 100,000 in adults who are 65 years or older [6]. The higher incidence of AML in elderly patients is almost entirely due to cases arising from age-related myelodys-plastic syndromes (MDS), which has led to rising rates of AML in the United States as the median age of the population has risen [9].

In children (younger than 15 years of age), AML is far less common than ALL, compris-ing 15–20% of acute leukemia with a peak incidence in the first year of life. AML incidence rates then decrease between the ages 1 and 4 years and remain stable at a low rate of 0.8 per 100,000 throughout childhood and early adulthood [8,10]. In the first few years of life, the incidence of AML is threefold higher in whites than in blacks; however, older black children have slightly higher rates of AML.

7.3. Diagnostic Criteria

The French–American–British Group (FAB) classification scheme has defined AML as the presence of at least 30% blasts with some degree of myeloid differentiation, as counted on a 200-cell BM aspirate differential. In the FAB scheme, cytochemical stains are used to separate AML from other blastoid tumors (left side of Fig. 7-1). In the 2008 World Health Organization (WHO) classification, the blast threshold for AML was lowered to 20% or more myeloblasts and/or monoblasts/promonocytes and/or megakaryoblasts in the periph-eral blood or BM (Table 7-1). In addition, neoplasms bearing t(8;21)(q22;q22), inv(16) (p13q22), t(15;17)(q22;q12), or their variants are now diagnosed as AML regardless of the blast percentage.

The WHO scheme requires the use of cytogenetic analysis, molecular testing, and immu-nophenotype profiling as well as morphologic examination (right side of Fig. 7-1). Following the completion of all these studies, AML is subclassified into cases with recurrent cytoge-netic abnormalities (that produce characteristic gene fusions), AML with MDS-related changes (AML-MDS), therapy-related cases (t-AML), or AML not otherwise specified (NOS) if the other three features are not present [11]. However, as discussed below, these categories are overlapping, and the individual molecular and cytogenetic features of any given tumor are likely more important than subtype for risk prediction.

Cases of AML with recurrent chromosomal translocation/gene fusions comprise the major-ity of pediatric leukemias but their incidence decreases with age and they comprise only a small percentage of AML in the elderly. Such translocations are seen in 10–15% of t-AML. The oncogenes activated by these translocations are transcription factors that alter hemat-opoietic cell differentiation. In this group of AML, karyotypic changes besides the defining translocation are uncommon at diagnosis in contrast to the complexity that characterizes many cases of AML arising from MDS. Presenting features and outcomes is largely deter-mined by the particular gene fusion, ranging from extremely favorable for t(15;17)/PML-RARA (promyelocytic leukemia), moderately favorable for t(8;21)/RUNX1-RUNX1T1 and inv(16)/t(16;16)/CBFB-MYH11, and extremely poor for AML with translocations involving the MLL gene at chr 11q23 (Table 7-2).

Treatment-related (t)-AMLs are those cases that arise following cytotoxic chemotherapy and/or radiation therapy and are grouped with t-MDS and treatment-related myelodysplastic/myeloproliferative neoplasms (t-MDS/MPN), since all have poor outcome [12,13]. Excluded from this category is blast phase of an underlying MPN, since it is often not possible to determine if leukemic transformation is a function of disease evolution or prior therapy. The majority of t-AML/MDS/MPN follows treatment of cancers with DNA-damaging chemo-therapeutic agents, particularly topoisomerase inhibitors and multiagent regimens containing antimetabolites or alkylating agents. The time between treatment and t-AML/MDS onset is variable (1–10 years), with the shortest intervals seen with use of topoisomerase inhibitors

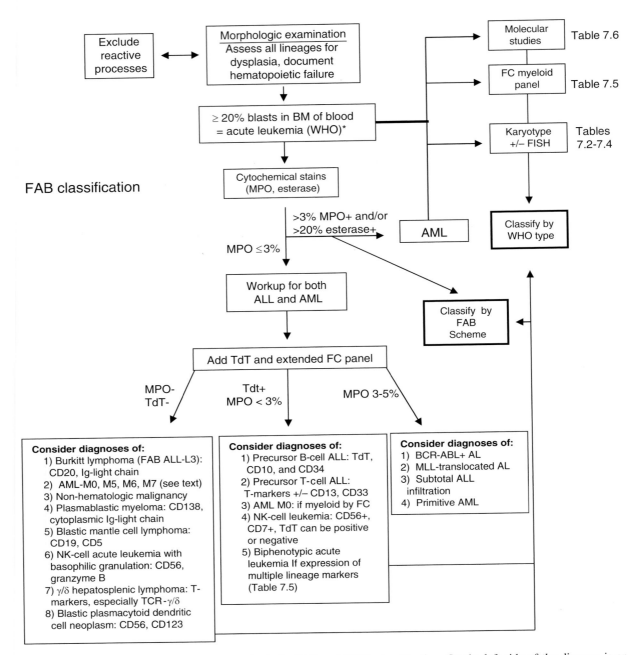

Fig. 7-1. Algorithmic approach to AML diagnosis using both the FAB and WHO classification. On the left side of the diagram is an approach using cytochemical stains in association with morphologic findings to narrow the differential in neoplasms presenting with blastoid cells. On the right of the figure, the WHO approach utilizing cytogenetic, molecular, and FC immunophenotyping to classify cases with more than 20% myeloblasts [43]

(often 6 months to 2 years). The frequent presence of multilineage dysplasia and high-risk karyotypic changes in t-AML/MDS is similar to AML-MDS (Table 7-3) [14,15].

AML-MDS is diagnosed if myelodysplasia is noted in the maturing hematopoiesis at the time of diagnosis, or if there is a prior history of MDS or MDS/MPN, or if one of the

Table 7-2. Genotypic-clinical correlations in AML with specific initiating chromosomal translocations.

Balanced structural rearrangements	Gene(s) involved	Median age (range), M:F	Phenotypic features	Risk group	Therapy	5-year OS
t(15;17) (q22;q12–21)	PML-RARA	47 (3–77), 0.9:1	Abnormal promyelocytes, hypergranular or microgranular, bilobed nuclei. 100% reactivity with MPO (FAB M3)	Favorable	ATRA + Arsenic trioxide	70–91%
t(8;21)(q22;q22)	RUNX1-RUNX1T1	43 (16–60), 1.1–1.4:1	Maturation in the granulocytic lineage; orange-pink granules (FAB M2)	Favorable	High sensitivity to anthracyclines. The incorporation of repetitive cycles of high-dose cytarabine as post-remission therapy has improved the outcome	50–60%
inv(16)(p13q22) or t(16;16)(p13;q22)	CBFB-MYH11	42 (17–60), 1.2:1	Monocytic and granulocytic differentiation. Abnormal eosinophils with basophilic granules (FAB M4Eo)	Favorable		50–60%
t(9;11)(p22;q23)	MLLT3-MLL	42, 2.2:1	Disseminated intravascular coagulation, extramedullary monocytic sarcomas (FAB M5)	Intermediate		70%
inv(3)(q21q26.2) or t(3;3)(q21;q26.2)	RPN1-EVI1	43.5, 2.3:1	Thrombocythemia, increased blasts, multilineage dysplasia, and dysplastic monolobated megakaryocytes (FAB M1, M4, or M7)	Unfavorable		<10%
t(6;9)(p23;q34)	DEK-NUP214	51 (20–76), 1:5	Basophilia, multilineage dysplasia and blasts with prominent azurophilic granules (FAB RAEB-T, M2-M4)	Unfavorable		<10%
t(6;11)(q27;q23)	MLL-MLLT4		Hyperleukocytosis, CNS disease, and skin involvement, FAB M4 or M5	Unfavorable		<10%
t(11;19)(q23;p13.1)	MLL-MLLT1		FAB M4 or M5	Unfavorable		<10%

Table 7-3. Frequency of cytogenetic abnormalities in de novo and therapy-related myelodysplasia (MDS) and acute myeloid leukemia (AML).

AML type	Balanced chromosomal translocations[a]	Chromosomal copy number changes[b] and other structural changes[c]	Diploid
de novo MDS	Rare	15–25	50–60
t-MDS	Rare	50–70	5–10
de novo AML	15–20	15–25	40–50
t-AML	15–20	40–50	10–15

[a] Including translocation involving 11q23 (MLL), 21q22 (RUNX1), 17q21 (RARA), or 16q22 (CBFB)
[b] High-risk changes include –5, –7, –17, –18, and –20 intermediate risk changes include –Y, +8, +11, +13, and +21
[c] High-risk changes include del(5q) (entire long arm), and del(7q), i(17q)/del(17p); intermediate risk changes include del(9q), del(11q) and del(20q)
Percentages are as reported in Pedersen-Bjergaard et al.[42].

MDS-associated cytogenetic changes is detected (Table 7-4) [16]. These cases comprise the vast majority of AML in the elderly and have chromosome abnormalities which are similar to those found in high-grade MDS including –7/del(7q), –5, and complex karyotypes [16]. AML with t(3;5)(q25;q32–33) or other translocations involving chr 5q32–33 are the exception

Table 7-4. Cytogenetic abnormalities sufficient to diagnose AML with myelodysplasia-related features when 20% PB and/or BM blasts are present.

Balanced translocations	Other clonal chromosomal abnormalities	Complex karyotypes
t(11;16)(q23;p13.3)[a]	−5/del(5q)	>3 unrelated abnormalities, none of which are included in the AML with recurrent translocation subgroup (Those listed in Table 7.2)
t(3;21)(q26.2;q22.1)[a]	−7/del(7q)	
t(1;3)(p36.3q21.1)	i(17q)/t(17p)	
t(2;11)(p21;q23)[a]	−13/del(13q)	
t(5;12)(q33;p12)	del(11q)	
t(5;7)(q33;q11.2)	del(12p)/t(12p)	
t(5;17)((q33;p13)	del(9q)	
t(5;10)(q33;q21)	idic(X)(q13)	
t(3;5)(q25;q34)		

[a]These abnormalities most commonly occur in therapy-related disease and therapy-related AML should be excluded before using these abnormalities as evidence for a diagnosis of AML with myelodysplasia-related features16

presenting at a younger age.17 Those AML cases remaining after exclusion of the t-AML, AML-MDS, and the recurrent translocation group are diagnosed as AML-NOS and subtyped according to differentiation states similarly to the FAB classification.

7.4. Morphological Features of AML

Given the importance of recognition of underlying myelodysplasia for subclassification of AML, careful morphological examination of all hematopoietic lineages in the BM aspirate is critical. For the diagnosis of AML-MDS, dysplasia must be present in at least 50% of cells from at least two lines, including: granulocytes with agranular or hypogranular cytoplasm or hyposegmented nuclei; erythroid forms with nuclear irregularities, cytoplasmic vacuolization (or globular PAS positivity), or nuclear-cytoplasmic dyssynchrony (megaloblastoid change); or megakaryocytic abnormalities including micromegakaryocytes, large monolobate forms, or those with multiple, widely separated nuclei [18].

Accurate blast enumeration is critical to diagnosis but is not always straightforward. In addition to agranular classical myeloblasts, reniform/bilobed progranulocytes, promonocytes, monoblasts, and megakaryoblasts are all counted as "blast equivalents" to meet the 20% threshold for AML (Fig. 7-2). The small lymphoid-appearing megakaryoblasts seen in infantile AML, AML-MDS [16], or in t-AML [19] are particularly difficult to recognize. AML with extensive fibrosis can be difficult to diagnose because aspirate smears often lack spicules, in which case immunostaining of the BM core biopsy or clot section for CD34 of CD117 can be used for blast enumeration (Fig. 7-3) [20]. In fibrotic AML, reticulin stain should also be done to grade the degree of marrow fibrosis since it has prognostic significance [21,22]; a commonly used scoring system for BM fibrosis is provided in Chap. 5 (Table 5-5). Given their paucicellular BM aspirates, cases of hypocellular AML may be misdiagnosed as aplastic anemia, and the diagnosis should be excluded by careful examination of the BM biopsy in any patient with a hypoplastic marrow and severe pancytopenia (Fig. 7-4).

Blast enumeration in erythroid-predominant BM is not straightforward. For example, in clear cases of MDS or AML, pronormoblasts should be included in the blast count, whereas in cases with a demonstrable reactive etiology they should not be. This is a particularly important consideration in those patients receiving hematopoietic growth factors, particularly erythropoietin, which may produce both left-shifted hematopoiesis and marked erythroid hyperplasia. In erythroid-predominant BM samples with fewer than 10% myeloblasts, minimal dysplasia, and/or a normal diploid karyotype, resampling of the BM after discontinuation of growth factor for several weeks is recommended before diagnosing MDS.

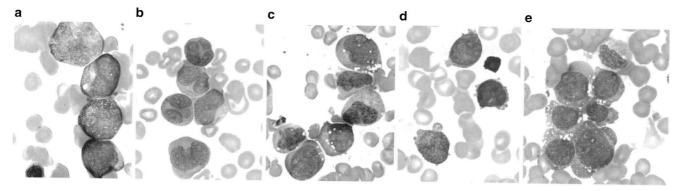

Fig. 7-2. Morphology of myeloblasts and blast equivalents. (**a**) Classical agranular and granular myeloblasts, some with Auer rods; (**b**) bilobed classical progranulocytes which are counted as a blasts in acute promyelocytic leukemia; (**c**) Monoblasts and promonocytes which are both included in the blast counts for myelomonocytic and monocytic leukemias; (**d**) Megakaryoblasts with cytoplasmic blebs; (**e**) pronormoblasts which are counted as blasts in erythroleukemia

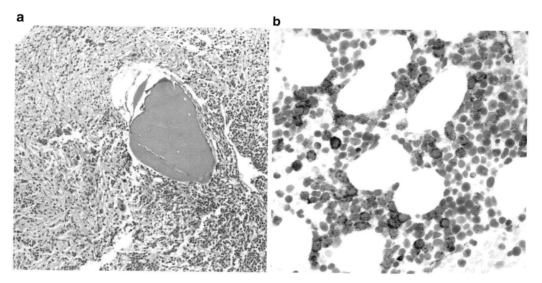

Fig. 7-3. Fibrotic AML. (**a**) Bone marrow biopsy showing extensive fibrosis, with interstitial blasts. (**b**) CD34 immunostain is helpful in accurate blast enumeration given the frequently cell-poor marrow aspirates

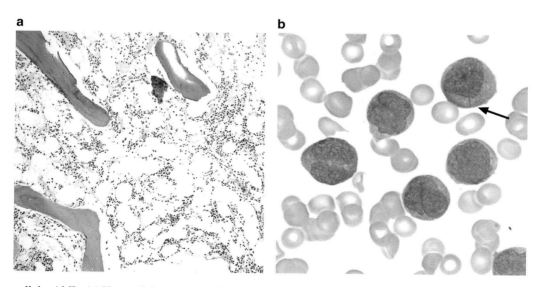

Fig. 7-4. Hypocellular AML. (**a**) Hypocellular marrow with scattered blasts simulating aplastic anemia. (**b**) The recognition of Auer rods in blasts on hypocellular marrow aspirate smear assists in diagnosis (*arrow*)

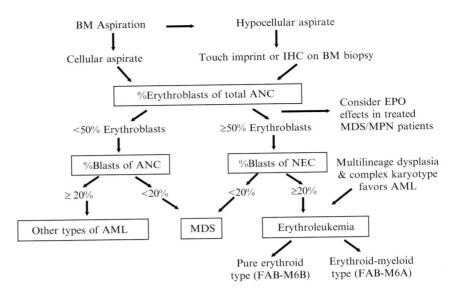

Fig. 7-5. Algorithmic approach to diagnosis of leukemias with erythroid predominance or erythroblasts. Abbreviations: *ANC* all nucleated cells, *NEC* non-erythroid cells

AMLs with an increased erythroid component or erythroid differentiation in the blasts may be difficult to distinguish from high-grade MDS, with the diagnostic criteria still evolving in this area [23. Although the algorithmic outline presented in Fig. 7-5 is helpful in separating erthyroid-predominant MDS from erythroleukemia, in some cases this distinction is arbitrary. In that regard, acute erythroleukemia is commonly associated with a previous diagnosis of MDS and a high-risk MDS-type cytogenetic changes supporting its close association with erythroid-predominant MDS [24]. Also, since high-grade MDS with erythroid predominance is often nearly as aggressive as erythroleukemia (and treated similarly), cytogenetic risk stratification may be more critical than blast count.

7.5. Blast Phenotyping by Cytochemical Methods and Flow Cytometry

Either cytochemical stains or flow cytometric (FC) immunophenotyping can be used to determine blast lineage in AML. Cytochemical stains, usually performed on unstained BM aspirate smears, include myeloperoxidase (MPO), nonspecific esterase (alpha-naphthyl butyrate), and periodic acid-schiff (PAS). Butyrate/nonspecific esterase positivity is characterized by a weak-to-strong brown cytoplasmic blush in monoblasts, promonocytes, and monocytes [18]. Cytochemical staining, which is required for FAB subclassification, can determine terminal myeloid and monocytic differentiation but is less sensitive for typing early-stage or poorly differentiated myeloblasts or the lymphoid lineage so has been gradually replaced by FC analysis.

Nonetheless, cytochemical stains still have great value as rapid and inexpensive tests for diagnosing AML. For example, if 3% or more of the blasts on a BM aspirate or blood smear are positive for MPO (or if Auer rods are highlighted by the stain), the diagnostic criteria for AML have been fulfilled and therapy can be initiated. The percentage of MPO-positive blasts is also a strong independent prognostic factor in most subtypes of AML. For example, AML with strong MPO cytochemical positivity (positive in >50% of blasts) showed better survival even in intermediate cytogenetic risk and normal diploid karyotype groups where molecular stratification is complex [25].

If the cytochemical stains are negative or not done, lineage determination in AML is based on the predominant pattern of antigen expression detected by FC. Blasts markers, including

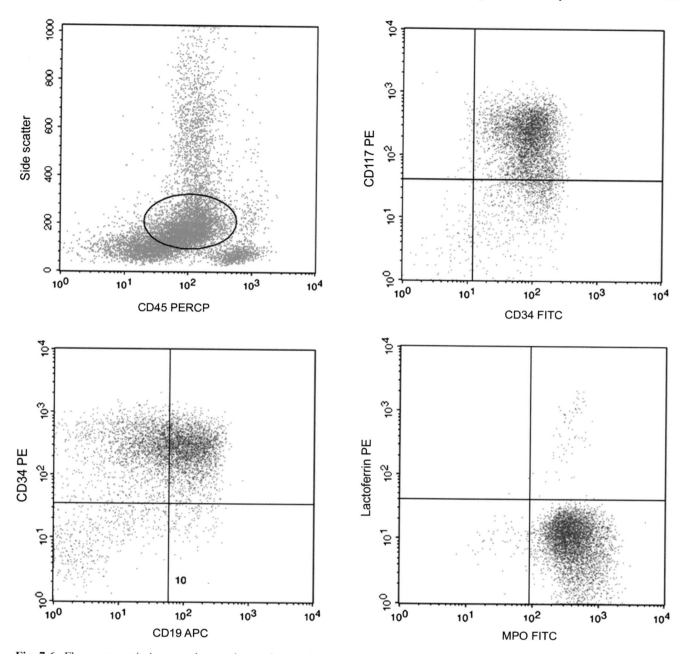

Fig. 7-6. Flow cytometric immunophenotyping to detect minimal residual AML. The characteristic immunophenotype of AML with t(8;21)(q22;q22) with aberrant expression of CD19 in the CD34+ blasts (*lower left panel*) allows sensitivity detection of residual AML

CD34, CD38, and CD117 (bright) (Fig. 7-6), and are typically used in conjunction with the forward and side light scatter properties of the cells to locate the blast population for further immunophenotype (see Chap. 3). Commonly employed FC markers to detect the myeloid (MPO, CD13, CD33, CD117), monocyte (CD14, CD64), erythroid (glycophorin A), and megakaryocytic (CD41, CD42b, and CD61) lineages are combined with markers to exclude lymphoid leukemia (Table 7-5). Expression of CD7, CD9, and CD56 are also frequently assessed on the blasts, and can have prognostic importance in certain settings.

Table 7-5. Common markers used in AML.

	Markers assessed (method/s)	Specificity
Blast markers	CD34, CD117-bright (FC/IHC) CD38, CD45RA (FC)	All types of AML except APL and monocytic variants, CD38 is most broadly expressed
Unequivocal myeloid	MPO (FC, IHC or cytochemistry) CD117 (FC, IHC)	Cytochemical MPO positivity is most specific for definitive myeloid differentiation
Myeloid-associated	CD13, CD15, CD33 (FC)	Also seen in t(9;22) in ALL and leukemias of ambiguous lineage and other tumor types
Monocyte-associated	NSE (cytochemistry) CD11c, CD14, CD64 (FC) Lysozyme (IHC)	Lysozyme and NSE positivity are the most specific for definitive monocytic differentiation
Megakaryocyte-associated	CD41, CD42 (FC) CD61 (IHC, FC)	CD61 IHC is the easiest to interpret in finding megakaryoblasts due to AML-associated fibrosis
Erythroid-associated	CD36-bright (FC), Glycophorin-A/CD235, hemoglobin (IHC, FC)	Can have high background
Usually lymphoid-associated	CD19, CD79a	B-cell markers seen in t(8;21) or other myeloid-type AMLs
	PAX5 (IHC)	B-cell markers seen in t(8;21) and t(15;17) AML
	Surface CD3 (flow), or Cytoplasmic CD3	T-cell markers seen in some AML and acute leukemia of ambiguous Lineage
	CD2	T-cell markers seen in inv(16) and t(15;17) AML

FC: Usually detected by flow cytometry; IHC: Usually detected by immunohistochemistry; see Table 3.1 for further information on each marker

Dysplastic features in the nonblast hematopoietic elements can also be assessed by FC, and used to detect cases of AML-MDS [26]. FC-detected dyspoiesis also confers an increased risk of relapse after allogeneic hematopoietic stem cell transplantation in AML [27, 28]. Proposed criteria for myeloid dysplasia by FC include asynchronous shift to the left in the granulocytes detected by the scattergram (or abnormal granularity by side scatter), abnormal decrease in CD45 expression, presence of bright HLA-DR, lack of CD11b, abnormal relationship between CD13 and CD16, expression of CD56 on a subpopulation, lack of CD33 expression, presence of lymphoid antigens, or increased CD34 expression [26]. For the monocytic lineage, commonly observed FC abnormalities include abnormal granularity, abnormal CD11b or HLA-DR expression, loss of CD13 or CD16, presence of CD56, lack of CD33 or CD14, presence of CD34, or lymphoid antigen expression [26].

7.6. Use of Conventional Cytogenetics and Fluorescence In Situ Hybridization (FISH)

An adequate G-banded karyotype is required for subclassification of AML in the WHO schema and should be performed on BM aspirate samples in all patients. The presence of any of the defining recurrent chromosomal translocations (Table 7-2) can also be detected by FISH using breakapart probes (e.g., for MLL translocation) or dual fusion probes (see Chap. 4). Given the large number of chromosomal copy number alterations and structural rearrangements that have prognostic significance in AML-MDS/t-AML (Tables 7-2 and 7-3), genomic analysis by FISH is not a realistic possibility for all cases of AML. However, in those cases, in which routine karyotyping has not done (or was suboptimal due to a hypocellular sample or a technical problem), a panel of FISH probes directed against the most commonly altered chromosome locations can be used (e.g., 5q, 7q, chr 8, chr 17 and chr 21). It is important to recognize that the finding of normal diploid karyotype may reflect a suboptimal karyotype study (e.g., failure of tumor cells to divide, or poor resolution of the G-banding). Some of the common reciprocal chromosomal translocations in AML can also be difficult to detect on G-banded karyotypes [particularly inv(16) and some MLL translocations], so selective use of additional FISH probes and molecular testing should be considered.

Whole genome profiling methods, such as array comparative genomic hybridization (CGH) and single nucleotide polymorphism (SNP) arrays, show promise in providing a more unbiased and high-resolution view of the chromosomal changes in AML than the G-banded karyotype. While these techniques have much higher resolution for detecting small chromosomal changes, they are typically less sensitive than FISH analyses and mostly do not detect reciprocal chromosomal translocations. For these reasons, they are still largely investigational in AML but can be used when karyotypic studies are suboptimal. CGH and SNP have also yielded important new insights into the genomics of AML, including the frequent presence of uniparental disomy at certain loci, which may be indicative of common underlying defects in genome instability and DNA repair.

7.7. Molecular Testing

7.7.1. Current Use of Molecular Testing in AML Workup

Molecular testing is playing an increasing role in the routine workup of AML. Detection of mutation/alteration in the FLT3 and duplications in NPM1 are now performed in almost all cases of normal karyotype and intermediate cytogenetic-risk AML where they provide important prognostic information. Multiplex detection of the fusion transcripts produced by reciprocal chromosomal translocation using quantitative reverse-transcription polymerase chain reaction (RQ-PCR) is also emerging as a more cost-effective and sensitive method for AML classification than FISH.

7.7.2. Molecular Markers for Prognosis

A summary of the most common genetic alterations affecting the clinical outcome of diploid AML patients is shown in Table 7-7. Gene mutations or deregulated expression of genes or sets of genes now allow us to dissect the diversity present in cytogenetically-defined subsets of AML. Such genetic alterations appear to fall into different classes of mutations [29]. One group (termed "class I mutations") comprises genetic changes that activate signal transduction pathways resulting in enhanced cell proliferation and/or survival (Fig. 7-7). Examples include mutations in the receptor tyrosine kinase genes and their effectors, such as FLT3, RAS, KIT, and PIK3C2B, and are frequently detected in AML with a normal diploid karyotype and core binding factor leukemias. So-called "class II mutations" affect transcription factors (RUNX1, RARA, EVI1, NPM1, TAL1, GATA1, EKLF, WT1, etc.) or components of the transcriptional co-activation complex, resulting in impaired differentiation. Recurring gene fusions resulting from balanced translocations, or mutations in CEBPA or other genes are examples of this category.

7.7.3. Expression Profiling of AML

Oligonucleotide or cDNA microarray technology to detect transcriptional changes reflecting genetically-determined growth pathway activation may provide an alternative and extension to conventional karyotyping and fluorescence in situ hybridization (FISH) in routine

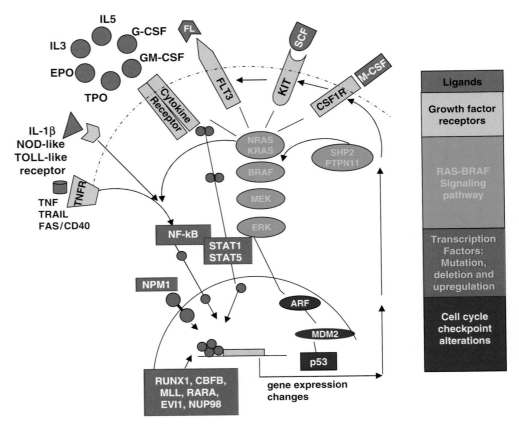

Fig. 7-7. Genetic pathways involved in AML. Genetic alterations in AML fall into several common categories including activating mutations in growth factor receptors (*highlighted in yellow*), common signaling molecular (*green*), altered differentiation-associated transcription factors (*red*), and loss or dysregulation of factors involved in the G1-S cell cycle checkpoint (*blue*). A shift from paracrine to autocrine growth factor signaling is likely a critical early stage transition in AML changing its interactions with the BM microenvironment (*highlighted in purple*)

diagnosis of AML. Several groups have demonstrated that gene signatures can be more than 90% sensitivity and specific for differentiating certain genetic subgroups of de novo AML and t-AML [30–32]. Common to each of the subgroups are gene expression patterns typical of arrested differentiation in early progenitors cells, but the range of genes expressed in each genetic category is different.

Gene expression studies may be particularly useful in highlighting commonalities and differences in AML with complex karyotype changes, particularly therapy-related cases. For example, t-AML with –5/del(5q) and complex karyotypes have a higher expression of genes involved in cell cycle control (CCNA2, CCNE2, CDC2), mitotic checkpoints (BUB1), or growth control (MYC). A second subgroup of t-AML (including –7, normal diploid karyotype, or those with rarer cytogenetic abnormalities) is characterized by downregulation of transcription factors involved in early hematopoiesis (TAL1, GATA1, and EKLF) and overexpression of proteins involved in signaling pathways in myeloid cells (FLT3) and cell survival (BCL2) [31]. Based on these types of studies, Pedersen-Bjergaard et al. have proposed that t-AML can be subdivided into at least eight genetic pathways that correlate (to some degree) with etiology and biologic characteristics (Table 7-7) [33].

7.7.4. Epigenetic Profiling of AML

A recently-recognized dimension of complexity in AML has been highlighted by the analysis of alterations in the epigenome. It has become clear that changes in epigenetic signatures comprising aberrant methylation and histone deacetylation are common modifications in various types of leukemia. Since both DNA methylation and histone deacetylation are reversible processes, they have become attractive targets for epigenetic therapy.

Recently, the discovery of a novel class of gene regulators, named microRNAs (miRs), has changed the landscape of human genetics. miRs are 22-nucleotide noncoding RNAs that regulate gene expression by binding to the 3'untranslated (3'UTR) regions of a range of mRNAs. If perfect complementarity between the miR and mRNA is present, the RNA complex is cleaved and degraded, whereas translational silencing is the main miR regulatory mechanism in the case of imperfect base pairing [34]. The 3'UTR of a single miRNA can bind multiple miRs [35]. As a result, the regulation of gene expression by miRNA is complex, with many of 500 or so known miRs influencing the transcript levels of tens to hundreds of genes. Extensive miRNAs deregulation has been observed in leukemias and mechanistic studies support a role for miRs in the pathogenesis of AML (Table 7-4) [34, 36–38]. For example, Nervi C et al. recently reported a link between the differentiation block of leukemia and the epigenetic silencing of the microRNA-223 gene by the AML1/ ETO oncoprotein [39].

In some cases, the clinical features and phenotypes in AML are highly correlated with the presence of a particular genetic or epigenetic alteration. This is best exemplified by AML with NPM1 duplication which usually has a normal diploid karyotype, absence of CD34 expression in the blasts, and no prior history of MDS. However, the distribution of different genetic and epigenetic changes does not always correlate with existing AML subtypes. For example, multilineage dysplasia is prevalent in FLT3-ITD-negative AML and equally distributed between AML with and without NPM1 mutation [14]. Cases with multilineage dysplasia may carry NPM1 and/or FLT3 mutations [40].

7.8. Overlaps Between Secondary AML and AML-MDS

Myelodysplasia (MDS) and acute myeloid leukemia (AML) are heterogeneous and, closely associated diseases that may arise de novo or following chemotherapy with alkylating agents, topoisomerase II inhibitors, or after radiotherapy. While de novo MDS and AML are almost always subclassified according to their cytogenetic characteristics, therapy-related MDS (t-MDS) and therapy-related AML (t-AML) are often considered to be closely-related entities and are not subdivided. Alternative genetic pathways have been previously proposed for t-MDS and t-AML based on their cytogenetic characteristics [33, 41–43]. An increasing number of gene mutations are now observed to cluster differently in these pathways with an identical pattern noted in de novo cases and in t-MDS and t-AML (Tables 7-6 and 7-7) [43, 44]. An association is observed between activating mutations of genes in the tyrosine kinase *RAS-BRAF* signal transduction pathway (Class I mutations) and inactivating mutations of genes encoding hematopoietic transcription factors (Class II mutations). Point mutations of *RUNX1/AML1* and RAS seem to cooperate and predispose to progression from t-MDS to t-AML. Recently, critical genetic effects underlying del(5q)/-5 and del(7q)/-7 have been proposed [43]. Their association and cooperation with point mutations of *TP53* and *RUNX1*, respectively, extend the range of cooperating genetic abnormalities in MDS and AML [43]. The p53 tumor suppressor directs the cellular response to DNA-damaging agents and is selected against during the pathogenesis of t-AML. The data indicate that MDM2 and TP53 variants interact to modulate responses to genotoxic therapy and are determinants of risk for t-AML [45, 46].

Table 7-6. Comparison of genetic alterations in de novo and therapy-related MDS and AML.

Genetic alteration	% MDS, de novo	% t-MDS	%AML, de novo	%t-AML
TP53 point mutation	5–10	25–30	10–15	20–25
FLT3 internal tandem duplication	Rare	Rare	35–50	10
JAK2 point mutation	2–5	2–5	Rare	Rare
KRAS/NRAS point mutation	10	10	10	10
PTPN11 point mutation	3–5	3–5	3–5	3–5
RUNX1chimeric rearrrangement	Rare	2	7–10	5–7
CBFB chimeric rearrangement	Rare	Rare	5–8	2–3
MLL chimeric rearrangement	Rare	Rare	5–7	5–7
RARA chimeric rearrangement	Rare	Rare	5–10	2–3
EVI1 chimeric rearrangement	Rare	Rare	2–3	2–3
RUNX1 point mutation	10–15	15–30	5–10	2–3
NPM1 point mutation	Rare	4–5	40–50	15
CEBPA point mutation	Rare	Rare	15–20	Rare

Percentages as in Pedersen-Bjergaard et al. [42].

Table 7-7. A delineation of the most commonly altered genetic pathways in secondary AML and MDS.

Initiating chromosomal change	Other chromosomal changes	Most common molecular change	Other molecular changes	Epigenetic changes
Alkylating agents (chromosomal breakage)				
-7/7q-	None	RUNX1 mutation	RAS mutations, TP53	Frequent CDKN2B
-5/5q-	-7/7q- 17p- complex karyotype	TP53 mutation	MLL and RUNX1 amplification/duplication	Promoter methylation
Topoisomerase II inhibitors (gene fusions)				
11q23 rearrangement		MLL rearrangement	Ras mutation, BRAF mutation	↓miR-29b
21q22/or 16q22 loci	-7/7q-	RUNX1 or CBFB gene fusions	KIT mutation RUNX3 downregulation	Frequent CDKN2B promoter methylation
t(15;17)(q22;q12–21)	None	RARA gene fusion	FLT3 ITD	
11p15 defects	None	NUP98 gene fusion	?	
"De novo" (unclear initiation event)				
Normal diploid karyotype	None	FLT3, RAS mutation MLL partial tandem duplication	RUNX1 mutation NF-kB activation	↓miR-181a Infrequent CDKN2B Promoter methylation
+8, other defects	None	NPM1 mutation		↑miR-191, ↑miR199a ↓miR-204

Schema as in Pedersen-Bjergaard et al. [41].

7.9. Differential Diagnosis of AML

The most problematic distinction encountered after routine diagnostic studies have been performed is between minimally-differentiated AML, acute lymphoblastic leukemia (ALL), and primitive leukemias with biphenotypic or bilineal components. Our approach to these cases is summarized in Fig. 7.1 and relies on extensive immunophenotypic and cytochemical studies.

These are extremely important clinical distinctions because the therapy for ALL and AML is currently different. Other blastoid neoplasms presenting in the BM, including mantle cell lymphoma, hepatosplenic T-cell lymphoma, blastoid plasmacytoid dendritic cell neoplasm, and natural killer (NK)-cell malignancies can be morphologic mimics but are immunophenotypically distinct.

A major issue in AML with atypical features is distinguishing de novo cases from the blast phase of an underlying MPN [19]. This distinction should be considered in any case that has a background myeloid hyperplasia (possibly reflecting CML, PV, or PMF), marked megakaryocytic hyperplasia/dysplasia (seen in CML, ET, or PMF), a pre-existing history of marked splenomegaly, fibrosis, osteosclerosis, and/or eosinophilia (possibly CMML, CML, or ETV6-PDGFRB MPN), or basophilia (suggesting CML). With the advent of routine molecular testing, an increase of such de novo presentations of MPN blast crisis are being recognized based on the findings of CML-type BCR-ABL transcripts, or JAK2 or MPL mutations (see Chap. 9), or chromosomal fusions involving tyrosine kinases such as PDGFB. If such cases are not recognized at diagnosis, they may be revealed by a follow-up BM biopsy that shows reversion to the chronic phase of the MPN.

7.10. Pathogenesis of AML and Patterns of Progression/ Transformation

The mechanisms responsible for the evolution of early MDS to advanced MDS and AML often result in decreased apoptosis and increased cell proliferation, a shift which highlights different options for therapy. The transcription factor RELA/NFKB1 and the FLT3/PI3KC2A/AKT1 pathways seem to play a key inter-related role in such processes [40, 47–50]. As a result, FLT3 receptor inhibition can reduce constitutive RELA/NFKB1 activation in high-risk MDS and AML [51]. The proteasome inhibitor bortezomib can influence DNA hypomethylation that silence transcription of growth regulators by regulating levels of Sp1/NFKB1-dependent DNA methyltransferase activity in AML [52]. This may be an effective therapeutic strategy since a number of AML cases show alteration in the promotor methylation status of multiple genes, suggesting a general disturbance of epigenetic memory similar to the CpG island methylator phenotype (CIMP) seen in colon cancer [53] in AML [54–57]. Such hypermethylation of multiple genes is associated with poor prognosis in older patients with high-risk MDS and AML following MDS [58]. Furthermore, CpG methylation levels may be increased in most patients with relapsed AML, [59] even in those with a stable karyotype, suggesting that epigenetic instability may drive disease progression independent of karyotypic changes.

Chromosome instability is another driving force for AML progression and likely interacts with epigenetic changes, as we and other have noted that promoter methylation patterns are different in AML with unstable karyotypes. Understanding the nature and extent of DNA methylation and other epigenetic alterations in AML will help us develop strategies for the use of DNA-demethylating and histone-modifying agents in the treatment of AML. A direct implication of our findings is that hypomethylating agents may be useful in AML at remission to prevent the emergence of hypermethylated (and possibly drug-resistant) clones.

7.11. Monitoring After Treatment

The recommended workups and monitoring of minimal residual disease (MRD) for various stages of AML is shown in Table 7-8. The term "minimal residual disease" usually refers to the persistence of leukemic cells not detectable by microscopic examination of the BM. The goal of MRD analysis is to anticipate an impending hematological relapse, which would allow for a timely therapeutic intervention. In most AML subtypes lacking an initiating chromosomal translocation, flow cytometry remains the dominant modality for MRD

Table 7-8. Recommended workups for various stages of AML.

	Morphology/ immunophenotying	Cytogenetics/FISH	Molecular testing
New diagnosis	Morphology, cytochemical stains	Conventional karyotype	FLT3
			NPM1 (if intermediate-risk)
	Flow immunophenotyping (FC) to evaluate blasts and background hematopoiesis for dysplasia	FISH for translocations, as needed	KIT (if CBF leukemias)
			CEBPA
			Chromosome translocation screen[a]
MRD assessment	Morphology	FISH for AML-specific change (if molecular test is not available)[c]	RQ-PCR for AML-specific translocation[d]
	MRD by FC with acquisition of at least 10,000 cells[b]		
Overt relapse	Morphology, cytochemical stains, extended FC panel	Convertional karyotype (or CGH or SNP array)	FLT3

[a] RT-PCR based multiplex screens including all of the common reciprocal translocations is an increasingly practical and cost-effective method of avoid multiple FISH testing and assist in selection of additional testing required for classification in the WHO schema. Anti-PML immunofluorescence stain can also be used as a rapid diagnostic aid in cases of suspected acute promyelocytic leukemia
[b] MRD by FC focusing on identifying residual blasts with the previously identified AML-associated aberrant immunophenotype
[c] Either FISH or [d] RQ-PCR for translocation-associated AML can be used depending on availability, although RQ-PCR is preferred given its greater dynamic range and faster turnaround time

assessment (Fig. 7-6). RQ-PCR to assess the transcript levels of genes highly expressed in leukemic blasts, such as WT1, shows promise as an MRD tool in AML but is not yet widely used.

7.12. Future Directions in Diagnosis and Classification

The WHO classification of AML represents a work in progress, with the older morphologic and immunophenotypic classification approaches merging with genetic and molecular data. Because of our understanding of the critical role of gross genomic aberrations, epigenetic changes (miR and promoter DNA methylation status), and activating and inactivating mutations, the complexity involved in the diagnostic workup of AML is currently greater than any other neoplasm. However, more remains to be done, and the complexity of AML diagnostics will likely only increase in the coming years. In particular, since epigenetic alterations do not change the DNA sequences and are pharmacologically reversible, they are promising therapeutic targets, necessitating the incorporation of DNA methylation status and miR profiles into routine AML profiling

Thus, rather than defining a specific disease entity, every case of AML is rightly regarded as its own unique constellation of genomic and molecular aberrations and functional dependencies. The individualized risk score that results from this approach points toward a set of targeted therapies that would be most efficient for any given patient. For instance, a cytogenetically intermediate-risk AML with FLT3 mutation, but no NPM1 mutation, currently has a different treatment plan than a morphologically identical leukemia with an NPM1 mutation. The move toward individualized risk assessment and therapy selection in AML provides a window into the complexity of stratification that will likely occur in other neoplasms. As a result of the codification of the diagnostic algorithm for AML, it is clear that subclassification schema are only a theoretical scheme for understanding and that each patient's neoplasm is unique.

Suggested Readings

Pedersen-Bjergaard J et al., Leukemia, 2008; 22:240–8
- Reviews the genetic pathways that are altered in the pathogenesis of acute myeloid leukemia

Mrozek K et al., Hematology, 2006;111:169–77
- Comprehensive review of chromosomal aberrations, gene mutations, and expression changes and prognosis in adult acute myeloid leukemia

Scholl C et al., Semin Oncol, 2008;35:336–45
- Survey of deregulation of signaling pathways in acute myeloid leukemia

References

1. Hope KJ, Jin L, Dick JE. Acute myeloid leukemia originates from a hierarchy of leukemic stem cell classes that differ in self-renewal capacity. Nat Immunol 2004;5:738–43.
2. Brunning RD ME, Harris NL, Flandrin G, Vardiman J, Bennett J, Head D. Acute Myeloid Leukemia. In: Jaffe ES, Harris NL, Stein H, Vardiman JW, eds. The World Health Organization classification of tumours: pathology and genetics of tumors of haematopoietic and lymphoid tissues. Lyon, France: IARC Press, 2001:75–107.
3. Vardiman JW, Harris NL, Brunning RD. The World Health Organization (WHO) classification of the myeloid neoplasms. Blood 2002;100:2292–302.
4. Wang JC, Dick JE. Cancer stem cells: lessons from leukemia. Trends Cell Biol 2005;15:494–501.
5. Warner JK, Wang JC, Takenaka K, et al. Direct evidence for cooperating genetic events in the leukemic transformation of normal human hematopoietic cells. Leukemia 2005;19:1794–805.
6. Ries LAG, Eisner MKC. SEER cancer statistics review, 1973–1999. Bethesda, MD: National Cancer Institute, 2002.
7. Hernandez JA, Land KJ, McKenna RW. Leukemias, myeloma, and other lymphoreticular neoplasms. Cancer 1995;75:381–94.
8. Deschler B, Lubbert M. Acute myeloid leukemia: epidemiology and etiology. Cancer 2006;107:2099–107.
9. Kinlen LJ. Leukaemia. Cancer Surv 1994;19–20:475–91.
10. Yamamoto JF, Goodman MT. Patterns of leukemia incidence in the United States by subtype and demographic characteristics, 1997–2002. Cancer Causes Control 2008;19:379–90.
11. Vardiman JW, Brunning RD, Arber DA, et al. Introduction and overview of the classification of the myeloid neoplasms. In: Swerdlow SH, Campo E, Harris NL, et al. eds. The World Health Organization (WHO) classification of tumours of haematopoietic and lymphoid tissues. Lyon, France: IARC Press, 2008:110–44.
12. Smith SM, Le Beau MM, Huo D, et al. Clinical-cytogenetic associations in 306 patients with therapy-related myelodysplasia and myeloid leukemia: the University of Chicago series. Blood 2003;102:43–52.
13. Guillem V, Tormo M. Influence of DNA damage and repair upon the risk of treatment related leukemia. Leuk Lymphoma 2008;49:204–17.
14. Wandt H, Schakel U, Kroschinsky F, et al. MLD according to the WHO classification in AML has no correlation with age and no independent prognostic relevance as analyzed in 1766 patients. Blood 2008;111:1855–61.
15. Haferlach T, Schoch C, Loffler H, et al. Morphologic dysplasia in de novo acute myeloid leukemia (AML) is related to unfavorable cytogenetics but has no independent prognostic relevance under the conditions of intensive induction therapy: results of a multiparameter analysis from the German AML Cooperative Group studies. J Clin Oncol 2003;21:256–65.
16. Arber DA, Brunning RD, Orazi A, et al. Acute myeloid leukemia with myelodysplasia-related changes. In: Swerdlow SH, Campo E, Harris NL, et al. eds. The World Health Organization (WHO) classification of tumours of haematopoietic and lymphoid tissues. Lyon, France: IARC Press, 2008:124–6.
17. Arber DA, Chang KL, Lyda MH, et al. Detection of NPM/MLF1 fusion in t(3;5)-positive acute myeloid leukemia and myelodysplasia. Hum Pathol 2003;34:809–13.
18. Konoplev S, Bueso-Ramos CE. Advances in the pathologic diagnosis and biology of acute myeloid leukemia. Ann Diagn Pathol 2006;10:39–65.
19. Oki Y, Kantarjian HM, Zhou X, et al. Adult acute megakaryocytic leukemia: an analysis of 37 patients treated at M.D. Anderson Cancer Center. Blood 2006;107:880–4.

20. Orazi A. Histopathology in the diagnosis and classification of acute myeloid leukemia, myelo-dysplastic syndromes, and myelodysplastic/myeloproliferative diseases. Pathobiology 2007;74: 97–114.

21. Vardiman JW, Brunning RD, Arber DA, et al. Introduction and overview of the classification of the myeloid neoplasms. In: Swerdlow SH, Campo E, Harris NL, et al. eds. The World Health Organization (WHO) classification of tumours of haematopoietic and lymphoid tissues. Lyon, France: IARC Press, 2008:18–30.

22. Della Porta MG, Malcovati L, Boveri E, et al. Clinical relevance of bone marrow fibrosis and CD34-positive cell clusters in primary myelodysplastic syndromes. J Clin Oncol 2009;27: 754–62.

23. Selby DM, Valdez R, Schnitzer B, et al. Diagnostic criteria for acute erythroleukemia. Blood 2003;101:2895–6.

24. Lessard M, Struski S, Leymarie V, et al. Cytogenetic study of 75 erythroleukemias. Cancer Genet Cytogenet 2005;163:113–22.

25. Matsuo T, Kuriyama K, Miyazaki Y, et al. The percentage of myeloperoxidase-positive blast cells is a strong independent prognostic factor in acute myeloid leukemia, even in the patients with normal karyotype. Leukemia 2003;17:1538–43.

26. Wells DA, Benesch M, Loken MR, et al. Myeloid and monocytic dyspoiesis as determined by flow cytometric scoring in myelodysplastic syndrome correlates with the IPSS and with outcome after hematopoietic stem cell transplantation. Blood 2003;102:394–403.

27. Scott BL, Wells DA, Loken MR, et al. Validation of a flow cytometric scoring system as a prog-nostic indicator for posttransplantation outcome in patients with myelodysplastic syndrome. Blood 2008;112:2681–6.

28. van de Loosdrecht AA, Westers TM, Westra AH, et al. Identification of distinct prognostic sub-groups in low- and intermediate-1-risk myelodysplastic syndromes by flow cytometry. Blood 2008;111:1067–77.

29. Kelly LM, Gilliland DG. Genetics of myeloid leukemias. Annu Rev Genomics Hum Genet 2002;3:179–98.

30. Haferlach T, Kohlmann A, Schnittger S, et al. Global approach to the diagnosis of leukemia using gene expression profiling. Blood 2005;106:1189–98.

31. Qian Z, Fernald AA, Godley LA, et al. Expression profiling of CD34+ hematopoietic stem/ pro-genitor cells reveals distinct subtypes of therapy-related acute myeloid leukemia. Proc Natl Acad Sci U S A 2002;99:14925–30.

32. Tsutsumi C, Ueda M, Miyazaki Y, et al. DNA microarray analysis of dysplastic morphology asso-ciated with acute myeloid leukemia. Exp Hematol 2004;32:828–35.

33. Pedersen-Bjergaard J, Andersen MK, Christiansen DH, et al. Genetic pathways in therapy-related myelodysplasia and acute myeloid leukemia. Blood 2002;99:1909–12.

34. Garzon R, Croce CM. MicroRNAs in normal and malignant hematopoiesis. Curr Opin Hematol 2008;15:352–8.

35. Zhang W, Dahlberg JE, Tam W. MicroRNAs in tumorigenesis: a primer. Am J Pathol 2007;171:728–38.

36. Fabbri M, Garzon R, Andreeff M, et al. MicroRNAs and noncoding RNAs in hematological malig-nancies: molecular, clinical and therapeutic implications. Leukemia 2008;22:1095–105.

37. Debernardi S, Skoulakis S, Molloy G, et al. MicroRNA miR-181a correlates with morphological sub-class of acute myeloid leukaemia and the expression of its target genes in global genome-wide analysis. Leukemia 2007;21:912–6.

38. Marcucci G, Radmacher MD, Maharry K, et al. MicroRNA expression in cytogenetically normal acute myeloid leukemia. N Engl J Med 2008;358:1919–28.

39. Nervi C, Fazi F, Grignani F. Oncoproteins, heterochromatin silencing and microRNAs: a new link for leukemogenesis. Epigenetics 2008;3:1–4.

40. Bacher U, Haferlach T, Kern W, et al. A comparative study of molecular mutations in 381 patients with myelodysplastic syndrome and in 4130 patients with acute myeloid leukemia. Haematologica 2007;92:744–52.

41. Pedersen-Bjergaard J, Christiansen DH, Desta F, et al. Alternative genetic pathways and cooperat-ing genetic abnormalities in the pathogenesis of therapy-related myelodysplasia and acute myeloid leukemia. Leukemia 2006;20:1943–9.

42. Pedersen-Bjergaard J, Andersen MT, Andersen MK. Genetic pathways in the pathogenesis of therapy-related myelodysplasia and acute myeloid leukemia. Hematology Am Soc Hematol Educ Program 2007;2007:392–7.

43. Pedersen-Bjergaard J, Andersen MK, Andersen MT, et al. Genetics of therapy-related myelodysplasia and acute myeloid leukemia. Leukemia 2008;22:240–8.

44. Bernasconi P. Molecular pathways in myelodysplastic syndromes and acute myeloid leukemia: relationships and distinctions – a review. Br J Haematol 2008;142:695–708.

45. Ellis NA, Huo D, Yildiz O, et al. MDM2 SNP309 and TP53 Arg72Pro interact to alter therapy-related acute myeloid leukemia susceptibility. Blood 2008;112:741–9.

46. Bueso-Ramos CE, Yang Y, deLeon E, et al. The human MDM-2 oncogene is overexpressed in leukemias. Blood 1993;82:2617–23.

47. Bueso-Ramos CE, Rocha FC, Shishodia S, et al. Expression of constitutively active nuclear-kappa B RelA transcription factor in blasts of acute myeloid leukemia. Hum Pathol 2004;35:246–53.

48. Braun BS, Archard JA, Van Ziffle JA, et al. Somatic activation of a conditional KrasG12D allele causes ineffective erythropoiesis in vivo. Blood 2006;108:2041–4.

49. Kerbauy DM, Lesnikov V, Abbasi N, et al. NF-kappaB and FLIP in arsenic trioxide (ATO)-induced apoptosis in myelodysplastic syndromes (MDSs). Blood 2005;106:3917–25.

50. Guzman ML, Neering SJ, Upchurch D, et al. Nuclear factor-kappaB is constitutively activated in primitive human acute myelogenous leukemia cells. Blood 2001;98:2301–7.

51. Grosjean-Raillard J, Ades L, Boehrer S, et al. Flt3 receptor inhibition reduces constitutive NFkappaB activation in high-risk myelodysplastic syndrome and acute myeloid leukemia. Apoptosis 2008;13:1148–61.

52. Liu S, Liu Z, Xie Z, et al. Bortezomib induces DNA hypomethylation and silenced gene transcription by interfering with Sp1/NF-kappaB-dependent DNA methyltransferase activity in acute myeloid leukemia. Blood 2008;111:2364–73.

53. Issa JP. CpG island methylator phenotype in cancer. Nat Rev Cancer 2004;4:988–93.

54. Toyota M, Kopecky KJ, Toyota MO, et al. Methylation profiling in acute myeloid leukemia. Blood 2001;97:2823–9.

55. Roman-Gomez J, Jimenez-Velasco A, Agirre X, et al. Lack of CpG island methylator phenotype defines a clinical subtype of T-cell acute lymphoblastic leukemia associated with good prognosis. J Clin Oncol 2005;23:7043–9.

56. Roman-Gomez J, Jimenez-Velasco A, Agirre X, et al. CpG island methylator phenotype redefines the prognostic effect of t(12;21) in childhood acute lymphoblastic leukemia. Clin Cancer Res 2006;12:4845–50.

57. Bueso-Ramos C, Xu Y, McDonnell TJ, et al. Protein expression of a triad of frequently methylated genes, p73, p57Kip2, and p15, has prognostic value in adult acute lymphocytic leukemia independently of its methylation status. J Clin Oncol 2005;23:3932–9.

58. Grovdal M, Khan R, Aggerholm A, et al. Negative effect of DNA hypermethylation on the outcome of intensive chemotherapy in older patients with high-risk myelodysplastic syndromes and acute myeloid leukemia following myelodysplastic syndrome. Clin Cancer Res 2007;13:7107–12.

59. Kroeger H, Jelinek J, Estecio MR, et al. Aberrant CpG island methylation in acute myeloid leukemia is accentuated at relapse. Blood 2008;112:1366–73.

Chapter 8

Treatment of Acute Myeloid Leukemia and Myelodysplastic Syndromes

Farhad Ravandi

Abstract/Scope of Chapter Recent advances in understanding the mechanisms and pathways leading to the pathogenesis of myeloid neoplasms, acute myeloid leukemia (AML) and myelodysplastic syndromes (MDS), have led to the identification of numerous molecular abnormalities that may be responsible for leukemogenesis and are resulting in progress in the clinical management of these disorders. In AML, large prospective trials conducted over the last 20–30 years have established standard regimens combining cytotoxic agents, in particular cytarabine and anthracyclines. Current research in AML is attempting to better stratify patients by identifying the risk factors responsible for chemotherapy resistance, and ways to incorporate newer agents with specific and targeted activity into the standard regimens. Treatment of MDS has been problematic and until recently no effective drugs were available for managing patients with these disorders. However, the identification of epigenetic modifiers and immunomodulatory agents has now improved outcomes in MDS. New agents and combinations aim to improve on the results obtained with the currently available drugs.

Keywords Acute myeloid leukemia (AML), treatment • Acute myeloid leukemia, induction therapy • Cytarabine (ara-C) • Anthracyclines • Acute myeloid leukemia, risk stratification • Core-binding factor leukemias, treatment • Promyelocytic leukemia, treatment • All-trans retinoic acid (ATRA) • FLT3, prognostic impact of mutations • FLT3, kinase inhibitors • MLL, partial tandem duplication • Myelodysplastic syndrome (MDS), treatment • Demethylating agents, decitabine and azacitidine • Immune response modulators, lenalidomide

8.1. The Need for Improved Therapies in AML

For over 20 years, standard frontline treatment of the most common types of acute myeloid leukemia (AML) in adults has involved combination chemotherapy with cytarabine (ara-C) and anthracyclines such as idarubicin and daunorubicin (Table 8-1). The approaches to timing of induction, consolidation and reinduction therapy have been similarly unchanged (Fig. 8-1). With the exception of the uncommon good prognostic AML subgroups described below, this is not because standard therapy has produced long remission rates, since the 5-year survival rates for intermediate and high-risk AML are 45% and 10%, respectively.

Despite several large, randomized clinical trials assessing the addition of different cytotoxic agents to this traditional regimen, few have shown significant, if any, additive benefit. Even variations in the dose of standard agents have not improved survival, with the exception of the use of high-dose cytarabine in younger patients with favorable cytogenetics.

From: *Neoplastic Hematopathology*: Contemporary Hematology,
Edited by: D. Jones, DOI 10.1007/978-1-60761-384-8_8,
© Humana Press, a part of Springer Science+Business Media, LLC 2010

Table 8-1. Standard therapies for AML subtypes.

Type	Therapy	Mechanism	Response rates, long term survival
AML-M3 (acute promyelocytic leukemia)	ATRA, with chemotherapy (typically idarubicin)	Action of ATRA in relieving PML-RARA transcriptional block and allowing promyelocyte maturation	Over 90%, over 75%
Intermediate and high-risk AML types	Cytarabine and anthracyclines	Synergistic effects of these two classes of compounds on inhibiting DNA replication	50–60%, 10–45%
Core binding factor (CBF) AML	As above with additional courses of cytarabine-based consolidation	High sensitivity of blasts with altered CBF proteins to these drugs	Over 80%, over 60%

ATRA all-trans retinoic acid

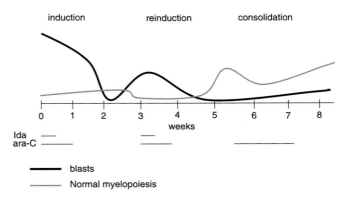

Fig. 8-1. *Timing of standard cytotoxic chemotherapy in AML.* The role of induction is to minimize the immediate life-threatening complications of the disease. Consolidation is given to reduce the disease burden further, hence decreasing the possibility of relapse. A second induction is given variably between 2 and 5 weeks after the first course, depending the intensity of the first course and response to it. Maintenance therapy has not been part of standard therapy of AML particularly in the US

The contribution of allogeneic stem cell transplantation (SCT) following consolidation therapy has been difficult to assess since few randomized trials have been conducted and the retrospective studies often are skewed by biases due to preferential recruitment of patients with tumors that have good genetic features. It is only within the last few years that understanding of the molecular and cellular changes in the common AML types has led to the identification of molecular alterations that provide new targets for therapeutic intervention.

8.2. DNA-Damaging Cytotoxic Chemotherapy in AML

Randomized clinical trials have established daunorubicin at 45–60 mg/m² daily for 3 days plus cytarabine 100–200 mg/m² daily for 7 days as the current standard induction regimen for AML. Variations studied have involved the use of high-dose cytarabine, and the addition of other agents such as etoposide, chlorodeoxyadenosine, and fludarabine. The main controversies have been with respect to the optimal dose and choice of daunorubicin versus idarubicin, the value of high-dose cytarabine during induction, and the possible inclusion of new agents. Although improvements in CR rate and survival have been reported for idarubicin over daunorubicin in some studies, differences in the efficacy of the two anthracyclines may not be demonstrable if a higher dose of daunorubicin is used (e.g., 60 or 90 mg/m^2 daily for 3 days).

High-dose cytarabine (HIDAC) (generally considered as doses ≥ 1 g/m^2/dose), as part of induction therapy, was associated with longer remission duration and event-free survival in the younger patients. Kern and Estey performed a pooled analysis of data from randomized clinical trials that compared HIDAC with standard-dose cytarabine (SDAC, ≤ 0.2 g/m^2/dose) during induction in patients with AML [1]. No differences were noted with regards to CR rates. However, the use of HIDAC was associated with better long-term disease control and improved survival in adults younger than 60 years of age.

The use of high doses of cytarabine for consolidation in younger patients has been evaluated and found to be beneficial particularly for those patients with favorable-risk cytogenetic abnormalities, such as the t(8;21)- and inv(16)-bearing core binding factor (CBF) AML [2]. Even in younger patients with intermediate risk AML, there is a definite benefit for intermediate- or high-dose cytarabine consolidation. However, the role of higher doses of cytarabine for consolidation in older patients and those with poor-risk cytogenetics is limited. Maintenance therapy is not routinely used for AML treatment in most centers, although a number of large studies from Germany have suggested that there may be a benefit for maintenance therapy with cytotoxic agents in prolonging disease-free survival.

Recombinant myeloid growth factors, such as granulocyte-colony stimulating factor (G-CSF) and granulocyte-macrophage-colony stimulating factor (GM-CSF) have been extensively evaluated as adjuncts to the various chemotherapeutic regimens [3]. They have been used to decrease the duration of chemotherapy-induced neutropenia and thereby reduce the incidence and severity of infections, as well as to recruit dormant leukemia cells into the S-phase of cell cycle in order to increase their susceptibility to cytarabine. Multiple prospective randomized trials have examined the benefit and safety of the addition of growth factors before, during, and after chemotherapy. The most consistent finding has been a reduction in the duration of neutropenia; whereas stimulation of leukemia cells has not typically been observed. However, few studies have reported a benefit in prolonging the duration of disease-free or overall survival with addition of growth factors.

Several new cytotoxic agents are under evaluation. Clofarabine, a purine nucleoside anti-metabolite, was recently approved by the United States Food and Drug Administration (FDA) for the treatment of pediatric patients with refractory or relapsed acute lymphoblastic leukemia (ALL), and is now being evaluated as monotherapy (or in combination) for the treatment of older patients with AML. Faderl et al. reported the results of a phase II study of clofarabine (40 mg/m^2, 1-h infusion, days 2–6) plus intermediate-dose cytarabine (1 g/m^2 daily, 2-h infusion for 5 days) in patients with newly-diagnosed AML who are 50 years or older [4]. The overall response rate was 60% (52% CR, 8% partial CR); myelosuppression was frequent; toxicities were mostly grade 2 or lower; and four patients (7%) died during induction. In another randomized phase II study, clofarabine in addition to low dose subcutaneous cytarabine was superior to clofarabine alone as the induction regimen for patients with AML older than 60 [5]. Most recently, in a large phase II study of clofarabine in older patients with AML (median age, 71 years), who are unlikely to tolerate or benefit from traditional chemotherapy, an overall response rate of 46% (38% CR and 8% CRi) was reported.

8.3. Clinical and Cytogenetic Risk Models of AML

Clinical predictors of response and survival in AML can be divided into three groups: (1) patient-related factors such as age, performance status, and presence or absence of organ dysfunction; (2) tumor-associated (genetic and epigenetic) changes producing inherent resistance to existing therapies; and (3) treatment-related factors which predict which therapies will be effective (Table 8-2). As described in Chap. 7, the morphologically-based FAB classification of AML has served clinicians well for two decades, but encodes limited prognostic information with the exception of the good outcome in the uncommon AML-M3 subtype (acute promyelocytic leukemia) due to the effectiveness of all-trans retinoic acid (ATRA) in inducing maturation and complete eradication of the neoplastic clone. The 2008 World Health Organization (WHO) classification of AML now incorporates some of the most prognostically important genetic changes into distinctive diagnostic subtypes.

Nearly, all retrospective studies of AML have identified similar demographic and clinical predictors of poor outcome with standard therapy including advanced age, [6] complex karyotype, poor performance status, renal and hepatic organ dysfunction, presence of antecedent hematological disorders, and white blood cell count (WBC) at presentation.

The importance of bone marrow cytogenetics in predicting the outcome of patients with AML is well-established (Table 8-3). Several large retrospective studies conducted by the cooperative oncology groups (i.e., CALGB, ECOG, and SWOG) have stratified patients with AML receiving standard cytotoxic chemotherapy into three risk groups based on specific findings on routine karyotyping [7–10]. Such cytogenetic risk assessment has already led to the tailoring of treatment strategies. For example, patients with favorable-risk AML other than APL (i.e., CBF AML) are highly sensitive to cytarabine, and therefore receive multiple courses of high-dose cytarabine (usually 3–4 cycles), which has significantly improved survival [2].

Table 8-2. Predictors of prognosis in AML.

Patient-related
  Age
  Performance status
  Organ function
  Presence of comorbidities
Disease-related
  Cytogenetics
  De novo versus secondary AML
  MDR expression
  Molecular abnormalities
Therapy-related
  Efficacy of available therapy (e.g., ATRA in APL)
  Toxicity of available therapy (e.g., allogeneic stem cell transplant)
  Donor availability

Table 8-3. Selected large studies of the role of cytogenetics as predictor of prognosis in AML.

Study	Patients (n)	Age (years)	5-year survival by cytogenetic risk group (%)[a]		
			Favorable	Intermediate	Unfavorable
MRC	1,612	<55	65	41	14
MRC	1,065	44–91	34	13	2
CALGB	1,213	15–86	55	24	5
SWOG/ECOG	609	<56	55	38	11

[a]Minor variations are seen in different studies in definitions of the cytogenetic risk groups for less common genetic changes but the core binding factor AMLs are always regarded as favorable, diploid AML as intermediate risk, and -5, -7 and complex karyotypes as unfavorable

However, clinical and genetic prediction factors are not independent of each other. The association of older age as an important determinant of poor outcome in AML is likely complex related to the specific (genetic) and dysplastic features of AML types that are common in the elderly as well as these patients' limited ability to tolerate the traditional cytotoxic agents. In a study combining data from 968 patients enrolled in five Southwest Oncology Group (SWOG) clinical trials, increasing age was associated with less favorable cytogenetic changes, poorer performance status scores, lower white blood cell counts, and a lower percentage of marrow blasts [6]. Favorable cytogenetic changes were present in 17% of patients younger than 55 years but in only 4% of those older than 75 years. Conversely, unfavorable cytogenetic changes were present in 3% of the youngest group and 51% of the oldest group. Increasing age was also associated with a higher incidence of early death after induction therapy, a lower CR rate, and shorter survival.

The increasingly routine use of molecular diagnostics has now led to the identification of one widely-accepted marker of adverse outcome which is an activating mutation in the receptor tyrosine kinase FLT3 by internal tandem duplication (ITD). FLT3 mutations are associated with a poor prognosis in most genetic subtypes, most especially when FLT3 ITD is seen in conjunction with loss of the second FLT3 allele by gene deletion [11].

8.4. Complex Molecular Genetic Models of Outcome in Diploid AML

Since AML with a normal diploid karyotype constitutes the largest single cytogenetic group, much effort has been focused on identifying predictors in this subtype (Table 8-4). Most such patients have a high likelihood of achieving CR with standard induction regimens but initial responses and relapse rates are variable and have been correlated with the presence of specific genetic changes and expression levels of leukemia-associated genes [12]. These studies are briefly reviewed below.

Partial tandem duplication (PTD) of the MLL gene (located at chromosome 11q23) was the first molecular abnormality to be preferentially associated with diploid karyotype AML, occurring in approximately 5–10% of cases. In those cases, the duration of remission was shorter if MLL PTD was present [13]. MLL PTD also occurs in conjunction with the poor cytogenetic risk group but much less commonly in the good prognostic groups (i.e., AML-M3 and CBF AML). Mutation of the CEBPA gene, which include insertions and deletions that lead to non-functional or dominant-negative proteins, occurs preferentially in diploid AML being identified in 15% of such tumors. It is associated with longer remissions and

Table 8-4. Selected molecular abnormalities in AML and their role as predictors of outcome.

Molecular abnormality	AML subtype	Disease-free survival	Overall survival
MLL PTD	Diploid, trisomy 11	Shortened	None
FLT3 ITD	Diploid	Shortened	Shortened
↑ BAALC mRNA	Diploid	Shortened	Shortened
CEBPA mutation	Diploid	Prolonged	Prolonged
NPM mutation	Diploid	Prolonged	Prolonged
↑WT-1 mRNA	All subtypes	NR	Shortened
NRAS mutation	All subtypes	None	None
KIT mutation	inv(16), t(8;21)	Shortened	Shortened
↑ ERG mRNA	Diploid	Shortened	Shortened

MLL PTD mixed lineage leukemia partial tandem duplication, *FLT3 ITD* FMS-like tyrosine kinase-3 internal tandem duplication, *BAALC* brain and acute leukemia cytoplasmic, *CEBPα* CCAAT/enhancer binding protein-α, *NPM* nucleophosmin, *WT-1* Wilm's tumor-1, *ERG* ETS-related gene, *AML* acute myeloid leukemia, *APL* acute promyelocytic leukemia, *NR* not reported

improved survival [14]. CEBPA encodes the CCAAT/enhancer binding protein α (C/EBPα), a transcription factor involved in the regulation of myelopoiesis. Studies using knock-out mice have shown that C/EBPα is essential for stem cell commitment to the granulocytic lineage.

Mutations in the nucleophosmin (NPM1) gene, usually 4-base pair duplications in exon 12 leading to an out-of-frame truncated protein, are seen in 40%–60% of diploid AML [15]. Cases with NPM1 mutation are associated with a higher CR rate, longer survival, and improved event-free survival. NPM1 mutations occur frequently along with FLT3 mutations in the same tumor but rarely with MLL PTD or CEBPA or ras mutations. In tumors with both NPM1 and FLT3 ITD mutation, the negative prognostic effects of FLT3 ITD predominate. The unmutated nucleophosmin protein is a transcriptional regulator that shuttles other proteins between the cell nucleus and cytoplasm and these mutations lead to its retention in the cytoplasm with a dominant-negative effect on myeloid maturation.

There have been several attempts to integrate the effects of all of these different mutations on outcome in diploid AML. In one study, molecular alterations in 872 adults younger than 60 with normal diploid karyotype AML who had been treated in one of four German AML trials were evaluated [16]. The overall CR rate was 77%. Mutations were seen in NPM1 in 53%, FLT3 ITD in 31%, FLT3 tyrosine kinase domain point mutations (TKD) in 11%, CEBPA in 13%, MLL PTD in 7%, and NRAS point mutations in 13%. Multivariable analysis in a subset of 693 patients revealed that mutant CEBPA (odds ratio, 1.33; 95% confidence interval [CI], 1.01–1.74), and mutant NPM1 without FLT3-ITD (odds ratio, 1.48; 95% CI, 1.21–1.80) represented the best outcome groups. Allogeneic SCT in first CR was beneficial for all groups of patients except for those with tumors that were mutated for NPM1 but lacked the FLT3 ITD [16].

Other molecular abnormalities with impact on outcome are now emerging for other cytogenetic subgroups. For example, the presence of activation mutations in the KIT tyrosine kinase predicts for worse outcome in patients with CBF leukemias [17]. Gene expression signatures have also been utilized to define prognostic groups in AML [18]. High expression of the BAALC gene has been shown to be an independent predictor of resistance ($p=.019$), high cumulative incidence of relapse ($p=.03$), and shorter survival ($P=.001$) in patients with normal diploid AML [19]. In one study, patients with both high levels of BAALC expression and FLT3 mutations had the worst survival, whereas patients with neither change did best. In another recent report, using microRNA expression profiling, samples of leukemia cells from adults younger than 60 years with normal karyotype AML that had high-risk molecular features (i.e., FLT3-ITD and/or unmutated NPM1) were evaluated. A microRNA signature that was associated with improved event-free survival was identified [20]. Whether these mRNA or microRNA profiles will assist in the routine risk stratification or the identification of new molecular targets for therapy remains to be determined.

8.5. Targeted Therapy of AML

Given the large number of specific genetic alterations that have outcome implications, strategies to develop more targeted therapies for molecular subgroups of AML are now needed. These could include strategies to reverse drug resistance (e.g., multi-drug resistance inhibitors), monoclonal antibodies directed at myeloid antigen targets [e.g., gemtuzumab ozogamicin (GO) which is directed against CD33], agents directed at signaling and apoptosis pathways, and small molecular inhibitors which target the mutated tyrosine kinases in AML such as KIT and FLT3 (summarized in Table 8-5).

8.5.1. Antibody-Based Immunotherapy

Because of the generally poor outcome of elderly patients with AML, current research is focused on identifying less toxic and more effective agents to use in this setting. GO immunotherapy has been approved by the FDA for AML treatment in first relapse for patients 60 years or older who have had a first remission duration of greater than

Table 8-5. Novel and targeted therapies and their possible role in AML.

Agent	Status	Potential role
Monoclonal antibodies		Treatment of relapse in older AML, may be beneficial when added to chemotherapy
Gemtuzumab ozogumicin	Approved	
Anti-CD45 (radiolabeled)	Investigational	
FLT3 kinase inhibitors		May benefit patients with FLT3 mutations
CEP701 (Lesutarnib)	Investigational	
PKC412	Investigational	
Sorafenib	Approved in RCC and HCC	
Farnesyltransferase inhibitors	Investigational	Early studies in the elderly did not lead to FDA approval
Tipifarnib (Zarnestra)		
Epigenetic modulators	Approved in MDS	
5AZA, decitabine		Potential role in elderly AML, potential role in maintenance
SAHA		Potential role in elderly AML in combination with epigenetic agents
Signaling modulators, apoptosis inducers	Investigational	Pending the results of early studies

AML acute myeloid leukemia, *RCC* renal cell carcinoma, *HCC* hepatocellular carcinoma, *DAC* decitabine, *SAHA* the histone deacetylation inhibitor suberoylanilide hydroxamic acid

3 months [21]. GO has also been evaluated as frontline therapy for patients with AML. Preliminary results on the subset of patients treated in the United Kingdom AML15 trial which combined gemtuzumab with chemotherapy showed a high CR rate of 82%. This study has increased interest in combining low doses of gemtuzumab with chemotherapy in the treatment of AML.

8.5.2. Targeting FLT3-Mutated AML with Kinase Inhibitors

The FMS-like tyrosine kinase FLT3 is expressed by early hematopoietic progenitors and has a major role in both stem cell survival and myeloid differentiation. The FLT3 ITD results in constitutive activation of the FLT3 kinase, leading to the activation of multiple downstream signaling pathways including the JAK-STAT, RAS, and mitogen activation protein (MAP) kinases that mediate survival and proliferation [22]. As described above, FLT3 ITD has been uniformly identified as a poor prognostic factor and occurs in 20%–30% of AML, most frequently in the AML-M3, CBF, and normal diploid subtypes. FLT3 is also mutated at codons 835 and 836 in 5–7% of AML leading to similar ligand-independent kinase activation.

Several inhibitors of the FLT3 kinase are under clinical evaluation. Lestaurtinib (CEP701) is being evaluated in relapsed AML with patients with FLT3-ITD-bearing tumors randomized to receive treatment with chemotherapy with or without lestaurtinib [23]. Preliminary results indicate that the addition of this FLT3 inhibitor may improve the response rate. PKC412, a FLT3 kinase inhibitor with some single-agent activity in AML, has also shown a favorable CR rate in newly diagnosed AML in patients younger than 60 years when combined with daunorubicin and cytarabine [24]. A large multi-national, multi-institutional study incorporating PKC412 in induction chemotherapy regimens for those with FLT3-mutated AML is now underway. Sorafenib, a multi-kinase inhibitor approved for the treatment of renal cell and hepatocellular cancer, has been found to be a strong inhibitor of ITD-mutated FLT3, and a phase II study of sorafenib in combination with chemotherapy shows promising initial results [25].

8.6. Role of Allogeneic Stem Cell Transplantation in AML

The role of allogeneic SCT in AML therapy remains unclear despite numerous studies. In several prospective trials, patients younger than 55 years who had an HLA-matched sibling donor were assigned to receive allogeneic SCT in first CR. In such studies, those with no matched donor were usually randomized to receive an autologous SCT or further chemotherapy complicating the analysis. Overall, these trials suggested a possible advantage for allogeneic transplantation in patients with poor-risk cytogenetic changes [26–28]. However, there has been no clear differences in outcome in the other cytogenetic risk groups with the exception of those with CBF AML who did better with additional chemotherapy alone. As described above, a retrospective German study showed a strong benefit for allogeneic SCT in first CR for patients with intermediate-risk AML except for those who had mutated NPM1 without FLT3 ITD mutation [16].

8.7. Myelodysplastic Syndromes (MDS) and Their Relation to AML

Hematopoietic elements are constantly exposed to genotoxic stresses related to infections, chemical injury, auto-immune attack, and emergency regeneration and thus accumulate genetic changes over time. Clonal hematopoietic stem cell disorders, termed myelodysplastic syndromes (MDS), are the end-result of such chronic insults and are manifested by dysplasia and cytopenia in one or more of the three main hematopoietic cell lineages (see Chap. 6) [29].

The progressive development of the bone marrow failure state in MDS has been modeled as a balance between the excessive apoptosis of progenitor cells (i.e., ineffective hematopoiesis) and an increased rate of abnormal proliferation [29]. Overproduction of pro-apoptotic cytokines, such as tumor necrosis factor-alpha and soluble Fas ligand, may contribute to this excessive apoptosis and are most important in the earlier (hypoproliferative) phases of MDS. Mutation of growth regulators (e.g., FLT3 and NRAS), anti-apoptotic mechanisms (e.g., BCL2 overexpression), cell cycle dysregulation (e.g., CDKN2B/p15 silencing) and acquisition of genomic maintenance defects (e.g., TP53 mutations) characterize the later stages of MDS.

As a result of these later pro-proliferative genetic changes, progression of MDS into AML occurs in approximately in 35% of cases, and is mostly detected in those who present with increased numbers of blasts (i.e., high-risk MDS). The FAB and WHO classification systems as well as the International Prognostic Scoring System (IPSS) have been used to sub-classify patients with MDS into different groups with different expectations of survival as well as different risks of transformation into AML.

8.8. Overcoming Ineffective Hematopoiesis in MDS: Growth Factors and Supportive Measures

Although AML transformation represents a major clinical problem for some patients, the overall prognosis in MDS is more closely related to the degree of cytopenias and related clinical factors such as need for transfusions and degree of iron overload. Because such ineffective hematopoiesis represents the main determinant of morbidity and mortality, a principal goal of traditional therapies in MDS has been to support patients against the complications of worsening cytopenias. Such supportive care measures including regular transfusion of blood products, use of antibiotics to prevent infections due to neutropenia, and the use of exogenous hematopoietic growth factors [such as recombinant erythropoietin (EPO), GM-CSF and G-CSF] to drive hematopoiesis.

EPO can reduce transfusion requirements in up to 40% of patients with MDS [30], and responses are more likely in patients who have low-risk MDS (i.e., RA and RARS). The best responses for EPO treatment are achieved in patients who require less than 2 units of packed red blood cell transfusions per month and who have low endogenous serum erythropoietin levels (<100 mU/mL). Although G-CSF and GM-CSF improve neutropenia in 70–80% of patients, there have been limited data showing that they reduce episodes of infections, prolong survival, or influence the rate of transformation to AML. Their use appears reasonable in patients who have recurrent neutropenic febrile episodes, but they are not recommended for chronic prophylactic use. Nonetheless, combined therapy with EPO and G-CSF in low-risk MDS appears to increase the quality of life and may be associated with an improved outcome in a subset of patients.

8.9. Overcoming Ineffective Hematopoiesis in MDS: Epigenetic Therapy

Other than supportive growth factors, there were no approved therapies for treatment of MDS for many years. This situation has been changed in the last 5 years with the introduction of demethylating agents that alter gene expression in the (abnormal) hematopoietic elements in MDS and improve cytopenias and clinical outcomes. Methylation of DNA at CpG-rich regions around the promoters of genes (i.e., CpG islands) is a major cellular mechanism of transcriptional silencing and provides an alternative mechanism for loss of expression of tumor suppressor genes during cancer progression. Methylation of the promoters of several growth regulators such as CDKN2B (p15) has been associated with progression and adverse outcome in MDS. DNA demethylation thus provides a potential opportunity to reverse some of the deleterious changes in MDS. Azacitidine (5AZA, Vidaza) and decitabine (5-aza-2'-deoxycitidine, DAC) are pyrimidine analogs that inhibit DNA methyltransferases, the enzymes that methylate newly synthesized DNA. DAC or 5AZA treatment leads to hypomethylation of the promoters of tumor suppressor gene leading to their reactivation and promotion of cell maturation.

Use of 5AZA and DAC have now been clearly associated with improved outcomes [31, 32], and both have been approved by the FDA for the treatment of MDS. In a large prospective randomized trial conducted by the Cancer and Leukemia Group B (CALGB), treatment with 5AZA (75 mg/m^2/d subcutaneously for 7 days every 28 days) was compared with supportive care alone [31]. Patients in the supportive care arm whose disease worsened were allowed to cross over to 5AZA. Responses occurred in 60% of patients on the 5AZA arm (7% complete response, 16% partial response, 37% improved) compared with 5% (improved) receiving supportive care ($p < .001$). Median time to leukemic transformation or death was 21 months for 5AZA versus 13 months for supportive care ($p = .007$). Transformation to AML occurred as the first event in 15% of patients on the 5AZA arm and in 38% of the supportive care group ($p = .001$). A landmark analysis after 6 months showed median survival of an additional 18 months for 5AZA and 11 months for supportive care ($P = .03$). Quality-of-life assessments also found some significant major advantages in terms of physical function, symptoms, and psychological state in patients initially randomized to 5AZA. In a more recent study, treatment with 5AZA was shown to be superior to the conventional care strategies including the traditional AML-type chemotherapy in 358 patients with MDS.

In another study, a total of 170 patients with MDS were randomized to receive either decitabine at a dose of 15 mg/m^2 given intravenously over 3 h every 8 h for 3 days (at a dose of 135 mg/m^2 per course) and repeated every 6 weeks, or best supportive care [32]. Patients who were treated with decitabine achieved a significantly higher overall response rate (17%), including 9% complete responses, compared with supportive care only (0%) ($p < .001$). Responses were durable (median, 10.3 months) and were associated with transfusion independence. Patients treated with decitabine had a trend toward a longer median time to progression to AML or death, when compared with patients who received supportive care alone and this was particularly true for patients with IPSS intermediate II and high risk disease.

Demethylating agents are also being evaluated for the treatment of patients with AML. A recent re-analysis of data from three sequential CALGB trials of 5-azacytidine demonstrated that among 103 patients with AML at baseline (using WHO criteria), 48% had hematological improvement or even better responses [33].

8.10. Immune Modulation in Treatment of MDS

The hypoproliferative variants of early-stage MDS shares features with aplastic anemia and other bone marrow failure syndromes and has suggested that an auto-immune attack by cytotoxic T cells may be adding to marrow injury in some cases of MDS. This has led to the empirical use of immunosuppressive therapy (with anti-thymocyte or anti-lymphocyte globulins, cyclosporine A, and steroids) and the eventual identification of subsets of patients with MDS who may be responsive. Expression of HLA-DR15 (a serologic split of HLA-DR2 that is over represented in MDS, and aplastic anemia), younger age, and shorter duration of RBC transfusion-dependence have been identified in multivariate analysis as pretreatment characteristics that correlate with response to immunosuppressive therapy. The presence of a population of paroxysmal nocturnal hemoglobinuria (PNH)-type leukocytes has been demonstrated in some patients with MDS (as well as aplastic anemia, see Chap. 6) and has been associated with a greater probability of response to cyclosporine and ATG therapy.

Another approach has been the use of agents which influence the abnormal cytokine and angiogenic microenvironment in MDS marrow such as the immunomodulatory drug lenalidomide, which is a compound related to thalidomide. In a pivotal study, 148 patients with MDS subtypes that showed deletions of chromosome 5q (which is associated with severe anemia) received lenalidomide 10 mg either for 21 days every 4 weeks or every day [34]. Hematologic, bone marrow, and cytogenetic changes were assessed after 24 weeks of treatment by an intention-to-treat analysis. Among the 148 patients, 112 had a reduced need for transfusions (76%; 95% confidence interval [CI], 68–82) and 99 patients (67%; 95% CI, 59–74) no longer required transfusions, regardless of the karyotype complexity. The response to lenalidomide was rapid and sustained; the median duration of transfusion independence had not been reached after a median of 104 weeks of follow-up. The maximum hemoglobin concentration reached a median of 13.4 g per deciliter (range, 9.2–18.6), with a corresponding median rise of 5.4 g per deciliter (range, 1.1–11.4), as compared with the baseline nadir value before transfusion. Among 85 patients who could be evaluated, 62 had cytogenetic improvement, and 38 of the 62 had a complete cytogenetic remission. Moderate-to-severe neutropenia (in 55% of patients) and thrombocytopenia (in 44%) were the most common reasons for interrupting treatment or adjusting the dose of lenalidomide. Based largely on this study, lenalidomide has now been approved by the FDA for the treatment of MDS with chromosome 5q deletions. More recent data have demonstrated the potential benefit of lenalidomide in the other subsets of patients with low-risk MDS.

8.11. Current Problems and Future Directions in MDS and AML Therapy

The supportive, epigenetic and immunomodulatory therapies for lower-risk MDS rarely result in CRs instead producing improvements in hematologic indices and reduction of transfusion requirements. Nonetheless, the successes with hypomethylating and immunomodulatory agents in particular have shown that outcome and risk of progression can be significantly reduced. However, MDS with high-risk IPSS scores remain difficult to treat. In these subtypes, use of cytotoxic DNA-damaging chemotherapy and allogeneic stem cell transplantation are not well-tolerated in elderly patients (who comprise most cases) and are usually reserved for younger patients. Therefore, a major focus of current clinical trials in MDS is the comparison of combinations of the new agents described above to improve response rates in higher-risk MDS subtypes. Current efforts in AML therapeutics are focused on better risk stratification and identifying predictors of anthracycline resistance to select appropriate patients requiring targeted therapies such as kinase inhibitors in addition to the standard regimens.

References

1. Kern W, Estey EH. High-dose cytosine arabinoside in the treatment of acute myeloid leukemia: review of three randomized trials. Cancer 2006;107(1):116–24.
2. Bloomfield CD, Lawrence D, Byrd JC, et al. Frequency of prolonged remission duration after high-dose cytarabine intensification in acute myeloid leukemia varies by cytogenetic subtype. Cancer Res 1998;58(18):4173–9.
3. Ravandi F. Role of cytokines in the treatment of acute leukemias: a review. Leukemia 2006;20(4):563–71.
4. Faderl S, Verstovsek S, Cortes J, et al. Clofarabine and cytarabine combination as induction therapy for acute myeloid leukemia (AML) in patients 50 years of age or older. Blood 2006;108(1):45–51.
5. Faderl S, Ravandi F, Huang X, et al. A randomized study of clofarabine versus clofarabine plus low-dose cytarabine as front-line therapy for patients aged 60 years and older with acute myeloid leukemia and high-risk myelodysplastic syndrome. Blood 2008;112(5):1638–45.
6. Appelbaum FR, Gundacker H, Head DR, et al. Age and acute myeloid leukemia. Blood 2006; 107(9):3481–5.
7. Grimwade D, Walker H, Oliver F, et al. The importance of diagnostic cytogenetics on outcome in AML: analysis of 1,612 patients entered into the MRC AML 10 trial. The Medical Research Council Adult and Children's Leukaemia Working Parties. Blood 1998;92(7):2322–33.
8. Grimwade D, Walker H, Harrison G, et al. The predictive value of hierarchical cytogenetic classification in older adults with acute myeloid leukemia (AML): analysis of 1065 patients entered into the United Kingdom Medical Research Council AML11 trial. Blood 2001;98(5):1312–20.
9. Byrd JC, Mrozek K, Dodge RK, et al. Pretreatment cytogenetic abnormalities are predictive of induction success, cumulative incidence of relapse, and overall survival in adult patients with de novo acute myeloid leukemia: results from Cancer and Leukemia Group B (CALGB 8461). Blood 2002;100(13):4325–36.
10. Slovak ML, Kopecky KJ, Cassileth PA, et al. Karyotypic analysis predicts outcome of preremission and postremission therapy in adult acute myeloid leukemia: a Southwest Oncology Group/Eastern Cooperative Oncology Group Study. Blood 2000;96(13):4075–83.
11. Kottaridis PD, Gale RE, Frew ME, et al. The presence of a FLT3 internal tandem duplication in patients with acute myeloid leukemia (AML) adds important prognostic information to cytogenetic risk group and response to the first cycle of chemotherapy: analysis of 854 patients from the United Kingdom Medical Research Council AML 10 and 12 trials. Blood 2001;98(6):1752–9.
12. Mrozek K, Marcucci G, Paschka P, Whitman SP, Bloomfield CD. Clinical relevance of mutations and gene-expression changes in adult acute myeloid leukemia with normal cytogenetics: are we ready for a prognostically prioritized molecular classification? Bloods 2007;109:341–448.
13. Dohner K, Tobis K, Ulrich R, et al. Prognostic significance of partial tandem duplications of the MLL gene in adult patients 16 to 60 years old with acute myeloid leukemia and normal cytogenetics: a study of the Acute Myeloid Leukemia Study Group Ulm. J Clin Oncol 2002;20(15):3254–61.
14. Frohling S, Schlenk RF, Stolze I, et al. CEBPA mutations in younger adults with acute myeloid leukemia and normal cytogenetics: prognostic relevance and analysis of cooperating mutations. J Clin Oncol 2004;22(4):624–33.
15. Falini B, Mecucci C, Tiacci E, et al. Cytoplasmic nucleophosmin in acute myelogenous leukemia with a normal karyotype. N Engl J Med 2005;352(3):254–66.
16. Schlenk RF, Dohner K, Krauter J, et al. Mutations and treatment outcome in cytogenetically normal acute myeloid leukemia. N Engl J Med 2008;358(18):1909–18.
17. Paschka P, Marcucci G, Ruppert AS, et al. Adverse prognostic significance of KIT mutations in adult acute myeloid leukemia with inv(16) and t(8;21): a Cancer and Leukemia Group B Study. J Clin Oncol 2006;24(24):3904–11.
18. Bullinger L, Dohner K, Bair E, et al. Use of gene-expression profiling to identify prognostic subclasses in adult acute myeloid leukemia. N Engl J Med 2004;350(16):1605–16.
19. Baldus CD, Thiede C, Soucek S, Bloomfield CD, Thiel E, Ehninger G. BAALC expression and FLT3 internal tandem duplication mutations in acute myeloid leukemia patients with normal cytogenetics: prognostic implications. J Clin Oncol 2006;24(5):790–7.

20. Marcucci G, Radmacher MD, Maharry K, et al. MicroRNA expression in cytogenetically normal acute myeloid leukemia. N Engl J Med 2008;358(18):1919–28.

21. Sievers EL, Larson RA, Stadtmauer EA, et al. Efficacy and safety of gemtuzumab ozogamicin in patients with CD33-positive acute myeloid leukemia in first relapse. J Clin Oncol 2001;19(13):3244–54.

22. Gilliland DG, Griffin JD. The roles of FLT3 in hematopoiesis and leukemia. Blood 2002;100(5): 1532–42.

23. Levis M, Smith BD, Beran M, et al. A randomized, open-label study of lestaurtinib (CEP-701), an oral FLT3 inhibitor, administered in sequence with chemotherapy in patients with relapsed AML harboring FLT3 activating mutations: clinical response correlates with successful FLT3 inhibition. Blood 2005;106(11):121a.

24. Stone RM, Fischer T, Paquette R, et al. Phase IB study of PKC412, an oral FLT3 kinase inhibitor, in sequential and simultaneous combinations with daunorubicin and cytarabine (DA) induction and high-dose cytarabine consolidation in newly diagnosed patients with AML. Blood 2006;108(11):50a.

25. Mori S, Cortes J, Kantarjian H, Zhang W, Andreef M, Ravandi F. Potential role of sorafenib in the treatment of acute myeloid leukemia. Leuk Lymphoma 2008;49(12):2246–55.

26. Cassileth PA, Harrington DP, Appelbaum FR, et al. Chemotherapy compared with autologous or allogeneic bone marrow transplantation in the management of acute myeloid leukemia in first remission. N Engl J Med 1998;339(23):1649–56.

27. Archimbaud E, Thomas X, Michallet M, et al. Prospective genetically randomized comparison between intensive postinduction chemotherapy and bone marrow transplantation in adults with newly diagnosed acute myeloid leukemia. J Clin Oncol 1994;12(2):262–7.

28. Zittoun RA, Mandelli F, Willemze R, et al. Autologous or allogeneic bone marrow transplantation compared with intensive chemotherapy in acute myelogenous leukemia. European Organization for Research and Treatment of Cancer (EORTC) and the Gruppo Italiano Malattie Ematologiche Maligne dell'Adulto (GIMEMA) Leukemia Cooperative Groups. N Engl J Med 1995;332(4):217–23.

29. Nimer SD. Myelodysplastic syndromes. Blood 2008;111(10):4841–51.

30. Hellstrom-Lindberg E, Gulbrandsen N, Lindberg G, et al. A validated decision model for treating the anaemia of myelodysplastic syndromes with erythropoietin + granulocyte colony-stimulating factor: significant effects on quality of life. Br J Haematol 2003;120(6):1037–46.

31. Silverman LR, Demakos EP, Peterson BL, et al. Randomized controlled trial of azacitidine in patients with the myelodysplastic syndrome: a study of the Cancer and Leukemia Group B. J Clin Oncol 2002;20(10):2429–40.

32. Kantarjian H, Issa JP, Rosenfeld CS, et al. Decitabine improves patient outcomes in myelodysplastic syndromes: results of a phase III randomized study. Cancer 2006;106(8):1794–803.

33. Silverman LR, McKenzie DR, Peterson BL, et al. Further analysis of trials with azacitidine in patients with myelodysplastic syndrome: studies 8421, 8921, and 9221 by the Cancer and Leukemia Group B. J Clin Oncol 2006;24(24):3895–903.

34. List A, Dewald G, Bennett J, et al. Lenalidomide in the myelodysplastic syndrome with chromosome 5q deletion. N Engl J Med 2006;355(14):1456–65.

Chapter 9

Myeloproliferative Neoplasms

C. Cameron Yin and Dan Jones

Abstract/Scope of Chapter Protein tyrosine kinases (PTKs) have been shown to play a critical role in the pathogenesis of myeloproliferative neoplasms (MPNs). A range of chromosomal rearrangements or mutations in MPNs lead to constitutive activation of PTKs and downstream signal transduction pathways, and thus confer proliferative and survival advantage to the neoplastic clone over normal hematopoietic stem/precursor cells. Molecular abnormalities involving PTKs have been used for the diagnosis, classification, detection of minimal residual disease, as well as targeted therapy in MPNs. We describe Philadelphia chromosome-negative MPNs associated with mutations or rearrangements of tyrosine kinase genes, including PV involving JAK2 (V617F, exon 12 mutation), PMF involving JAK2 (V617F) and MPL (W515L/K), ET involving JAK2 (V617F) and MPL (W515L/K), mastocytosis involving KIT D816V, and myeloid neoplasms with eosinophilia involving PDGFRA, PDGFRB, or FGFR1.

Keywords Polycythemia vera • Essential thrombocythemia • Primary myelofibrosis • Myeloproliferative neoplasm, classification • Myeloproliferative neoplasm, JAK2 mutation • Myeloproliferative neoplasm, MPL mutation • JAK2, molecular analysis • Mastocytosis, KIT mutation • Hypereosinophilic syndrome • Platelet-derived growth factor receptor, chromosomal translocation • PDGFRA • PDGFRB • FGFR1 • Myeloid neoplasm with eosinophilia • Chronic myeloid leukemia, atypical, CBL mutation • Myeloid neoplasm, TET2 mutation

9.1. The Myeloproliferative Neoplasms: Shared Features

Myeloproliferative neoplasms (MPNs) comprise a variety of different chronic clonal hematopoietic stem cell disorders that show the proliferation of at least one hematopoietic cell type, including the myeloid, erythroid, and megakaryocytic lineages, with minimal defects in maturation (Table 9-1). The most common MPNs are the related polycythemia vera (PV), essential thrombocythemia (ET) and primary myelofibrosis (PMF), which share a common genetic origin (JAK2 mutation) in the majority of cases. Another group of MPNs have recurrent chromosomal translocations or point mutations that activate growth signaling tyrosine kinases (TKs), of which the t(9;22)(q34;q11)-bearing chronic myelogenous leukemia (CML) is the most common and the best-understood example.

Shared features of most MPNs include:

1. An indolent clinical course
2. Roughly equal gender predilection with a wide age range at presentation

From: *Neoplastic Hematopathology*: Contemporary Hematology,
Edited by: D. Jones, DOI 10.1007/978-1-60761-384-8_9,
© Humana Press, a part of Springer Science+Business Media, LLC 2010

Table 9-1. Growth-activating mutations in MPNs and their effects.

Disease type	Genes	Mechanism of transformation	Pathway(s) activated	Cells that proliferate
CML	BCR-ABL1	t(9;22)(q34;q11)	Dysregulated TK signaling nexus	All myeloid lineages, including basophils (p210 protein), lymphoid lineage (p190), monocytic lineage (altered p190)
PV, ET, PMF	JAK2, MPL	Activating point mutation (V617F or W515L/K)	Cytokine receptor signaling	Homozygous JAK2 mutation/LOH: erythroid > others
				Heterozygous/low-level JAK2 mutation: megakaryocyte > erythroid
Systemic mastocytosis	KIT	Activating point mutation (D816V)	Receptor TK in ras-MAPK pathway	Mast cells, and subsets of secondary myeloid MPNs that can develop
MPN with eosinophilia	PDGFRA-FIP1L1	Interstitial deletion at chromosome 4q12	Receptor TK in RAS-MAPK pathway	Eosinophils and mast cells, rarely appears to transform other lineages
MPN with eosinophilia	ETV6-PDGFRB	t(5;12)(q31-33;p13)	Receptor TK	Eosinophils > monocytes, mast cells
MPD with eosinophilia	FGFR1-ZNF198	t(8;13)(p11;q12)	Receptor TK	Eosinophils > other myeloid lineages

3. Initial development through a somatic genetic change that activates a growth-promoting signaling pathway (e.g., BCR-ABL1, JAK2, or PDGFR)
4. Sensitivity of the mutated hematopoietic clone to the growth inhibitory effects of interferon
5. Stepwise progression through chronic (indolent), accelerated, and blast phases due to the accumulation of shared genetic (or epigenetic) changes
6. Disruptions of the bone marrow (BM) microenvironment that lead to progressive myelofibrosis, or myelodysplasia/secondary leukemia from the resulting ineffective hematopoiesis
7. Minimal impact of currently known hereditary or germline genetic changes in their development

Each of the MPNs differs with respect to their presenting features, histogenesis, and the frequency with which they progress to accelerated/blast phases or a fibrotic end-stage. However, the above commonalities highlight the critical elements that drive hematopoiesis which will be the focus of this chapter. The clinical presentation, workup, and treatment algorithms for CML and PV/ET/PMF are discussed in Chap. 11. The pathologic and genetic features of CML are discussed in Chap. 10.

9.2. PV, ET and PMF

9.2.1. Disease Presentation: Overlaps and Differences

Long before the identification of the JAK2 V617F mutation, it was apparent that PV, ET, and PMF (formerly known as idiopathic myelofibrosis or agnogenic myeloid metaplasia) were biologically related. For example, cultured marrow from all three of these neoplasms is hypersensitive to stimulation by exogenous growth factors that bind to JAK-STAT-linked cytokine receptors, including erythropoietin (EPO), thrombopoietin (TPO), granulocyte-macrophage colony stimulating factor (GM-CSF), and granulocyte colony-stimulating factor (G-CSF).

Also, many of the presenting signs, symptoms, and laboratory findings are overlapping with nearly all patients presenting with palpable splenomegaly to varying degrees. The defining feature of PV is increased red blood cell (RBC) mass, but abnormalities of coagulation or platelet dysfunction are also seen in some patients producing hemorrhage or thrombotic episodes. The defining feature of ET is an elevated platelet count, detected incidentally during routine exam in 30% or in a workup for fatigue (due to anemia), and less commonly due to thrombosis or hemorrhage. However, presentations of ET with leukocytosis or marked splenomegaly are also seen. Finally, PMF usually presents with abdominal pain (due to massive splenomegaly) or fatigue (due to anemia) but can present incidentally with thrombocytosis. Also given that ET and PV are often discovered incidentally on routine exam or during workup for other conditions, the differential manifestations may reflect the disease stage in which each case is diagnosed.

The overlapping clinical and biologic features of PV, ET and PMF are now known to reflect the occurrence early in the disease course of a mutation in the JAK2 kinase in a majority of cases. This kinase mediates activation of the receptors for all of the cytokines described above. Therefore, the differing clinical presentations of PV, ET and PMF are likely due to the stem cell stage at which the JAK2 mutation arises, the host genetic background, and most importantly the complementing genetic events that arise with disease progression. Given this overlap and the common treatments employed, JAK2-mutated PV, ET and PMF may be better regarded as a spectrum disorder with a unitary molecular origin. However, largely because approximately half of ET and PMF cases lack JAK2 mutation, the distinctions between these neoplasms are still based on hematologic and clinical criteria (Table 9-2).

Diagnosis of PV requires the demonstration of increased RBC mass (i.e., high hematocrit) with a demonstrable JAK2 mutation, or at least exclusion of other causes of erythrocytosis [1]. Diagnosis of ET requires a platelet count of at least 450×10^9/L, an absence of fully developed PV or PMF, and either JAK2/MPL mutation or exclusion of secondary causes

Table 9-2. Diagnostic criteria of PV, ET and PMF.

Type	Major criteria	Minor criteria	Diagnostic criteria
PV	(1) Hgb >18.5 g/dL (men), >16.5 g/dL (women), or increased red cell mass by another method (2) JAK2 V617F or similar mutation (e.g. JAK2 exon 12)	(1) Hypercellular BM with panmyelosis (2) Decreased serum erythropoietin level (3) Endogenous erythroid colony formation in vitro	2 major and 1 minor, or 1 major and 2 minor
ET	(1) Sustained PB platelets ≥450×10^9/L (2) JAK2/MPL mutation or exclusion of secondary thrombocytosis (3) Increased large mature megakaryocytes in BM (4) Absence of granulocytosis or erythrocytosis (i.e., no signs of PV, PMF or other MPNs)		All 4 major
PMF	(1) Atypical megakaryocytic hyperplasia with BM fibrosis, or granulocytic hyperplasia (2) Presence of JAK2/MPL mutation, other characteristic genetic changes, or exclusion of secondary causes of BM fibrosis (3) No signs of other myeloid neoplasms	(1) Leukoerythroblastic PB (2) Increased serum LDH (3) Anemia (4) Splenomegaly	All 3 major and 2 minor

of thrombocytosis. The diagnosis of PMF requires the presence of marrow fibrosis, or in those pre-fibrotic cases, the presence of myeloid and megakaryocytic hyperplasia usually accompanied by anemia [2]. The diagnosis of any of the other MPNs with specific molecular genetic definitions (i.e., BCR-ABL1+ CML, PDGFRA/PDGFRB/FGFR1-translocated HES or KIT-mutated mastocytosis) takes precedence over PV, ET, and PMF, which are still officially regarded as diagnoses of exclusion.

9.2.2. Presenting Features and Clinical Course

PV, ET, and PMF present with roughly equal incidence in men and women, and have a cumulative incidence higher than any other MPN type (Table 9-3) [3,4]. The presenting signs and symptoms relate to the degree of erythrocytosis, blood viscosity and platelet dysfunction that produce weakness, fatigue, headache, tinnitus, visual disturbance, pruritis, and erythromelalgia, and the degree of marrow infiltration producing bone pain. Venous or arterial thrombosis occurs in approximately 20% of patients with PV including abdominal vein thrombosis (e.g., Budd-Chiari syndrome) and obstruction of the portal, mesenteric, and/or spleen circulation. Similarly to ET, thrombotic consequences can be macrocirculatory (e.g., stroke, transient ischemic attack, myocardial infarction, peripheral arterial thrombosis, deep venous thrombosis, Budd-Chiari syndrome) or microcirculatory (producing headache, visual disturbance, or erythromelalgia). The most frequent site of hemorrhage is the gastrointestinal (GI) tract [3].

The natural history of PV includes an early phase with mild erythrocytosis, followed by marked polycythemia, and a myelofibrotic phase with cytopenias associated with BM fibrosis (Fig. 9-1), extramedullary hematopoiesis, and hypersplenism. The median survival is more than 10 years, with most disease-associated mortality due to thrombosis or hemorrhage [5]. Older age at diagnosis and a previous history of thrombosis are the most well-established negative prognostic factors, with higher leukocyte count and increased JAK2 mutation burden also recognized as adverse predictors [6]. ET is generally more indolent with a median survival of over 20 years [6]. but may also progress to myelofibrosis at a frequency of ~10% after 10 years [7]. Advanced age, higher leukocyte count or hemoglobin level, and prior history of thrombosis are independent predictors of inferior survival in ET [7,8]. Cases with JAK2 or MPL mutation have an increased risk of thrombosis [9].

The clinical course of PMF is more aggressive with a median survival of only 4 years [5]. Presentation with marked BM fibrosis and extramedullary hematopoiesis producing significant hepatosplenomegaly is most common; however, presentation at prefibrotic stage with myeloid and megakaryocytic hyperplasia in the BM also occurs (Fig. 9-1). Factors at diagnosis that adversely affect prognosis include age >70 years, hemoglobin <10 g/dL, platelet $<100 \times 10^9$/L, abnormal karyotype, and increased BM fibrosis [8]. The major causes of morbidity and mortality in PMF are infection, hemorrhage, thrombosis, portal hypertension, cardiac failure, and transformation to acute leukemia [2].

Some patients with PV, ET, and especially PMF develop a coincident myelodysplastic syndrome (MDS) or acute myeloid leukemia (AML). The incidence of AML at 10 years is

Table 9-3. Comparison of demographic and clinical features of PV, ET, and PMF.

Type	Median age (years)	Gender	Incidence per 100,000 (US/ Europe)	Median survival (years)	Progression to MF at 10 years	Incidence of AML at 10 years	Comments
PV	~70	M≥F	0.02–2.8	>10	5–10%	~5%	
ET	~55	M=F	1.5–2.5	>20	5–10%	1–2%	Variants presenting in younger women
PMF	~60	M=F	0.4–1.5	~4	not applicable	5–30%	

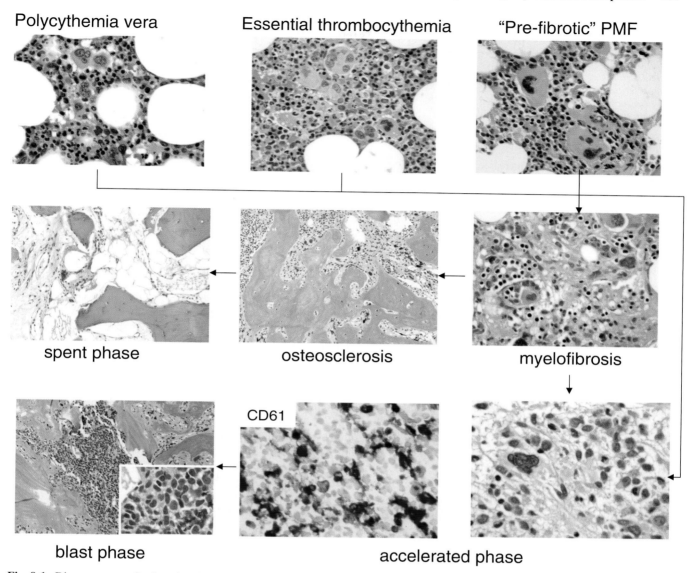

Polycythemia vera Essential thrombocythemia "Pre-fibrotic" PMF

spent phase osteosclerosis myelofibrosis

CD61

blast phase accelerated phase

Fig. 9-1. Disease stages of polycythemia vera (PV), essential thrombocythemia (ET) and primary myelofibrosis (PMF). The progression of PV and ET to myelofibrosis, and of all three neoplasms to accelerated and blast phases is illustrated

2–5% for PV, 1–2% for ET, and 5–30% for PMF. MDS/AML is increased in those treated with cytotoxic agents (e.g., hydroxyurea) consistent with secondary leukemia rather than MPN progression in some cases [2]. This is also supported by the absence of JAK2 mutation in many of these treatment-related acute leukemias [10]. The effect of increasing marrow fibrosis and the resulting ineffective marrow microenvironment on driving genetic instability and marrow dysplasia is suggested.

9.2.3. Pathologic Features and Useful Laboratory Testing

The bone marrow findings in PV, ET and PMF show a wide spectrum, with the most common findings summarized in Table 9-4. Two primary diagnostic problems arise; diagnosis of

Table 9-4. Comparison of bone marrow findings in PV, ET, and PMF.

Feature	PV[a]	ET	PMF-cellular phase	PMF-fibrotic phase
Cellularity	Increased	Normal or mildly increased	Increased	Decreased
Reticulin fibrosis	Minimal	Minimal	Minimal	Marked
Osteosclerosis	Minimal	Minimal	Minimal	Marked
Megakaryocyte number	Increased, scattered	Increased, small clusters	Increased	Increased
Megakaryocyte morphology	Minimally atypical	Large and hyperlobated with typical chromatin	Markedly atypical (hyperchromatic, staghorn, shaped nuclei with cloud-like chromatin) Dense clusters of megakaryocytes adjacent to sinuses or bone trabeculae	
Granulocytes	Increased	Normal	Increased	Decreased
Erythrocytes	Increased	Normal	Decreased	Decreased
Iron storage	Depleted	Present	Present	Present

[a] Indicates pre-polycythemic or polycythemic phase. It is usually difficult to distinguish post-polycythemic myelofibrotic phase and PMF based solely on morphologic features

early stage lesions (without significant fibrosis) and distinguishing PV, ET, and PMF once BM fibrosis is evident.

In classical PV, PB shows increased normochromic, normocytic red blood cells, slightly left-shifted mild neutrophilia, and often prominent thrombocytosis. The BM in PV is usually hypercellular with panmyelosis, especially in the erythroid and megakaryocytic lineages; the megakaryocytes show minimal atypia and occasional loose clusters. Iron stores are often depleted. Multi-color flow cytometry shows promise in identifying myeloid maturation defects in early-stage PV [11]. The BM in ET is usually normocellular and shows a predominance of enlarged megakaryocytes with hyperlobated nuclei and abundant cytoplasm. Special stain usually shows normal to slightly increased reticulin fibers in the early stages of PV and ET.

PMF will show a uniformly hypercellular BM with granulocytic and megakaryocytic hyperplasia and relative erythroid hypoplasia in the "pre-fibrotic" phase when leukocytosis predominates. Atypical megakaryocytes often form dense clusters around the sinuses, and have "staghorn" nuclear contours with "cloud-like" chromatin. In the fibrotic (spent) phase, fully developed myelophtisis is seen with leukoerythroblastosis (circulating marrow elements including blasts) and dacrocytosis (tear-drop shaped RBCs). BM shows great variability with empty areas alternating with areas of dense reticulin and/or collagen fibrosis, accompanied by osteosclerosis, dilated sinuses, and intrasinusoidal hematopoiesis. Cytogenetic studies are extremely useful in the evaluation of pre-fibrotic PMF that lacks JAK2/MPL mutations, as up to one-third of cases will show a characteristic clonal abnormality (Table 9-5).

As disease progresses, PV and ET show increasing fibrosis (and associated osteosclerosis) eventually becoming indistinguishable from PMF. Most of the fibrosis is believed to result from abnormal megakaryocytic proliferation, which is more pronounced in ET. Clonogenic involvement of endothelial and stromal elements may also contribute, as JAK-STAT signaling through EPO and other cytokine receptors is active in these cell types [15].

The most important role for BM biopsy after diagnosis is the detection of accelerated phase (10–19% blasts), blast transformation, and secondary MDS/AML. This is often a diagnostic challenge because the fibrosis in advanced PV, ET and especially PMF precludes obtaining an adequate aspirate. Therefore, use of CD34 immunostaining is recommended for an accurate blast enumeration. The phenotype of blasts in accelerated phase typically have a myeloid phenotype, with AML cases showing the full range of FAB phenotypes.

9.2.4. Detection of JAK2 and MPL Mutations at Diagnosis

The presence of a valine to phenylalanine substitution mutation at codon 617 of the JAK2 kinase was reported simultaneously by three groups in 2005, and was subsequently shown by many centers to occur in ~95% of PV, and 40-50% of ET and PMF (Table 9-5) [16–21].

Table 9-5. Genetic features of PV, ET and PMF.

Type	% JAK2 V617F	% MPL W515L/K	%TET2 mutations [12]	% with karyotype changes at diagnosis	Chromosomal changes
PV	95[a]	0	15–20	20	del(20q), +8, +9
ET	45	5	5	10	As above, chr1q changes
PMF	50	5	15–20	40	As above, del(13q), +1

[a]JAK2 exon 12 mutations seen in the majority of the rare PV cases that are negative for V617F [13,14]

Homozygous V617F mutation (usually arising through uniparental disomy) [22] increased mutated gene dosage due to trisomy 9, and heterozygous mutation with deletion of the other JAK2 locus occur frequently, particularly in PV [18]. Subsequent studies have identified JAK2 exon 12 deletions in the rare PV cases without JAK2 V617F, [13,14,23] and W515L or W515K activating mutations in the thrombopoietin receptor (MPL/TPOR) in 5–10% of ET and PMF lacking the JAK2 V617F [24,25]. MPL mutations may occur concurrently with JAK2 V617F in a small number of cases, suggesting that these mutations could be functionally complementing [13].

For diagnosis of PV, ET, and PMF, initial assessment for JAK2 V617F followed by detection of either JAK2 exon 12 mutation for patients with suspected PV, or MPL W515L/K mutation for patients with suspected ET or PMF is a reasonable approach. However, the appropriate sample source and testing method are still far from clear. Both RNA and DNA have been used to detect the levels of JAK2-mutated transcript versus gene copy number, respectively. Some studies have recommended using BM over PB, and sorting of granulocytes or megakaryocytes to improve detection. In our experience, levels of JAK2 V617F mutation in unsorted PB and BM are similar and are not likely to alter detection rates except when very low mutation burdens are present (see below).

In contrast, the choice of a detection assay can greatly influence the detection frequency and how the results are interpreted. Most of the initial studies on JAK2/MPL mutation frequency utilized the relatively insensitive and non-quantitative restriction-fragment length polymorphism (RFLP) or direct Sanger sequencing method which has a lower limit of sensitivity of 20%. Quantitation of mutation levels, using pyrosequencing (lower limit 1%) or mutation-specific quantitative PCR (lower limit 0.01%), has revealed that PV almost always has higher mutation burden at diagnosis than ET [18] and PMF and these differences can be helpful in diagnosis. Low levels of JAK2 mutations (e.g., 5–20% of the level of unmutated DNA) are common in early ET and in patients presenting with isolated splanchnic vein thrombosis [26]. Extremely low levels of JAK2 mutation can be detected in 10% to 30% of healthy individuals if qPCR is used [5]. These results suggest that the optimal JAK2 and MPL mutation assays should have a minimum diagnostic sensitivity of around 1% and provide quantitation to exclude reporting false-positive results seen in healthy individuals.

9.2.5. Role of JAK2 and MPL Mutation in MPN Transformation

JAK2, located at chromosome 9p24, encodes the Janus kinase 2 which binds to a membrane proximal proline-rich region of the cytokine receptors EPO, TPO, GM-CSF, and G-CSF following cytokine-induced conformational changes. JAK2 phosphorylates the receptor, STAT5, and other SH2-containing recruited signaling proteins (Fig. 9-2). STAT5 then homo- and heterodimerizes via its phosphorylated SH2 domains and translocates to the cell nucleus to act as a transcriptional factor for many genes involved in hematopoietic cells growth and differentiation. The phosphorylated cytokine receptors also bind signaling molecules such as the SHP phosphatases and phosphatidylinositol 3-kinase (PI3K) which activates the AKT signaling cascade (Fig. 9-2).

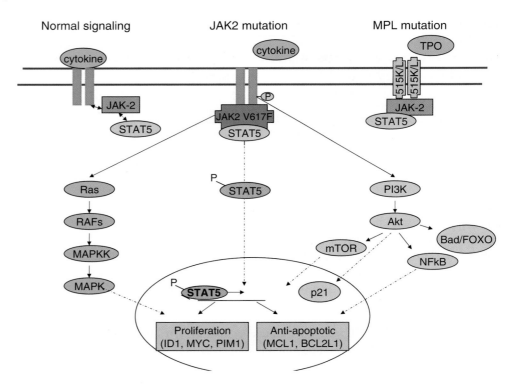

Fig. 9-2. Cytokine signaling alterations in myeloproliferative neoplasms. Hypersensitivity cytokine receptor signaling following the activating V617F mutation in JAK2 is illustrated in the center. The normal growth factor-induced association of JAK-STAT with cytokine receptors is illustrated on the left side. The association of MPL codon 515 point mutation with hyperactive JAK2-STAT signaling of the thrombopoietin receptor seen in some cases of ET and PMF is shown on the right side. Phosphorylation of STAT5 by JAK2 leads to its disassociation from membrane complexes and migration to the nucleus where it binds to promoter DNA sequences and drives transcription of numerous growth and anti-apoptotic genes.

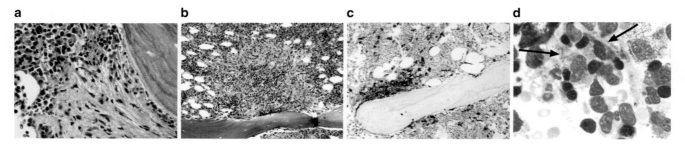

Fig. 9-3. Systemic mastocytosis, bone marrow findings. (**a**) Typical spindled appearance of neoplastic mast in a paratrabecular location in bone marrow. (**b**) Zonated appearance of mast cell aggregates with central core of small lymphocytes. (**c**) CD117 immunostain highlights mast cell aggregates and scattered interstitial forms. (**d**) Appearance of neoplastic hypergranular mast cells on BM aspirate (arrows)

The V617F mutation occurs in the negative regulatory domain of JAK2 allowing it to bind and phosphorylate the cytokine receptors more avidly following autophosphorylation. As a result, the JAK2 V617F mutation induces hypersensitive or even EPO-independent growth and activation of STAT5, PI3K, and ERK in cell lines [18]. The association of JAK2 V617F mutation with a particular JAK2 haplotype further supports functional cooperativity between somatic mutation development and genetic polymorphisms in the JAK-STAT pathway in development of JAK2-mutated MPNs [59].

MPL mutations leads to constitutive JAK-STAT signaling through MPL/TPOR. Introduction of W515L mutation into MPL in cell lines confers cytokine-independent growth and TPO hypersensitivity, with constitutive autophosphorylation of JAK2. Mouse models of JAK2 and MPL mutation have also confirmed their role in MPN transformation, and replicated some but not all of the various disease manifestations of PV, ET and PMF. Mice receiving bone marrow transplant with stem cells containing the JAK2 V617F mutation develop erythrocytosis [27,28]. Expression of MPL W515L in murine bone marrow transplant models leads to an MPN with certain features of human PMF [25].

The clinical characteristics of MPN with JAK2 mutation differ from those without any detectable mutations. For example, cases of ET with JAK2 V617F mutation are associated with older age, higher leukocyte and hemoglobin levels, as well as an increased risk of thrombosis [7,9]. Cases of ET with MPL mutations may have higher platelet counts than JAK/MPL-unmutated cases, [29] but risk of thrombosis, major hemorrhage, myelofibrotic transformation appears independent of mutation status [29,30]. However, JAK2 and MPL mutational status do not appear to be strong independent predictors of inferior survival. This may be due to similar dysregulated JAK-STAT cytokine signaling by other mechanisms in MPNs without JAK2 and MPL mutations. Promoter methylation silencing of SOCS3, SOCS1 and PTPN6, which are negative regulators of JAK signaling, likely represents one such alternative mechanism [31]. Overexpression of TPO, producing repression of the GATA1 transcription factors, may shift the balance toward overexpression of fibrogenic cytokines such as TGFβ, PDGF, basic FGF, and VEGF [32].

9.2.6. Other Genetic Changes in PV, ET and PMF

The absence of germline JAK2 mutations in patients with a familial/inherited MPNs suggests that there must be other mechanisms of tumor initiation [33,34]. The variability in the outcome among MPNs with the same JAK2 mutation also strongly supports the importance of other genetic changes in determining phenotype [35]. Further evidence that PV, ET and PMF exist along the same disease spectrum can be seen by the presence of both distinct and shared genomic changes in PV, ET, and PMF. Cytogenetic aberrations are found at diagnosis in approximately 20% of patients with PV and include del(20q), +8, and +9 (increasing gene dosage for JAK2) [36]. Although less common, these same changes with the addition of chromosome 1q and 1p34-35 (spanning the MPL locus) rearrangements also occur in ET [37]. Finally, cytogenetic changes are much more common in PMF at diagnosis and include the same changes with the addition of del(13q), +1, and chromosome 1q21 rearrangements [31,38].

The mechanisms of transformation in MPNs lacking JAK2/MPL mutation are still under investigation. Recently, loss of function mutations in the tumor suppressor TET2 have been reported in 5-20% of MPNs, including both JAK2-mutated and unmutated cases [12]. As with del(20q) changes, TET2 mutations can precede or follow JAK2 mutations suggesting independent transforming activities, as does their common finding in MDS and AML [39]. Mutations in the ubiquitin ligase CBL occur frequently in the MPNs with atypical features (e.g., atypical CML) [40].

9.2.7. Differential Diagnoses

JAK2-mutated MPN should be distinguished from other myeloid neoplasms, including Ph-positive CML, other Ph-negative MPN, chronic myelomonocytic leukemia (CMML), and MDS with isolated del(5q) that sometimes produces marked thrombocytosis. Screening for the presence of BCR-ABL1 fusion transcript and JAK2 V617F, JAK2 exon 12, as well as MPL W515L/K mutation is recommended for all new presentations of possible MPN or MDS/MPN (See screening algorithm presented in Fig. 11-1). Significant dyserythropoiesis or dysgranunolopoiesis suggest a diagnosis of MDS. There are two clinically distinct myeloid diseases which can have JAK2 V617F mutation; RARS-T is similar to ET but has dysplastic features, and may just be MDS that has acquired a JAK2 mutation [41]. CMML, regarded as an overlap MDS/MPN disorder, may rarely show JAK2 mutation, and often shows TET2 mutations like MPNs, but will have isolated peripheral blood monocytosis.

9.3. Mastocytosis

9.3.1. Mastocytosis and Its Variants

The WHO classification schema for tumors arising from mast cells has been made unnecessarily difficult (Table 9-6). This unfortunate complexity has impeded the simple observation that mast cell tumors (like any other neoplasm) can have localized and systemic presentations and varying degrees of clinical aggressiveness.

Infiltrates restricted to the dermis of skin (cutaneous mastocytosis, CM) show one of the three patterns, including the common maculopapular rash known as urticaria pigmentosa (UP), rare cases with diffuse rash, and the extremely rare tumor-forming solitary mastocytoma seen in young children [42]. CM typically involves the trunk and extremities with a tendency to spare sun-exposed areas. Mast cell degranulation after physical stimulation or exposure to heat producing swelling and redness is a diagnostic clue ("Darier's sign"). Pure CM is rare in adults and childhood cases usually resolve spontaneously by puberty suggesting most may be driven by allergic reactions to exogenous antigen.

In contrast, adult-onset systemic mastocytosis (SM) involving the BM, skin, and other sites has features of a clonal BM disorder that does not regress without treatment.

Table 9-6. Diagnostic criteria for mastocytosis and its variants.

Diagnostic criteria	Description of criteria
Localized or tumor-forming mast cell proliferations	
Cutaneous mastocytosis	Limited to skin, with urticaria pigmentosa, diffuse and mastocytoma types
Extracutaneous mastocytoma	Unifocal, non-destructive growth pattern, low-grade cytology
Mast cell sarcoma	Unifocal, destructive growth pattern, high-grade cytology
Systemic mastocytosis (SM)	
Diagnosis of SM requires major and 1 minor, or 3 minor criteria	*Major*: Multifocal, dense infiltrates of mast cells ($\geq$15 mast cells in aggregate) in BM and/or other extra-cutaneous organ
	Minor:
	1. Atypical morphology in >25% of the mast cells
	2. Detection of an activating point mutation at codon 816 of KIT
	3. Coexpression of CD2 and/or CD25 in addition to normal mast cell markers
	4. Persistently elevated serum tryptase level of >20 ng/mL
Aggressive SM with one or more "C" findings	1. One or more cytopenia (ANC < 1.0×10^9/L, Hb < 10 g/dL, or platelets < 100×10^9/L)
	2. Palpable splenomegaly with hypersplenism
	3. Palpable hepatomegaly with impairment of liver function
	4. Skeletal involvement with large osteolytic lesions and/or pathological fractures
	5. Malabsorption with weight loss due to GI mast cell infiltrates
SM with associated clonal haematological non-mast cell lineage disease (AHNMD)	Common associated neoplasms are CMML, MDS or hypereosinophilic syndrome
Indolent SM	No "C" findings
	No evidence of AHNMD
Mast cell leukaemia (MCL)	Leukemic mast cells $\geq$10% of cells in blood (or $\geq$20% on BM aspirate)
	"Aleukemic" variant if <10% of cells in blood

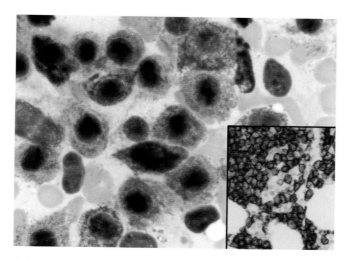

Fig. 9-4. Mast cell leukemia. Epithelioid mast cells with densely granular cytoplasm in BM aspirate and in peripheral blood (not shown). All tumor cells were strongly immunopositive for CD117 (inset) and mast cell tryptase (not shown) on BM core biopsy

Skin lesions are seen in 50% of adult patients with SM [42]. Major symptoms in SM are related to the release of mast cell mediators and destructive mast cell infiltration, and include constitutional symptoms, flushing, syncope, hypotension, tachycardia, GI distress, abdominal pain, and bone and muscle pain. SM is generally diagnosed after the second decade of life, with a male-to-female ratio varying from 1:1 to 1:3, and the majority of patients have an indolent course with a normal life expectancy [43].

However, one of the most intriguing aspects of SM is its association in a subset of patients with other clonal haematological non-mast cell lineage diseases (SM-AHNMD). These conditions can include HES, MDS, and CMML as well as various cytopenias not meeting the criteria for a distinct neoplasm [35]. Most of the associated neoplasms appear to be clonally related to the mast cell clone, as they often share KIT mutation [44]. Patients with SM-AHNMD generally have a shorter survival attributable to the SM-associated neoplasm. Rare patients with a leukemic form of SM usually have a rapid clinical course with a median survival of approximately 6 months (Fig. 9-4) [43].

9.3.2. Pathologic Features and Useful Laboratory Testing

The mast cell infiltrates in CM are often minimally atypical and show dense band-like, perivascular or periadnexal dermal infiltration without epidermal infiltration. Toluidine blue stain may be helpful in highlighting the mast cell granules. In SM, the BM is almost always involved and demonstrates multifocal, sharply demarcated clusters of enlarged and spindled mast cells with sparse and atypical cytoplasmic granules that don't resemble normal mast cells (Fig. 9-3). Mast cells with bilobed or multilobated nuclei may also be seen. The frequently paratrabecular mast cell aggregates in BM often have a central core of lymphocyte with eosinophils at the periphery and marked reticulin fibrosis. Other organs involved in SM include spleen, lymph node, liver, and gastrointestinal tract [43]. Circulating mast cells in SM and mast cell leukemia (Fig. 9-4, diagnosed when mast cells comprise 20% of cellularity on BM aspirate, and/or 10% of circulating leukocytes) is an ominous sign.

Flow cytometric detection using a sequential gating strategy is a highly sensitive method of detecting the SM mast cells in BM aspirate samples. This is because, in addition to CD117, neoplastic mast cells express CD25 and/or CD2, both of which are rarely uniformly expressed in nonneoplastic mast cells [45]. Elevation of serum (mast cell) tryptase levels (≥20 ng/mL) is also helpful in the diagnosis and residual disease detection in SM. Serum tryptase levels are normal to slightly elevated in most patients with CM limiting its utility in skin presentations [43]. Mast cell tryptase and CD117 immunostains can be used to detect CM and SM in tissue biopsies (Figs. 9-3 and 9-4).

9.3.3. KIT Mutation: Pathogenesis and Detection Methods

The KIT gene, located at chromosome 4q12, encodes a receptor tyrosine kinase that has a central role in myeloid, mast cell, neural crest (melanocyte), and gamete development [46,47]. Upon binding to its ligand, stem cell factor (SCF), KIT signals through multiple signaling pathways including PI3K-AKT, phospholipase Cγ, JAK-STAT, and RAS-MAPK [48]. Activating mutations of KIT, which occur in AML, SM, germ cell tumors, and gastrointestinal stromal tumors result in constitutive, ligand-independent KIT autoactivation. In mast cell disease, KIT mutations are largely restricted to codon 816 in exon 17 (usually D816V) and occur in 50-95% of adults with SM and 30-50% of pediatric patients with cutaneous mastocytosis [49,50]. The detection of KIT mutations in other cell lineages in SM may explain the increased association with other hematopoietic tumors (i.e., SM-AHNMD) [51]. Other rare sites of KIT mutation in SM include D820G, E839K, F522C, and V560G [48]. Although the kinase inhibitor imatinib (Gleevec) is active against the KIT kinase, the D816V mutation is largely resistant, and the other inhibitors such as dasatinib or PKC412 have shown more clinical activity [52].

Although rates of KIT codon 816 mutation rates as high as 100% have been reported in some series of SM, [53] our experience and that of others is closer to an incidence of 75% [37]. These discrepancies may be explained by varying diagnostic criteria or the differing

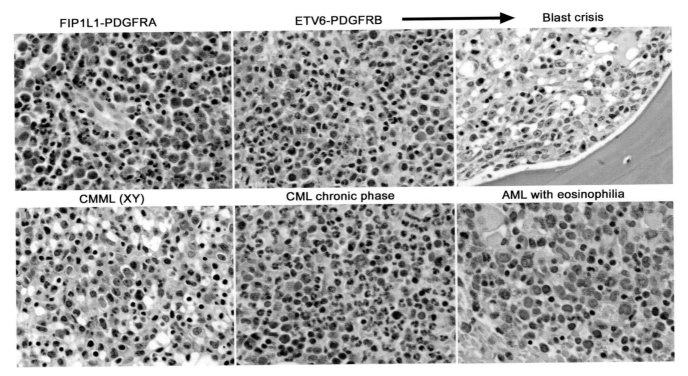

Fig. 9-5. Bone marrow findings in various types of hypereosinophilic syndrome. Chronic eosinophilic leukemia with FIP1L1-PDGFRA gene fusion shows a predominance of eosinophilic forms (*top left*). In contrast, MPN with t(5;12)(q33;p13)/ETV6-PDGFRB shows pan-myeloid hyperplasia (*top middle*),with more rapid progression. In this case, blast crisis/AML occurred within 4 months of presentation accompanied by clonal evolution (+8 and +11, in this case) (*top right*). Eosinophilia is also seen with other stem cell leukemias such as CMML (*bottom left*), CML (*bottom middle*) and AML (*bottom right*)

Table 9-7. Partner genes involved in the rearrangements of PDGFRA, PDGFRB, and FGFR1.

Tyrosine kinase gene	Chromosome location	Partner gene (most common partner is first)	Chromosome location
PDGFRA	4q12	FIP1L1	4q12
		STRN	2p24
		CDK5RAP2	9q33
		KIF5B	10p11
		ETV6	12p13
		BCR	22q11
PDGFRB	5q31-33	ETV6/TEL	12p13
		TPM3	1q21
		PDE4DIP	1q22
		WDR48	3p22
		GOLGA4	3p22
		PRKG2	4q21
		HIP1	7q11
		CCDC6/H4	10q21
		GPIAP1	11p13
		GIT2	12q24
		NIN	14q24
		KIAA1509	14q32
		TRIP11/CEV14	14q32
		TP53BP1	15q22
		NDE1	16p13
		SPECC1	17p11
		RABEP1	17p13
FGFR1	8p11	ZNF198/RAMP/FIM	13q12
		FGFR1OP/FOP	6q27
		TIF1	7q34
		CEP110	9q33
		FGFR1OP2	12p11
		MYO18A	17q11
		LOC113386/HERV-K	19q13
		BCR	22q11

sensitivity of techniques for mutation detection. Given the focal nature of mast cell aggregates in SM (and their poor sampling in BM aspirates due to tumor-associated fibrosis), direct Sanger sequencing is not recommended for mutation detection. We favor the use of pyrosequencing (lower limit of sensitivity of 1%) or mutation-specific quantitative PCR (lower sensitivity of 0.01%) on DNA extracted from grossly-microdissected, involved BM biopsy or skin samples [44]. Testing can also be done on mast cells sorted from bone marrow aspirate samples. Use of non-quantitative mutation-specific PCR is not recommended given the difficulties in ensuring adequate assay specificity with this technique. To date, mutations and chromosomal rearrangements involving genes other than KIT are rare in SM, and generally occur when an AHNMD is also present.

9.4. Hypereosinophilic Syndromes

9.4.1. Overview

Eosinophilia has the most complex workup among all of the MPNs [54]. Reactive causes of eosinophilia, such as drug reaction, parasite infection, allergic states, and T-cell lymphoma or Hodgkin lymphoma are far more common than the primary hematopoietic disorders. Common myeloid neoplasms associated with eosinophilia include acute myelomonocytic leukemia, CML, and CMML (Fig. 9-5).

Extremely rare but genetic distinct MPNs that produce eosinophilia are due to activation of the receptor tyrosine kinases PDGFRA, PDGFRB, and FGFR1, by gene fusion through chromosome rearrangements. Multiple fusion gene partners have been reported, with the most common being FIP1L1, ETV6/TEL, and ZNF198 for PDGFRA, PEGFRB, and FGFR1, respectively (Table 9-7) [55]. These fusion proteins produce constitutive kinase activation, and upregulation of growth and survival pathways but there appears to be considerable heterogeneity in the cell populations affected [55,56]. PDGFRA rearrangements usually present as chronic eosinophilic leukemia (CEL) with or without mast cell proliferations [52] whereas PDGFRB- and FGFR1-translocated cases produce stem cell leukemias, with mixed cell proliferations, and are more likely to progress to AML (Fig. 9-5) [56,57].

All PDGFR/FGFR1-translocated MPNs show BM hypercellularity with eosinophilia including hyposegmented and abnormally granulated dysplastic forms, leukocytosis, and spleen infiltration [56]. Factors generally associated with unfavorable outcome include marked splenomegaly, elevated blasts in blood or BM, dysplastic features in other myeloid lineages, and additional cytogenetic abnormalities. The most common molecular abnormality in this group is the cytogenetically occult FIP1L1-PDGFRA fusion resulting from ~800 kilobase interstitial deletion at 4q12, which is best detected by FISH using a probe against the CHIC2 gene located between FIP1L1 and PDGFRA which is deleted by the translocation [58]. Karyotyping or FISH can be used to detect PDGFRB- or FGFR1-translocated cases.

Selected Reviews

Cross NCP, Reiter A. Fibroblast growth factor receptor and platelet-derived growth factor receptor abnormalities in eosinophilic myeloproliferative disorders. Acta Haematol 2008;119:199–206.

Lim K, Pardanani A, Tefferi A. *KIT* and mastocytosis. Acta Haematol 2008;119:194–8.

Tefferi A. JAK and MPL mutations in myeloid malignancies. Leuk Lymphoma 2008;49:388–97.

References

1. Thiele J, Kvasnicka HM, Orazi A, Tefferi A, Birgegard G. Polycythaemia vera. In: Swerdlow SH, Campo E, Harris NL, et al., eds. WHO classfication of tumours of haematopoietic and lymphoid tissues. Lyon: IARC, 2008:40–3.
2. Thiele J, Kvasnicka HM, Tefferi A, Barosi G, Orazi A, Vardiman JW. Primary myelofibrosis. In: Swerdlow SH, Campo E, Harris NL, eds. WHO classification of tumours of haematopoetic and lymphoid tissues. Lyon, France, IARC Press. 2008:44–7.
3. Finazzi G. Essential thrombocythemia. Cancer Treat Res 2008;142:51–68.
4. Johansson P. Epidemiology of the myeloproliferative disorders polycythemia vera and essential thrombocythemia. Semin Thromb Hemost 2006;32(3):171–3.
5. Silver RT. Polycythemia vera and other polycythemia syndromes. Cancer Treat Res 2008; 142:1–27.
6. Steensma DP, Tefferi A. Cytogenetic and molecular genetic aspects of essential thrombocythemia. Acta Haematol 2002;108(2):55–65.
7. Wolanskyj AP, Lasho TL, Schwager SM, et al. JAK2 mutation in essential thrombocythaemia: clinical associations and long-term prognostic relevance. Br J Haematol 2005;131(2):208–13.
8. Cervantes F, Passamonti F, Barosi G. Life expectancy and prognostic factors in the classic BCR/ABL-negative myeloproliferative disorders. Leukemia 2008;22(5):905–14.
9. Dahabreh IJ, Zoi K, Giannouli S, Zoi C, Loukopoulos D, Voulgarelis M. Is JAK2 V617F mutation more than a diagnostic index? A meta-analysis of clinical outcomes in essential thrombocythemia. Leuk Res 2009;33(1):67–73.
10. Theocharides A, Boissinot M, Girodon F, et al. Leukemic blasts in transformed JAK2–V617F-positive myeloproliferative disorders are frequently negative for the JAK2–V617F mutation. Blood 2007;110(1):375–9.
11. Kussick SJ, Wood BL. Four-color flow cytometry identifies virtually all cytogenetically abnormal bone marrow samples in the workup of non-CML myeloproliferative disorders. Am J Clin Pathol 2003;120(6):854–65.

12. Tefferi A, Pardanani A, Lim KH, et al. TET2 mutations and their clinical correlates in polycythemia vera, essential thrombocythemia and myelofibrosis. Leukemia 2009;23(5):905–11.

13. Pardanani A, Lasho TL, Finke C, Hanson CA, Tefferi A. Prevalence and clinicopathologic correlates of JAK2 exon 12 mutations in JAK2V617F-negative polycythemia vera. Leukemia 2007;21(9):1960–3.

14. Pietra D, Li S, Brisci A, et al. Somatic mutations of JAK2 exon 12 in patients with JAK2 (V617F)-negative myeloproliferative disorders. Blood 2008;111(3):1686–9.

15. Oppliger Leibundgut E, Horn MP, Brunold C, et al. Hematopoietic and endothelial progenitor cell trafficking in patients with myeloproliferative diseases. Haematologica 2006;91(11):1465–72.

16. Baxter EJ, Scott LM, Campbell PJ, et al. Acquired mutation of the tyrosine kinase JAK2 in human myeloproliferative disorders. Lancet 2005;365(9464):1054–61.

17. James C, Ugo V, Le Couedic JP, et al. A unique clonal JAK2 mutation leading to constitutive signalling causes polycythaemia vera. Nature 2005;434(7037):1144–8.

18. Jones AV, Kreil S, Zoi K, et al. Widespread occurrence of the JAK2 V617F mutation in chronic myeloproliferative disorders. Blood 2005;106(6):2162–8.

19. Kralovics R, Passamonti F, Buser AS, et al. A gain-of-function mutation of JAK2 in myeloproliferative disorders. N Engl J Med 2005;352(17):1779–90.

20. Levine RL, Wadleigh M, Cools J, et al. Activating mutation in the tyrosine kinase JAK2 in polycythemia vera, essential thrombocythemia, and myeloid metaplasia with myelofibrosis. Cancer Cell 2005;7(4):387–97.

21. Steensma DP, Dewald GW, Lasho TL, et al. The JAK2 V617F activating tyrosine kinase mutation is an infrequent event in both "atypical" myeloproliferative disorders and myelodysplastic syndromes. Blood 2005;106(4):1207–9.

22. Kawamata N, Ogawa S, Yamamoto G, et al. Genetic profiling of myeloproliferative disorders by single-nucleotide polymorphism oligonucleotide microarray. Exp Hematol 2008;36(11):1471–9.

23. Scott LM, Tong W, Levine RL, et al. JAK2 exon 12 mutations in polycythemia vera and idiopathic erythrocytosis. N Engl J Med 2007;356(5):459–68.

24. Pardanani AD, Levine RL, Lasho T, et al. MPL515 mutations in myeloproliferative and other myeloid disorders: a study of 1182 patients. Blood 2006;108(10):3472–6.

25. Pikman Y, Lee BH, Mercher T, et al. MPLW515L is a novel somatic activating mutation in myelofibrosis with myeloid metaplasia. PLoS Med 2006;3(7):e270.

26. Kiladjian JJ, Cervantes F, Leebeek FW, et al. The impact of JAK2 and MPL mutations on diagnosis and prognosis of splanchnic vein thrombosis: a report on 241 cases. Blood 2008;111(10):4922–9.

27. Zaleskas VM, Krause DS, Lazarides K, et al. Molecular pathogenesis and therapy of polycythemia induced in mice by JAK2 V617F. PLoS ONE 2006;1:e18.

28. Wernig G, Mercher T, Okabe R, Levine RL, Lee BH, Gilliland DG. Expression of Jak2V617F causes a polycythemia vera-like disease with associated myelofibrosis in a murine bone marrow transplant model. Blood 2006;107(11):4274–81.

29. Vannucchi AM, Antonioli E, Guglielmelli P, et al. Clinical profile of homozygous JAK2 617V>F mutation in patients with polycythemia vera or essential thrombocythemia. Blood 2007;110(3):840–6.

30. Beer PA, Campbell PJ, Scott LM, et al. MPL mutations in myeloproliferative disorders: analysis of the PT-1 cohort. Blood 2008;112(1):141–9.

31. Dingli D, Grand FH, Mahaffey V, et al. Der(6)t(1;6)(q21-23;p21.3): a specific cytogenetic abnormality in myelofibrosis with myeloid metaplasia. Br J Haematol 2005;130(2):229–32.

32. Chou JM, Li CY, Tefferi A. Bone marrow immunohistochemical studies of angiogenic cytokines and their receptors in myelofibrosis with myeloid metaplasia. Leuk Res 2003;27(6):499–504.

33. Liu K, Kralovics R, Rudzki Z, et al. A de novo splice donor mutation in the thrombopoietin gene causes hereditary thrombocythemia in a Polish family. Haematologica 2008;93(5):706–14.

34. Skoda R, Prchal JT. Lessons from familial myeloproliferative disorders. Semin Hematol 2005;42(4):266–73.

35. Li S, Kralovics R, De Libero G, Theocharides A, Gisslinger H, Skoda RC. Clonal heterogeneity in polycythemia vera patients with JAK2 exon12 and JAK2–V617F mutations. Blood 2008;111(7):3863–6.

36. Westwood NB, Gruszka-Westwood AM, Pearson CE, et al. The incidences of trisomy 8, trisomy 9 and D20S108 deletion in polycythaemia vera: an analysis of blood granulocytes using interphase fluorescence in situ hybridization. Br J Haematol 2000;110(4):839–46.

37. Tefferi A. Primary myelofibrosis. Cancer Treat Res 2008;142:29–49.

38. Hussein K, Van Dyke DL, Tefferi A. Conventional cytogenetics in myelofibrosis: Literature review and discussion. Eur J Haematol 2009;82(5):329–38.

39. Jankowska AM, Szpurka H, Tiu RV, et al. Loss of heterozygosity 4q24 and TET2 mutations associated with myelodysplastic/myeloproliferative neoplasms. Blood 2009;113(25)):6403–10.

40. Grand FH, Hidalgo-Curtis CE, Ernst T, et al. Frequent CBL mutations associated with 11q acquired uniparental disomy in myeloproliferative neoplasms. Blood 2009;113(24):6182–92.

41. Schnittger S, Bacher U, Kern W, Haferlach T, Haferlach C. JAK2V617F as progression marker in CMPD and as cooperative mutation in AML with trisomy 8 and t(8;21): a comparative study on 1103 CMPD and 269 AML cases. Leukemia 2007;21(8):1843–5.

42. Horny HP, Akin C, Metcalfe DD, et al. Matocytosis. In: Swerdlow SH, Campo E, Harris NL, et al., eds. WHO classfication of tumours of haematopoietic and lymphoid tissues. Lyon: IARC, 2008:54–63.

43. Pardanani A, Akin C, Valent P. Pathogenesis, clinical features, and treatment advances in mastocytosis. Best Pract Res Clin Haematol 2006;19(3):595–615.

44. Zhao W, Bueso-Ramos CE, Verstovsek S, Barkoh BA, Khitamy AA, Jones D. Quantitative profiling of codon 816 KIT mutations can aid in the classification of systemic mast cell disease. Leukemia 2007;21(7):1574–6.

45. Escribano L, Orfao A, Diaz-Agustin B, et al. Indolent systemic mast cell disease in adults: immunophenotypic characterization of bone marrow mast cells and its diagnostic implications. Blood 1998;91(8):2731–6.

46. D'Auriol L, Mattei MG, Andre C, Galibert F. Localization of the human c-kit protooncogene on the q11–q12 region of chromosome 4. Hum Genet 1988;78(4):374–6.

47. Yarden Y, Kuang WJ, Yang-Feng T, et al. Human proto-oncogene c-kit: a new cell surface receptor tyrosine kinase for an unidentified ligand. Embo J 1987;6(11):3341–51.

48. Lim KH, Pardanani A, Tefferi A. KIT and mastocytosis. Acta Haematol 2008;119(4):194–8.

49. Furitsu T, Tsujimura T, Tono T, et al. Identification of mutations in the coding sequence of the proto-oncogene c-kit in a human mast cell leukemia cell line causing ligand-independent activation of c-kit product. J Clin Invest 1993;92(4):1736–44.

50. Nagata H, Worobec AS, Oh CK, et al. Identification of a point mutation in the catalytic domain of the protooncogene c-kit in peripheral blood mononuclear cells of patients who have mastocytosis with an associated hematologic disorder. Proc Natl Acad Sci USA 1995;92(23):10560–4.

51. Yavuz AS, Lipsky PE, Yavuz S, Metcalfe DD, Akin C. Evidence for the involvement of a hematopoietic progenitor cell in systemic mastocytosis from single-cell analysis of mutations in the c-kit gene. Blood 2002;100(2):661–5.

52. Akin C. Molecular diagnosis of mast cell disorders: a paper from the 2005 William Beaumont Hospital Symposium on Molecular Pathology. J Mol Diagn 2006;8(4):412–9.

53. Tan A, Westerman D, McArthur GA, Lynch K, Waring P, Dobrovic A. Sensitive detection of KIT D816V in patients with mastocytosis. Clin Chem 2006;52(12):2250–7.

54. Bacher U, Reiter A, Haferlach T, et al. A combination of cytomorphology, cytogenetic analysis, fluorescence in situ hybridization and reverse transcriptase polymerase chain reaction for establishing clonality in cases of persisting hypereosinophilia. Haematologica 2006;91(6):817–20.

55. Cross NC, Reiter A. Fibroblast growth factor receptor and platelet-derived growth factor receptor abnormalities in eosinophilic myeloproliferative disorders. Acta Haematol 2008;119(4):199–206.

56. Bain BJ, Gilliland DG, Horny HP, Vardiman JW. Myeloid and lymphoid neoplasms with eosinophilia and abnormalities of PDGFRA, PDGFRB or FGFR1. In: Swerdlow SH, Campo E, Harris NL, et al., eds. WHO classfication of tumours of haematopoietic and lymphoid tissues. Lyon: IARC, 2008:68–73.

57. Bain BJ, Fletcher SH. Chronic eosinophilic leukemias and the myeloproliferative variant of the hypereosinophilic syndrome. Immunol Allergy Clin North Am 2007;27(3):377–88.

58. Cools J, DeAngelo DJ, Gotlib J, et al. A tyrosine kinase created by fusion of the PDGFRA and FIP1L1 genes as a therapeutic target of imatinib in idiopathic hypereosinophilic syndrome. N Engl J Med 2003;348(13):1201–14.

59. Jones AV, Chose A, Silver RT et al. JAK2 haplotype is a mager risk factor for the development of myeloproliferative neoplasms Nature Genetics 2009;41:446–449.

Chapter 10

Chronic Myelogenous Leukemia

Robert P. Hasserjian

Abstract Chronic myelogenous leukemia, BCR-ABL1+ (CML), is a myeloproliferative neoplasm defined by the presence of the BCR-ABL fusion gene produced by the t(9;22) (q32;q11) cytogenetic abnormality. CML manifests clinically as leukocytosis with circulating immature granulocytic precursors and splenomegaly. When untreated, its natural history is that of inexorable progression to an acute leukemia (blast crisis) after a prolonged chronic phase. The recent development of inhibitors of BCR-ABL tyrosine kinase activity have dramatically altered the clinical course of CML, with long-term remissions in most patients treated early in the course of disease.

Keywords Chronic myelogenous leukemia (CML) • Philadelphia chromosome, BCR-ABL, kinase in CML • Chronic myelogenous leukemia, accelerated phase (definition) • Chronic myelogenous leukemia, blast phase/crisis • Chronic myelogenous leukemia, prognostic models (Sokol score) • Chronic myelogenous leukemia • Use of cytogenetics • Chronic myelogenous leukemia, use of PCR • Chronic myelogenous leukemia • Use of FISH • Imatinib (Gleevec), resistance (definitions) • Imatinib, primary resistance • Chronic myelogenous leukemia, BCR-ABL point mutation • Chronic myelogenous leukemia, imatinib (Gleevec) resistance • Chronic myelogenous leukemia, genetic progression

10.1. Definition and Historical Overview

Chronic myelogenous leukemia, BCR-ABL1+ (CML, synonyms: chronic myeloid leukemia and chronic myelocytic leukemia), is a myeloproliferative neoplasm defined by the presence of the BCR-ABL fusion gene that is usually associated with the t(9;22)(q34;q11) cytogenetic abnormality. When untreated, its natural history is that of inexorable progression to an acute leukemia (blast crisis) after a prolonged chronic phase.

The molecular etiology of CML has been revealed, and highly effective targeted therapies have been developed: the eventful history of these inspiring scientific advances spans a half century. Nowell and Hungerford first reported a small chromosome in the leukemic cells of two CML patients in 1960 [1]. This was termed the 'Philadelphia chromosome' according to the convention at the time to name abnormal chromosomes and proteins after the city of their discovery or origin (a tradition that is still preserved in the nomenclature of abnormal hemoglobin proteins today). The Philadelphia chromosome was the first genetic abnormality associated with a malignancy and helped establish the hypothesis proposed by Boveri in 1914 that cancers resulted from the expansion of a single genetically altered cell [2]. Subsequent

From: *Neoplastic Hematopathology*: Contemporary Hematology,
Edited by: D. Jones, DOI 10.1007/978-1-60761-384-8_10,
© Humana Press, a part of Springer Science+Business Media, LLC 2010

demonstration that the Philadelphia chromosome was the product of a reciprocal translocation between chromosomes 9 and 22 by Rowley in 1973 [3] and identification of the ABL1 proto-oncogene at this site in 1984 [4] set the stage for revealing the definitive link between a gene and a tumor: the introduction of BCR-ABL, the fusion gene resulting from the t(9;22), into hematopoietic cells caused CML in murine models [5]. The triumphant and gratifying culmination of this chapter in cancer research was the development of pharmacologic inhibitors of BCR-ABL that have dramatically improved the survival of CML patients since 2000. CML thus represents both the first cancer in which the genetic culprit was revealed and the first cancer to advance into the era of targeted molecular therapy as the treatment of choice; one hopes that the CML story will represent a paradigm for other cancers in which the molecular pathogenesis is still being solved.

10.2. Incidence and Demographics

The annual incidence of CML is 1.6/100,000 adults, with a slight male predominance; [6] the disease is rare in children and its incidence increases with age [7]. The median age at diagnosis is 65. There is no known geographic or familial disposition. The only known risk factor associated with the development of CML is ionizing radiation exposure; [8,9] some investigators have also noted a higher incidence in individuals exposed to benzene or alkylating agents [10].

10.3. Clinical Features and Diagnosis

The typical diagnostic features of CML are shown in Table 10-1. The main clinical manifestations of the disease are leukocytosis with increased circulating immature granulocytic precursors, basophilia, and splenomegaly. The peripheral blood features of CML are illustrated in Fig. 10-1. Patients typically present with clinical symptoms related to the increased white cell mass, including fatigue, weight loss, and/or abdominal discomfort due to splenomegaly; however, the disease is discovered incidentally in asymptomatic patients in up to 50% of cases [11,12].

The bone marrow biopsy in CML patients at diagnosis is markedly hypercellular, usually approaching 100% (Fig. 10-2). There is a marked predominance of maturing myeloid elements with a relative decrease in erythroid forms. Megakaryocytes are often increased and are usually smaller than normal with hypolobated nuclei, a feature that distinguishes them from the typical megakaryocyte morphology of other myeloproliferative neoplasms (MPNs), such as essential thrombocythemia and primary myelofibrosis. This is an important distinction because the bone marrow in CML may exhibit varying degrees of reticulin fibrosis,

Table 10-1. Typical features of chronic myelogenous leukemia in chronic phase.

Peripheral blood findings	Bone marrow findings	Molecular genetic findings
– Leukocytosis (median 100×10^9/L)	– Hypercellularity (usually 100%)	– Karyotype: t(9;22)(q34:q11) translocation or complex translocation involving 9q32 and 22q11 loci
– Increased immature myeloid precursors	– Increased myeloid:erythroid ratio (typically ~10:1)	
– Eosinophilia	– Increased myelocytes	– FISH: Fusion of BCR and ABL1 loci
– Basophilia	– Basophilia	
– Often thrombocytosis	– Small, hypolobated megakaryocytes	– RT-PCR: Fusion transcript of BCR and ABL1
	– Lack of morphologic dysplasia of erythroid and myeloid elements	

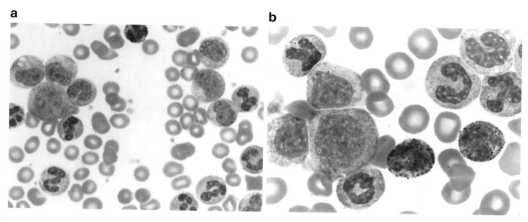

Fig. 10-1. *CML in chronic phase, peripheral blood.* (**a**) Marked leukocytosis present with a spectrum of maturing granulocytic elements. (**b**) Granulocytic elements show normal nuclear morphology and granulation; basophils are increased

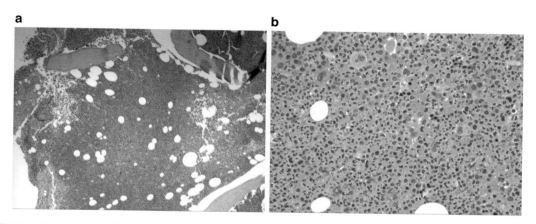

Fig. 10-2. *CML in chronic phase, bone marrow biopsy* (**a**) The marrow is markedly hypercellular. (**b**). Markedly increased myeloid to erythroid ratio present with numerous band and segmented granulocytes; erythroid elements are sparse

either at diagnosis or upon progression, potentially mimicking primary myelofibrosis. The bone marrow in CML also shows increased vascular density. The fibrosis and neoangiogenesis in CML appear to be due to cytokines elaborated by the CML hematopoietic cells, including PDGFRβ, FGFRβ, and TGFβ [13]. The bone marrow aspirate shows an elevated myeloid to erythroid ratio with a spectrum of all stages of granulocytic maturation represented (Fig. 10-3). Basophils and eosinophils are often increased. Unless in an advanced phase of disease, blasts comprise <10% of the marrow and peripheral blood cells and there is no significant morphologic dysplasia in erythroid and myeloid cells.

A bone marrow examination including biopsy, aspiration, and cytogenetics is recommended at diagnosis; flow cytometry has no current role in the diagnosis of CML in chronic phase, but is useful in determining the blast phenotype (lymphoid, myeloid, or biphenotypic) in blast crisis. The BCR-ABL translocation and t(9;22) can be readily detected in peripheral blood, and peripheral blood testing is acceptable for most disease monitoring on therapy. However, a pretherapy bone marrow sample is desirable, since bone marrow blast count is an important determinant of CML stage and may be higher than the peripheral blood blast count and adverse cytogenetic markers of clonal evolution are more readily detected in bone marrow than peripheral blood samples. Finally, the bone marrow biopsy may show reticulin

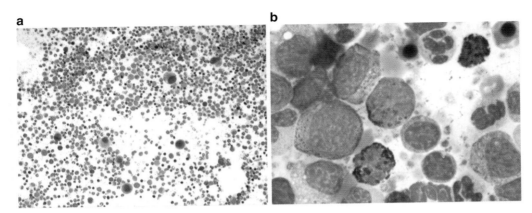

Fig. 10-3. *CML in chronic phase, bone marrow aspirate* (**a**) Aspirate smear is hypercellular with numerous small megakaryocytes with hypolobated and round nuclei. (**b**) A spectrum of nondysplastic maturing granulocytic elements and increased basophils present

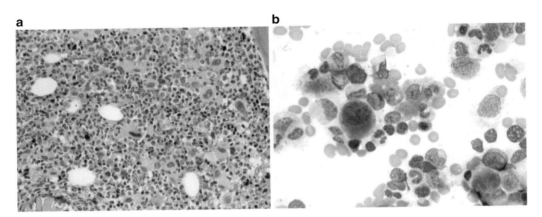

Fig. 10-4. *CML with marked thrombocytosis mimicking essential thrombocythemia.* Patient presented with platelet count of $1{,}093 \times 10^9$/L and only minimal leukocytosis, and showed t(9;22) by cytogenetic analysis. (**a**) Markedly hypercellular marrow with small, hypolobated megakaryocytes unlike the enlarged megakaryocytes with complex nuclear lobation seen in essential thrombocythemia. (**b**) Aspirate smear shows the relative myeloid hyperplasia and small megakaryocytes typical of CML

fibrosis, providing both prognostic information as well as a baseline to measure the reduction in reticulin fibrosis that occurs in most patients responding to imatinib [14].

Although the characteristic peripheral blood and bone marrow findings allow a presumptive diagnosis of CML in most cases, the BCR-ABL fusion gene is the defining feature of the disease [15]. Moreover, CML may present with atypical features, such as blunted leukocytosis due to concomitant metabolic deficiencies, marked eosinophilia, or prominent thrombocytosis (Fig. 10-4). Given the highly effective targeted therapies available to treat CML, molecular genetic testing should be performed to exclude this diagnosis in any suspected myeloproliferative process. Demonstration of a t(9;22)(q34;q11) translocation by karyotype or BCR-ABL fusion by reverse-transcriptase PCR (RT-PCR) or fluorescence in situ hybridization (FISH) is required to confirm a diagnosis of CML (Fig. 10-5). The absence of BCR-ABL effectively excludes CML, although in cases that are highly suspicious for CML and are unexpectedly negative for BCR-ABL by cytogenetics, FISH, or RT-PCR, an additional test, should be performed to exclude the occasional false negative results that can occur with any of these tests. A classical t(9;22) translocation is present in 95% of CML patients at diagnosis. The remaining cases (by definition) also bear a BCR-ABL fusion gene, but lack a classic t(9;22) due to a variant translocation involving additional chromosome(s) or, less commonly, a cryptic BCR-ABL fusion lacking abnormalities at the 9q34 or 22q11 loci

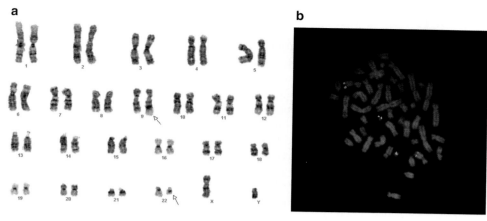

Fig. 10-5. Molecular genetics of CML (**a**) CML in chronic phase showing the typical t(9;22)(q34;q11) abnormality (arrows). (**b**) Metaphase FISH using the Vysis LSI ES Dual-Color Translocation probe set illustrates an intact chromosome 9 with a red (ABL1, 9q34) signal, an intact chromosome 22 with a green (BCR, q22q11.2) signal, and a Philadelphia chromosome (derivative 22) with a *green/red* BCR-ABL fusion signal, as well as the smaller *orange* signal on the derivative 9 chromosome

Table 10-2. Types of BCR-ABL fusion transcripts

Breakpoint in BCR gene	Fusion transcript	Fusion protein size (KDa)	Percentage of CML cases	Clinical features
M-bcr	e13a2	p210	99%	Typical CML
	e14a2			
M-bcr with ABL1 a3 breakpoints	e13a3	p210	1%	Uncertain
	e14a3			
m-bcr	e1a2	p190	<1%	Monocytosis
	e1a3 also occur very rarely			
μ-bcr	e19a2	p230	<1%	Less prominent myeloid immaturity
ν−bcr	e6a2	~p190	Very rare	May be more aggressive

on routine karyotyping. FISH or RT-PCR are not required in cases with a typical t(9;22) finding on cytogenetics, but they can help prove BCR-ABL fusion in cases with complex variant translocations or in the rare cytogenetically cryptic cases [16].

BCR-ABL fusion transcripts are named by the exons that span the 9q32 and 22q11 breakpoints. The most common types and their associated fusion proteins are listed in Table 10-2. In the vast majority of CML cases, the BCR breakpoints occur in the relatively small (5.8 kb) major breakpoint cluster region (M-bcr), located after either BCR exon 13 (e13, previously termed b2) or BCR exon 14 (e14, previously termed b3) [17] and result in a 210 kDa fusion protein (p210). While the breakpoint region within ABL1 is much more variable, spanning up to 300 kb [17,18], in almost all cases, this is located in a large intron before exon 2 (a2). The resulting fusion transcript thus contains most of the 3′ portion of the ABL1 gene (missing only exon 1 that eliminates a critical regulatory domain of ABL kinase function) fused to the 5′ portion of the BCR gene. About 1% of BCR-ABL translocations that utilize the M-bcr breakpoint involve ABL1 exon 3 (e13a3 and e14a3), thereby excluding the regulatory Src homology domain of ABL1 located in exon 2 [19]. These cases respond to imatinib, but their clinical behavior compared to the more common e13a2/e14a2 cases is uncertain [20].

Rare CML cases (about 0.3%) have a breakpoint in the minor breakpoint cluster region (m-bcr), resulting in an e1a2 transcript and a p190 fusion protein [21]. The latter has greater kinase activity that favors stem cell differentiation toward lymphoid rather than myeloid lineage in vitro; indeed, the p190 fusion protein is far more common in Ph+ B-ALL than in CML [22]. The extremely rare CML cases with p190 fusion protein often present with prominent monocytosis and usually lack splenomegaly but can show an altered RNA sequence [21], which may explain the absence of lymphoid blast crisis [23], In rare CML cases, the breakpoint occurs at the micro breakpoint cluster region (μ-bcr), generating an e19a2 transcript and a p230 fusion protein. Due to differential splicing, more than one transcript may be present in some cases, [24, 25] with most p210 cases expressing very low levels of the e1a2 transcript and many expressing both e13a2 and e14a2 transcripts. Long template qualitative RT-PCR can detect nearly all of these variants and thus represents the most sensitive method of detecting BCR-ABL in putative CML cases at diagnosis [26, 27]. The extremely rare e6a2 variant (involving the so-called "nano-BCR" breakpoint) may escape detection by even long template RT-PCR, requiring multiplex PCR utilizing a primer sequence from BCR exon 6 [28–30] FISH can also help confirm BCR-ABL fusion in these and other rare cases that are falsely negative by RT-PCR [31].

10.4. Pathogenesis of Chronic Phase Disease

The ABL1 gene is the human homologue of the Abelson murine leukemia virus oncogene and encodes a nonreceptor tyrosine kinase that shuttles between the nucleus and the cytoplasm [32]. ABL promotes cell growth and differentiation by its regulated kinase activity. Fusion with BCR (the breakpoint cluster region gene, a serine-threonine kinase) produces a constitutively active chimeric protein with aberrant cytoplasmic localization. BCR-ABL promotes neoplastic transformation via dysregulated phosphorylation of various substrates and activates the RAS, PI3K, and JAK-STAT pathways, among others (reviewed in [33, 34]). This genetic event affects an early hematopoietic stem cell and ultimately leads to the uncontrolled expansion of a myeloid neoplasm that replaces normal hematopoiesis in the bone marrow, but (unlike acute leukemias) maintains differentiation. The most characteristic features of CML hematopoiesis are a differentiation pattern that favors the granulocytic lineage over the erythroid lineage; deregulated proliferation, growth factor independence, and defective apoptosis that contribute to bone marrow hypercellularity and defective adhesion of immature cells to marrow stromal cells, resulting in their inappropriate entry into the peripheral blood and their colonization of extramedullary tissues such as the spleen [35, 36].

10.5. Patterns of Progression

The natural history of CML is characterized by evolution through three clinical phases of disease. Patients usually present in the chronic phase of disease (CML-CP), characterized by indolent and clinically stable features. However, in the absence of effective therapy, patients inexorably progress to an acute leukemia termed blast crisis (CML-BC). The median time to progression from CML-CP to CML-BC in untreated patients or in patients treated with older therapies such as hydroxyurea ranged from 3–5 years [37]. Blast crisis is typically preceded by an intermediate accelerated phase of disease (CML-AP) by a period of 4–6 months [38], but up to 25% of CML-BC cases develop without any clinically evident preceding accelerated phase, [39] usually due to acquisition of an AML-type second chromosomal translocation or a high-activity BCR-ABL kinase mutation.

According to the 2008 WHO Classification, elevated bone marrow and peripheral blood blast counts, increased peripheral blood basophil, and high or low platelet counts unresponsiveness to cytoreductive therapy, and cytogenetic evaluation are the parameters used to define CML-AP [15] (see Table 10-3 and Fig. 10-6). Dysplasia of peripheral blood granulocytes

Table 10-3. Staging system for chronic myelogenous leukemia (WHO Classification 2008).

Feature	Chronic phase	Accelerated phase	Blast crisis
Blast % in blood or bone marrow	<10%	10–19%	≥20%
Basophil % in blood	<20%	≥20%	NA
Thrombocytosis (×10⁹/L)	≤1000 or responsive to therapy if >1000	>1000, unresponsive to therapy	NA
Thrombocytopenia (×10⁹/L)	≥100 or related to therapy if <100	<100, unrelated to therapy	NA
Leukocytosis (×10⁹/L)	≤10 or responsive to therapy if >10	>10, unresponsive to therapy	NA
Splenomegaly	Responsive to therapy	Persistent or increasing, unresponsive to therapy	NA
Extramedullary blast tumor (chloroma)	Absent	Absent	Present
New cytogenetic changes that develop after the initial bone marrow karyotype[a]	Absent	Present	NA

[a]Most frequently observed changes of cytogenetic evolution are additional Philadelphia chromosome, isochromosome 17q, trisomy 8, and trisomy 19

NA: not applicable

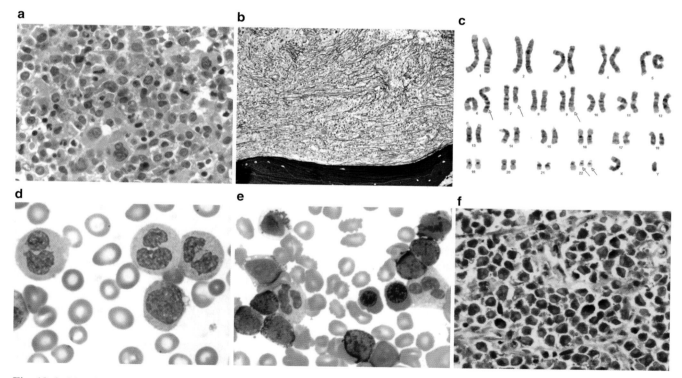

Fig. 10-6. *Morphologic and genetic progression in CML.* (**a**) CML-AP shows markedly left-shifted myeloid maturation with a paucity of mature forms; megakaryocytes are small with hypolobated nuclei. (**b**) Silver stain shows moderate reticulin fibrosis, a feature associated with progression to accelerated phase. (**c**) CML-AP with acquisition of an additional Philadelphia chromosome and a t(6;7)(q23-24;q11.2) abnormality. (**d**) CML-AP shows abnormal, bilobed dysplastic granulocytes. (**e**) CML in myeloid blast crisis shows numerous large blasts with a near absence of myeloid maturation. (**f**) A pelvic mass biopsy with sheets of blasts with myeloid phenotype by flow cytometry representing blast crisis of long-standing CML

(hypogranulation and nuclear hypolobation) can also be associated with CML-AP and may precede its diagnosis by conventional criteria [40]. Although not a defining feature of CML-AP in the WHO Classification, marked reticulin and/or collagen fibrosis in the bone marrow accompanied by a prominent increase in megakaryocytes is also associated with disease progression and was used as a defining feature of CML-AP according to International Bone Marrow Transplant Registry criteria [41]. Some clinicians and investigators use the criteria of Kantarjian et al to define CML-AP and CML-BC. These criteria differ somewhat from the WHO criteria, using higher blast count thresholds (15–29% for CML-AP and >30% for CML-BC) and taking into account the percentage of promyelocytes as well as blasts [42]. The CML staging systems have not been extensively validated in the current era of TKI therapy. One recent study suggests that patients with 20–29% blasts (classified as CML-BC according to WHO Classification criteria) and treated with imatinib have a prognosis similar to CML-AP rather than other CML-BC patients [43]. About 10% of CML patients present in advanced phases (CML-AP or CML-BC) without a clinically diagnosed chronic phase [44].

The progression to advanced phases of disease is caused by the development of genetic lesions in addition to BCR-ABL; secondary cytogenetic changes are identified in 85% of patients by the time of progression to CML-BC [45]. The most frequent secondary cytogenetic changes in advanced phase CML are trisomy 8, one or more additional Philadelphia chromosomes (derivative 22), and an isochromosome 17 [46]. Rare cases of CML may develop a concurrent inv(16)(p13q22) abnormality associated with transformation to CML-BC and often associated with abnormal eosinophils resembling those seen in de novo AML with inv(16) [47, 48]. In contrast to the relative simplicity of the link between BCR-ABL and CML development, the molecular events associated with CML progression are complex and appear to be variable among different patients (reviewed in reference [49]). This is not surprising, as one of the consequences of BCR-ABL expression is genetic instability and impaired DNA repair mechanisms [49–51]. In addition to cytogenetic aberrations, BCR-ABL amplification, gene mutations, and epigenetic changes such as gene methylation also appear to play a role in disease progression [52]. Gene expression profiling of CML cases reveals distinct expression patterns in CML-CP and advanced phase CML. However, the expression patterns in CML-AP and CML-BC are similar, suggesting that genetic progression in CML is a two-stage process and that CML-AP merely represents a clinical transitional phase reflecting molecularly evolved disease [53].

The additional genetic alterations in advanced phase CML eventually cause an arrest of maturation and the expansion of a blast population that fulfills diagnostic features of an acute leukemia. CML-BC may also manifest as an extramedullary tumor-forming proliferation of blasts, and in such situations is diagnosed as blast crisis irrespective of the peripheral blood or bone marrow blast count [15,54]. Supporting the primitive nature of the postulated CML stem cell, this blast crisis may exhibit a myeloid (about 60% of cases), lymphoid (20–30% of cases), or mixed myeloid-lymphoid phenotype (10–25% of cases) [55–57]. Many myeloid-phenotype CML-BC cases show "promiscuous" rearrangement of immunoglobulin genes, a feature that can also be seen in de novo AML [57]. The blast population in CML-BC appears to derive from a more committed hematopoietic progenitor than the stem cell of chronic phase CML; presumably this committed progenitor acquires additional genetic and epigenetic changes that promote self-renewal and maturation arrest [53,58].

Although blast crisis can be morphologically indistinguishable from an acute myeloid leukemia (AML) or acute lymphoblastic leukemia (ALL), the terms AML, ALL, or acute biphenotypic leukemia should not be used in cases that develop in a patient previously diagnosed with CML. These cases should be diagnosed as CML-BC with further designation as myeloid, lymphoid, or biphenotypic type according to standard lineage definitions for acute leukemias. The prognosis of CML-BC with lymphoid versus myeloid phenotype is uncertain in the era of TKI therapy. However, different blast crisis phenotypes have been be associated with unique patterns of molecular evolution: ABL kinase domain mutations that confer resistance to TKI occur frequently in lymphoid blast crisis, while myeloid blast crisis is more commonly associated with cytogenetic evolution. BCR-ABL amplification is seen in about one third of both myeloid and lymphoid blast crisis cases [21].

Recent data suggest that underlying molecular mechanisms behind CML progression may precede the typical defining features of CML-AP [53]. Moreover, the features of CML-AP in patients progressing on TKI therapy are still poorly defined. For these reasons, disease progression in CML is currently defined more practically in terms of responsiveness to TKI therapy [59]. Therefore, evidence of therapeutic refractoriness should elicit a clinical intervention whether or not this is accompanied by standard features of CML-AP or CML-BC. While therapeutic refractoriness to imatinib is often associated with cytogenetic evolution, between 2–4% of CML patients treated with imatinib develop clonal cytogenetic abnormalities in non-CML cells lacking a t(9;22) [60,61]. The abnormalities include changes often associated with myelodysplastic syndromes, such as trisomy 8 (the most frequently observed), deletion 7q, and deletion 20q; however, only rare patients develop myelodysplastic syndromes and these changes are often transient [62]. The etiology of these cytogenetic abnormalities is uncertain: normal hematopoiesis following successful TKI therapy has been shown to be polyclonal in most patients and imatinib does not appear to be mutagenic in vitro [63,64]. Further follow-up is required to determine the incidence and significance of these cytogenetic changes in TKI-treated patients.

10.6. Monitoring Algorithms to Detect Therapy Resistance

Imatinib therapy is highly effective in treating CML, but its effectiveness is limited in some patients by the development of disease resistance. Primary resistance to TKIs is infrequent and is usually related to drug efflux mechanisms or BCR-ABL amplification that overcomes the inhibitory effects of the drug. Secondary resistance, occurring after an initial response to TKI, is more common and is frequently due to mutations in the BCR-ABL kinase domain (KD) that abrogate the inhibitory activity of imatinib and/or other TKIs [65]. These KD mutations develop as a result of selection pressure and correlate with progression to advanced phases and shortened survival. Thus, early identification of imatinib resistance is critical to allow the use of other effective therapies, such as second-generation TKIs and/or stem cell transplantation. Cytogenetic analysis and molecular genetic testing to quantify the disease burden are the cornerstones of disease monitoring of CML patients on TKI therapy.

The hematologic, cytogenetic and molecular criteria for responses to TKI therapy are shown in Table 10-4. Imatinib and other TKIs induce a complete hematological remission (CHR, defined by normalization of the leukocyte count and spleen size) in nearly all patients

Table 10-4. Definitions of response of CML to imatinib and therapeutic targets [59,117].

Milestones to obtain by 3 months of imatinib therapy[a]		
CHR	Complete hematologic response	Normalization of leukocyte count and differential and normalization of spleen size
Milestone to obtain by 6 months of imatinib therapy[a]		
MCR	Major cytogenetic response	<35% of Ph+ metaphases on bone marrow cytogenetics
Milestone to obtain by 12 months of imatinib therapy[a]		
CCR	Complete cytogenetic response	0% Ph+ metaphases (at least 20 cells counted) on bone marrow cytogenetics
Milestones to obtain by 18 months of imatinib therapy[a]		
MMR	Major molecular response	≥3-log reduction in BCR-ABL transcript ratio[b] in blood compared to pretreatment reference level
CMR	Complete molecular response	Negativity for BCR-ABL by sensitive (at least 4.5 log) RQ-PCR assay

[a]Failure to meet expected therapeutic targets indicates a suboptimal response, and should elicit TKI-resistance mutation analysis
[b]BCR-ABL transcript ratio = ratio of BCR-ABL transcript level to transcript level of a reference gene, as assessed by real-time quantitative RT-PCR (RQ-PCR)

treated in chronic phase. CHR is usually accompanied by normalization of bone marrow cellularity, myeloid to erythroid ratio, megakaryocyte number and morphology, and reduction of any reticulin fibrosis that was present prior to therapy [14]. These changes are accompanied by increased apoptosis of CML cells and are maintained with long-term imatinib therapy, provided that a cytogenetic response persists [66]. Cytogenetic responses are measured by the percentage of at least 20 bone marrow metaphases that bear the t(9;22) translocation (Ph+ metaphases): a major cytogenetic response (MCR) represents <35% (<7/20) Ph+ metaphases, with a partial response being 1-34% Ph+ metaphases and a complete response (CCR) being 0% Ph+ metaphases.

In the first year of TKI therapy, complete hematologic responses and morphologic normalization of marrow may occur even in patients lacking a cytogenetic response, underscoring the need to monitor residual disease using genetic and/or molecular genetic techniques [14]. Most imatinib-treated CML-CP patients achieve CCR; failure to achieve a MCR is associated with increased risk of progression to advanced phases of disease and shortened survival [67]. Although cytogenetic analysis of bone marrow is considered to be the "gold standard" of cytogenetic responsiveness, interphase FISH analysis of peripheral blood to detect BCR-ABL appears to correlate well with cytogenetic responsiveness and is used in lieu of bone marrow cytogenetic analysis at some centers [68]. Dual-color FISH can identify colocalization of 5′ BCR and 3′ ABL1 fluorescent probes in cases of CML. Double-FISH using both 3′ and 5′ BCR and 3′ and 5′ ABL1 probes FISH is more sensitive and specific than dual-color FISH and also allows detection of der(9) deletions that have been associated with an adverse prognosis with earlier CML therapies [69,70]. FISH is more sensitive than cytogenetics as it routinely analyzes 200 rather than 20 cells, can detect cryptic BCR-ABL fusions, and can easily detect BCR-ABL fusion in peripheral blood specimens that may be difficult to karyotype [68]. However, unlike cytogenetics, interphase FISH indiscriminately examines cells that are not necessarily proliferating and cannot detect all the potential cytogenetic changes of clonal evolution. Thus, while FISH on peripheral blood may be a reasonable substitute for bone marrow cytogenetics in assessing some timepoints on TKI therapy, periodic bone marrow cytogenetics to confirm CCR and to assess for clonal evolution are still indicated [71].

While the achievement of a CCR is a desirable goal with imatinib therapy, real-time quantitative RT-PCR (RQ-PCR) currently represents the "gold standard" to detect and quantify low levels of persistent CML. Molecular response by RQ-PCR is defined as the detectable BCR-ABL transcript ratio (ratio of the BCR-ABL transcript level to the level of a reference gene transcript, usually BCR, ABL1, or GUSB) as a percentage of the average BCR-ABL transcript ratio of a control group of pretherapy CML cases, established at each laboratory [59]. BCR-ABL transcript levels can be determined on blood or bone marrow. Although a quantitative technique, RQ-PCR results may be variable between and within laboratories and are subject to a high coefficient of variation (reviewed in [72]). Variables that can affect the result include different sample types (blood versus bone marrow), RNA quality, reverse transcription efficiency, and PCR amplification efficiency. Ideally, RQ-PCR analyses on a given patient should be done consistently on the same type of sample (usually blood) and in the same laboratory over the course of his/her treatment [72]. Current efforts are focusing on standardizing the BCR-ABL transcript scale between laboratories so that molecular responses can be more meaningfully evaluated across different centers [73]. Major molecular response (MMR) represents a decrease in the BCR-ABL transcript ratio of at least 3-logs from the baseline (i.e. 0.1% of the transcript level present at initial diagnosis).

Achieving MMR is the goal of imatinib therapy, and is attained in 50–60% of CML patients by 12 months of therapy and in up to 80% of patients after 4 years of therapy [33]. Patients achieving MMR have excellent progression-free survival with continued imatinib therapy and rapid attainment of MMR is particularly associated with long-term responsiveness to imatinib [74]. Surprisingly, low-level detectable BCR-ABL transcripts persist in the vast majority of CML patients enjoying MMR, in spite of continued imatinib therapy and long-term disease free progression, and only 10–40% of patients achieve a complete molecular response (CMR),which is defined as undetectable BCR-ABL transcript in a RQ-PCR assay that has at least 4–5 log dynamic range [71,75]. The reasons for this persistent low-level disease are uncertain. It has been postulated that this may reflect a persistent CML stem cell population that expresses high levels of BCR-ABL that allow it to circumvent the effects of imatinib inhibition. A less distressing possibility is that the transcript resides in a differentiated, nonproliferating cell compartment such as pseudo-Gaucher histiocytes [76]; however, a persistent CML stem cell appears more likely, as most patients even in CCR relapse following cessation of imatinib therapy. Nevertheless, the durability of MMR in most patients indicates that imatinib can keep this small residual CML population in a quiescent state with low likelihood of secondary resistance development and very low incidence of progression to advanced phase disease. Further follow-up studies are needed to determine how long imatinib can maintain this "sleeping dragon" in its state of docile hibernation. In contrast, CMR represents an important therapeutic goal following allogeneic stem cell transplantation, as it is predictive of remaining disease-free posttransplant [77]. The prognostic value of CMR in current protocols that combine stem cell transplant with TKI therapy is unknown.

Although there is some variability in practice, most current centers monitor disease by RQ-PCR in blood every 3 months during the first 12 months of TKI therapy, then every 6 months once CCR is attained. Bone marrow cytogenetic studies should be performed prior to initiating TKI therapy and every 6 to 12 months until CCR, then every 1–2 years. These frequent periodic cytogenetic and molecular response assessments are performed in order to reveal patients that respond suboptimally to imatinib therapy (see Table 10-4); as therapy continues to evolve, it is likely that these monitoring algorithms will also change. Suboptimal response, defined by a failure to achieve specific cytogenetic and/or molecular response targets at the designated timepoints in Table 10-4, correlates with resistance to imatinib and warrants an investigation for ABL kinase domain (KD) mutations. Loss of CCR or hematologic relapse in a previously responding patient should also elicit resistance mutation analysis. A confirmed rise in the BCR-ABL transcript level by RQ-PCR should also elicit mutation analysis testing [59], but interpretation of a small rise in transcript ratio by RQ-PCR is more difficult due to some variability in this technique and the ability of TKI to control for many years such fluctuating but relatively low-level disease. A sustained or increasing rise in transcript level of two to fivefold even at very low disease levels has been associated with an increased likelihood of detecting TKI-resistance mutations [78, 79], but most centers use a tenfold increase in transcript levels above MMR to trigger mutation analysis only when a change in therapy is seriously contemplated [80].

The most common mechanism of secondary resistance to TKI is KD mutation in BCR-ABL. KD mutations can be detected by several methods, including pyrosequencing, mutation-specific RQ-PCR, liquid bead arrays, and denaturing high performance liquid chromatography (HPLC), but direct sequencing is by far the most common [81]. Although it is the least sensitive method, direct sequencing is the most routinely available and reliable method to cover all possible mutation sites and has been recommended for BCR-ABL mutation analysis by an international consensus panel [73]. More than 70 different KD mutations involving 57 different amino acids have been reported, but 15 amino acid substitutions account for 80–90% of the reported TKI-resistance mutations [81]. These resistance-conferring mutations cluster in four critical regions in the BCR-ABL KD, involving ATP binding (P-loop), imatinib-binding, catalytic activity, and kinase activation (A-loop). Mutations vary in their ability to inhibit the currently available TKI and thus the specific mutation type can help guide the use of a TKI that is active against a particular mutation. The mutation at amino acid 315 in the imatinib-binding site (T315I mutation) confers resistance to imatinib, dasatinib, and nilotinib by preventing access of these drugs to the ATP-binding pocket.

The mechanisms by which these mutations develop are poorly understood. KD mutations can be present at low-levels in CML cases prior to exposure to TKI therapy. However, these small mutant clones do not necessarily confer an adverse prognosis and resistant clones may not expand even under the "selection pressure" of TKI therapy [82,83]. For these reasons, upfront assessment for KD mutations is not recommended prior to the institution of TKI therapy, as it may not predict resistance to TKI therapy. Gene expression profiling (see Sect. 10.7) appears to hold more promise than KD mutation analysis in predicting whether patients will respond to TKI therapy upfront. Secondary resistance to TKIs due to KD mutations usually occurs within the first two years of TKI therapy and is much more common in CML-AP and CML-BC than CML-CP [75]. Although KD mutations are a common cause of secondary resistance to TKI therapy, about half of the resistance occurrences are due to other mechanisms [84]. These include BCR-ABL overexpression (due to amplification at the genomic level or other mechanisms) and rare mutations outside the KD. Mechanisms of resistance not directly involving BCR-ABL are often associated with cytogenetic evolution that results in the activation of oncogenes and/or loss of tumor suppression genes. Gene expression profiling may be helpful in identifying target genes associated with KD-mutation-independent TKI resistance [85]. Alteration in drug metabolic kinetics is usually a mechanism of primary TKI resistance to TKI and only rarely a cause of secondary TKI resistance.

10.7. Prognosis

Even with the advent of TKI therapy, the phase of disease remains an important prognostic factor in CML [84]. However, several other clinicopathologic parameters have been identified at the time of diagnosis that correlate with time to progression and survival. The Sokal score was based on a multivariate analysis on the prognosis of CML-CP patients treated with earlier therapies (hydroxyurea and busulfan). The significant factors include age (in years), spleen size (in centimeters), platelet count ($\times 10^9$/L), and blast percentage in the peripheral blood which are combined into a hazard ratio combining using the following equation:

$$\text{Hazard ratio (HR)} = \text{EXP} [0.116(\text{Age} - 43.4) + 0.0345(\text{Spleen size} - 7.51) + ([\text{Platelet count}/700]^2 - 0.563) + 0.0887(\text{Blast count} - 2.10)].$$

The HR (Sokal score) stratifies patients into high risk (HR < 0.08), intermediate risk (HR = 0.8–1.2), and low risk (HR > 1.2) groups, with median survival ranging from 58 months in the low risk group to 31 months in the high risk group [86]. The Hasford score was devised to establish prognostic groups in interferon-treated patients and uses the same four variables as the Sokal score as well as peripheral eosinophil and basophil counts [87]. The European Group for Blood and Bone Marrow transplantation developed yet another risk-stratifying scheme for patients undergoing stem cell transplantation for CML that includes age, interval from diagnosis to transplant, disease phase, donor-recipient sex match, and donor type [88]. The Sokal scoring system retains its prognostic significance even in TKI-treated CML patients [75]. Increased bone marrow reticulin fibrosis in CML is associated with other features of disease progression and is an independent adverse prognostic risk factor in interferon and hydroxyurea-treated patients [89]. While pretreatment increased reticulin was associated with a lower rate of cytogenetic remission in imatinib-treated CML patients, this did not appear to be an independent risk factor; however, increasing reticulin fibrosis on imatinib therapy was independently associated with treatment failure [90].

While the development of additional chromosomal abnormalities in CML-CP patient represents disease progression and is diagnostic criterion of CML-AP, the significance of chromosomal abnormalities additional to t(9;22) at the time of diagnosis is uncertain. Additional chromosomal abnormalities present at diagnosis were associated with a poor prognosis in earlier studies, but not in more recent studies examining interferon- or imatinib-treated patients [91–93]. In contrast, the acquisition of new cytogenetic abnormalities in patients treated with imatinib is associated with loss of response and poor prognosis [93,94]. FISH appears to increase the yield of identifying the most common additional chromosomal abnormalities associated with disease progression, but it is unclear if these small clones with secondary abnormalities have clinical relevance [95]. Thus, the use of FISH to examine for additional secondary changes that are not evident on routine karyotype is not currently indicated.

Imatinib-treated CML patients with variant translocations that produce BCR-ABL fusion but involve three or more chromosomes have a similar prognosis to patients with a classic t(9;22) [96]. The small subset CML cases with a cryptic (invisible on standard metaphase preparations) BCR-ABL fusion also have the same prognosis and clinicopathologic features as CML with t(9;22) [97]. At the molecular level, CML cases with variant transcripts that encode p190 and p230 fusion proteins may show distinct clinical features (see Table 10-2), but do respond to imatinib. The prognosis of these cases compared with classic p210 CML when treated with TKI is uncertain, but some recent studies suggest that the rare p190 CML cases may have a poorer outcome [98, 99]. Variable large (several megabase) deletions of the derivative chromosome 9 of the t(9;22) translocation are present in 10-15% of CML patients at diagnosis [69]. These deletions eliminate the reciprocal ABL-BCR fusion gene that has been shown to be transcribed in most CML cases, but is not expressed as protein and whose function is unclear [100, 101]. Although deletion of a tumor suppressor gene or regulatory region at this site has been postulated, no specific candidate gene has been identified and any potential role of the der(9) deletions in CML pathogenesis remains uncertain. Der(9) deletion is independently associated with adverse outcome in CML-CP patients treated with hydroxyurea and interferon [102, 103]. However, it is controversial whether der(9) deletions have prognostic significance in patients treated with imatinib and examination for these deletions is not routine in current diagnostic practice [104–107].

Gene expression profiling shows promise in risk-stratifying CML patients treated with TKI. In one study, microarray analysis of CD34+ progenitor cells in CML-CP cases revealed differential gene expression in patients with indolent disease from those who rapidly progressed to CML-BC; specifically, lower expression of CD7 and higher expression of proteinase 3 or elastase were associated with a more indolent course [108]. CD7 expression in CD34+ CML blasts detected by flow cytometry has also been independently associated with adverse prognosis in CML-CP [109,110]. Several studies have also shown differential gene expression between peripheral blood leukocytes from CML cases that subsequently respond or do not respond to imatinib [111–113]. One recent study showed differential expression of a single drug metabolism gene, PTGS1/COX1, in CML cases that had primary resistance to TKI therapy; in contrast, the signature of secondary TKI resistance that did not involve the common ABL KD mutations was more complex, including up to 11 different genes [85]. These studies suggest that gene expression profiling in the future may obviate the current 'trial-and-error' practice of using molecular monitoring to guide the use of TKI versus alternative therapies for CML.

10.8. Differential Diagnosis

Leukocytosis due to an infection or as a paraneoplastic phenomenon to nonmyeloid neoplasms can be marked and can be accompanied by immature granulocytic precursors and eosinophilia mimicking CML. Leukocyte alkaline phosphatase (LAP) activity is markedly reduced in CML granulocytes and is usually increased in reactive leukocytosis [114]. LAP testing is no longer used in most centers, as clinical history usually helps resolve this differential; molecular genetic and/or FISH testing of peripheral blood for BCR-ABL can diagnose or exclude CML in clinically ambiguous cases.

CML cases may exhibit an increased absolute monocyte count, raising the differential diagnosis of chronic myelomonocytic leukemia (CMML). This is an important distinction, as CMML (as defined by the WHO 2008 Classification) does not respond to therapy with the current tyrosine kinase inhibitors (TKI) used to treat CML. The monocytes are part of the neoplastic clone in CML and participate in the unregulated myeloid proliferation; however, monocytes only rarely comprise >10% of all peripheral blood leukocytes in CML, as is seen in almost all CMML cases (see Chap. 6). The rare CML cases with >10% peripheral monocytes that may mimic CMML are often associated with a p190 (e1a2) BCR-ABL. Atypical CML, BCR-ABL negative (referred to in earlier publications as "Philadelphia-negative CML") also presents with leukocytosis and immature myeloid elements, but lacks basophilia. Moreover, morphologic dysplasia is often present in both atypical CML and in CMML but is usually absent in CML except in advanced phases. Chronic neutrophilic leukemia (CNL) is a rare MPN that also presents with leukocytosis, but lacks significant circulating immature granulocytic elements or basophilia. CML patients with p230 BCR-ABL may present with a mature neutrophilia resembling CNL or with prominent thrombocytosis mimicking essential thrombocythemia [115]. Most importantly, atypical CML, BCR-ABL negative, CMML, CNL, and other non-CML MPNs all lack BCR-ABL by definition, thus molecular genetic testing is the most reliable method to distinguish among these entities.

Rarely, CML patients may present in blast crisis (CML-BC), mimicking a de novo Philadelphia-chromosome positive (Ph+) AML or ALL. In contrast to Ph+ ALL that usually bears the e1a2 p190 BCR-ABL variant, only very rare cases of CML show the e1a2 variant [21]. Distinguishing rare cases of de novo Ph+ AML from CML-BC may be more difficult, as p210 BCR-ABL characterizes both. Unlike CML-BC, Ph+ AML usually lacks basophilia and is less likely to manifest massive splenomegaly [116]. Cases of presumed acute leukemia treated with induction chemotherapy in which the postinduction bone marrow shows no acute leukemia, but morphologically resembles CML-CP and continues to show a t(9;22) by conventional cytogenetics, likely represent cases of CML presenting in blast crisis. Now that adjuvant TKI therapy is standard for induction of Ph+ acute leukemias, cases of CML-BC mimicking de novo ALL or AML may be more difficult to recognize postinduction.

References

1. Nowell P, Hungerford D. A minute chromosome in human chronic granulocytic leukemia. Science 1960;132:1497–501.
2. Boveri T. Zur Frage der Entstehung maligner Tumoren. Gustav Fischer, Jena, Germany 1914:64.
3. Rowley JD. Identification of a translocation with quinacrine fluorescence in a patient with acute leukemia. Ann Genet 1973;16:109–12.
4. Groffen J, Stephenson JR, Heisterkamp N, de Klein A, Bartram CR, Grosveld G. Philadelphia chromosomal breakpoints are clustered within a limited region, bcr, on chromosome 22. Cell 1984;36:93–9.
5. Daley GQ, Van Etten RA, Baltimore D. Induction of chronic myelogenous leukemia in mice by the P210bcr/abl gene of the Philadelphia chromosome. Science 1990;247:824–30.
6. Jemal A, Tiwari RC, Murray T, et al. Cancer statistics, 2004. CA. Cancer J Clin 2004;54:8–29.
7. Deininger MW, Goldman JM, Melo JV. The molecular biology of chronic myeloid leukemia. Blood 2000;96:3343–56.
8. Bizzozero OJ Jr, Johnson KG, Ciocco A, Kawasaki S, Toyoda S. Radiation-related leukemia in Hiroshima and Nagasaki 1946–1964. II. Ann Intern Med 1967;66:522–30.
9. Corso A, Lazzarino M, Morra E, et al. Chronic myelogenous leukemia and exposure to ionizing radiation–a retrospective study of 443 patients. Ann Hematol 1995;70:79–82.
10. Aksoy M, Erdem S, DinCol G. Leukemia in shoe-workers exposed chronically to benzene. Blood 1974;44:837–41.
11. Faderl S, Talpaz M, Estrov Z, O'Brien S, Kurzrock R, Kantarjian HM. The biology of chronic myeloid leukemia. N Engl J Med 1999;341:164–72.
12. Kantarjian HM, Smith TL, McCredie KB, et al. Chronic myelogenous leukemia: a multivariate analysis of the associations of patient characteristics and therapy with survival. Blood 1985;66:1326–35.
13. Aguayo A, Kantarjian H, Manshouri T, et al. Angiogenesis in acute and chronic leukemias and myelodysplastic syndromes. Blood 2000;96:2240–5.
14. Hasserjian RP, Boecklin F, Parker S, et al. ST1571 (imatinib mesylate) reduces bone marrow cellularity and normalizes morphologic features irrespective of cytogenetic response. Am J Clin Pathol 2002;117:360–7.

15. Vardiman JW MJ, Baccarani M, Thieke J. Chronic myelogenous leukemia, BCR-ABL1 positive. In: Swerdlow SH CE, Harris NL, Jaffe ES, Pileri SA, Stein H, Thiele J, Vardiman JW, ed. WHO Classification of Tumours of Haematopoietic and Lymphoid Tissues. 4th ed. Lyon: International Angency for Research on Cancer (IARC); 2008:32–7

16. Mark HF, Sokolic RA, Mark Y. Conventional cytogenetics and FISH in the detection of BCR/ABL fusion in chronic myeloid leukemia (CML). Exp Mol Pathol 2006;81:1–7.

17. Melo JV. The diversity of BCR-ABL fusion proteins and their relationship to leukemia phenotype. Blood 1996;88:2375–84.

18. Laurent E, Talpaz M, Kantarjian H, Kurzrock R. The BCR gene and philadelphia chromosome-positive leukemogenesis. Cancer Res 2001;61:2343–55.

19. Iwata S, Mizutani S, Nakazawa S, Yata J. Heterogeneity of the breakpoint in the ABL gene in cases with BCR/ABL transcript lacking ABL exon a2. Leukemia 1994;8:1696–702.

20. Snyder DS, McMahon R, Cohen SR, Slovak ML. Chronic myeloid leukemia with an e13a3 BCR-ABL fusion: benign course responsive to imatinib with an RT-PCR advisory. Am J Hematol 2004;75:92–5.

21. Jones D, Luthra R, Cortes J, et al. BCR-ABL fusion transcript types and levels and their interaction with secondary genetic changes in determining the phenotype of Philadelphia chromosome-positive leukemias. Blood 2008;112:5190–2.

22. Lugo TG, Pendergast AM, Muller AJ, Witte ON. Tyrosine kinase activity and transformation potency of bcr-abl oncogene products. Science 1990;247:1079–82.

23. Ravandi F, Cortes J, Albitar M, et al. Chronic myelogenous leukaemia with p185(BCR/ABL) expression: characteristics and clinical significance. Br J Haematol 1999;107:581–6.

24. Lichty BD, Keating A, Callum J, et al. Expression of p210 and p190 BCR-ABL due to alternative splicing in chronic myelogenous leukaemia. Br J Haematol 1998;103:711–5.

25. Branford S, Hughes TP, Rudzki Z. Dual transcription of b2a2 and b3a2 BCR-ABL transcripts in chronic myeloid leukaemia is confined to patients with a linked polymorphism within the BCR gene. Br J Haematol 2002;117:875–7.

26. Luthra R, Sanchez-Vega B, Medeiros LJ. TaqMan RT-PCR assay coupled with capillary electrophoresis for quantification and identification of bcr-abl transcript type. Mod Pathol 2004;17:96–103.

27. Branford S, Hughes T. Diagnosis and monitoring of chronic myeloid leukemia by qualitative and quantitative RT-PCR. Methods Mol Med 2006;125:69–92.

28. Burmeister T, Reinhardt R. A multiplex PCR for improved detection of typical and atypical BCR-ABL fusion transcripts. Leuk Res 2008;32:579–85.

29. Schultheis B, Wang L, Clark RE, Melo JV. BCR-ABL with an e6a2 fusion in a CML patient diagnosed in blast crisis. Leukemia 2003;17:2054–5.

30. Hochaus A, Reiter A, Skladny H, et al. A novel BCR-ABL fusion gene (e6a2) in a patient with Philadelphia chromosome-negative chronic myelogenous leukemia. Blood 1996;88:2236–40.

31. Dessars B, El Housni H, Lambert F, Kentos A, Heimann P. Rational use of the EAC real-time quantitative PCR protocol in chronic myelogenous leukemia: report of three false-negative cases at diagnosis. Leukemia 2006;20:886–8.

32. Taagepera S, McDonald D, Loeb JE, et al. Nuclear-cytoplasmic shuttling of C-ABL tyrosine kinase. Proc Natl Acad Sci USA 1998;95:7457–62.

33. Druker BJ, O'Brien SG, Cortes J, Radich J. Chronic myelogenous leukemia. Hematology Am Soc Hematol Educ Program 2002:111–35

34. Ren R. Mechanisms of BCR-ABL in the pathogenesis of chronic myelogenous leukaemia. Nat Rev Cancer 2005;5:172–83.

35. Gordon MY, Dowding CR, Riley GP, Goldman JM, Greaves MF. Altered adhesive interactions with marrow stroma of haematopoietic progenitor cells in chronic myeloid leukaemia. Nature 1987;328:342–4.

36. Goldman JM, Melo JV. Chronic myeloid leukemia–advances in biology and new approaches to treatment. N Engl J Med 2003;349:1451–64.

37. Sokal JE, Baccarani M, Russo D, Tura S. Staging and prognosis in chronic myelogenous leukemia. Semin Hematol 1988;25:49–61.

38. Griesshammer M, Heinze B, Hellmann A, et al. Chronic myelogenous leukemia in blast crisis: retrospective analysis of prognostic factors in 90 patients. Ann Hematol 1996;73:225–30.

39. Kantarjian HM, Deisseroth A, Kurzrock R, Estrov Z, Talpaz M. Chronic myelogenous leukemia: a concise update. Blood 1993;82:691–703.

40. Xu Y, Dolan MM, Nguyen PL. Diagnostic significance of detecting dysgranulopoiesis in chronic myeloid leukemia. Am J Clin Pathol 2003;120:778–84.

41. Speck B, Bortin MM, Champlin R, et al. Allogeneic bone-marrow transplantation for chronic myelogenous leukaemia. Lancet 1984;1:665–8.

42. Kantarjian HM, Keating MJ, Smith TL, Talpaz M, McCredie KB. Proposal for a simple synthesis prognostic staging system in chronic myelogenous leukemia. Am J Med 1990;88:1–8.

43. Cortes JE, Talpaz M, O'Brien S, et al. Staging of chronic myeloid leukemia in the imatinib era: an evaluation of the World Health Organization proposal. Cancer 2006;106:1306–15.

44. Quintas-Cardama A, Cortes JE. Chronic myeloid leukemia: diagnosis and treatment. Mayo Clin Proc 2006;81:973–88.

45. Gribble SM, Sinclair PB, Grace C, Green AR, Nacheva EP. Comparative analysis of G-banding, chromosome painting, locus-specific fluorescence in situ hybridization, and comparative genomic hybridization in chronic myeloid leukemia blast crisis. Cancer Genet Cytogenet 1999;111:7–17.

46. Johansson B, Fioretos T, Mitelman F. Cytogenetic and molecular genetic evolution of chronic myeloid leukemia. Acta Haematol 2002;107:76–94.

47. Wu Y, Slovak ML, Snyder DS, Arber DA. Coexistence of inversion 16 and the Philadelphia chromosome in acute and chronic myeloid leukemias: report of six cases and review of literature. Am J Clin Pathol 2006;125:260–6.

48. Merzianu M, Medeiros LJ, Cortes J, et al. inv(16)(p13q22) in chronic myelogenous leukemia in blast phase: a clinicopathologic, cytogenetic, and molecular study of five cases. Am J Clin Pathol 2005;124:807–14.

49. Melo JV, Barnes DJ. Chronic myeloid leukaemia as a model of disease evolution in human cancer. Nat Rev Cancer 2007;7:441–53.

50. Salloukh HF, Laneuville P. Increase in mutant frequencies in mice expressing the BCR-ABL activated tyrosine kinase. Leukemia 2000;14:1401–4.

51. Calabretta B, Perrotti D. The biology of CML blast crisis. Blood 2004;103:4010–22.

52. Asimakopoulos FA, Shteper PJ, Krichevsky S, et al. ABL1 methylation is a distinct molecular event associated with clonal evolution of chronic myeloid leukemia. Blood 1999;94:2452–60.

53. Radich JP, Dai H, Mao M, et al. Gene expression changes associated with progression and response in chronic myeloid leukemia. Proc Natl Acad Sci U S A 2006;103:2794–9.

54. Jacknow G, Frizzera G, Gajl-Peczalska K, et al. Extramedullary presentation of the blast crisis of chronic myelogenous leukaemia. Br J Haematol 1985;61:225–36.

55. Saikia T, Advani S, Dasgupta A, et al. Characterisation of blast cells during blastic phase of chronic myeloid leukaemia by immunophenotyping–experience in 60 patients. Leuk Res 1988;12:499–506.

56. Cortes JE, Talpaz M, Kantarjian H. Chronic myelogenous leukemia: a review. Am J Med 1996;100:555–70.

57. Khalidi HS, Brynes RK, Medeiros LJ, et al. The immunophenotype of blast transformation of chronic myelogenous leukemia: a high frequency of mixed lineage phenotype in "lymphoid" blasts and A comparison of morphologic, immunophenotypic, and molecular findings. Mod Pathol 1998;11:1211–21.

58. Jamieson CH, Ailles LE, Dylla SJ, et al. Granulocyte-macrophage progenitors as candidate leukemic stem cells in blast-crisis CML. N Engl J Med 2004;351:657–67.

59. Baccarani M, Saglio G, Goldman J, et al. Evolving concepts in the management of chronic myeloid leukemia: recommendations from an expert panel on behalf of the European LeukemiaNet. Blood 2006;108:1809–20.

60. Terre C, Eclache V, Rousselot P, et al. Report of 34 patients with clonal chromosomal abnormalities in Philadelphia-negative cells during imatinib treatment of Philadelphia-positive chronic myeloid leukemia. Leukemia 2004;18:1340–6.

61. Loriaux M, Deininger M. Clonal cytogenetic abnormalities in Philadelphia chromosome negative cells in chronic myeloid leukemia patients treated with imatinib. Leuk Lymphoma 2004;45:2197–203.

62. Jabbour E, Kantarjian HM, Abruzzo LV, et al. Chromosomal abnormalities in Philadelphia chromosome negative metaphases appearing during imatinib mesylate therapy in patients with newly diagnosed chronic myeloid leukemia in chronic phase. Blood 2007;110:2991–5.

63. Bumm T, Muller C, Al-Ali HK, et al. Emergence of clonal cytogenetic abnormalities in Ph- cells in some CML patients in cytogenetic remission to imatinib but restoration of polyclonal hematopoiesis in the majority. Blood 2003;101:1941–9.

64. McMullin MF, Humphreys M, Byrne J, Russell NH, Cuthbert RJ, O'Dwyer ME. Chromosomal abnormalities in Ph- cells of patients on imatinib. Blood 2003;102:2700–1. author reply 1.

65. Branford S, Rudzki Z, Walsh S, et al. High frequency of point mutations clustered within the adenosine triphosphate-binding region of BCR/ABL in patients with chronic myeloid leukemia or Ph-positive acute lymphoblastic leukemia who develop imatinib (STI571) resistance. Blood 2002;99:3472–5.

66. Thiele J, Kvasnicka HM, Schmitt-Graeff A, et al. Bone marrow changes in chronic myelogenous leukaemia after long-term treatment with the tyrosine kinase inhibitor STI571: an immunohisto-chemical study on 75 patients. Histopathology 2005;46:540–50.

67. Rosti G, Testoni N, Martinelli G, Baccarani M. The cytogenetic response as a surrogate marker of survival. Semin Hematol 2003;40:56–61.

68. Landstrom AP, Tefferi A. Fluorescent in situ hybridization in the diagnosis, prognosis, and treatment monitoring of chronic myeloid leukemia. Leuk Lymphoma 2006;47:397–402.

69. Sinclair PB, Nacheva EP, Leversha M, et al. Large deletions at the t(9;22) breakpoint are common and may identify a poor-prognosis subgroup of patients with chronic myeloid leukemia. Blood 2000;95:738–43.

70. Dewald GW, Wyatt WA, Juneau AL, et al. Highly sensitive fluorescence in situ hybridization method to detect double BCR/ABL fusion and monitor response to therapy in chronic myeloid leukemia. Blood 1998;91:3357–65.

71. Kantarjian H, Schiffer C, Jones D, Cortes J. Monitoring the response and course of chronic myeloid leukemia in the modern era of BCR-ABL tyrosine kinase inhibitors: practical advice on the use and interpretation of monitoring methods. Blood 2008;111:1774–80.

72. Branford S, Cross NC, Hochhaus A, et al. Rationale for the recommendations for harmonizing current methodology for detecting BCR-ABL transcripts in patients with chronic myeloid leukaemia. Leukemia 2006;20:1925–30.

73. Hughes T, Deininger M, Hochhaus A, et al. Monitoring CML patients responding to treatment with tyrosine kinase inhibitors: review and recommendations for harmonizing current methodology for detecting BCR-ABL transcripts and kinase domain mutations and for expressing results. Blood 2006;108:28–37.

74. Wang L, Pearson K, Ferguson JE, Clark RE. The early molecular response to imatinib predicts cytogenetic and clinical outcome in chronic myeloid leukaemia. Br J Haematol 2003;120:990–9.

75. Druker BJ, Guilhot F, O'Brien SG, et al. Five-year follow-up of patients receiving imatinib for chronic myeloid leukemia. N Engl J Med 2006;355:2408–17.

76. Anastasi J, Musvee T, Roulston D, Domer PH, Larson RA, Vardiman JW. Pseudo-Gaucher histiocytes identified up to 1 year after transplantation for CML are BCR/ABL-positive. Leukemia 1998;12:233–7.

77. Radich JP, Gehly G, Gooley T, et al. Polymerase chain reaction detection of the BCR-ABL fusion transcript after allogeneic marrow transplantation for chronic myeloid leukemia: results and implications in 346 patients. Blood 1995;85:2632–8.

78. Press RD, Love Z, Tronnes AA, et al. BCR-ABL mRNA levels at and after the time of a complete cytogenetic response (CCR) predict the duration of CCR in imatinib mesylate-treated patients with CML. Blood 2006;107:4250–6.

79. Branford S, Rudzki Z, Parkinson I, et al. Real-time quantitative PCR analysis can be used as a primary screen to identify patients with CML treated with imatinib who have BCR-ABL kinase domain mutations. Blood 2004;104:2926–32.

80. Cortes J, Talpaz M, O'Brien S, et al. Molecular responses in patients with chronic myelogenous leukemia in chronic phase treated with imatinib mesylate. Clin Cancer Res 2005;11:3425–32.

81. Jones D, Kamel-Reid S, Bahler D, et al. Laboratory practice guidelines for detecting and reporting BCR-ABL drug resistance mutations in chronic myelogenous leukemia and acute lymphoblastic leukemia: a report of the Association for Molecular Pathology. J Mol Diagn 2009;11:4–11.

82. O'Hare T, Eide CA, Deininger MW. Bcr-Abl kinase domain mutations, drug resistance, and the road to a cure for chronic myeloid leukemia. Blood 2007;110:2242–9.

83. Willis SG, Lange T, Demehri S, et al. High-sensitivity detection of BCR-ABL kinase domain mutations in imatinib-naive patients: correlation with clonal cytogenetic evolution but not response to therapy. Blood 2005;106:2128–37.

84. Jabbour E, Kantarjian H, Jones D, et al. Frequency and clinical significance of BCR-ABL mutations in patients with chronic myeloid leukemia treated with imatinib mesylate. Leukemia 2006;20:1767–73.

85. Zhang WW CJ, Yao H, Zhang L, Reddy NG, Jabbour E, Kantarjian HM, Jones D. Predictors of primary imatinib resistance in chronic myeloid leukemia are distinct from those in secondary imatinib resistance. J Clin Oncol 2009;27:3642–3649.

86. Sokal JE, Cox EB, Baccarani M, et al. Prognostic discrimination in "good-risk" chronic granulocytic leukemia. Blood 1984;63:789–99.

87. Hasford J, Pfirrmann M, Hehlmann R, et al. A new prognostic score for survival of patients with chronic myeloid leukemia treated with interferon alfa. Writing Committee for the Collaborative CML Prognostic Factors Project Group. J Natl Cancer Inst 1998;90:850–8.

88. Gratwohl A, Hermans J, Niederwieser D, et al. Bone marrow transplantation for chronic myeloid leukemia: long-term results. Chronic Leukemia Working Party of the European Group for Bone Marrow Transplantation. Bone Marrow Transplant 1993;12:509–16.

89. Buesche G, Hehlmann R, Hecker H, et al. Marrow fibrosis, indicator of therapy failure in chronic myeloid leukemia - prospective long-term results from a randomized-controlled trial. Leukemia 2003;17:2444–53.

90. Buesche G, Ganser A, Schlegelberger B, et al. Marrow fibrosis and its relevance during imatinib treatment of chronic myeloid leukemia. Leukemia 2007;21:2420–7.

91. Sokal JE, Gomez GA, Baccarani M, et al. Prognostic significance of additional cytogenetic abnormalities at diagnosis of Philadelphia chromosome-positive chronic granulocytic leukemia. Blood 1988;72:294–8.

92. Farag SS, Ruppert AS, Mrozek K, et al. Prognostic significance of additional cytogenetic abnormalities in newly diagnosed patients with Philadelphia chromosome-positive chronic myelogenous leukemia treated with interferon-alpha: a Cancer and Leukemia Group B study. Int J Oncol 2004;25:143–51.

93. Cortes JE, Talpaz M, Giles F, et al. Prognostic significance of cytogenetic clonal evolution in patients with chronic myelogenous leukemia on imatinib mesylate therapy. Blood 2003;101:3794–800.

94. O'Dwyer ME, Mauro MJ, Blasdel C, et al. Clonal evolution and lack of cytogenetic response are adverse prognostic factors for hematologic relapse of chronic phase CML patients treated with imatinib mesylate. Blood 2004;103:451–5.

95. Wang Y, Hopwood VL, Hu P, Lennon A, Osterberger J, Glassman A. Determination of secondary chromosomal aberrations of chronic myelocytic leukemia. Cancer Genet Cytogenet 2004;153:53–6.

96. El-Zimaity MM, Kantarjian H, Talpaz M, et al. Results of imatinib mesylate therapy in chronic myelogenous leukaemia with variant Philadelphia chromosome. Br J Haematol 2004;125:187–95.

97. Shtalrid M, Talpaz M, Blick M, et al. Philadelphia-negative chronic myelogenous leukemia with breakpoint cluster region rearrangement: molecular analysis, clinical characteristics, and response to therapy. J Clin Oncol 1988;6:1569–75.

98. Lee JJ, Kim HJ, Kim YJ, et al. Imatinib induces a cytogenetic response in blast crisis or interferon failure chronic myeloid leukemia patients with e19a2 BCR-ABL transcripts. Leukemia 2004;18:1539–40.

99. Verma D, Kantarjian HM, Jones D, et al. Chronic myeloid leukemia (CML) with p190 BCR-ABL: analysis of characteristics, outcomes and prognostic significance. Blood 2009;114:2232–5.

100. de la Fuente J, Merx K, Steer EJ, et al. ABL-BCR expression does not correlate with deletions on the derivative chromosome 9 or survival in chronic myeloid leukemia. Blood 2001;98:2879–80.

101. Melo JV, Gordon DE, Cross NC, Goldman JM. The ABL-BCR fusion gene is expressed in chronic myeloid leukemia. Blood 1993;81:158–65.

102. Cohen N, Rozenfeld-Granot G, Hardan I, et al. Subgroup of patients with Philadelphia-positive chronic myelogenous leukemia characterized by a deletion of 9q proximal to ABL gene: expression profiling, resistance to interferon therapy, and poor prognosis. Cancer Genet Cytogenet 2001;128:114–9.

103. Huntly BJ, Reid AG, Bench AJ, et al. Deletions of the derivative chromosome 9 occur at the time of the Philadelphia translocation and provide a powerful and independent prognostic indicator in chronic myeloid leukemia. Blood 2001;98:1732–8.

104. Huntly BJ, Guilhot F, Reid AG, et al. Imatinib improves but may not fully reverse the poor prognosis of patients with CML with derivative chromosome 9 deletions. Blood 2003;102:2205–12.

105. Yoong Y, VanDeWalker TJ, Carlson RO, Dewald GW, Tefferi A. Clinical correlates of submicroscopic deletions involving the ABL-BCR translocation region in chronic myeloid leukemia. Eur J Haematol 2005;74:124–7.

106. Quintas-Cardama A, Kantarjian H, Talpaz M, et al. Imatinib mesylate therapy may overcome the poor prognostic significance of deletions of derivative chromosome 9 in patients with chronic myelogenous leukemia. Blood 2005;105:2281–6.

107. Kreil S, Pfirrmann M, Haferlach C, et al. Heterogeneous prognostic impact of derivative chromosome 9 deletions in chronic myelogenous leukemia. Blood 2007;110:1283–90.

108. Yong AS, Szydlo RM, Goldman JM, Apperley JF, Melo JV. Molecular profiling of CD34+ cells identifies low expression of CD7, along with high expression of proteinase 3 or elastase, as predictors of longer survival in patients with CML. Blood 2006;107:205–12.

109. Martin-Henao GA, Quiroga R, Sureda A, Garcia J. CD7 expression on CD34+ cells from chronic myeloid leukaemia in chronic phase. Am J Hematol 1999;61:178–86.

110. Kosugi N, Ebihara Y, Nakahata T, Saisho H, Asano S, Tojo A. CD34+CD7+ leukemic progenitor cells may be involved in maintenance and clonal evolution of chronic myeloid leukemia. Clin Cancer Res 2005;11:505–11.

111. Kaneta Y, Kagami Y, Katagiri T, et al. Prediction of sensitivity to STI571 among chronic myeloid leukemia patients by genome-wide cDNA microarray analysis. Jpn J Cancer Res 2002;93:849–56.

112. Ohno R, Nakamura Y. Prediction of response to imatinib by cDNA microarray analysis. Semin Hematol 2003;40:42–9.

113. McLean LA, Gathmann I, Capdeville R, Polymeropoulos MH, Dressman M. Pharmacogenomic analysis of cytogenetic response in chronic myeloid leukemia patients treated with imatinib. Clin Cancer Res 2004;10:155–65.

114. Rosner F, Schreiber ZR, Parise F. Leukocyte alkaline phosphatase. Fluctuations with disease status in chronic granulocytic leukemia. Arch Intern Med 1972;130:892–4.

115. Pane F, Frigeri F, Sindona M, et al. Neutrophilic-chronic myeloid leukemia: a distinct disease with a specific molecular marker (BCR/ABL with C3/A2 junction). Blood 1996;88:2410–4.

116. Soupir CP, Vergilio JA, Dal Cin P, et al. Philadelphia chromosome-positive acute myeloid leukemia: a rare aggressive leukemia with clinicopathologic features distinct from chronic myeloid leukemia in myeloid blast crisis. Am J Clin Pathol 2007;127:642–50.

117. Deininger M. Resistance and relapse with imatinib in CML: causes and consequences. J Natl Compr Canc Netw 2008;6(Suppl 2):S11–21.

Chapter 11

Treatment of Myeloproliferative Neoplasms

Starla Sweany and Elias Jabbour

Abstract/Scope of Chapter The treatment of chronic myeloproliferative neoplasms, including chronic myelogenous leukemia, polycythemia vera, primary myelofibrosis, and essential thrombocythemia are summarized. The indications for supportive care versus chemotherapy versus targeted (kinase inhibitor) therapy and stem cell transplantation are compared.

Keywords Myeloproliferative neoplasms, workup • Leukoerythroblastosis • Myeloproliferative neoplasms, thrombotic risk • Chronic myelogenous leukemia, treatment • Tyrosine kinase inhibitors, imatinib and next generation compounds, polycythemia vera, treatment • Primary myelofibrosis, treatment • Essential thrombocythemia, treatment • MPL (thrombopoietin receptor, mutation • JAK2, inhibitors

11.1. Workup of MPNs at Time of Diagnosis

Myeloproliferative neoplasms (MPNs) comprise a group of indolent tumors with growth-activating genetic changes in hematopoietic progenitors that drive overproduction of one more cell lineages. In contrast to myelodysplastic syndromes (MDS) or acute leukemias, there are minimal effects on hematopoietic maturation. However, all MPNs can transform (at varying frequency) to acute leukemia, often progressing through an accelerated phase with increased blasts or marrow fibrosis. In the 2008 WHO classification [1], MPNs are subcategorized as polycythemia vera (PV), essential thrombocythemia (ET), primary myelofibrosis (PMF), chronic myeloid leukemia (CML), and the less common chronic neutrophilic leukemia (CNL), hypereosinophilic syndrome (HES), and systemic mastocytosis. Clinical, hematologic and molecular features that differentiate CML, PV, ET and PMF are summarized in Table 11-1, and a diagnostic algorithm is presented in Fig. 11-1.

CML should be suspected whenever marked leukocytosis with increased basophils is detected in the blood, as basophilia is rare in any reactive condition. Bone marrow biopsy and aspirate to detect the t(9;22)(q34;q11) [i.e. the Philadelphia chromosome, (Ph)] by FISH or G-banded karyotype is essential for diagnosis. The blood platelet level and number of blasts and basophils in blood and bone marrow are used to distinguish the chronic, accelerated, and blast phases of disease (See Chap. 10, Table 10-3). The degree of splenomegaly and the hematologic parameters are combined to generate the Sokal outcome prediction score (defined in Chap. 10.7), which appears to still be prognostically useful in the imatinib-treatment era [2].

A majority of patients with PV are diagnosed incidentally when a high hemoglobin or hematocrit is discovered on routine blood work without other presenting signs and symptoms [3].

From: *Neoplastic Hematopathology*: Contemporary Hematology,
Edited by: D. Jones, DOI 10.1007/978-1-60761-384-8_11,
© Humana Press, a part of Springer Science+Business Media, LLC 2010

Table 11-1. Findings in specific MPN types.

CML	PV	ET	PMF
BM findings			
• >90% cellular, myeloid predominant • Variable increases in blast and basophil % • t(9;22)(q34;q11) by karyotype	• Typically not needed, but can be variably cellular	• Fibrosis variable on reticulin and trichrome stains • JAK2/MPL mutation: in 50%	• Fibrosis variable on reticulin and trichrome stains • JAK2/MPL mutation in 40–50%
Laboratory findings			
• Basophilia on CBC • High BCR-ABL on RQ-PCR (baseline level)	• Serum EPO: low/normal • RBC mass: increased • Positive for JAK2 V617F mutation	• Platelet counts > 450×10^9/L	• Leukoerythroblastic CBC • Negative ANA, RF, and Coombs test
History and physical findings			
• B-symptoms • Variable splenomegaly	• Neurologic symptoms related to hyperviscosity • History of venous or arterial thrombosis • Microvascular-based swelling of extremities (erythromelagia) • Variable splenomegaly	• Assess for hemorrhagic and thrombotic sequelae • Mild splenomegaly	• B-symptoms • Splenomegaly, often marked

BM bone marrow, *CBC* complete blood count, *RQ-PCR* reverse transcription polymerase chain reaction, B-symptoms: night sweats, weight loss, fevers, *EPO* erythropoietin, *RBC* red blood cell, *ANA* anti-nuclear antibody, *RF* rheumatoid factor

Demonstration of an increased red blood cell (RBC) mass is important to distinguish PV from elevated hematocrit due to plasma volume contraction, as is the finding of a low to normal erythropoietin (EPO) level which excludes reactive erythrocytosis that has elevated EPO. With the discovery that an activating point mutation in codon 617 of the Janus-associated kinase-2 (JAK2) is found in nearly all cases of PV, molecular criteria for diagnosis have now been incorporated into screening algorithms [1,4]. Bone marrow biopsy is not commonly performed at the time of diagnosis because specific morphologic features of PV are lacking, and marrow fibrosis or karyotypic changes are rare until later in the disease course [5].

Most patients with ET are incidentally noted to have elevated platelet counts during routine medical care [3]. Diagnosis of essential thrombocythemia (ET), which was formerly a diagnosis of exclusion, can now be made definitively when persistent thrombocytosis ($>450 \times 10^9$ platelets/L) is accompanied by the detection of either a JAK2 codon 617 or MPL codon 515 point mutation [6]. ET with MPL mutation often shows higher platelet counts (and more microthrombotic sequelae) than cases with JAK2 mutation [7] and have higher mutation levels [34]. Diagnosis of the 50% of ET cases without detectable JAK2 or MPL mutation depends on an algorithmic workup to exclude other MPNs or reactive causes of thrombocytosis, with both karyotyping and additional molecular studies useful in classification (Fig. 11-1). In, particular, evaluation for t(9;22)(q34;q11) (or the BCR-ABL fusion transcript) is essential to exclude CML, and the other genetic changes, such as del(13q), del(20q), and del(5q), which are associated with PMF or MDS subtypes (e.g., refactory anemia with ring sideroblasts and thrombocytosis/RARS-T).

PMF has a variety of different clinical presentations, including abdominal pain due to splenomegaly or B-symptoms due to cytopenias. The diagnosis of PMF can be suspected whenever splenomegaly is accompanied by a leukoerythroblastic or myelophtisic peripheral smear (i.e. circulating BM elements along with teardrop erythrocytes). However, given that other marrow infiltrative tumors (e.g. metastatic carcinomas and storage diseases) can produce similar blood findings, bone marrow biopsy with reticulin/trichrome stains, JAK2/MPL

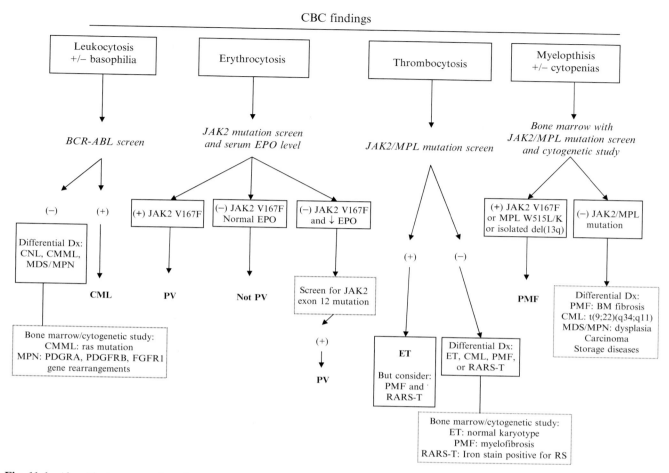

Fig. 11-1. *Algorithmic approach to diagnosis of chronic myeloproliferative neoplasms.* The use of BCR-ABL transcript profiling and of JAK2 and MPL mutation testing following the detection of peripheral blood abnormalities is highlighted. Abbreviations are as in the text

mutational analysis and cytogenetic studies is essential for diagnosis. JAK2 or MPL mutations will be detected in 40–50% of patients with PMF [8], with clonal karyotypic abnormalities seen in an additional 10–15%. Although, there are some subtle bone marrow morphologic changes in the initial stages of PMF, early diagnosis in the absence of overt fibrosis or a characteristic cytogenetic change remains difficult [1]. Array comparative genomic hybridization shows promise in identifying clonal changes in other cases [9]. Some PMF cases also show marrow dysplastic features (and transfusion or growth factor requirements) and may be better regarded as mixed MPN-MDS. Finally, secondary myelofibrotic transformation of an underlying ET or PV should always be considered, especially when presentation is atypical or a past history of unspecified hematologic abnormalities is reported [10].

11.2. Therapy Options in MPNs for Newly Diagnosed and Refectory Cases

11.2.1. Treatment of CML

The course of treatment for CML has drastically changed in the 10 years since the introduction of imatinib mesylate, a small molecule inhibitor of the BCR-ABL kinase. At a dose of 400 mg/day for chronic phase and 600 mg/day for advanced phases of CML, imatinib rapidly and selectively inhibits BCR-ABL-expressing hematopoiesis. Imatinib induces complete cytogenetic response in 87% of patients by 18 months, with most of the remaining patients having suboptimal responses or dose-limiting toxicities [11]. Criteria for defining suboptimal response or failure to imatinib have now been promulgated by the European Leukemia Net [12] and subsequently adopted by the National Comprehensive Cancer Network [13] (Tables 11-2 and 11-3), and are used as the criteria for either imatinib dose-escalation or switch to a new therapy [14]. Second generation tyrosine kinase inhibitors (TKIs), like dasatinib and nilotinib, are approved for patients with imatinib resistance. Both agents induce complete cytogenetic response rates in 45-55% of patients [15,16] and are currently being assessed as replacements for imatinib as frontline therapy.

Table 11-2. Criteria for imatinib failure in CML.

	Response	
Time (months)	Failure	Suboptimal
3	No HR[a]	No CHR
6	No CHR No CgR (Ph+>95%)	Less than PCgR (Ph+ ≥ 35%)
12	Less than PCgR (Ph+ ≥ 35%)	Less than CCgR (Ph+ > 0%)
18	Less than CCgR (Ph+ > 0%)	No MMR (<3-log decrease in BCR-ABL)
Any	Loss of CHR[b]	Clonal Evolution[d]
	Loss of CCgR[c]	Loss of MMR[d]
	High-risk BCR-ABL mutation	BCR-ABL mutation

HR hematologic response, *CHR* complete HR, *CgR* cytogenetic response, *PCgR* Partial cytogenetic response, *CCgR* compete cytogenetic response, *MMR* major molecular response
[a]Stable disease or disease progression
[b]Confirmed on 2 occasions, unless associated with progression to accelerated or blast phase
[c]Confirmed on 2 occasions, unless associated with CHR loss or progression to accelerated or blast phase
[d]Confirmed on 2 occasions, unless associated with CHR or CCgR loss

Table 11-3. Definitions of respone criteria in CML.

Hematologic response	
Complete	Normalization of peripheral blood counts
	• WBC < 10 × 10⁹/L, Platelets < 450 × 10⁹/L
	• Disappearance of all CML signs and symptoms, including splenomegaly
Partial	Criteria similar to complete response except for:
	• Presence of immature cells (blasts, promyelocytes, myelocytes)
	• Presence of splenomegaly, but <50% of pretreatment of size
	• Platelets > 450 × 10⁹/L, but <50% of pretreatment count
Cytogenetic Response[a]	
Complete	0% Ph(+) metaphases
Partial	1–35% Ph(+) metaphases
Major	0–35% Ph(+) metaphases (complete + partial)
Minor	>35–95% Ph(+) metaphases
Molecular Response	
Complete	Undetectable BCR-ABL transcripts by PCR in an assay with at least 4.5-log sensitivity
Major	≥ 3-log reduction in BCR-ABL transcripts

[a] Minimum of 20 metaphases must be analyzed

Other options for treatment of imatinib-resistant CML include combination therapies, and allogeneic hematopoietic stem cell transplant (HSCT) in selected patients. Since the approval of imatinib therapy for chronic phase CML, the use of upfront allogeneic HSCT for patients in chronic and accelerated phase has diminished significantly. Current guidelines recommend that HSCT be considered in patients who are resistant to available TKI therapy and/or those harboring pan-resistant mutations in BCR-ABL (e.g., T315I) [12]. For patients with CML in blast crisis, TKI therapy with or without cytotoxic chemotherapy can serve as a bridge to allogeneic HSCT.

11.2.2. Treatment of Other MPNs

PV is generally an indolent disorder, with the decision to treat based on risk stratification (Table 11-4). Patients with low-risk disease, i.e. those with no history of thrombosis, age less than 60 years, or platelets below $1,000 \times 10^9$/L, are usually treated with phlebotomy and/or aspirin [17,18]. The goal of phlebotomy is to keep the hematocrit level below 45% in men and below 42% in women [3]. Initially, phlebotomy is used to reduce hyperviscosity by decreasing the red cell mass, with subsequent phlebotomies timed to maintain the red cell mass in a normal range. For patients with high-risk features, i.e. history of thrombosis or age greater than 60 years, the range of treatments include phlebotomy, aspirin, and/or cytoreductive therapy with hydroxyurea [17,19].

Given its typically indolent course, the primary goal of treatment in patients with ET is the prevention of complications from thrombocytosis, such as microvascular disturbances or hemorrhagic events caused by acquired von Willebrand disease. Aspirin therapy is often used to reduce microvascular symptoms for patients in all risk categories (Table 11-4) [20,21] To reduce platelet counts, use of hydroxyurea in combination with low-dose aspirin has been shown to decrease the risk of arterial thrombosis in patients with high-risk ET, such as those older than 60 years, with platelets $>1,000 \times 10^9$/L, hypertension, diabetes requiring treatment, or ischemia, thrombosis, embolism, or hemorrhage related to ET [22].

For ET patients whose platelet counts are refractory to therapy with aspirin or other salicylates, therapy with interferon-alpha (INF-α) (including in pegylated preparations), anagrelide, or hydroxyurea can be used [23]. Anagrelide, originally developed to prevent platelet aggregation, was subsequently found to reduce platelet counts in ET and PMF by blocking megakaryocytic maturation when used at low dose.

PMF has a much more aggressive course than ET and PV; treatments include androgen preparations (e.g. fluoxymesterone or danazol), corticosteroids, erythropoietin (EPO), and lenalidomide [8]. Splenectomy is considered for patients with portal hypertension, anemia due to splenic sequestration, or for symptomatic relief of abdominal pain or problems with alimentation [3,24]. Radiation therapy to control splenomegaly may be beneficial for palliative relief however a significant increase in the risk of neutropenia and infection is seen [3,25–27]. Allogeneic HSCT is considered the only curable treatment option for patients with PMF. This option should be considered in young patients with intermediate/high-risk

Table 11-4. Risk for thrombosis in patients with ET and PV.

Category	Definitions	Treatment		
		ASA	Cytoreduction chemotherapy	Phlebotomy (in PV patients)
Low-risk	Age < 60 *and* no history of thrombosis *and* platelets $< 1000 \times 10^9$/L	Yes	No	Yes
Intermediate-risk	Platelets $> 1000 \times 10^9$/L	Yes	No	Yes
High-risk	Age $\geq$ 60 years *or* previous thrombosis	Yes	Yes	Yes

PMF [28]. For patients more older than 60 years of age, a reasonable option would be HSCT following a reduced-intensity conditioning regimen [23].

For PV, ET, and PMF, studies are ongoing to assess if one or more JAK kinase inhibitors will provide clinical benefit and eventually change the course of the disease [29].

11.3. How Responses are Assessed

11.3.1. CML

Response to TKI treatment in CML is based on the combination of hematologic, cytogenetic and molecular criteria (Table 11-3). Therefore, it is very important to establish baseline levels of BCR-ABL transcript levels as well as the number of Ph+ cells detected by G-banded karyotype or FISH at diagnosis to evaluate therapy success. Standardized protocols include the use of hematologic monitoring and BCR-ABL PCR in blood and cytogenetic studies in bone marrow every 3 months for the first year of treatment, and then BCR-ABL and hematologic monitoring every 6–12 months thereafter. Use of routine bone marrow biopsy with cytogenetics to evaluate for secondary TKI resistance after initial response has been achieved is more variable [30]. Criteria for the triggering testing of the BCR-ABL transcript to detect resistance mutations are also somewhat variable [31].

11.3.2. Monitoring of Other MPNs

Hematologic criteria and/or changes in spleen size are used to assess the response to treatment in PV, ET and PMF. Response to therapy in ET also can be evaluated by the decreased incidence of microvascular complications. Normalization of platelet counts is not essential nor does it completely prevent the risk of thrombosis. For those patients with ET, PMF, or PV with JAK2 or MPL mutation, serial quantitiative mutational analysis can be used to monitor the treatment responses. Quantitative reductions in JAK2 mutations levels have been observed with interferon [32], and lenalidomide [33].

Suggested Readings

Jabbour E, Cortes JE, Kantarjian HM. Molecular monitoring in chronic myeloid leukemia: response to tyrosine kinase inhibitors and prognostic implications. Cancer 2008;112:2112–2118.
Tefferi A. JAK2 mutations and clinical practice in myeloproliferative neoplasms. Cancer J 2007;13:366–371.

References

1. Tefferi A, Thiele J, Orazi A, et al. Proposals and rationale for revision of the World Health Organization diagnostic criteria for polycythemia vera, essential thrombocythemia, and primary myelofibrosis: recommendations from an ad hoc international expert panel. Blood 2007;110:1092–7.
2. Larson RA, Druker BJ, Guilhot F, et al. Imatinib pharmacokinetics and its correlation with response and safety in chronic-phase chronic myeloid leukemia: a subanalysis of the IRIS study. Blood 2008;111:4022–8.
3. Spivak JL. Polycythemia vera and other myeloproliferative diseases. In: Harrison's principles of internal medicine. New York: McGraw-Hill, 2005:626-31.
4. Tefferi A. Polycythemia vera: a comprehensive review and clinical recommendations. Mayo Clin Proc 2003;78:174–94.
5. Andrieux J, Demory JL, Caulier MT, et al. Karyotypic abnormalities in myelofibrosis following polycythemia vera. Cancer Genet Cytogenet 2003;140:118–23.
6. Sanchez S, Ewton A. Essential thrombocythemia: a review of diagnostic and pathologic features. Arch Pathol Lab Med 2006;130:1144–50.
7. Vannucchi AM, Antonioli E, Guglielmelli P, et al. Characteristics and clinical correlates of MPL 515W>L/K mutation in essential thrombocythemia. Blood 2008;112:844–7.

8. Tefferi A. Myelofibrosis with myeloid metaplasia. N Engl J Med 2000;342:1255–65.

9. Tefferi A, Sirhan S, Sun Y, et al. Oligonucleotide array CGH studies in myeloproliferative neoplasms: Comparison with JAK2V617F mutational status and conventional chromosome analysis. Leuk Res 2009;33:662–4.

10. Passamonti F, Malabarba L, Orlandi E, et al. Polycythemia vera in young patients: a study on the long-term risk of thrombosis, myelofibrosis and leukemia. Haematologica 2003;88:13–8.

11. Druker BJ, Guilhot F, O'Brien SG, et al. Five-year follow-up of patients receiving imatinib for chronic myeloid leukemia. N Engl J Med 2006;355:2408–17.

12. Baccarani M, Saglio G, Goldman J, et al. Evolving concepts in the management of chronic myeloid leukemia: recommendations from an expert panel on behalf of the European LeukemiaNet. Blood 2006;108:1809–20.

13. Chronic Myelogenous Leukemia. Clinical practice guidelines in oncology. In: Version 2.2009 ed: 2006 National Comprehensive Cancer Network, Inc.

14. Kantarjian HM, Larson RA, Guilhot F, et al. Efficacy of imatinib dose escalation in patients with chronic myeloid leukemia in chronic phase. Cancer 2009;115:551–60.

15. le Coutre P, Ottmann OG, Giles F, et al. Nilotinib (formerly AMN107), a highly selective BCR-ABL tyrosine kinase inhibitor, is active in patients with imatinib-resistant or -intolerant accelerated-phase chronic myelogenous leukemia. Blood 2008;111:1834–9.

16. Hochhaus A, Kantarjian HM, Baccarani M, et al. Dasatinib induces notable hematologic and cytogenetic responses in chronic-phase chronic myeloid leukemia after failure of imatinib therapy. Blood 2007;109:2303–9.

17. Tefferi A, Spivak JL. Polycythemia vera: scientific advances and current practice. Semin Hematol 2005;42:206–20.

18. Landolfi R, Marchioli R, Kutti J, et al. Efficacy and safety of low-dose aspirin in polycythemia vera. N Engl J Med 2004;350:114–24.

19. Fruchtman SM, Mack K, Kaplan ME, Peterson P, Berk PD, Wasserman LR. From efficacy to safety: a Polycythemia Vera Study group report on hydroxyurea in patients with polycythemia vera. Semin Hematol 1997;34:17–23.

20. Tefferi A, Gangat N, Wolanskyj AP. Management of extreme thrombocytosis in otherwise low-risk essential thrombocythemia; does number matter? Blood 2006;108:2493–4.

21. Harrison CN, Campbell PJ, Buck G, et al. Hydroxyurea compared with anagrelide in high-risk essential thrombocythemia. N Engl J Med 2005;353:33–45.

22. Finazzi G, Ruggeri M, Rodeghiero F, Barbui T. Second malignancies in patients with essential thrombocythaemia treated with busulphan and hydroxyurea: long-term follow-up of a randomized clinical trial. Br J Haematol 2000;110:577–83.

23. Tefferi A. Essential thrombocythemia, polycythemia vera, and myelofibrosis: current management and the prospect of targeted therapy. Am J Hematol 2008;83:491–7.

24. Lofvenberg E, Wahlin A. Management of polycythaemia vera, essential thrombocythaemia and myelofibrosis with hydroxyurea. Eur J Haematol 1988;41:375–81.

25. Tefferi A, Jimenez T, Gray LA, Mesa RA, Chen MG. Radiation therapy for symptomatic hepatomegaly in myelofibrosis with myeloid metaplasia. Eur J Haematol 2001;66:37–42.

26. Steensma DP, Hook CC, Stafford SL, Tefferi A. Low-dose, single-fraction, whole-lung radiotherapy for pulmonary hypertension associated with myelofibrosis with myeloid metaplasia. Br J Haematol 2002;118:813–6.

27. Elliott MA, Chen MG, Silverstein MN, Tefferi A. Splenic irradiation for symptomatic splenomegaly associated with myelofibrosis with myeloid metaplasia. Br J Haematol 1998;103:505–11.

28. Kroger N, Mesa RA. Choosing between stem cell therapy and drugs in myelofibrosis. Leukemia 2008;22:474–86.

29. Pesu M, Laurence A, Kishore N, Zwillich SH, Chan G, O'Shea JJ. Therapeutic targeting of Janus kinases. Immunol Rev 2008;223:132–42.

30. Kantarjian H, Schiffer C, Jones D, Cortes J. Monitoring the response and course of chronic myeloid leukemia in the modern era of BCR-ABL tyrosine kinase inhibitors: practical advice on the use and interpretation of monitoring methods. Blood 2008;111:1774–80.

31. Jones D, Kamel-Reid S, Bahler D, et al. Laboratory practice guidelines for detecting and reporting BCR-ABL drug resistance mutations in chronic myelogenous leukemia and acute lymphoblastic leukemia: a report of the Association for Molecular Pathology. J Mol Diagn 2009;11:4–11.

32. Quintas-Cardama A, Kantarjian H, Manshouri T, et al. Pegylated interferon alfa-2a yields high rates of hematologic and molecular response in patients with advanced essential thrombocythemia and polycythemia vera. J Clin Oncol 2009;27:5418–24.

33. Tefferi A, Cortes J, Verstovsek S, et al. Lenalidomide therapy in myelofibrosis with myeloid metaplasia. Blood 2006;108:1158–1164.

34. Millecker L, Lennon P, Verstovsek S, et al. Distinct patterns of cytogenetic and clinical progression in chronic myeloproliferative neoplasms with or without JAK2 or MPL mutations. Cancer Genet Cytogenet 2010;196.

Section 3

Tumors of the Lymph Node and Extranodal Tissues

Chapter 12

Lymph Node Biology and Lymphadenitis

Roberto N. Miranda

Abstract/Scope of Chapter The lymph node and other secondary lymphoid tissues, such as the tonsil/Waldeyer's ring and Peyer's patches, are the sites in the immune system, where B cells encounter antigen and expand to produce effector and memory B cells and plasma cells, with the assistance of T cells. B-cell expansion and maturation then occurs mainly in the germinal center and T-cell expansion and activation occurs both in the germinal center and the interfollicular or paracortical regions. Reactive lymphadenitis has many causes, with some histologic patterns that may resemble lymphoma. Depending on the inciting cause, one or several lymph node compartments may be expanded with distinctive follicular, paracortical, sinusoidal or medullary, and mixed patterns. For example, expansion of the follicles with prominent germinal centers is due to factors that promote B-cell expansion, whereas progressive transformation of germinal centers and follicular lysis represent follicular expansions associated with dissolution and termination of the germinal center reaction.

Keywords Lymph node, anatomy • Lymph node, cortex • Lymph node, medulla • Lymph node, paracortex • Lymphoid follicle • Lymph node, primary follicle • Lymph node, secondary follicle • Germinal center • Affinity maturation • Somatic hypermutation • Immunoglobulin class switch • Tingible body macrophage • Antigen-presenting cell • B-cell receptor • Centroblast • Centrocyte • Immunoblast • Follicular dendritic cell • Fibroblastic reticular cell • High endothelial venule • Lymph node, perifollicular sinus • Progressive transformation of germinal center • Follicular hyperplasia • Follicle lysis • Castleman disease • Toxoplasmosis • Immunoblastic proliferation, viral • Lymph node • Drug reaction • Paracortical hyperplasia • Dermatopathic lymphadenitis • Vascular transformation of lymph node sinuses • Kaposi's sarcoma

12.1. Introduction

Lymph node (LN) enlargement can be a function of normal immune response, autoimmune disease, or colonization by lymphoma or other tumors. Understanding the normal function of the lymph node is therefore essential for accurate diagnosis. This chapter reviews this function and some of the helpful patterns that distinguish reactive lymphadenitis from lymphoma. A full discussion of non-neoplastic hematopathology is beyond the goals of this textbook. Also omitted are the differences between LN and the other secondary lymphoid organs such as the spleen, Peyer's patches, and Waldeyer's ring tissue. Instead, we focus here on general immune system dynamics that may expand various compartments of the lymph node and

From: *Neoplastic Hematopathology*: Contemporary Hematology,
Edited by: D. Jones, DOI 10.1007/978-1-60761-384-8_12,
© Humana Press, a part of Springer Science+Business Media, LLC 2010

provide some examples of each pattern. However, in truth, the specific cause(s) of any given case of lymphadenitis is rarely identified, and little is known currently about the genetic factors that lead to dramatic lymph node enlargement in one patient and not another.

12.2. Lymph Node Structure

The compartments of the lymph node (LN) include the *cortex*, comprised of B-cell-rich lymphoid follicles and their germinal centers (GCs) and surrounding mantle zones; the *interfollicular* or *paracortical* areas rich in T cells; the *medulla*, which is organized into cords rich in histiocytes, plasma cells, and the larger blood vessels; and the *sinus system* which drains the lymph (Fig. 12-1). Immunostaining with lineage-specific antibodies can be used to highlight the different subsets of B cells and T cells, and the dendritic cells (DCs), and macrophages that represent the *antigen-presenting cells* (APCs), as well as the resident stromal cells, blood vessels, and lymphatics (Table 12-1) [1,2].

The lymph node is a dynamic structure with temporal shifts of cell populations between various compartments depending on the stage of the immune reaction. There are two opposing flows through the LN bringing growth factors (cytokines), chemokines, and soluble and cell-bound antigens from lymph into contact with lymphocytes and APCs arriving from the blood. In one direction, afferent lymphatic vessels drain lymph containing APCs, antigens, and soluble growth factors from surrounding skin and mucosa into the LN. There are two pathways for this lymph, with bulk flow moving into the subcapsular sinus, then branching to the interfollicular sinuses and cords, before exiting into efferent vessels to move to the next lymph node in the chain. A parallel pathway for lymph is along the *fibroblastic reticular cell* (FRC) network, which connects the sinuses to the blood vessels through a branching conduit of *reticular fibers* draped with FRCs to create small channels (Fig. 12-2) [3].

Cells flow through the LN in the opposite direction exiting from the blood at sites within the paracortex. Blood vessels enter through the nodal hilum, branch in the medulla, and ramify through each section of the lymph node cortex before returning in a counter-circulation similar to tubules in the kidney. Blood vessels with prominent endothelial linings, located at the cortical-paracortical junction, known as *high-walled endothelial venules* (HEVs) are the primary site of egress of lymphocytes and APCs (Fig. 12-2). HEVs display selectin ligand adhesion molecules such as the HECA-452 epitope which slow circulating leukocytes, and adhesion molecules which trap and permit transmigration of leukocytes

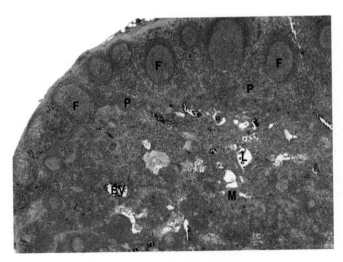

Fig. 12-1. Compartments of the lymph node. H&E stain of reactive node displays cortex with lymphoid follicles (F), minimally expanded paracortex (P), and medulla (M) with blood vessels (BV) and efferent lymphatics (L)

Table 12-1. Comparison of immune cell types in the lymph node.

Type of cell	Markers expressed	Role in immunity	Maturation sites
B cells	CD19, CD20, CD22	Humoral response	Bone marrow
Mantle cells	IgD, CD72	Naive and memory lymphocytes	
Follicular center cells	CD10, BCL6-high	Clonal expansion after antigen exposure	
T cells	CD2, CD3, CD5, CD7	Cellular response	Bone marrow to thymus
Helper T cell subset	CD4	Boost B-cell response (Th2 type)	
		Secrete cytokines	
Follicular helper subsets	BCL6, CD4, CD10, CD57, CD134, CXCR5	Boost B-cell expansion within the germinal center	
Cytotoxic subset	CD8, granzyme B, perforin	Lysis of foreign or infected cells	
Regulatory subset (Tregs)	CD25, FOXP3	Inhibition of T helper expansion	
Antigen-presenting cells			
Interdigitating dendritic cells	S100	Soluble antigen to T cells	Bone marrow to other tissues
Langerhans cells	S100, CD1a, langerin	Trapping of skin antigens and comigration with lymphocytes	Bone marrow to skin
Sinusoidal histiocytes	CD68, ±S100	Nonsoluble antigen presentation	Bone marrow to tissues
Follicular dendritic cells	CD21, CD23, CD35	Antigen presentation	Likely mesenchymal origin
Antigen-processing cells			
Macrophages	CD68, CD164, lysozyme	Phagocytosis of particulate antigens	Bone marrow precursor
Stromal cells			
Endothelial cells	CD34, VCAM-1 HECA-452 (HEV)	Source of cytokines, mediates leukocyte migration	Mesenchymal origin
Fibroblastic reticular cells	Actin, vimetin, ±desmin, ±keratin type 8/18	Soluble antigen transport	Mesenchymal origin

across HEVs into the nodal parenchyma. Antigen presentation takes place between lymph-borne DCs that migrate across the lymphatics and meet circulating lymphocytes in the vicinity of HEVs. Finally, there are typically compressed *perifollicular lymphatics* encircling the GCs which may, under certain conditions, expand and drive B-cell and follicular T-cell expansion (Fig. 12-3) [4].

The two opposing lymphatic and HEV-mediated LN flows are regulated in parallel [5]. For example, activation of the HEV to permit more leukocyte binding and egress is accomplished by endothelial stimulation by cytokines of the tumor necrosis factor family that are delivered to the adluminal surface of the HEV by the FRC conduits of lymph draining from sites of inflammation (Fig. 12-2). In this way, there is coordinate regulation of all compartments of the lymph node. There is also segmental anatomy of most lymph nodes so that one lobule of a node can have an activated cortex/paracortex, while an adjacent one might be more quiescent depending on regional patterns of lymph flow.

12.3. Functional Biology of the Germinal Center

The germinal center (GC) is the principal site where expansion of B cells occurs in response to antigen [1,6]. The role of the GC is to generate short-lived effector B cells, long-lived memory B cells, and antibody-secreting plasma cells that all have high affinity immunoglobulin for the

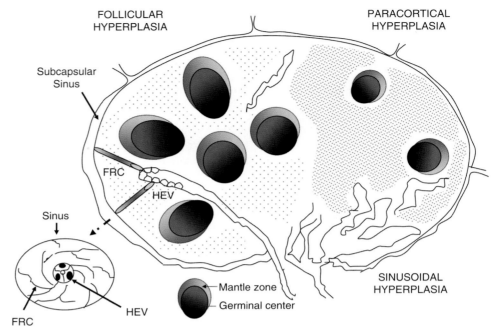

Fig. 12-2. Compartments of the lymph node. Diagram of a reactive lymph node displays expansion of the cortex, paracortex, and the sinuses. Displayed on the left are the fibroblastic reticular cell (FRC) conduits that connect the subcapsular sinus with a high-walled endothelial venule (HEV)

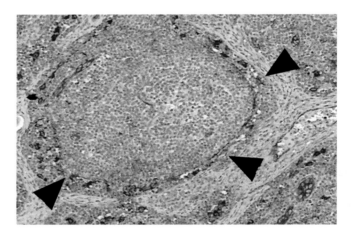

Fig. 12-3. Relationship of the germinal center to the paracortex. The stromal marker transglutaminase highlights the perifollicular sinus (*black arrowheads*) nearly encircling the germinal center with a small collar connecting the follicles to the paracortex. In most tissue sections of lymph node, the perifollicular sinus is partially collapsed and difficult to visualize without the use of lymphatic immunomarkers

specific inciting antigen. These goals are achieved through the interconnected processes of somatic hypermutation, affinity maturation, and immunoglobulin class switch (Fig. 12-4).

The early stages of B-cell maturation are summarized in Chap. 31, whereby immature B cells (lymphoblasts) move from the bone marrow to the peripheral blood. Such circulating antigen-naïve mature B cells then enter the lymph node and colonize the mantle zones of pre-existing *secondary follicles* or form aggregates known as *primary follicles*. Upon

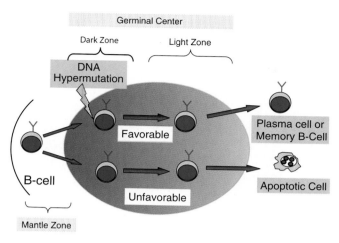

Fig. 12-4. The processes of lymphocyte migration, somatic hypermutation, and affinity maturation in the lymphoid follicle. Diagram showing the dark and light zone compartments within the germinal center where somatic hypermutation, immunoglobulin class switch, and clonal expansion occur during B-cell maturation

encountering the appropriate APC-bound antigen for their surface immunoglobulin/B-cell receptor (BCR), each B cell becomes activated and migrates into a developing GC to undergo *clonal expansion*. The location of initial B-cell activation by antigen is still under study. In one model, APCs such as the S100+ and CD1a+ Langerhans cell (LC) migrating from lymph and resident LN interdigitating dendritic cells (IDCs) encounter and stimulate helper T cells in the paracortex and these activated T cells then cooperate in initial B-cell activation.

Growth and persistence of B cells within the GC is supported by specialized subsets of T cells and a dense meshwork of stromal cells known as follicular dendritic cells (FDCs). FDCs bind and trap immune complexes which they acquire from circulating lymph to their surface through Ig Fc and complement receptors [1]. FDC-bound immune complexes are long-lived and can provide sustained B-cell stimulation. FDCs also secrete chemokines which attract B cells and growth factors which inhibit B-cell apoptosis [1]. It is believed that each GC is populated by a small number of founder B cells, but B cells may travel from GC to GC and reactivate clonal expansion a number of times [6,7]. Experimental models suggest that initial development of the GC is dependent on expression of multiple members of the *tumor necrosis factor* (TNF) gene family, including TNF-alpha, lymphotoxin-alpha, and lymphotoxin-beta [6]. In animal models, continued development of the GC is dependent on helper T cells which shift the balance between B-cell proliferation and apoptosis.

The GC has a polarized structure (Fig. 12-5) whereby proliferation of B cells occurs predominantly in the *dark zone,* a cell-dense area with highly proliferative lymphocytes termed *B-blasts*. At this time of rapid cell division, the process of *somatic hypermutation* is activated, which is a form of error-prone DNA replication that produces additional nucleotide substitutions in the immunoglobulin genes. From a single progenitor B cell thus emerges a range of B cells, some with nonfunctional or lower affinity BCRs, and others with a higher affinity BCRs for a particular inciting antigen. These mutated B cells then encounter FDC-bound antigen and undergo testing of the signaling fitness of the altered BCR (Fig. 12-4). B cells with lower affinity BCR undergo apoptotic cell death through a FAS-mediated process, [7] and are continuously phagocytised producing *tingible body macrophages* that have numerous lymphocyte fragments in their cytoplasm. Apoptosis also occurs in B cells that acquire BCR that are auto-reactive against self-antigens [2]. B cells with higher affinity for the target antigen proliferate and may undergo successive rounds of somatic hypermutation. Through such *affinity maturation,* B cells with BCR that most avidly bind the inciting antigen survive,

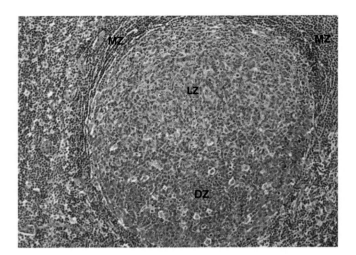

Fig. 12-5. Reactive germinal center in a case of follicular lymphoid hyperplasia. H&E stain displays germinal center surrounded by well-defined mantle zone (MZ). Dark zone (DZ) with tingible bodies in the *lower half*, and light zone (LZ) in the *upper half*

proliferate, and differentiate further in the *light zone*. These B cells assume different sizes and shapes, that include the *centrocytes* or *small cleaved* lymphocytes and the proliferating large *centroblasts*, and upon further antigen stimulation may acquire large, vesicular nuclei and abundant, basophilic cytoplasm and are termed *immunoblasts* (Fig. 12-6).

The process of *immunoglobulin class switch* also occurs in the GC, whereby a subset of B cells change from expressing surface IgM (with or without IgD) to IgG, IgA, or IgE. This switch, which is produced by a DNA recombination event, happens in parallel with and using some of the same enzymes as somatic hypermutation. Further maturation of B cells occurs upon their movement out of the GC, with some B cells migrating back to the mantle zone, others forming a recirculating memory pool, and some differentiating into plasma cells that home to nodal sinuses, extranodal lymphoid aggregates, and the bone marrow.

Polarization of the GC into dark zones and light zones is also a reflection of the differential distribution of T cells and FDCs [6]. Like GC B cells, follicle-homing T cells also express CD10 and BCL6 and migrate into the developing follicle after upregulation of the homing chemokine receptor CXCR5 [6,8,9]. Follicle-associated T cells and FDCs also produce the chemokine ligand for CXCR5 (CXCL13) that drives GC B-cell recruitment. A different subset of CD4+CD57+ T cells are mainly located at the apex of the light zone where they mediate CD40–CD40 ligand interactions that promote B-cell survival [6]. Although T cells in the GC do not undergo somatic hypermutation, they do undergo expansion through T-cell receptor (TCR) binding to FDC-bound antigen and thus provide antigen-specific recirculating CD4+ memory T cells [6]. While most FDC subsets promote GC B-cell proliferation, some subsets can express ligands that drive apoptosis of B cells, [7] and there are varying densities of trapped antigen on FDCs due to differential expression of complement receptors (CD21, CD35) and Fc (CD23) receptors.

12.4. Regression of the Germinal Center

Following an immune assault, there is a variable persistence of GCs probably related to previous antigen exposure, current antigen dose, and exposure duration [6]. As discussed above, specialized GC helper T cells are critical for GC persistence and their activity is regulated by *CD25+ FOXP3+ regulatory T cells*, which can be found in great numbers in the LN at various stages of the immune response. The function of regulatory T cells tends to decline with age

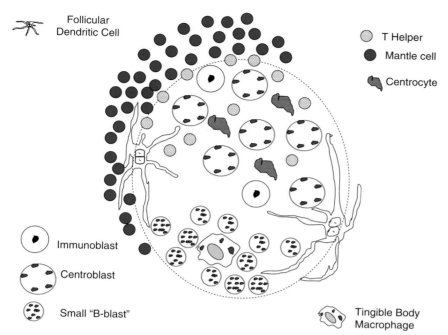

Fig. 12-6. Microarchitecture of the lymphoid follicle. Diagram showing cell types and distribution pattern within a reactive germinal center

and with iatrogenic and viral-associated immuosuppression and thus affects GC persistence. The altered GC dynamics seen in patients with germline mutations in FAS or FASL in *autoimmune lymphoproliferative syndrome* (ALPS) indicates that abnormal function of growth regulatory cytokines or their receptors also influences the rate of GC formation and dissolution, and may be an under-recognized driving force for some persistent lymphadenitis.

12.5. Follicular Hyperplasia with or Without Plasmacytosis

Follicular hyperplasia (FH) with prominent GCs can be produced by a variety of different stimuli. Common non-neoplastic causes of *localized FH* include persistent bacterial infection such as *mesenteric lymphadenitis* seen with gastrointestinal pathogens, protozoal cervical lymphadenitis due to *Toxoplasma gondii* infection (Fig. 12-7), and *hyaline vascular Castleman disease*, discussed below. Generalized FH can occur with primary or reactivating viral infections (e.g., herpesviruses or human immunodeficiency virus), autoimmune diseases (particularly rheumatoid arthritis), or with drug reactions.

FH may be confused with follicular lymphoma (Fig. 12-8), or other lymphomas with a nodular pattern, such as mantle cell and marginal zone lymphoma. Features that favor FH over follicular lymphoma include the preservation of all LN compartments, a predominance of follicles restricted to the cortex, and most importantly preservation of the polarity of mantle zones and the light and dark zones of the GC (Table 12-2). Overexpression of the anti-apoptotic protein BCL-2 in B cells within the follicles, which is not seen in reactive GCs, strongly supports a diagnosis of lymphoma. In difficult cases, immunophenotyping to exclude monotypic kappa or lambda Ig light chain expression can be done by flow cytometry or by frozen section immunoperoxidase. Lymphomas that can show colonization of reactive GC by tumor cells include the floral variant of follicular lymphoma, some marginal zone lymphomas, and the nodular variant of mantle cell lymphoma.

A particular etiology of generalized FH with associated plasmacytosis is due to reactivated infection of human herpesvirus 8 and is known as *multicentric plasma cell Castleman*

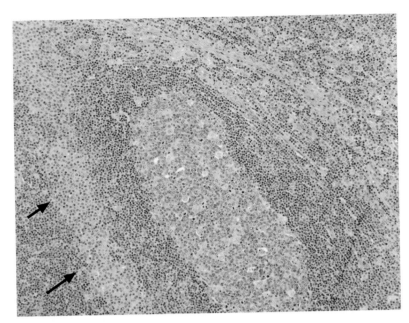

Fig. 12-7. Reactive lymphoid follicles in a case of toxoplasmosis. Florid follicular hyperplasia with perifollicular sheets of monocytoid B cells (*arrows*) are characteristic of this typically self-limited protozoan infection. Serologic confirmation of *T. gondii* antibody titers is diagnostic

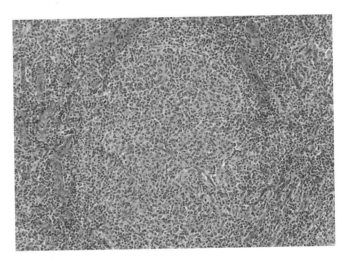

Fig. 12-8. Neoplastic lymphoid follicle in a case of follicular lymphoma. H&E stain displays an ill-defined follicle surrounded by a faint mantle zone. There is a monomorphous cytomorphology and absence of polarity throughout the entire follicle

disease [10]. This lesion, seen in immunodeficient and elderly patients from HHV8-endemic areas, is often a precursor lesion to Kaposi sarcoma, or monoclonal plasma cell proliferations associated with the *POEMS syndrome* (*p*olyneuropathy, *o*rganomegaly, *e*ndocrinopathy, *m*onoclonal gammopathy, and *s*kin changes), or plasmablastic lymphoma (see Chap. 17). In contrast, localized FH with plasmacytosis (i.e., *localized plasma cell Castleman disease*) is almost always a benign lesion, but can occur in draining LNs adjacent to those involved by Hodgkin's lymphoma (HL) or other cytokine-producing tumors (See Chap. 20).

Table 12-2. Features of follicular hyperplasia versus follicular lymphoma.

Feature	Follicular hyperplasia	Follicular lymphoma
Clinical findings	Any age, autoimmune, inflammatory or infectious symptomatology	Older population, long-standing adenopathy, multiple sites
Nodal architecture	All compartments present	Effaced with loss of some compartments
Density of follicles	Mainly in cortical region	Throughout lymph node
Appearance of follicles	Polarity detected; dark and light zones seen	Loss of polarity, uniform cellularity
Mantle zone around follicles	Prominent and polarized	Thin or inconspicuous
Cell composition	Mixture of small, intermediate, and large cells	Predominance of one type of cell
Tingible body macrophages	Frequent in dark zones	Absent or few
BCL-2 in GC B cells by immunohistochemistry	Negative in GC B cells	Uniformly positive in >90% of cases
FDC phenotype (CD21/CD23/CD35)	Similar in most follicles	Variable loss of FDC staining
Proliferation markers (e.g., Ki-67)	Positive in ~100% of cells in GC dark zone, very high in light zone	Usually low (<20%), but may be up to 70% in higher grade follicular lymphoma
Ig-kappa and Ig-lambda by flow cytometry or frozen section immunostain	Polyclonal	Monoclonal (i.e., kappa to lambda > 4:1 or lambda to kappa > 2:1)
Cytogenetic or molecular analysis	Normal	t(14;18) or BCL2/IGH detected in >85% of cases

Another reactive condition resulting in enlarged follicles is *progressive transformation of germinal centers (PTGC)*. In PTGC, perifollicular B cells with a mantle zone phenotype migrate into the GC, T cells spread from the light zone, and FDCs lose their fully differentiated state. This results in fragmentation and expansion of the follicle. T cells within the transformed follicle acquire CD57 and may express T-cell activation markers such as CD134/OX40 [6, 7, 11]. A small number of follicles with PTGC may occur in any immune reaction, but large numbers of them may indicate an underlying immune abnormality [12]. PTGC follicles resemble the expansive nodules in nodular lymphocyte predominant (NLP) HL requiring detailed examination of any case to look for the large CD20+ neoplastic (L&H or LP) cells that are the hallmark of this tumor (Chap. 20). Interestingly, some patients who develop NLPHL also have a propensity to show large numbers of PTGC follicles in uninvolved LNs, suggesting the two lesions may be pathogenetically related.

12.6. Contraction and Fragmentation of the Lymphoid Follicle

Some enlarged LNs show a predominance of secondary lymphoid follicles that are small, but still maintain the stromal organization of the GC. Such "Castlemanoid" or regressed follicles are composed predominantly of FDCs and are depleted of GC B cells and tingible body macrophages, suggesting that the process of follicular proliferation has largely ceased. Mantle zones are preserved or even prominent, and some cases show interfollicular immunoblastic proliferation indicative of ongoing antigenic stimulation. Causes of lymphadenitis with such prominent regressed follicles include nodal irradiation, prolonged immune stimulation, and the *hyaline vascular variant of Castleman disease* (HVCD), which is a benign but possibly clonal disorder of FDC. Definitive features of HVCD, in addition to localized lymphadenopathy and regressed follicles (Fig. 12-9), include prominent interfollicular HEV, proliferations of plasmacytoid DCs, and partial or complete loss of subcapsular sinuses due to expansile compression. One variant of follicular lymphoma, particularly common in intraabdominal and pelvic LNs, can show a predominance of regressed follicles simulating HVCD.

Other patterns of reactive GC dissolution include *follicular lysis*, necrosis of follicles, and formation of granulomas within GCs. Follicular lysis is usually found in HIV+ patients with high viral titers and is characterized by invasion of CD8+ cytotoxic T cells into the GC. Necrosis of follicles is occasionally seen in children with severe bacterial infections, probably caused by cytolytic attack against lymphocytes or APCs containing bacterial antigens.

12.7. Paracortical (Interfollicular) Expansions

In general, immune reactions due to soluble antigens recognized by B cells (i.e., humoral immunity) lead to follicular hyperplasia, whereas immune reactions handled by T-cell-mediated immunity without B cells selectively expand the LN paracortex [1].

One such T-cell-mediated condition is *dermatopathic-type lymphadenitis*, which is characterized by expansion of T cells in the interfollicular or subcapsular regions along with marked DC or Langerhans cell infiltration. This results in a low-magnification "mottled" appearance (Fig. 12-10). If the infiltrate is due to lymph drainage from sites of skin breakdown, melanin-laden histiocytes/DCs will also be prominent [13,14]. Mycosis fungoides and other cutaneous lymphomas frequently produce dermatopathic lymphadenitis and careful examination for lymphocyte atypia along with flow cytometric characterization of the T cells is often required to distinguish benign from neoplastic causes (Table 12-3 and Chap. 24) [15,16].

Another difficult pattern of paracortical lymphadenitis to distinguish from lymphoma is *interfollicular immunoblastic proliferations* that occur with hypersensitivity reactions to vaccines or drugs (e.g., phenytoin), or with prolonged viral infections (most commonly EBV-driven infectious mononucleosis or cytomegalovirus infection) (Fig. 12-11). Such *immunoblastic reactions* may distort or obliterate normal LN architecture, but there is usually a polymorphous lymphoid infiltrate. Admixed plasma cells, neutrophils, eosinophils, or histiocytes are also often present [13]. Reactive immunoblasts can have very prominent nucleoli or be binucleated like the Reed–Sternberg cells seen in HL, although reactive immunoblasts are variably positive for CD20 and CD3, and do not have the uniformly strong CD30 and CD15 positivity seen in HL. A malignant process, such as large B-cell lymphoma or peripheral T-cell lymphoma, is favored when the architecture is completely

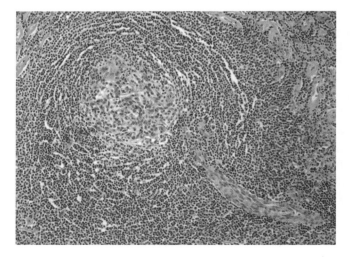

Fig. 12-9. Regressed follicle in a case of hyaline vascular Castleman's disease. H&E stain displays a compact germinal center composed predominantly of follicular dendritic cells surrounded by a prominent mantle zone containing a thick-walled penetrating arteriole ("lollipop" appearance)

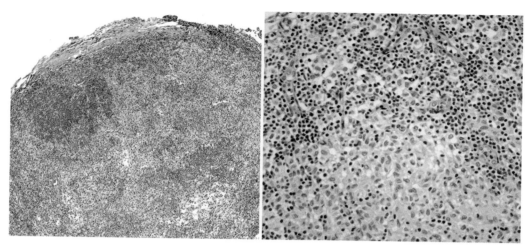

Fig. 12-10. Paracortical expansion in a case of dermatopathic lymphadenitis. H&E stain displays expanded paracortical region with a "mottled" appearance (*left*). There are admixed small lymphocytes and epithelioid histiocytes (*right*)

Table 12-3. Features distinguishing reactive dermatopathic lymphadenitis from nodal involvement by mycosis fungoides.

Feature	Dermatopathic lymphadenitis	Mycosis fungoides
Clinical findings	Any age, skin itching, chronic dermatosis	Older population, skin tumor, history of mycosis fungoides
Nodal architecture	Preserved; it is possible to identify all compartments	Similar to dermatopathic
Lymphoid follicles	Pushed apart due to interfollicular expansion	Pushed apart due to interfollicular expansion
Interfollicular region	"Mottled" appearance	"Mottled" appearance
Cell composition	Mixture of small, round lymphocytes, interdigitating dendritic cells, and melanin laden histiocytes	Similar to dermatopathic in early (N1) disease; cerebriform or large nucleolated cells in later stages (N2/N3)
Flow cytometric phenotype	Majority are CD3+CD4+ T cells, with partial or complete loss of CD7, but no change in CD3 or CD4 surface density	Predominantly CD3+CD4+ T cells with altered density of surface staining and complete CD26 loss in a subpopulation
T-cell receptor genes by PCR or Southern blot analysis	Polyclonal or oligoclonal pattern	Clonally rearranged

effaced or when there is asymmetrical expansions of "immunoblasts" with monomorphous cytomorphology (Table 12-4). Most lymphomas increase in incidence with age and emerge over many weeks to months, whereas immunoblastic reactions are common in children and develop rapidly over days to weeks.

Reactive LN conditions that produce histiocytic infiltration include *Kukuchi–Fujimoto disease* (subacute or histiocytic necrotizing lymphadenitis), which shows zonal collections of crescentic histiocytes (with C-shaped nuclei) with associated necrosis but an absence of neutrophils, and is a self-limited lymphadenitis often seen in younger woman with systemic lupus erythematosus. *Cat-scratch disease* (*Bartonella henselae* infection) produces stellate-shaped abscesses with frequent neutrophils and cellular debris, as well as surrounding follicular hyperplasia and collections of plasmacytoid B cells.

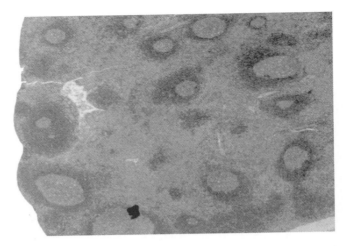

Fig. 12-11. Benign immunoblastic proliferation. Marked expansion of the interfollicular areas of the lymph node and associated follicular hyperplasia

Table 12-4. Most helpful features in distinguishing benign interfollicular lymphadenitis from lymphoma.

Feature	Benign/reactive lymphadenitis	Large cell lymphoma (EBV+ or −)
Clinical findings	Young age, recent onset fever, neck node enlargement	Older population, generalized adenopathy, history of lymphoma
Node architecture	Marked uniform expansion of interfollicular regions	Asymmetrical interfollicular expansions or diffuse effacement in areas
Lymphoid follicles	Often reactive, but displaced by interfollicular expansion	Infiltrated or displaced by sheet-like interfollicular expansion
Cell composition	Mixture of small, intermediate, and large lymphocytes with immunoblasts	Sheets or clusters of atypical cells with clear cytoplasm (in T-cell lymphoma) or uniform plasmablastic or immunoblastic appearance (large B-cell lymphoma)
Immunophenotyping	Polytypic B lymphocytes and mixed population of T cells	Aberrant loss of normal B-cell and T-cell populations (many large B-cell lymphomas lack surface Ig)
EBV in situ hybridization	Negative or scattered positivity	Absent or uniformly positive

12.8. Disorders Involving the Lymph Node Sinuses and Medulla

Prominent or distended LN sinuses are common in prolonged immune reactions, but may be associated with infiltration by solid tumors, lymphomas, or intrinsic tumors of the lymph node vessels and stroma. There are great regional variations in lymph flow at different lymph node sites producing varying levels of sinus distension and sometimes *vascular transformation of sinuses*, especially in abdominal and pelvic locations. Most cases of sinus engorgement represent reactive histiocytosis due to lymph drainage from inflammatory processes. Such activated histiocytes and DCs can have prominent nucleoli and a cohesive appearance; however, sinus infiltrates that have necrosis, marked atypia, or numerous mitoses should raise the differential diagnosis of metastatic carcinoma (Fig. 12-12), anaplastic large cell lymphoma, or Langerhans cell histiocytosis (Chap. 26). Massive expansion of

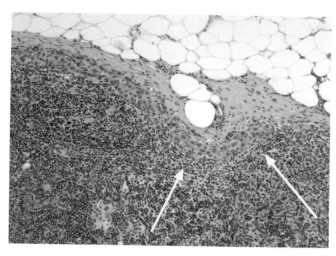

Fig. 12-12. Lymph node with distended sinuses in a case of metastatic breast carcinoma. Infiltrating breast cancer cells are seen within lymph node sinuses (*arrows*)

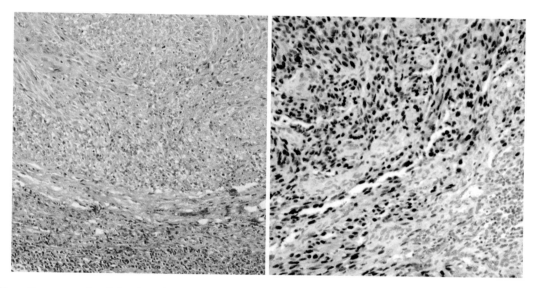

Fig. 12-13. Kaposi's sarcoma involving lymph node. A spindle cell proliferation emanating from the sinus shows entrapped red blood cells in vascular slits and a sharp border with surrounding lymph node (*left*). Immunostain for HHV8 LNA-1 is positive in all spindle cells (*right*)

the LN by benign-appearing sinus histiocytes with lymphocyte engulfment should raise the diagnosis of Rosai–Dorfman disease (Chap. 26).

Lesions that may involve the medullary region of the LN include vascular lesions such as the reactive *angiomyomatous hamartoma* seen in pelvic LNs (likely due to pressure changes), hemangioma, angiomatosis, and *Kaposi's sarcoma* (KS). KS usually involves the LN capsule and subcapsular sinus initially and then extends inward along the sinuses. The most common appearance is that of a cellular spindle cell proliferation with increased mitoses. Slit-like spaces, intracellular erythrocytes, and hemosiderin deposition are characteristic. Tumor cells are positive for the endothelial markers CD31, Factor VIII, and CD34, and the diagnosis can be confirmed by immunohistochemistry for HHV8 latent nuclear antigen (LNA-1) (Fig. 12-13).

Bacillary angiomatosis is a vascular lesion, usually caused by *Bartonella henselae* or *Bartonella quintana* bacterial infections, and involves the interfollicular or medullary LN regions. It is characterized by open, edematous, medium-sized vessels surrounded by edema and inflammatory cells [13]. Diagnosis of *Bartonella* infections may be confirmed by serologic and microbiologic cultures of blood or tissues. Warthin–Starry or Steiner silver-impregnation stains, immunohistochemistry using antibodies against *Bartonella* antigens, or PCR can also be used to confirm diagnosis in tissues. Cat scratch disease and bacillary angiomatosis are two disease manifestations of *Bartonella* infection, with the granulomatous suppurative reaction of the former occurring mainly in immunocompetent patients, and the vasculoproliferative reaction of the latter usually occurring among immunocompromised patients.

12.9. Open Lymph Node Biopsy versus Fine Needle Aspiration

The wealth of reactive and neoplastic lesions of the LN described in this section of the text are best diagnosed in reference to the LN microanatomy. Even in the era of fine needle aspiration and flow cytometry, open lymph node biopsy is still a much more valuable tool to determine causes of lymphadenopathy. In the last several years, we have begun to appreciate that there are host genetic factors [revealed by single nucleotide polymorphisms (SNPs) or chromosomal copy number variations (CNVs), and even undiagnosed inherited immune defects] which present as subtle distortions of normal LN architecture and which sometimes obscure the distinctions between lymphoma, pre-neoplastic states, and immune alterations. Therefore, as understanding of these genetically-determined immune variations increases, open LN biopsies will become even more important in the workup of lymphadenopathy. A thorough morphologic examination coupled with an understanding of the normal dynamics of the LN is thus essential in distinguishing between overt lymphoma and the various abnormal but non-neoplastic immune states that can produce LN enlargement.

Suggested Readings

Gretz JE, Anderson AO, Shaw S. Cords, channels, corridors and conduits: critical architectural elements facilitating cell interactions in the lymph node cortex. Immunol Rev 1997;156:11–24.
  • This forward-thinking model integrating all compartments of the lymph node has been largely confirmed by recent in vivo imaging and functional studies.
King C, Tangye SG, Mackay CR. T follicular helper (TFH) cells in normal and dysregulated immune responses. Annu Rev Immunol 2008;26:741–66.
  • A recent review of the emerging importance of the follicular-associated T cell subsets.

References

1. Delves P, Martin S, Burton D, Roitt IM. Roitt's essential immunology. 11th ed. Massachusetts: Blackwell, 2006.
2. van der Valk PMC. Reactive lymph nodes. In: Sternberg SS, ed. Histology for pathologists. Philadelphia: Lippincott-Raven, 1997.
3. Gretz JE, Norbury CC, Anderson AO, Proudfoot AE, Shaw S. Lymph-borne chemokines and other low molecular weight molecules reach high endothelial venules via specialized conduits while a functional barrier limits access to the lymphocyte microenvironments in lymph node cortex. J Exp Med 2000;192:1425–40.
4. Ottaviani G, Bueso-Ramos CE, Seilstad K, Medeiros LJ, Manning JT, Jones D. The role of the perifollicular sinus in determining the complex immunoarchitecture of angioimmunoblastic T-cell lymphoma. Am J Surg Pathol 2004;28:1632–40.
5. Thomazy VA, Vega F, Medeiros LJ, Davies PJ, Jones D. Phenotypic modulation of the stromal reticular network in normal and neoplastic lymph nodes: tissue transglutaminase reveals coordinate regulation of multiple cell types. Am J Pathol 2003;163:165–74.
6. Jones D. Dismantling the germinal center: comparing the processes of transformation, regression, and fragmentation of the lymphoid follicle. Adv Anat Pathol 2002;9:129–38.

7. Hur DY, Kim DJ, Kim S, et al. Role of follicular dendritic cells in the apoptosis of germinal center B cells. Immunol Lett 2000;72:107–11.

8. Dupuis J, Boye K, Martin N, et al. Expression of CXCL13 by neoplastic cells in angioimmunoblastic T-cell lymphoma (AITL): a new diagnostic marker providing evidence that AITL derives from follicular helper T cells. Am J Surg Pathol 2006;30:490–4.

9. Grogg KL, Attygalle AD, Macon WR, Remstein ED, Kurtin PJ, Dogan A. Expression of CXCL13, a chemokine highly upregulated in germinal center T-helper cells, distinguishes angioimmunoblastic T-cell lymphoma from peripheral T-cell lymphoma, unspecified. Mod Pathol 2006;19:1101–7.

10. Amin HM, Medeiros LJ, Manning JT, Jones D. Dissolution of the lymphoid follicle is a feature of the HHV8+ variant of plasma cell Castleman's disease. Am J Surg Pathol 2003;27:91–100.

11. Lin P, Medeiros LJ, Wilder RB, Abruzzo LV, Manning JT, Jones D. The activation profile of tumour-associated reactive T-cells differs in the nodular and diffuse patterns of lymphocyte predominant Hodgkin's disease. Histopathology 2004;44:561–9.

12. Ferry JA, Zukerberg LR, Harris NL. Florid progressive transformation of germinal centers. A syndrome affecting young men, without early progression to nodular lymphocyte predominance Hodgkin's disease. Am J Surg Pathol 1992;16:252–8.

13. Ioachim HM, Medeiros LJ. Ioachim's lymph node pathology. 4th ed. Philadelphia: Wolters Kluwer/Lippincott Williams&Wilkins, 2009.

14. Gould E, Porto R, Albores-Saavedra J, Ibe MJ. Dermatopathic lymphadenitis. The spectrum and significance of its morphologic features. Arch Pathol Lab Med 1988;112:1145–50.

15. Zinzani PL, Ferreri AJ, Cerroni L. Mycosis fungoides. Crit Rev Oncol Hematol 2008;65:172–82.

16. Hoppe RT, Wood GS, Abel EA. Mycosis fungoides and the Sezary syndrome: pathology, staging, and treatment. Curr Prob Cancer 1990;14:293–371.

17. Jaffe ES, Harris NL, Stein H, Isaacson PG. Classification of lymphoid neoplasms: the microscope as a tool for disease discovery. Blood 2008;112:4384–99.

18. Lukes RJ, Collins RD. Immunologic characterization of human malignant lymphomas. Cancer 1974;34(Suppl):1488–503.

19. Mann RB, Jaffe ES, Berard CW. Malignant lymphomas – a conceptual understanding of morphologic diversity. A review. Am J Pathol 1979;94:105–92.

Chapter 13

Lymphoblastic Leukemia and Lymphoma

Andrea M. Sheehan

Abstract/Scope of Chapter This chapter covers T and B lymphoblastic neoplasms, including acute lymphoblastic leukemia (ALL) and lymphoblastic lymphoma (LBL). Morphologic, immunophenotypic, and cytogenetic features are discussed along with the parameters of various modalities used in their diagnosis. The techniques and utility of minimum residual disease (MRD) measurement after therapy is discussed, as are new insights into the molecular biology of leukemogenesis gleaned from recent studies using gene expression profiling and copy number analysis via microarray techniques.

Keywords Lymphoblastic leukemia • Lymphoblastic lymphoma • Acute lymphoblastic leukemia • Pharmacogenetics, lymphoblastic leukemia • HOX genes • Gene expression profiling, acute lymphoblastic leukemia

13.1. Historical Overview, Pathogenesis, and Current Classification

The improved outcome in pediatric acute lymphoblastic leukemia (ALL) has been one of the great success stories in oncology. With the refinement of multiagent chemotherapy protocols, the cure rate has gone from less than 10% fifty years ago to greater than 80% today. However, the same degree of success has yet to be achieved in adults with ALL where the long-term remission rate is currently only 30–40%.

As outcomes have improved, the classification schemas for ALL and its tissue-based counterpart lymphoblastic lymphoma (LBL) have also been refined (Table 13-1). The first systematic approach to diagnose ALL, the French-American-British (FAB) classification, was developed during the late 1970's and early 1980's and defined L1, L2, and L3 subtypes based on the morphologic appearance of the blasts. Cytochemical stains were used to distinguish ALL from other types of acute leukemia. The association of precursor T-cell ALL/LBL with the thymus and precursor B-cell ALL with the bone marrow (BM) had been recognized for many years but only when immunophenotyping by flow cytometry (FC) became more common was there a shift toward an immunophenotypic classification of ALL/LBL. This approach was based on mapping ALL/LBL to the stages of lymphocyte maturation, defining pro-B, common, pre-B and Burkitt/mature B-cell types of B-ALL, and similar subsets for T-ALL/LBL (Table 13-2). The World Health Organization (WHO) classification of 2001 unified ALL and LBL, diagnosed whenever the percentage of lymphoblasts in BM or peripheral blood (PB) is less than 25%, into the categories of precursor B- and precursor T-lymphoblastic leukemia/LBL.

From: *Neoplastic Hematopathology*: Contemporary Hematology,
Edited by: D. Jones, DOI 10.1007/978-1-60761-384-8_13,
© Humana Press, a part of Springer Science+Business Media, LLC 2010

Table 13-1. Common cytogenetic and molecular subtypes of B-ALL/LBL and T-ALL/LBL.

Subtype	Genetic alteration	Frequency in children	Frequency in adults	Unique features	Prognosis
B-ALL/LBL with t(9;22) (q34;q11.2)	BCR-ABL1 fusion	2–4%	25%	coexpression of myeloid antigens CD13 and CD33 relatively common	Poor
B-ALL/LBL with t(v;11q23)	MLL rearranged; t(4;11) (q21;q23) AFF1/AF4-MLL most common	most common abnormality in infants <1 year old	less common than in infants, but gradually increases with age	CD19+, CD10+, CD15+	Poor
B-ALL/LBL with t(12;21) (p13;q22)	ETV6-RUNX1 (TEL-AML1) fusion	20–25%	Rare	often cryptic, requiring FISH or PCR, CD25+, coexpression of myeloid antigens, especially CD13 common	Good
B-ALL/LBL with hyperdiploidy	>50 chromosomes	25–30%	Rare	none	Good; excellent if "triple trisomy" positive (+4, +10, +17)
B-ALL/LBL with hypodiploidy	<46 chromosomes	5%; 1% for <45	5%, 1% of <45	none	Intermediate for 45 chromosomes; worse prognosis if <45 chr
B-ALL/LBL with near haploidy	23–29 chromosomes	Rare	almost never seen	none	very poor
B-ALL/LBL with t(5;14) (q31;q32)	IL3-IGH fusion	Rare	Rare	peripheral eosinophilia	unknown; requires further study
B-ALL/LBL with t(1;19) (q23;p13.3)	TCF3-PBX1 (E2A-PBX1) fusion	5–6%	3%	CD19+ CD10+, mu-chain+, CD34-	Intermediate
T-ALL/LBL with t(10;14) (q24;q11) or t(7;10) (q35;q24)	TLX1 (HOX11)-TCRA/D or TCRB-TLX1 (HOX11), respectively	4–7%	30%	none	
T-ALL/LBL with t(5;14) (q35;q32)	TLX3 (HOX11L2)-BCL11B	20%	10–15%	cryptic	
T-ALL/LBL with 1p32	SIL/TAL1	9–30%	decreases with age	cryptic	
T-ALL/LBL with t(10;11) (p13;q14) deletion	CALM/AF10	10%	10%	often cryptic	
T-ALL/LBL with del (9) (p21)	CDKN2A (p16)	65%	15%	cryptic	

Percentages are from references[1,7–9]

Table 13-2. Common immunophenotypic markers used in the diagnosis of ALL/LBL and their correlation with maturational stages.

Modality	Flow Cytometry	Immunohistochemistry	Maturational stage	Notes
B-ALL/LBL	Positive for CD19, CD22, CD20 (dim to negative), CD10, HLA-DR, cCD79a, cCD22, cytoplasmic mu chain (some cases), CD34 (variable), CD38 (variable) CD45 (variable), TdT, and myeloid antigens (CD13, CD33, CD15) in some cases	CD79a, PAX-5, TdT	*Pro-B:* CD10 negative, cytoplasmic mu-negative *Common ALL:* CD10 positive, cytoplasmic mu-negative *Pre-B:* CD10 positive, cytoplasmic mu-positive *Mature B:* CD10 positive, CD20 positive, surface IgM positive	CD10 negativity along with CD15 positivity suggest MLL rearrangement; the majority of cases are negative for surface light chain expression
T-ALL/LBL	Positive for CD7 (bright), CD2, CD5, CD3 (often surface negative but cytoplasmic positive), CD4 (variable), CD8 (variable), CD1a, CD10 (uncommon), CD34 (variable), CD45 (usually dim), TdT, and myeloid antigens (CD13, CD33, CD15, CD36, CD117) in some cases	CD3, CD99, TdT	*Pro-T:* cCD3 positive, CD7 positive, CD2 negative, CD1a negative, CD34 +/-, CD4 negative, CD8 negative *Pre-T:* cCD3 positive, CD7 positive, CD2 positive, CD5 positive, CD1a negative, CD34 +/-, CD4 negative, CD8 negative *Cortical T:* cCD3 positive, CD7 positive, CD2 positive, CD5 positive, CD1a positive CD34 negative, CD4 positive, CD8 positive *Medullary T:* cCD3 positive, surface CD3 positive, CD7 positive, CD2 positive, CD5 positive, TCR positive, CD4 or CD8 positive, CD1a negative,	Bright CD7 is the most sensitive marker; TdT expressed in majority of cases but can be negative; most cases are either CD4 and CD8 double-negative or double-positive but occasionally cases are single positive; surface expression of TCR $\alpha\beta$ or $\gamma\delta$ follows CD3 and is usually negative; although T-ALL/LBL may loosely follow the maturational stages of normal thymocytes, there is often overlap between stages and aberrant phenotypes

In parallel, the prognostic power of cytogenetic subgroups of ALL/LBL was being recognized as the molecular events underlying these chromosomal rearrangements were uncovered. This improved understanding of the pathogenesis of ALL/LBL is reflected in the current 2008 WHO classification that divides B lymphoblastic neoplasms into molecular subgroups based on their central cytogenetic (or molecular) findings [1]. More sophisticated interrogation of the leukemia genome through gene expression profiling, single nucleotide polymorphism (SNP) arrays, and gene copy number analysis has further validated these cytogenetic subgroups [2] and identified new pathways involved in leukemogenesis including the regulators of B-cell development PAX-5 and IKZF [3]. Similar studies in T-ALL/LBL have demonstrated the importance of NOTCH1, [4] HOX11, TAL1, and LYL1 [5].

As a result, B ALL/LBL is now classified based on the presence or absence of characteristic recurrent cytogenetic abnormalities (Table 13-1). The recognized recurrent cytogenetic abnormalities include t(9;22)(q34;q11.2) BCR-ABL1, t(v;11q23) MLL rearranged, t(12;21)(p13;q22) ETV6-RUNX1 (formerly TEL-AML1), t(5;14)(q31;q32) IL3-IgH, and t(1;19)(q23;p13.3) TCF2-PBX1 (formerly E2A-PBX1) [6,7]. Another group of B-LBL/ALL lack chromosomal translocations, but show characteristic chromosome copy number alterations and are divided into a hyperdiploid (>50 and usually <66 chromosomes) group and a hypodiploid group (<46 chromosomes) with fewer than 44 or 45 chromsomes correlating with poor outcome.

The range of recurrent chromosomal translocations associated with T LBL/ALL is broader and comprises 50–70% of all cases. Approximately, 30–35% of patients have translocations involving the TCRA/D, TCRB, or TCRG T-cell receptor genes at chromosome regions 14q11-q13, 7q32-q35, and 7p15, respectively, bringing transcription of the translocation partner gene under the control of the T-cell receptor enhancers [8]. The identified partner genes are numerous and include mostly transcription factors such as TLX1 (HOX11), TLX3 (HOX11L2), the HOXA cluster, TAL1, TAL2, LYL1, BHLHB1, LMO1, and LMO2, or growth regulators such as LCK, NOTCH1, and CCND2. Other translocations identified in T-ALL/LBL create fusion proteins. Common examples include chromosome 1p32 interstitial deletion producing STIL-TAL1 fusions (9-30% of cases in children, less in adults), t(10;11) (p13;q14)/CALM-AF10 (~10% of cases), and chromosome 11q23 rearrangements producing MLL gene fusions (~8% of cases). Deletions of the cell cycle regulator CDKN2A (p16) at chromosome 9p21 are also common [8]. Because the range of pathogenetic features associated with any particular translocation is still poorly understood (given the relative rarity of each), genetic subclassification of T-LBL/ALL is not part of the current WHO approach.

13.2. Comparison of ALL/LBL in Children and Adults

ALL and LBL occur in all age groups, but the vast majority of cases occur in children, with ALL representing the most common pediatric malignancy. B-ALL represents 85% of childhood ALL and approximately 75% of cases of adult ALL, with most of the remaining cases being of T-cell lineage. LBL/ALL of natural killer (NK) cell or null lineage as well as primitive and bilineal immunophenotypes represent approximately 1–2% of ALL/LBL. Although most cases of ALL are of B-cell lineage, the majority (approximately 85–90%) of LBL are conversely of T-cell lineage, regardless of the age of the patient.

A slight male predominance has been noted for both ALL and LBL. In children, most cases of B-ALL present before 10 years of age, whereas T-ALL/LBL more frequently occurs in older children and adolescents. With B-ALL, patients commonly present with fever, bone pain, lymphadenopathy, and hepatosplenomegaly, whereas patients with T-ALL usually have a mediastinal mass with or without pleural effusions and variable levels of PB and BM involvement. Among adults, B-LBL becomes more common in the elderly, often presenting in skin, and may have an indolent course without systemic dissemination. T-ALL/ LBL in younger adults is similar to children with a mediastinal/thymic origin, whereas in older adults lymph node-based tumors, and mixed T-LBL/myeloid (stem cell) malignancies become more common. In both adults and older children, some cases of ALL/LBL represent cryptic de novo blast crisis of myeloproliferative neoplasms, particularly chronic myelogenous leukemia (CML).

13.3. Morphologic Features

Tumor cells in both B- and T-ALL/LBL are usually small to medium-sized with very high nuclear to cytoplasmic ratios, somewhat coarse but evenly dispersed chromatin (sometimes described as "powdery"), and indistinct to small nucleoli (Fig. 13-1). The nuclear contours of the tumor cells may be folded or notched and the cytoplasm tends to be basophilic and rather scant, sometimes containing a few cytoplasmic vacuoles. Occasionally, the blasts are larger with more abundant cytoplasm, prominent nucleoli, and fine chromatin resembling myeloblasts. Some cases of ALL have a discrete pseudopodal extension of cytoplasm resembling a hand mirror and occasional cases can have cytoplasmic granules. Infantile ALL, especially those with MLL gene fusions often show a subpopulation of larger blasts with more abundant cytoplasm.

The BM in ALL is usually diffusely replaced by sheets of blasts with few remaining normal hematopoietic elements (Fig. 13-2a); necrosis can be seen. In tissue sections, lymphoblasts infiltrate in a single file fashion or as diffuse sheets, and in thin sections may have "mosaic" or "puzzle piece" interlocking of the blast contours (Fig. 13-2b). Mitotic figures are common, and some cases may show abundant tingible body macrophages, giving a "starry sky" appearance similar to what is seen in Burkitt lymphoma. Lymph nodes that are partially involved by LBL may show paracortical or T-zone infiltration with residual germinal centers; extracapsular extension of blasts is also common.

Certain cytogenetic subgroups of ALL/LBL can be associated with admixed eosinophils or basophils, but large numbers of nonneoplastic lymphocytes and neutrophils are uncommon. The 8p11 stem cell leukemia with FGFR1 chromosomal rearrangements shows T-lymphoblasts admixed with myeloid proliferations containing neoplastic eosinophils, or an associated discrete hypereosinophilic syndrome (See Chap. 9) [90].

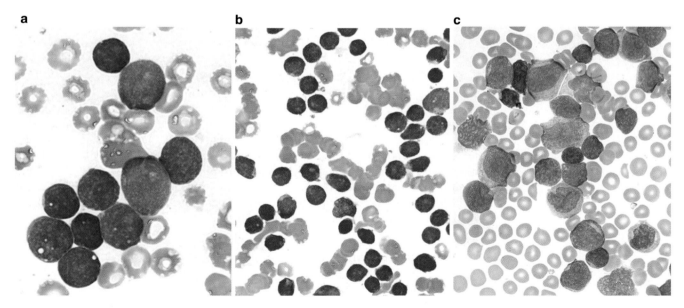

Fig. 13-1. *B-lymphoblastic leukemia.* (**a**) Typical lymphoblasts with scant cytoplasm, fine chromatin, small nucleoli, and one to two small cytoplasmic vacuoles (BM aspirate). (**b**) Smaller lymphoblasts with dispersed but coarse chromatin (BM aspirate). (**c**) Infantile ALL with t(4;11)/MLL-rearrangement showing classical morphology. Dual populations of smaller lymphoblasts and larger monoblasts are present (peripheral blood)

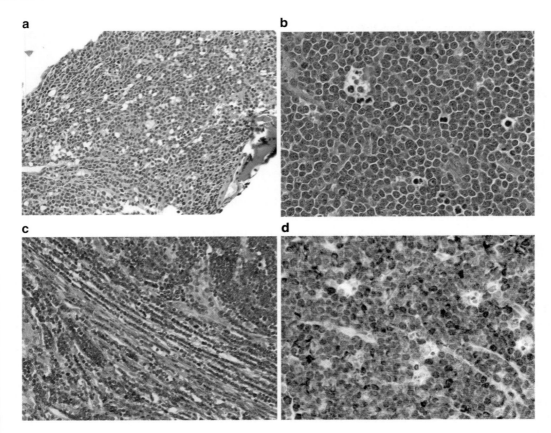

Fig. 13-2. *Lymphoblastic leukemia/lymphoma in tissue sections.* (**a**) Appearance of B-ALL in BM biopsy. (**b**) T-LBL in lymph node: Sheets of monotonous lymphoblasts with "mosaic pattern," show numerous mitoses, and are admixed with tingible body macrophages. (**c**) T-LBL in lymph node: Lymphoblasts demonstrate a linear pattern of infiltration in the adjacent capsule and soft tissue. (**d**) TdT immunohistochemical stain in T-LBL

13.4. Use of Laboratory Testing for Diagnosis

The diagnosis of ALL/LBL requires integration of data from a variety of modalities, including morphology, immunophenotyping by FC, or occasionally by immunohistochemistry (IHC), G-banded karyotype, fluorescence in situ hybridization (FISH), and increasingly molecular genetic testing. Although cytochemical stains were a major part of the previous FAB classification, the utility of cytochemistry is currently limited since stains such as periodic acid-schiff (PAS) and acid phosphatase are neither sensitive nor specific enough to identify lymphoblasts. The most common antigenic markers employed to diagnose and subclassify ALL/LBL by FC or IHC are summarized in Table 13-2.

13.5. Differential Diagnosis

ALL/LBL must be distinguished from the other neoplasms that have blastic or blastoid morphologic appearance including poorly differentiated/small cell carcinomas and lymphomas in adults, blastoid sarcomas in children, and acute myeloid leukemia (AML) in both groups. A comprehensive approach to this differential diagnosis is presented in Chaps. 2 and 7 (Tables 2-6 and 7-1).

13.5.1. Differential Diagnosis of B-ALL/LBL

Burkitt lymphoma/leukemia (formerly diagnosed as ALL-L3 in the FAB classification) is a high-grade, blastoid mature B-cell lymphoma with the expression of surface immunoglobulin. Distinction of ALL/LBL from BL is based on the expression of TdT in the former, and of activating translocations of the MYC locus in the latter (See Chap. 17). Cases of AML/ myeloid sarcoma may express TdT (especially by FC), or co-express B-cell markers CD19 and PAX-5 (particularly t(8;21)-bearing AML) but will also express myeloid markers such as myeloperoxidase and CD117. Mantle cell lymphoma may have a leukemic presentation and an immature/blastoid morphology in tissue sections, but will show strong and bright expression of CD20 and surface immunoglobulin and aberrant co-expression of CD5 and cyclin D1.

13.5.2. Differential Diagnosis of T-ALL/LBL

In children, other "small round blue cell" tumors such as rhabdomyosarcoma and Ewing's sarcoma (or peripheral/primitive neuroectodermal tumor) represent the primary differential with tissue-based T-LBL. Ewing's sarcoma expresses CD99, which is also expressed in T-ALL/LBL, but will be negative for TdT. The expression of CD3 and other T-cell markers will distinguish T-ALL/LBL from the poorly differentiated/blastoid sarcomas. In adults with a mediastinal mass, the primary differential diagnosis of T-ALL/LBL is with thymomas, which always have admixed tumor-associated immature thymocytes. These thymocytes may cause diagnostic confusion especially when only cytologic preparation and FC analysis is done, making the thymic epithelial cell proliferation difficult to appreciate. The uniformly blastoid cytologic appearance and expression of CD4, CD7 (subset), CD43, CD45RA, CD56, and TdT are the overlapping features of T-ALL/LBL with blastic plasmacytoid dendritic cell neoplasm. However, nearly all cases of T-ALL/LBL express cytoplasmic (and occasionally surface) CD3 and CD5, which are absent in the blastic plasmacytoid dendritic cell neoplasm.

The differential diagnosis of T-ALL/LBL with mature T-cell lymphomas and leukemias can be problematic especially when TdT is negative or only focally expressed. Some mature peripheral T-cell lymphomas can have infiltrative growth patterns, blastoid cytologic features, and a high mitotic rate and should be considered in any blastoid T-cell tumor presenting outside of the mediastinum. In particular, hepatosplenic T-cell lymphomas presenting in BM usually have a blastoid appearance, and their typical immunophenotype (CD4-CD8- dim TCR-γ/δ+) may suggest T-ALL/LBL. In these cases, immunophenotyping with the other markers of immature T-cells, such as CD1a, TdT, and CD34, is most helpful. Finally, T-prolymphocytic leukemia can be CD4-CD8- or CD4+CD8+ simulating T-ALL/LBL, but will have a more mature lymphocyte appearance and express TCL1, which is absent in nearly all cases of T-ALL/LBL.

13.6. Prognostic Schemes and Markers

In pediatric ALL/LBL, there are widely-utilized models for risk stratification that can be used to tailor therapy and predict outcome. The most important parameters include age, presenting white blood cell (WBC) count, and type of cytogenetic abnormality. A comprehensive analysis of more than 6,000 children treated on Children's Cancer Group (CCG) and Pediatric Oncology Group (POG) protocols during the 1980s and 1990s defined low, standard, high, and very high risk groups [6]. Low-risk parameters include age between 1 and 10 years old, presenting WBC count less than 50×10^9/L, "triple trisomies" (i.e. hyperdiploidy with trisomy 4, 10, and/or 17), or the presence of t(12;21)/ETV6-RUNX1. High-risk findings include age older than 10 years and/or presenting WBC greater than 50×10^9/L; very high-risk parameters include presence of t(9;22)/BCR-ABL1 or MLL chromosomal translocations, and hypodiploidy with fewer than 44 chromosomes that correlates with a DNA index in the tumor of less than 0.81. The presence of a t(1;19)/E2A-PBX1 chromosomal translocation was initially regarded as a high-risk feature but outcomes have improved with current treatment regimens [7].

The persistence of minimal residual disease (MRD) after the first cycle of treatment has been shown to have an important influence on outcome. Morphologically-identifiable persistent BM involvement at day 29 (or >1% MRD detected by FC) identifies patients at very high risk for relapse, whereas FC-MRD levels < 0.1% indicates low risk of relapse. In addition to the basic clinical characteristics at presentation and the genetic abnormalities of the tumors themselves, several recent studies have shown that germline polymorphisms in cytokine and drug metabolism genes can impact response to chemotherapy and risk of residual leukemia. These genetic factors have included particular SNPs in interleukin-15 [10] and the particular genotype pf the GSTM1 and TYMS genes [11]. These results are intriguing and will require further study on additional cohorts of patients.

Adults with B-ALL/LBL have lower cure rates, in part due to the higher incidence of the poor-risk t(9;22)/BCR-ABL1 ALL and the virtual absence of the low-risk cytogenetic ALL subgroups found in children, such as triple trisomies or t(12;21)/ETV6-RUNX1. The reasons why there should be such differences in molecular pathogenesis between pediatric and adult ALL are not clear. However, given the rarity of adult ALL, effective, intensive chemotherapy protocols for adult B-ALL/LBL have only recently been optimized and prognostic factors are less clear. A promising development has been the addition of kinase inhibitors such as imatinib (Gleevec) for BCR-ABL1+ B-ALL/LBL, which has improved outcomes. A more indolent subset of B-LBL in adults that has a localized, extramedullary/extranodal presentation has also been identified [20].

T-ALL/LBL in adults and children has a generally worse outcome than B-cell cases, with adverse predictors being older age and high WBC count at diagnosis. Given the large number of genetic alterations in T-ALL/LBL, and the frequent absence of genetic data on tissue-based tumors, prognostic models incorporating genetic features are not yet widely used.

13.7. Monitoring After Treatment

As discussed above, the importance of achieving a complete response early following induction chemotherapy has been shown to be predictive of both relapse and outcome. But the definition of remission in ALL is highly dependent on the method used to assess disease levels. Morphologic detection of ALL in BM samples is not accurate below 5% of the cellularity and even above that level differentiation between leukemic lymphoblasts and hematogones can be problematic. Routine cytogenetics has a similar sensitivity of 5%, since 20 cells are usually counted; however this method is not informative for MRD assessment if the original tumor has a normal diploid karyotype. FISH for a tumor-specific aberration increases the sensitivity to 1–2% (because 200 cells are usually counted) but is applicable only to certain genetic subgroups. As a result, patients with ALL/LBL in apparent remission based on these tools may still harbor millions of leukemia cells. Thus, while these low-sensitivity methods may be useful as screening tools, they are limited in their ability to predict who will ultimately relapse.

The advent of highly sensitive FC and PCR-based MRD assays has redefined the concept of remission in ALL/LBL and such assays are now widely employed in pediatric patients where high rates of initial complete response are typically obtained. The optimal MRD assay in ALL/LBL should be quantitative over a wide range of disease levels, have a sensitivity of at least 1 in 10^{-4} to 10^{-5} (i.e. able to detect 1 leukemia cell in 100,000 total cells), be applicable to the majority of patients, and be reproducible within and between laboratories. Although no single assay fitting all of these criteria currently exists for ALL/LBL, the three best MRD methods in wide use are reverse transcription quantitative (RQ)-PCR for translocation-specific fusion transcripts, clone-specific quantitative PCR for ALL-associated TCR and/or IgH gene rearrangements, and multiparameter FC tracking the leukemia-specific blast immunophenotype.

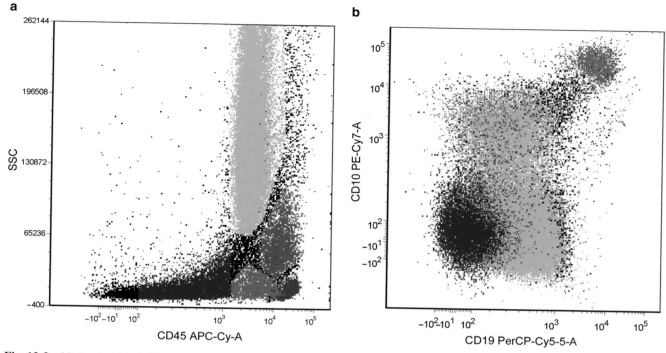

Fig. 13-3. *Minimal residual disease analysis by flow cytometry findings.* (**a**) CD45 versus side scatter histogram highlights the different populations present in the BM after treatment for B-ALL. The fuchsia-colored population represents the blast gate. (**b**) CD19 versus CD10 histogram shows that 1.5% of the analyzed events are CD19+ CD10+ lymphoblasts consistent with residual leukemia (images provided by Mike Cubbage)

MRD by FC is the most commonly-used method since it is rapid, relatively inexpensive, and broadly applicable to most cases of T- and B-ALL/LBL (Fig. 13-3). Initial FC panels using 3- and 4-color assays are being gradually replaced by 6-color methods, which have improved sensitivity (typically at least 10^{-4}) and are only slightly less sensitive than PCR assays [12]. MRD by FC is most easily applied to T-ALL since TdT+ T cells are not normally present in BM and their detection is thus indicative of residual disease. Detecting small number of B-ALL tumor cells by FC is more challenging since nonneoplastic immature B-cell populations (hematogones) are normally present in BM, especially in young children and in older patients after chemotherapy or hematopoietic stem cell transplantation [12,13]. The qualitatively abnormal phenotypes (i.e. aberrant expression of antigens not normally expressed) or quantitatively abnormal phenotypes i.e. (abnormally bright or dim expression of normally expressed antigens) on most B-ALL/LBL allows for focused testing of the follow-up samples for the specific abnormalities identified in the original clone [14]. However, there is evidence that these ALL-associated aberrations may shift over time or at relapse as a result of the effects of therapy selection. One retrospective study of the immunophenotypes in the blasts in 51 ALL cases at both diagnosis and relapse found multiple aberrancies in each case with 73% of cases showing loss of at least one of the identified aberrancies. However, 85.9% of the originally identified aberrancies were still present, and all cases remained multiply aberrant allowing distinction of the relapsed blasts from normal hematogone populations [15]. This study highlights the importance of using multiple sets of markers per patient when performing FC-MRD in ALL.

RQ-PCR analysis for leukemia-specific fusion transcripts has high sensitivity (i.e. 10^{-5} to 10^{-6}) and very high specificity given the absence of such chimeric transcripts in non-neoplastic BM. These assays are also rapid and relatively inexpensive. However, RQ-PCR can be applied only cases with fusion transcripts, such as ETV6-RUNX1 and BCR-ABL1 in B-ALL/LBL, and STIL-TAL1 or TLX3 (HOX11L2)-BCL11B in T-ALL/LBL. Also, specific primer-probes sets must be developed for each translocation and adequate quality control measures and sensitivity controls must be included (see Chap. 4) [12]. As with any

PCR-based assay, great care must also be taken to prevent cross contamination that would produce false-positive results.

Quantitative PCR analysis for leukemia-specific TCR and IGH rearrangements also offers high sensitivity (usually 10^{-4} to 10^{-6}), but it is a laborious and expensive method requiring sequencing of the original leukemic clone and design of at least one tumor-specific PCR primer or probe [13]. However, this method is more broadly applicable as the vast majority of ALL/LBL have at least one clonal IGH, TCRG, or TCRD gene rearrangement that can be used to generate a clone-specific primer-probe set. The IGK gene can also be used if no clonal rearrangement is detected at the other loci. One problem occasionally encountered is the subsequent recombination or deletion of the rearranged loci in the ALL/LBL at the time of relapse leading to failure of the original primer-probe set to bind and amplify. To avoid this issue, some laboratories recommend developing clone-specific assays against two IGH and/or TCR rearrangements for each tumor, which, of course, adds additional cost and complexity.

There have been several studies comparing FC and quantitative PCR in the detection of MRD in ALL, and the two methods often show high rates of correlation. One large series involving children receiving chemotherapy for B-lineage ALL found very good concordance between results of IGH PCR and FC in 1329 of 1375 (96.7%) samples. The authors of that report suggest that the combination of both methods should be applied to leukemia patients rather than relying solely on one method so that the impact on outcome of discrepant cases can be tracked [16].

13.8. Molecular Pathogenesis and Possible New Targets

Cytogenetic analysis has been central to defining the chromosomal copy number patterns and tumor-specific translocations that characterize B-ALL/LBL. More recently, the techniques of gene expression profiling (GEP) by microarrays has provided insights into how leukemic transformation differs from the normal lymphoblast maturation. In a landmark GEP study of 360 cases of pediatric ALL, investigators at St Jude's Children's Research Hospital demonstrated unique expression profiles corresponding to each of the already-known prognostically important ALL subtypes, as well as a new profile not previously recognized [2]. Similar results have been published in cohorts of adult patients as well,[17] although cases of B-ALL with t(9;22)/BCR-ABL1 have generally shown more heterogeneous expression patterns in adults than in children. Interestingly, many adult ALL cases that lack t(9;22) show increased transcript expression of the tyrosine kinases FLT3 and DDR1 which may provide a new use for kinase inhibitor therapy [18].

Genomic analyses of high-risk pediatric ALL, using array comparative genomic hybridization, have shown recurrent chromosomal deletions spanning genes involved in cell cycle regulation (CDKN2A/B and RB1), in the regulation of apoptosis (BTG1), in transcriptional regulation of hematopoiesis (ETV6), and in the transcriptional control of B-cell differentiation (PAX-5 and IKZF1). Deletion of the IKZF1 locus has been associated with poor outcome.[3]

Some of the initial studies utilizing gene expression profiling in T-ALL have found consistent overexpression of the T-cell oncogenes HOX11/TLX1, TAL1, LYL1, LMO1, and LMO2 in subsets of cases. Further studies have demonstrated unique gene expression signatures corresponding to stages of T-cell development: LYL1+ (early thymocyte), HOX11+ (early cortical thymocyte), and TAL1+ (late cortical thymocyte). These studies also identified HOX11L2 activation as a common event in T-cell leukemogenesis [5]. TAL1 is a basic helix-loop-helix (bHLH) protein and a transcriptional regulator necessary for hematopoiesis, and it is constitutively active in 25% of T-ALL. Mouse models have shown the activation of TAL1 is not sufficient to cause leukemia, but in combination with LMO1 or LMO2 results in the development of T-ALL [19]. LYL1 (lymphoblastic leukemia-derived sequence 1) is another bHLH protein that shares sequence identity with TAL1 and is expressed in hematopoietic cells. Taken together, these studies implicate bHLH and homeobox transcription factors as playing a similar role in T-cell leukemogenesis as they do in normal T-cell development and differentiation, with increased expression noted even in some T ALL/LBL without detectable chromosomal alterations at these loci [19].

In addition to alterations in the transcriptional regulators, more than 50% of T-ALL/LBL have activating mutations in NOTCH1 [4]. NOTCH1 is one of a family of proteins important in lymphocyte development that regulate the commitment of hematopoietic precursors to the T-cell lineage, and NOTCH1 has proven to be a key oncogene in T-ALL. Genes or pathways activated following NOTCH dysregulation include MYC, NF-kappa B, and cell metabolism and protein biosynthesis modulators. The central regulatory role of NOTCH1 has made it a promising potential therapeutic target, with several small molecule inhibitors blocking NOTCH activation now undergoing clinical trials in ALL/LBL. These types of agents, as well as kinase inhibitors and epigenetic modulators, will likely be routinely used as adjuvants to cytotoxic chemotherapy during induction/consolidation or as maintenance therapy in subsets of ALL/LBL in the near future.

Suggested Readings

Aifantis I, Raetz E, Buonamici S. Molecular pathogenesis of T-cell leukaemia and lymphoma. Nat Rev Immunol 2008;8:380-90.
- Overview of the currently-known molecular pathways deregulated in T-cell acute lymphoblastic leukemia/lymphoma and how they relate to normal T-cell development.

Mullighan CG, Downing JR. Genome-wide profiling of genetic alterations in acute lymphoblastic leukemia: recent insights and future directions. Leukemia 2009;23:1209-18.
- Most up-date review of the molecular alterations in B and T ALL identified thus far by microarray techniques

Nathwani BN, Diamond LW, Winberg CD, et al. Lymphoblastic lymphoma: a clinicopathologic study of 95 patients. Cancer 1981;48:2347-2357.
- Classic paper outlining the clinicopathologic features of mediastinal lymphoblastic lymphoma in a large series of patients

References

1. Borowitz MJ, Chan JKC. B lymphoblastic leukaemia/lymphoma, NOS, B lymphoblastic leukaemia/lymphoma with recurrent genetic abnormalities, and T lymphoblastic leukaemia/lymphoma. In: Swerdlow SH, Campo E, Harris NL, et al., eds. WHO Classification of Tumours of Haematopoietic and Lymphoid Tissues. 4th ed. Lyon, France: International Agency for Research on Cancer, 2008:168–78.
2. Yeoh EJ, Ross ME, Shurtleff SA, et al. Classification, subtype discovery, and prediction of outcome in pediatric acute lymphoblastic leukemia by gene expression profiling. Cancer Cell 2002;1:133–43.
3. Mullighan CG, Su X, Zhang J, et al. Deletion of *IKZF1* and prognosis in acute lymphoblastic leukemia. N Engl J Med 2009;360:470–80.
4. Weng AP, Ferrando AA, Lee W, et al. Activating mutations of *NOTCH1* in human T cell acute lymphoblastic leukemia. Science 2004;306:269–71.
5. Ferrando AA, Neuberg DS, Staunton J, et al. Gene expression signatures define novel oncogenic pathways in T cell acute lymphoblastic leukemia. Cancer Cell 2002;1:75–87.
6. Schultz KR, Pullen DJ, Sather HN, et al. Risk- and response-based classification of childhood B-precursor acute lymphoblastic leukemia: a combined analysis of prognostic markers from the Pediatric Oncology Group (POG) and Children's Cancer Group (CCG). Blood 2007;109:926–35.
7. Harrison CJ, Foront L. Cytogenetics and molecular genetics of acute lymphoblastic leukemia. Rev Clin Exp Hematol 2002;6:91–113.
8. Graux C, Cools J, Michaux L, et al. Cytogenetics and molecular genetics of T-cell acute lymphoblastic leukemia: from thymocyte to lymphoblast. Leukemia 2006;20:1496–510.
9. Vega F, Medeiros LJ, Davuluri R, et al. t(8;13) positive bilineal lymphomas: report of 6 cases. Am J Surg Path 2008;32:14–20.

10. Yang JJ, Cheng C, Yang W. Genome-wide interrogation of germline genetic variation associated with treatment response in childhood acute lymphoblastic leukemia. JAMA 2009;301:393–403.

11. Rocha JC, Cheng C, Liu W. Pharmacogenetics of outcome in children with acute lymphoblastic leukemia. Blood 2005;105:4752–8.

12. Szczepanski T. Why and how to quantify minimum residual disease in acute lymphoblastic leukemia? Leukemia 2007;21:622–6.

13. Campana D. Determination of minimum residual disease in leukaemia patients. Br J Haematol 2003;121:823–38.

14. Campana D, Coustan-Smith E. Detection of minimal residual disease in acute leukemia by flow cytometry. Cytometry (Communications in Clinical Cytometry) 1999;38:139–52.

15. Chen W, Karandikar NJ, McKenna RW, Kroft SH. Stability of leukemia-associated immunophenotypes in precursor B-lymphoblastic leukemia/lymphoma: a single institution experience. Am J Clin Path 2007;127:39–46.

16. Neale GAM, Coustan-Smith E, Stow P, et al. Comparative analysis of flow cytometry and polymerase chain reaction for the detection of minimal residual disease in childhood acute lymphoblastic leukemia. Leukemia 2004;18:934–8.

17. Kohlmann A, Shoch C, Shnittger S, et al. Pediatric acute lymphoblastic leukemia (ALL) gene expression signatures classify an idependent cohort of adult ALL patients. Leukemia 2004;18:63–71.

18. Chiaretti S, Li X, Gentleman R, et al. Gene expression profiles of B-lineage adult acute lymphoblastic leukemia reveal genetic patterns that identify lineage derivation and distinct mechanisms of transformation. Clin Cancer Res 2005;11:7209–19.

19. Aifantis I, Raetz E, Buonamici S. Molecular pathogenesis of T-cell leukaemia and lymphoma. Nat Rev Immunol 2008;8:380–90.

20. Lin P, Jones D, Dorfman DM, Medeiros LJ. Precursor B-cell lymphoblastic lymphoma: a predominantly extranodal tumor with low propensity for leukemic involvement. Am J Surg Pathol 2000;24:1480–90.

Chapter 14

Chronic Lymphocytic Leukemia and Small Lymphocytic Lymphoma

Ellen Schlette

Abstract/Scope of Chapter This chapter covers chronic lymphocytic leukemia (CLL) and its variants as well as its lymph node counterpart, small lymphocytic lymphoma (SLL). The role of well-established and more experimental immunophenotypic and molecular biomarkers in predicting outcome and need for treatment in CLL/SLL is summarized.

Keywords Chronic lymphocytic leukemia • Small lymphocytic leukemia • Prolymphocytes • Proliferation centers • Richter's transformation

14.1. Introduction

Chronic lymphocytic leukemia (CLL) and its lymph node counterpart, small lymphocytic lymphoma (SLL), are common low-grade and usually indolent B-cell lymphoproliferative disorders. Both CLL and SLL can arise from low-level pre-existing monoclonal and oligoclonal B-cell expansions and are unusual among B-cell malignancies in lacking characteristic reciprocal chromosomal translocations. CLL/SLL currently provides the best model among hematopoietic tumors for use of prognostic and predictive markers in shaping the decision to treat. CLL/SLL also provides a model for how to combine serum biomarkers with tumor immunophenotyping, using flow cytometry (FC), and immunohistochemistry (IHC), genomic profiling, typically by fluorescence in situ hybridization (FISH), and tumor histogenesis studies such as mutational status of the expressed immunoglobulin (Ig) genes. As with CML and ALL, minimal residual disease (MRD) monitoring by FC has also become routine in disease management following treatment.

14.2. Diagnostic Definitions and Clinical Features

CLL is a chronic B-cell lymphoproliferative disorder characterized by progressive lymphocytosis caused by the clonal accumulation of small, monomorphous, monoclonal B cells in peripheral blood (PB), bone marrow (BM), and lymphoid organs. Classically, the diagnosis of CLL requires an absolute lymphocytosis ($\geq 5 \times 10^9$/L) of at least 3-month duration, with a compatible immunophenotype (i.e. clonal B cells expressing CD5 and CD23). Updated diagnostic criteria have been incorporated into the 2008 WHO classification, [1] namely that CLL can be diagnosed when lymphocytosis is less than 5×10^9/L if cytopenias or disease-related symptoms are also present. In the absence of lymphadenopathy, organomegaly (as defined by physical examination or CT scans), cytopenias, or disease-related symptoms, the presence of

From: *Neoplastic Hematopathology*: Contemporary Hematology,
Edited by: D. Jones, DOI 10.1007/978-1-60761-384-8_14,
© Humana Press, a part of Springer Science+Business Media, LLC 2010

fewer than 5×10^9 monoclonal B cells/L of blood is defined as "monoclonal B-lymphocytosis" (MBL), which may progress to frank CLL at a rate of 1–2% per year [1].

In the United States and Europe, CLL is the most common leukemia in adults, occurring predominantly in elderly people. The incidence rate is approximately 2–6 cases per 100,000 persons per year, but increases with age, reaching 12.8 cases per 100,000 per year for those over 65 years. The male to female ratio is approximately 2:1. The incidence is very low in Asian countries, and in Asian populations following migration to Western countries, supporting constitutional genetic influences in its development.

The primary complication of aggressive and/or long-standing CLL is impaired hematopoiesis leading to progressive cytopenias, which is the basis of the clinical staging systems. A subset of CLL cases present with autoimmune hemolytic anemia, likely related to immune dysregulation induced by the CLL cells, or occasionally due to paraproteinemia. Small lymphocytic lymphoma (SLL) is the non-leukemic form (i.e. lymphocytosis $<5 \times 10^9$/L) presenting with lymphadenopathy and/or splenomegaly. Occasional lymphomas with typical morphology and immunophenotype may present exclusively at extranodal sites (e.g. gastrointestinal tract), but usually progress to typical CLL/SLL over time.

14.3. Morphologic and Histologic Features of CLL/SLL and Its Variants

CLL cells in BM aspirate and PB smears are characteristically small, mature lymphocytes with a narrow border of cytoplasm and a densely-stained nucleus (Fig. 14-1a). Gumprecht nuclear shadows, or smudge cells (fragmented cell remnants), are the other characteristic morphologic features seen on smear preparations. Small CLL cells are admixed with variable numbers of prolymphocytes, which are larger lymphoid cells with round nuclei and prominent nucleoli (Fig. 14-1b) and likely represent the proliferative components. Some CLL/SLL cases also have tumor cells resembling the circulating lymphoma cells, including those with nuclear folds and clefts or deeply basophilic cytoplasm [2].

Cases of CLL with increased numbers of larger or atypical forms may be true morphologic variants (Table 14-1) or evidence of progression in a tumor that began as typical CLL. Beginning with the French American British (FAB) classification, these cases were recognized and designated as either mixed cell type or CLL–PLL, for those having a dimorphic population of small lymphocytes and prolymphocytes comprising at least 10% but fewer than 55% of the circulating lymphocytes, or as atypical CLL, for those with a spectrum of

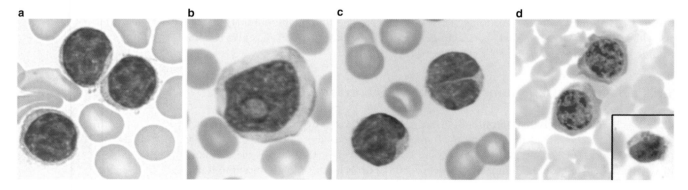

a   b   c   d

Fig. 14-1. CLL, morphologic appearances. (**a**) Classical morphology: Small, round cells with distinctly clumped chromatin and small amounts of cytoplasm. (**b**) Prolymphocytes: Larger cells with single prominent nucleolus and moderately abundant cytoplasm. (**c**) Lymphoma-like cells: Small but atypical cells with irregular nuclear contours and/or clefts. (**d**) Lymphoplasmacytoid forms: Mildly enlarged cells with clumped plasma cell-like chromatin and amphophilic cytoplasm. Some lymphoplasmacytoid variants of CLL show cytoplasmic immunoglobulin expression and can rarely express IgG (*inset*)

Table 14-1. Morphology and immunophenotype of CLL/SLL and its variants.

		Immunophenotype	
	Morphology	**Positive expression**	**Negative or minimal expression**
CLL/SLL	Homogeneous small lymphoid cells with: 1. Condensed/clumped nuclear chromatin 2. Smooth nuclear contours 3. Indistinct nucleoli 4. Scant cytoplasm	CD5 CD19 CD20(dim) CD23 CD79a CD43 BCL-2 IgM/IgD(dim) Monotypic surface Ig light chain	CD10 CD22 CD79b BCL-6 FMC-7 Cyclin D1
Atypical CLL	One or more of the following: 1. Larger size 2. Open nuclear chromatin 3. Irregular nuclear contours 4. Visible or prominent nucleoli 5. Variable amounts of cytoplasm	Either typical or atypical immunophenotype (see below)	
CLL with an atypical immunophenotype	Either typical or atypical morphology	CLL cells express markers that are usually negative or minimal in typical cases, such as: CD22 CD79b FMC-7 *and/or* Change in expression of one or more of the following markers: CD20(strong) CD23 negative	
CLL with increased prolymphocytes	>10–55% prolymphocytes present in PB or BM	Either typical or atypical immunophenotype	
(CLL/PLL) or mixed cell type De novo B-cell prolymphocytic leukemia[a]	Leukemia presents with >55% prolymphocytes in PB; usually >90%	*Positive* CD19 CD20 CD79a CD79b FMC-7 BCL-2 IgM/IgD Monotypic surface Ig light chain	*Variable (−/+)* CD5 CD23 *Negative* CD10 BCL-6 Cyclin D1

[a]De novo B-PLL is extremely rare and is only diagnosed if there is no antecedent history of another B-cell lymphoproliferative disorder such as CLL

small to large pleomorphic lymphocytes (Fig. 14-1c) but fewer than 10% prolymphocytes [3]. Another CLL/SLL variant has tumor cells with more abundant amphophilic cytoplasm and plasmacytoid appearance to the nuclei (Fig. 14-1d), which raises the possibility of lymphoplasmacytic lymphoma; however CLL/SLL usually lacks a large serum paraprotein. While such morphologic variation is noted, these subtypes are not classified as distinct subtypes in the 2008 WHO classification, despite studies linking some morphologic variants with poor prognosis [2·4].

Cases presenting with a CLL-like immunophenotype but with greater than 55% prolymphocytes at diagnosis are diagnosed in the WHO and FAB schemes as prolymphocytic leukemia (B-cell PLL), but are rare and should raise a differential diagnosis that includes large B-cell lymphoma and mantle cell lymphoma.

Bone marrow involvement is invariably present in CLL and (at lower levels) in approximately 70% of SLL at diagnosis, [5] and can show interstitial, nodular, or diffuse patterns of infiltration. Diffuse involvement is associated with more advanced disease stages and a poor outcome. CLL lymphoid aggregates are usually intertrabular, but can rarely be paratrabecular, as is usually seen in follicular lymphoma (FL). Sinusoidal BM involvement, while more typical of splenic marginal zone lymphoma (MZL), may rarely be seen in CLL.

Diagnosis of SLL is based on tissue sampling, most commonly by fine needle aspirate or biopsy of lymph node (LN) or splenectomy. The LN architecture is almost always effaced by diffuse, monotonous sheets of mostly small lymphocytes interspersed with vaguely nodular and pale-staining proliferation centers or pseudofollicles (Fig. 14-2), which contain the medium-sized nucleolated cells known as paraimmunoblasts which are the tissue counterparts of prolymphocytes. Mitotic figures are more frequent in proliferation centers although overall mitotic activity in SLL is usually low. LN sinuses are usually obliterated and infiltration of the capsule and extension into the perinodal adipose tissue is frequent. CLL cells also migrate to sites of pre-existing inflammation (e.g. prostatitis, dermatitis), so may incidentally involve biopsies taken for the other reasons.

14.4. Laboratory Testing for Diagnosis

By flow cytometry (FC), CLL cells characteristically coexpress CD5 (normally a T-cell antigen) along with the B-cell surface antigens CD19, CD20, and CD23, with restricted expression of clonotypic kappa or lambda immunoglobulin light chain. The expression levels

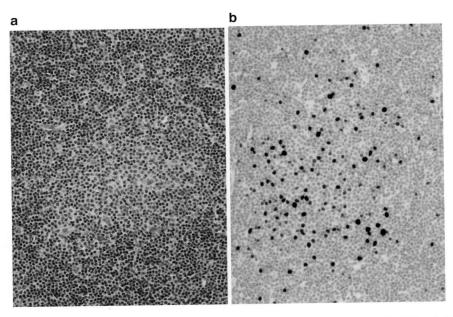

Fig. 14-2. The proliferation center. (**a**) A pseudonodular appearance is imparted in this diffuse infiltrate of SLL in lymph node by the presence of larger cells (paraimmunoblasts) among the small lymphocytes. (**b**) Ki-67 immunostain reveals that proliferation is largely restricted to the proliferation center

of surface immunoglobulin (usually IgM), CD20, and CD79b are characteristically low when compared with the normal circulating B cells and the other B-cell tumors. FMC7, an altered epitope of CD20, is also usually negative in CLL but expressed in other B-cell tumors. Most of these markers for CLL can also be performed routinely on fixed sections of the bone marrow biopsy or clot section. Although the immunophenotype sometimes deviates from the typical CLL pattern for one or more markers (see Table 14-1), such variations must be weighed against the clinical, laboratory and morphologic findings to exclude the other B-cell tumors.

14.5. Differential Diagnosis

It is important to verify that the patient has CLL/SLL rather than one of the other lymphoproliferative disorders that can mimic it, such as hairy cell leukemia, leukemic manifestations of MCL, nodal MZL, splenic MZL, or follicular lymphoma. Cases of CLL that do not meet the required blood tumor burden or the typical morphology and immunophenotype are discussed in more detail below. As the therapy and prognosis for other B-cell neoplasms, especially MCL, differ from that of CLL/SLL, it is vital to exclude them, especially if the cytomorphology, immunophenotype and/or molecular features are not typical of CLL/SLL. The identification of either t(11;14)(q13;q32) which is characteristic of MCL, or t(14;18)(q32;q21) seen in FL, would exclude the diagnosis of CLL/SLL.

14.6. Routinely Used Prognostic and Predictive Markers

The range of outcomes for CLL is very broad, as are the current therapeutic options including observation only, single agent chemotherapy (such as corticosteriods or alkylating agents), immunotherapy with anti-CD20 antibody (such as rituximab), two-, three- or four-drug combinations, or even stem cell transplantation. As a result, a large number of prognostic and therapy response predictive markers have been developed for CLL (and SLL to a lesser extent). However, the staging systems based on hematologic parameters remain the most important.

Clinicopathologic scoring: The two widely accepted hematologic-based staging methods, the Rai and the Binet systems (Table 14-2), are similar and used in both patient care and clinical trials. The current Rai classification is based upon PB lymphocytosis, platelet count, hemoglobin (Hb) level and the presence or absence of lymphadenopathy, and was reduced from five stages (0–IV) to three groups (low-, intermediate- and high-risk) that have distinct clinical outcomes with most current therapy regimens. The Binet staging

Table 14-2. The Rai and Binet staging systems for CLL.

		Rai stages		Binet stages	Median survival time (years)
Low risk	0	Lymphocytosis in PB and BM	A	Hb ≥ 10 g/dL, plts ≥ 100,000 ×10 E9/L ≤2 sites involved[a]	>10
Intermediate risk	I	Lymphocytosis and lymphadenopathy	B	Hb ≤ 10 g/dL, plts ≥ 100,000 ×10 E9/L ≥3 sites involved[a]	5–7
	II	Lymphocytosis and splenomegaly and/or hepatomegaly			
High risk	III	Lymphocytosis and Hb < 11.0 g/dL	C	Hb < 10 g/dL, plts < 100,000 ×10 E9/L	<3–4
	IV	Lymphocytosis and plts < 100,000 × 10 E9/L			

[a]Sites involved are liver, spleen and lymph nodes (either unilateral or bilateral) in inguinal, axillary and cervical regions

system is based on the number of involved areas, as defined by the presence of enlarged lymph nodes of greater than 1 cm in diameter, or organomegaly, and on whether there is anemia or thrombocytopenia. These two staging systems are simple, inexpensive, and can be applied by physicians worldwide. Both rely solely on a physical examination and standard laboratory tests and do not require ultrasound, computed tomography, or magnetic resonance imaging.

Genomic analysis: Reciprocal chromosomal translocations are rare in CLL but characteristic genomic losses and gains are frequent. These include deletions of chromosome (chr) 13(q14) in 50%, chr 11(q23) (spanning the ATM locus) in 19%, extra copies of chr 12 ("trisomy") in 20%, and alterations of the chr 17 resulting in loss of TP53 locus in 8% [6·7]. Detection of these aberrations by routine karyotyping of metaphase chromosomes is suboptimal given the low proliferative capability of most CLL cells and the small size or complex patterns of these changes, so FISH is the preferred method. Using a limited FISH panel comprising the four loci above, supplemented by the routine karyotyping, genetic aberrations are seen in over 80% of CLL [8]. Loss of TP53 and ATM are highly associated with poor outcome, and are usually seen in advanced or progressed CLL. Recently, whole genomic profiling using array-based comparative genomic hybridization (CGH) has been shown to be a cost-effective method to detect all of these aberrations and others in CLL/SLL [9].

Immunoglobulin heavy chain variable region (IgV$_H$) usage and mutation status: As described in Chap. 4, somatic hypermutation of the immunoglobulin variable gene segments occurs in the germinal center (GC) resulting in the introduction of sequence changes in the immunoglobulin genes that increase the expressed antibody's affinity for antigen. This mutation status is typically determined by PCR-based sequencing of IgV$_H$ from tumor RNA, and then compared to the reference sequence for that IGVH segment. It is generally accepted that if a B-cell tumor has somatically mutated IgV$_H$ genes then it arose from a post-GC, antigen-experienced B cell [10].

Approximately 50% of CLL have such mutated IgV$_H$ genes [11]. An association between mutated IgV$_H$ and favorable clinical outcome was first demonstrated in studies by Hamblin et al. and Damle et al. in 1999, [12·13] and then subsequently in large studies by many groups worldwide. Patients with CLL with unmutated IgV$_H$ genes have a significantly shorter median overall survival (usually around 10 years) compared to patients with tumors with mutated IgV$_H$ genes (usually greater than 20 years). In addition, "unmutated" or pre-GC CLL is associated with presentation as advanced stage disease, atypical morphology, ATM and TP53 deletions, and genomic progression.

Surface CD38, ZAP-70, TCL1 and B-cell receptor-associated biomarkers: Since IgV$_H$ mutational analysis is time-consuming, expensive, and requires isolation of tumor RNA; surrogate markers that correlate with mutation status and maturation stage have been identified. The best-characterized are surface CD38, 70-kDa zeta-associated protein (ZAP-70) and T-cell leukemia gene 1 (TCL1) [14] and are molecules involved in the surface antibody/B-cell receptor (BCR) signaling pathway. Each of them correlates, to varying degrees, with "unmutated" or pre-GC tumor status. The pre-GC/unmutated association is the strongest for TCL1 and ZAP70, which both also correlate with the ability of cultured CLL cells to grow in response to BCR-crosslinking.

The most widely used of these markers is ZAP-70, which was identified as a gene differentially expressed in pre-GC CLL, [15] and can be assessed by transcript levels, protein detected by Western blot, [16] IHC or FC [17]. Generally correlated best with shorter time-to-treatment, ZAP-70 is discordant with mutation status in 20–30% of cases, but may have more prognostic power than IgV$_H$ mutation status itself [17]. Problems in assay standardization, particularly in the FC assay, have limited the widespread use of ZAP70. Surface CD38 expression assessed by FC, typically uses a cutoff of 30% positive CLL cells, shows a poorer correlation with mutation status, and can show variation in the same tumor over time also limiting its routine use. TCL1 is a promising biomarker that correlates with pre-GC status,

Table 14-3. Prognostic markers for CLL/SLL in routine use.

Prognostic indicator		Method	Prognostic implication	References
Karyotypic abnormalities	del(13q13)	FISH	Stable disease with more favorable outcome than CLL with trisomy 12, del11q or del17p	[6, 26]
	Diploid		Stable disease with more favorable outcome than CLL with trisomy 12, del11q or del17p	
	Trisomy 12		Shorter OS	
	del (11q) (ATM loss)		Shorter OS	
	del (17p) (TP53 loss)		Rapid disease progression	
			Marked lymphadenopathy	
			Higher frequency of p53 dysfunction	
			Shorter OS	
			Resistance to conventional chemotherapy treatment	
IgV_H MS (unmutated)		PCR	Advanced stage disease	[12]
			Progressive disease	
V_H3-21 gene usage in mutated CLL			Shorter OS (comparable to unmutated IgV_H MS CLL)	[27]
			Higher frequency of p53 dysfunction	
ZAP70 expression		FC or IHC	Shorter time to progression (TTP)	[17, 28]
			OS	
			Treatment free survival (TFS)	
CD38 expression		FC	Shorter OS	[13, 29]
			TFS	
			Event free survival (EFS)	

Abbreviations as in text

poor OS and PFS and shows a strong association with the other adverse CLL markers and has been assessed by a variety of different methods [18].

As illustrated in Table 14-3, the adverse prognostic factors determined by genetic, immunophenotypic and functional profiling are highly related so that testing for all markers is probably not required or cost-effective. In most centers, the clinical staging remains the most important indication for treatment although genomic changes such as identification of TP53 and ATM loss are playing a significant role.

14.7. Less Commonly-Used Prognostic Markers

Proliferation markers: Markers of cell growth and turnover can provide additional prognostic information to the assessment of tumor load. These include serial measures of serum lactate dehydrogenase (LDH), beta-2 microglobulin (B2M) and lymphocyte doubling time (LDT), which is defined as the number of months it takes the absolute lymphocyte count to double in number in an untreated patient. Even in early-stage CLL, patients with a LDT of less than 12 months have been shown to have significantly shorter OS and treatment-free intervals than patients with longer LDTs. A drawback of LDT is that it can only be assessed retrospectively. Assessment of telomere length and telomerase activity also show promise as predictors of progression (Table 14-4).

Serum markers: Assessment of levels of secreted or shed soluble (s)CD23, sCD27, sCD44, and sCD138 and circulating (c)CD20 as well as the levels of interleukin (IL)-6, IL-8 and IL-10 and thrombopoietin (TPO) have been proposed as prognostic markers (Table 14-4). These markers presumably reflect the degree of immune activation in CLL and microenvironmental influences on growth. More direct assessment of the tissue microenvironment, such as measuring microvessel density in the bone marrow and lymph nodes, has also been linked

Table 14-4. Additional biomarkers with reported prognostic significance in CLL/SLL[30].

Prognostic indicator		Method	Associations	Prognostic implication
Serum markers	High B2M	Enzyme-linked immunosorbent assay (ELISA)	Bulky disease High CD38 expression High ZAP70 expression	High clinical stage
	High LDH		del(17p)/TP53 High CD38 expression High ZAP70 expression	Shorter survival time
	High thymidine kinase		Unmutated IgV$_H$ status	Advanced Rai stage Progressive disease
	Elevated circulating CD20 (cCD20)		High B2M levels High CD38 expression	Clinical stage Shorter OS Disease progression
	Elevated soluble CD23		Diffuse BM infiltration Short LDT High CD38 expression High ZAP70 expression	Shorter PFS
	Elevated soluble CD27		High B2M levels High LDH levels	Clinical stage
	Elevated soluble CD44		High B2M levels High LDH levels Splenomegaly	Advanced stage Need for therapy Shorter PFS
	Elevated soluble CD138 level			Shorter PFS Shorter OS
	Elevated interleukin levels (IL-6, IL-8, IL-10)		High β2-M levels High LDH levels	Clinical stage Shorter PFS Shorter OS
Telomere length and telomerase activity	Short telomere length and/or high telomerase activity	Quantitative polymerase chain reaction (qPCR)	del(11q)/ATM del(17p)/TP53 2 or more genomic aberrations Unmutated IgV$_H$ status	Worse TFS Shorter OS
	Long telomere length and/or low telomerase activity		Isolated del(13q)	

Abbreviations are as in text

to clinical stage and disease progression. CLL cells have also been shown to express and release pro-angiogenic molecules, such as VEGF (vascular endothelial growth factor) and bFGF (basic fibroblast growth factor), whose serum levels have been associated with the clinical stage and disease progression. CLL cells express VEGF receptors (VEGFR-1 and -2), further supporting the importance of angiogenic pathways for signaling.

14.8. Monitoring After Treatment

The development of potentially curative regimens for CLL/SLL, particularly 3- and 4-drug combinations of rituximab with conventional chemotherapy has created the need for more sensitive methods to assess for very low levels of residual disease. There are several approaches now available, the simplest and the most rapid being FC to track the numbers of CD5+ B cells expressing the same surface Ig light chain as the original tumor.

Improvements in quantification can be accomplished by using cluster analysis (see Chap. 3) with 4-color or 6-color panels that can routinely detect 1 in 1,000–10,000 residual CLL cells if adequate events are collected during the analysis [19]. Molecular analyses using standard non-quantitative PCR for the immunoglobulin heavy chain gene (IGH) can be used but lacks adequate sensitivity. Quantitative IGH PCR using primers designed specifically for each CLL case, also called "allele-specific qPCR" (see Chap. 4), have the highest sensitivity for MRD detection but is not routinely available. Unfortunately, the use of monitoring methods with widely differing sensitivities has made it difficult to compare the results from different studies.

14.9. Patterns of Progression/Transformation

CLL/SLL can progress or transform over time in several different ways, including commonly a step-wise clonal progression of the same tumor, and less commonly with the emergence of a genetically distinct B-cell neoplasm. The discrete transformation of CLL to large B-cell lymphoma (LBCL) has been termed Richter's syndrome or Richter's transformation, and occurs in 2–8% of CLL patients (Fig. 14-3). Secondary occurrence of classical Hodgkin lymphoma, [7] or other high-grade lymphoid malignancies is more rare, but has been labeled as Richter's transformation by some authors, adding to the confusion [20]. Such discrete large cell transformation is often characterized by sudden clinical deterioration and development of new systemic symptoms of fever and weight loss, associated with rapid enlargement of one or more nodal groups, particularly in the retroperitoneum. Elevated serum LDH, paraproteinemia, hypercalcemia (without lytic bone lesions), hepatosplenomegaly and new extranodal sites of involvement are the other common features.

In a recent longitudinal study of 186 patients, features at diagnosis that predicted for large cell transformation in univariate analyses included unmutated IgV_H status, IGH-V4-39 usage, absence of del(13q14), CD38 and ZAP70 expression, size and number of lymph nodes, advanced Binet stage, and increased LDH [21]. In multivariate analysis, however,

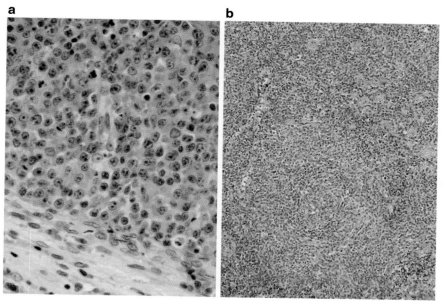

Fig. 14-3. Large cell transformation of CLL. (**a**) Diffuse infiltrate of large nucleolated tumor cells present in soft tissue. A stain for Epstein–Barr virus was negative (not shown). (**b**) Interfollicular large CD5+ B cells in a patient with CLL representing occult large cell transformation

only increased lymph node size (≥3 cm) and absence of chr 13q14 deletion were independent predictors. It is intriguing that many of these identified factors were distinct from those most highly associated with clinical progression and OS.

The finding of Epstein–Barr virus (EBV) in some cases of large cell transformation provides a clear pathogenetic mechanism since the known impairment of T-cell immunity in CLL (as well as the immunosuppressant effects of treatment) likely provides an opportunity for latent EBV to reemerge and initiate clonal B-cell expansions that terminate in lymphoma (see Chap. 30) [22]. In such a model, EBV infection could occur in either CLL cells or bystander lymphocytes. For example, Ansell et al. showed that 4 of 25 CLL patients with large cell transformation had EBV in the transformed tumor cells, including three with a B-cell phenotype expressing virally-encoded LMP1 and EBV-encoded RNAs (EBERs), and one with a T-cell phenotype positive only for EBERs [23]. Thornton and colleagues showed that the EBV+ lymphoma cells were clonally derived from the original CLL in 2 of 3 cases. Although secondary occurrence of EBV-driven B-cell malignancies is common in T-cell malignancies (which share a tumor-associated immunodeficient state), they occur rarely in B-cell neoplasms other than CLL/SLL. Therapy with fludarabine, which is known to impair T-cell immunity, [22,24] likely contributes to outgrowth of EBV-associated B-cell proliferation.

A pattern of disease progression in CLL unrelated to EBV is due to stepwise accumulation of genetic changes including loss of p53 and/or ATM function that lead to increased cell growth. This ultimately terminates in prolymphocytic transformation when more than 55% prolymphocytes are present, but also occurs in the other cases that don't meet this strict definition. Remarkably, this pattern of clonal progression is nearly entirely restricted to the pre-GC subset of CLL/SLL, [25] and probably accounts for the worse outcome of that subgroup. A clear delineation of the mechanism of transformation (i.e. classical clonal progression in the pre-GC subset versus secondary EBV transformation due to immunosuppression) is critically important to avoid confusing two entirely different processes. For this reason, we recommend that the imprecise and outdated term "Richter's transformation" be abandoned in favor of more precise histogenetic classification.

Suggested Readings

Hallek M, Cheson BD, et al. Guidelines for the diagnosis and treatment of chronic lymphocytic leukemia: a report from the International Workshop on Chronic Lymphocytic Leukemia updating the National Cancer Institute-Working Group 1996 guidelines. Blood 2008;111(12):5446–56.

Van Bockstaele F, Verhasselt B, et al. Prognostic markers in chronic lymphocytic leukemia: a comprehensive review. Blood Rev 2009;23(1):25–47.

References

1. Hallek M, Cheson BD, Catovsky D, et al. Guidelines for the diagnosis and treatment of chronic lymphocytic leukemia: a report from the International Workshop on Chronic Lymphocytic Leukemia updating the National Cancer Institute-Working Group 1996 guidelines. Blood 2008;111(12):5446–56.
2. Frater JL, McCarron KF, Hammel JP, et al. Typical and atypical chronic lymphocytic leukemia differ clinically and immunophenotypically. Am J Clin Pathol 2001;116(5):655–64.
3. Bennett JM, Catovsky D, Daniel MT, et al. Proposals for the classification of chronic (mature) B and T lymphoid leukaemias. French-American-British (FAB) Cooperative Group. J Clin Pathol 1989;42(6):567–84.
4. Schwarz J, Mikulenkova D, Cermakova M, et al. Prognostic relevance of the FAB morphological criteria in chronic lymphocytic leukemia: correlations with IgVH gene mutational status and other prognostic markers. Neoplasma 2006;53(3):219–25.
5. Nola M, Pavletic SZ, Weisenburger DD, et al. Prognostic factors influencing survival in patients with B-cell small lymphocytic lymphoma. Am J Hematol 2004;77(1):31–5.

6. Dohner H, Stilgenbauer S, Dohner K, Bentz M, Lichter P. Chromosome aberrations in B-cell chronic lymphocytic leukemia: reassessment based on molecular cytogenetic analysis. J Mol Med 1999;77(2):266–81.

7. Muller-Hermelink HK, Montserrat E, Catovsky D, Campo E, Harris NL, Stein H. WHO classification of tumours of haematopoietic and lymphoid tissues. Lyon: IARC, 2008.

8. Ripolles L, Ortega M, Ortuno F, et al. Genetic abnormalities and clinical outcome in chronic lymphocytic leukemia. Cancer Genet Cytogenet 2006;171(1):57–64.

9. Sargent R, Jones D, Abruzzo LV, et al. Customized oligonucleotide array-based comparative genomic hybridization as a clinical assay for genomic profiling of chronic lymphocytic leukemia. J Mol Diagn 2009;11(1):25–34.

10. Shaffer AL, Rosenwald A, Staudt LM. Lymphoid malignancies: the dark side of B-cell differentiation. Nat Rev 2002;2(12):920–32.

11. Fais F, Ghiotto F, Hashimoto S, et al. Chronic lymphocytic leukemia B cells express restricted sets of mutated and unmutated antigen receptors. J Clin Invest 1998;102(8):1515–25.

12. Hamblin TJ, Davis Z, Gardiner A, Oscier DG, Stevenson FK. Unmutated Ig V(H) genes are associated with a more aggressive form of chronic lymphocytic leukemia. Blood 1999;94(6):1848–54.

13. Damle RN, Wasil T, Fais F, et al. Ig V gene mutation status and CD38 expression as novel prognostic indicators in chronic lymphocytic leukemia. Blood 1999;94(6):1840–7.

14. Herling M, Patel KA, Hsi ED, et al. TCL1 in B-cell tumors retains its normal b-cell pattern of regulation and is a marker of differentiation stage. Am J Surg Pathol 2007;31(7):1123–9.

15. Rosenwald A, Alizadeh AA, Widhopf G, et al. Relation of gene expression phenotype to immunoglobulin mutation genotype in B cell chronic lymphocytic leukemia. J Exp Med 2001;194(11):1639–47.

16. Crespo M, Bosch F, Villamor N, et al. ZAP-70 expression as a surrogate for immunoglobulin-variable-region mutations in chronic lymphocytic leukemia. N Engl J Med 2003;348(18):1764–75.

17. Rassenti LZ, Huynh L, Toy TL, et al. ZAP-70 compared with immunoglobulin heavy-chain gene mutation status as a predictor of disease progression in chronic lymphocytic leukemia. N Engl J Med 2004;351(9):893–901.

18. Herling M, Patel KA, Khalili J, et al. TCL1 shows a regulated expression pattern in chronic lymphocytic leukemia that correlates with molecular subtypes and proliferative state. Leukemia 2006;20(2):280–5.

19. Rawstron AC, Villamor N, Ritgen M, et al. International standardized approach for flow cytometric residual disease monitoring in chronic lymphocytic leukaemia. Leukemia 2007;21(5):956–64.

20. Hamblin TJ. Richter's syndrome – the downside of fludarabine? Leuk Res 2005;29(10):1103–4.

21. Rossi D, Cerri M, Capello D, et al. Biological and clinical risk factors of chronic lymphocytic leukaemia transformation to Richter syndrome. Br J Haematol 2008.

22. Thornton PD, Bellas C, Santon A, et al. Richter's transformation of chronic lymphocytic leukemia. The possible role of fludarabine and the Epstein–Barr virus in its pathogenesis. Leuk Res 2005;29(4):389–95.

23. Ansell SM, Li CY, Lloyd RV, Phyliky RL. Epstein–Barr virus infection in Richter's transformation. Am J Hematol 1999;60(2):99–104.

24. Keating MJ, O'Brien S, Lerner S, et al. Long-term follow-up of patients with chronic lymphocytic leukemia (CLL) receiving fludarabine regimens as initial therapy. Blood 1998;92(4):1165–71.

25. Timar B, Fulop Z, Csernus B, et al. Relationship between the mutational status of VH genes and pathogenesis of diffuse large B-cell lymphoma in Richter's syndrome. Leukemia 2004;18(2):326–30.

26. Stilgenbauer S, Dohner H. Molecular genetics and its clinical relevance. Hematol Oncol Clin North Am 2004;18(4):827–48. viii.

27. Thorselius M, Krober A, Murray F, et al. Strikingly homologous immunoglobulin gene rearrangements and poor outcome in VH3-21-using chronic lymphocytic leukemia patients independent of geographic origin and mutational status. Blood 2006;107(7):2889–94.

28. Rassenti LZ, Jain S, Keating MJ, et al. Relative value of ZAP-70, CD38, and immunoglobulin mutation status in predicting aggressive disease in chronic lymphocytic leukemia. Blood 2008;112(5):1923–30.

29. Ibrahim S, Keating M, Do KA, et al. CD38 expression as an important prognostic factor in B-cell chronic lymphocytic leukemia. Blood 2001;98(1):181–6.

30. Van Bockstaele F, Verhasselt B, Philippe J. Prognostic markers in chronic lymphocytic leukemia: a comprehensive review. Blood Rev 2009;23(1):25–47.

Chapter 15

Marginal Zone Lymphomas

Rachel L. Sargent

Abstract/Scope of Chapter *Marginal zone lymphoma* (MZL) encompasses a heterogeneous group of small B-cell lymphomas, characterized by a predominance of tumor cells with a phenotype, homing pattern, and occasionally the appearance of the nonneoplastic *marginal zone B cells* that surround germinal centers and populate the white pulp of the spleen. Covered in this chapter are extranodal marginal zone lymphoma of mucosa-associated lymphoid tissue (MALT lymphoma), nodal marginal zone lymphoma (NMZL), and splenic B-cell marginal zone lymphoma (SMZL). Although the different subtypes of MZL share histologic and immunophenotypic features, they have divergent etiologies, molecular genetics, and clinical presentations. The pathogeneses of NMZL and SMZL are not yet clearly understood. The relationship of SMZL to hairy cell leukemia (HCL) and HCL-variant (HCL-v) is also discussed.

Keywords Marginal zone lymphoma • Monocytoid B cell • Extranodal marginal zone lymphoma of mucosa-associated lymphoid tissue • *Helicobacter pylori* • MALT lymphoma • Sjogren's syndrome • lymphoma • Hashimoto's thyroiditis • MALT lymphoma • Immunocytoma • MALT1 • translocations • BCL10 • MALT lymphoma • NF-kB • marginal zone lymphoma • Nodal marginal zone lymphoma • Lymphoplasmacytic lymphoma • lymph node • Splenic marginal zone lymphoma • Splenic lymphoma with villous lymphocytes • Splenic B-cell marginal zone lymphoma • sonic hedgehog signaling • Trisomy 3 • Splenic B-cell lymphoma/leukemia • unclassifiable • Hairy cell leukemia • Hairy cell leukemia-variant

15.1. The Three Types of Marginal Zone Lymphoma

Marginal zone lymphoma (MZL) encompasses a heterogeneous group of small B-cell lymphomas, characterized by a predominance of lymphocytes that show some morphologic or functional relationship to the nonneoplastic marginal zone B cells that surround germinal centers (GCs) in secondary lymphoid tissues and occur within a specialized microenvironment in the white pulp of the spleen. Some MZLs also resemble monocytoid B cells, which are a post-GC B-cell subset with abundant pale cytoplasm that arise following antigen stimulation. Although the different subtypes of MZL share histologic and immunophenotypic features, they have divergent etiologies, molecular genetics, and clinical presentations (Table 15-1). MZL, particularly extranodal marginal zone lymphoma of mucosa-associated lymphoid tissue (MALT lymphoma), also has the unique property (at least for B-cell lymphomas) of inducing the formation of reactive B-cell inflammation (e.g., germinal centers) adjacent to and within the clonal lymphomatous component [2].

From: *Neoplastic Hematopathology*: Contemporary Hematology,
Edited by: D. Jones, DOI 10.1007/978-1-60761-384-8_15,
© Humana Press, a part of Springer Science+Business Media, LLC 2010

Table 15-1. MZL lymphomas: Anatomical distribution and immunophenotypic, cytogenetic, and molecular features.

Type	Presumed cell of origin	Sites of involvement	Bone marrow involvement	Immunophenotype	Cytogenetic features	Role for antigen?
MALT	Post-GC B cell	Gastrointestinal tract, salivary glands, lung, ocular adnexa, skin, thyroid, breast	2–20%[a]	*Positive*: All pan-B-cell markers, surface or cytoplasmic Ig *Variable*: CD11c, CD43 *Negative*: CD5	+3, +18 and translocations as in Table 15-2	Strong association with underlying inflammatory state in the majority
NMZL	Post-GC B cell in majority	Lymph nodes	Rare (<10%)	As above	+3, +18, +7, del(6q21-q25)	Minimal VH antigen bias
SMZL	Pre-GC[b] & Post-GC	Spleen, splenic hilar lymph nodes, peripheral blood	Typically present	As above, except CD43- and IgD+	del(7q21-q36), +3	VH antigen bias (VH1-2, in ~50%)

[a]Most common in lung and ocular adnexa presentation, lowest in skin and stomach MALT lymphomas
[b]Absence of mutated VH could be explained by extrafollicular B-cell maturation (see text)

Our current understanding of the origin of MALT lymphomas emerged from the work of Isaacson and colleagues who demonstrated the role of persistent antigen stimulation and chronic inflammation in the development of gastric and bowel MALT lymphomas [3]. The subsequent identification of recurrent chromosomal translocations activating the nuclear factor kappa B (NF-kB) pathway has highlighted another etiologic mechanism of MALT lymphoma related to B-cell signaling. The pathogeneses of nodal marginal zone lymphoma (NMZL) and splenic B-cell marginal zone lymphoma (SMZL) are not yet clearly understood.

15.2. Extranodal Marginal Zone Lymphoma of Mucosa-Associated Lymphoid Tissue

15.2.1. Incidence and Clinical Features

MALT lymphoma occurs in adults with a slight female predominance and is the most common type of primary extranodal lymphoma (see Chap. 27) [2]. The etiology of MALT lymphoma varies between anatomic locations and is often associated with chronic immune stimulation secondary to bacterial colonization or an autoimmune disorder (Table 15-2) [4]. Patients with gastric MALT lymphoma often present with symptoms that resemble gastritis or peptic ulcer disease such as epigastric pain, nausea, or vomiting. Patients with MALT lymphoma at other sites usually present with symptoms related to the presence of a mass but without systemic symptoms [5]. Involvement of multiple extranodal sites at presentation occurs in up to 25% of gastric cases and 46% of extragastric cases. Lymph node involvement occurs in approximately 30% of cases, particularly in salivary gland MALT lymphoma associated with Sjögren syndrome and thyroid cases with Hashimoto thyroiditis. Bone marrow involvement is rare, presenting in approximately 10% of patients, most of whom have lung and ocular primaries [6,7].

15.2.2. Diagnostic Features and Subcategories

The gastrointestinal (GI) tract is the most common site of MALT lymphoma with the majority occurring in the stomach. Other anatomical sites (in descending order of frequency) are salivary gland, lung, ocular adnexa, skin, thyroid, and breast [8]. Regardless of the organ involved, there is typically an extensive inflammatory infiltrate representing the inciting immune reaction. The most common histological pattern is reactive GCs surrounded by monoclonal monocytoid B cells admixed with T cells. Follicular colonization and epithelial

Table 15-2. MALT lymphoma: anatomical distribution, etiology, and frequency of chromosomal aberrations.

Anatomic site	Histologic features	Etiologic agent in antigen-driven cases	Incidence of translocations (%)[a]			Aneuploidy incidence (%)	
			t(11;18) (q21;q21)	t(14;18) (q32;q21)	t(3;14) (p14.1;q32)	+3	+18
Stomach	GCs, LELs, MCB clusters	*Helicobacter pylori*	6–26	1–5	0	11	6
Intestine	Intramucosal plasma cells	*Campylobacter jejuni*	12–56	0	0	75	25
Salivary gland	Large GCs, LELs, sheets of MCB	Sjögren syndrome	0–5	0–16	0	55	19
Lung	Diffuse, LELs, GCs with MCB colonization	Sjögren syndrome (rarely)	31–53	6–10	0	20	7
Ocular adnexae	GCs with MCB colonization	*Chlamydia psittaci*	0–10	0–25	0–20	38	13
Skin	GCs with monotypic MCB/ plasma cells	*Borrelia burgdorferi*	0–8	0–10	0–10	20	4
Thyroid	Plasma cells, diffuse	Hashimoto thyroiditis	0–17	0	0–50	17	0

Abbreviations: GC: germinal center; LEL: lymphoepithelial lesion; MCB: monocytoid B cells

[a]Incidences of genetic changes as in the 2008 WHO classification. Rare cases of t(1;14)(p22;q32) are seen in intestinal, salivary gland, and lung MALT lymphomas [1]

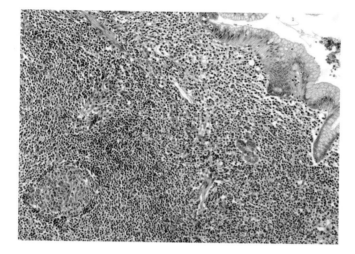

Fig. 15-1. *MALT lymphoma, stomach.* Mucosal infiltrate of reactive germinal centers surrounded by by sheets of small lymphocytes that are mostly B cells

infiltration by neoplastic lymphocytes (i.e., lymphoepithelial lesions) are common findings in MALT lymphoma of the GI tract (Fig. 15-1), lung (Fig. 15-2), and ocular adnexa. MALT lymphomas demonstrating one of the characteristic chromosomal translocations discussed below often have a more sheet-like diffuse B-cell infiltrate with less reactive inflammation. Extensive plasmacytic differentiation, simulating plasmacytoma, is common in MALT lymphoma of the small bowel and thyroid (Fig. 15-3). MALT lymphoma with plasma cell infiltrates expressing IgA or Ig heavy chain only present as immunoproliferative disease of the small bowel (IPSID or Mediterranean lymphoma), are associated with malabsorption and diarrhea and may respond to antibiotic treatment directed against *Campylobacter jejuni* infection [9]. Variants of cutaneous MALT lymphoma include Borrelioma, arising at sites of Lyme disease that are associated with typically densely sclerotic dermis (Fig. 15-4a, b), and immunocytoma, characterized by numerous nonneoplastic GCs with adjacent sheets of monotypic plasma cells or plasmacytoid lymphocytes (Fig. 15-4c).

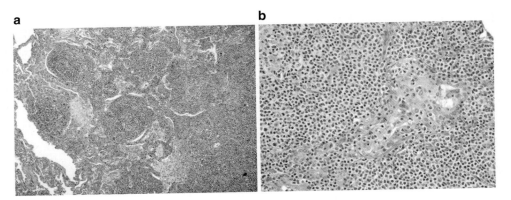

Fig. 15-2. *MALT lymphoma, lung.* (**a**) Nodular, dense lymphoid infiltrate with reactive germinal centers surrounded by intra-alveolar sheets of small B cells. (**b**) Some lesions show extensive monocytoid B-cell differentiation and destructive infiltration of lymphocytes into bronchial mucosa ("BALToma")

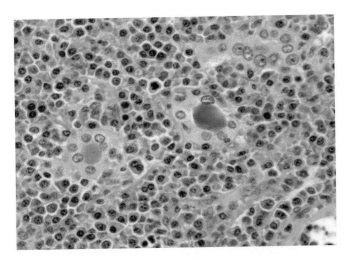

Fig. 15-3. *MALT lymphoma, thyroid.* Well-differentiated monoclonal plasma cells infiltrate between and into thyroid glands

15.2.3. Laboratory Testing for Diagnosis

Regardless of site, immunophenotyping in MALT lymphoma will reveal a mixture of T cells, polyclonal B cells, and monoclonal B cells that are negative for CD5 and CD10, usually express CD43, and show immunoglobulin (Ig) light chain restriction. Although most MALT lymphomas express surface IgM, cases with prominent plasmacytic differentiation can express IgG or IgA, particularly in the small bowel. Depending on the degree of monocytoid or plasmacytic differentiation, Ig heavy or light chain restriction may be demonstrable by paraffin-section immunohistochemistry or in situ hybridization, although the monotypic areas may be only focally present. Similarly, although clonal IGH gene rearrangements are usually detected by PCR or Southern blot analysis, a false-negative result can be seen due to the obscuring effects of the polyclonal reactive B cells, and careful selection of the areas used for DNA extraction prior to PCR is recommended. MALT lymphomas always show mutated IGH variable regions consistent with a post-GC B-cell derivation [5].

MALT lymphomas may also show recurrent reciprocal chromosomal translocations including t(11;18)(q21;q21) producing a fusion of the MALT1 and API2 genes, and t(14;18)

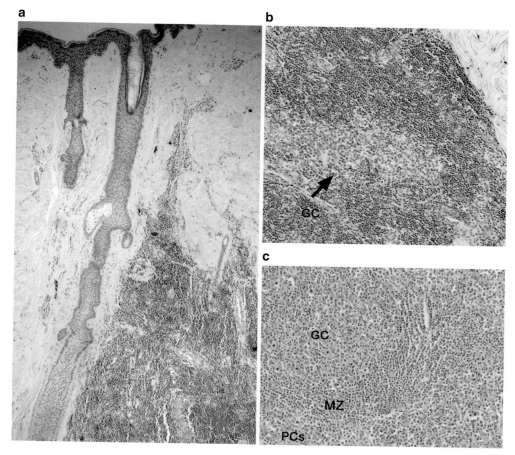

Fig. 15-4. *MALT lymphoma, skin.* (**a** and **b**) Skin of back shows dermal fibrosis with a multifocal deep dermal B-cell infiltrate surrounding adnexa. This 53-year old male patient showed serologic evidence of Borrelia infection. (**c**) Immunocytoma pattern of cutaneous MALT lymphoma shows a reactive germinal center (GC) with expanded mantle zone (MZ), surrounded by a monotypic infiltrate of plasmacytoid lymphocytes (PCs)

(q32;q21) and t(3;14)(p14.1;q32) which drive overexpression of the MALT1 and FOXP1 genes, respectively, by juxtaposition to the IGH enhancer. The rare t(1;14)(p22;q32), usually seen in thyroid or lung MALT lymphomas, activates the BCL10 gene through the IGH enhancer [2,4]. These translocations are readily detected by fluorescence in situ hybridization (FISH) on tissue sections using IGH and/or MALT1 breakapart probes, and their incidences vary between anatomic locations (Table 15-2).

15.2.4. Differential Diagnosis

The differential diagnosis of MALT lymphoma includes nonneoplastic inflammatory processes, other low-grade B-cell lymphomas, and extranodal large B-cell lymphoma. Bowel and thyroid MALT lymphomas are typically extensively plasmacytic and should not be diagnosed as plasmacytoma or lymphoplasmacytic lymphoma (a prominent M-spike is usually lacking). CD10+ follicular lymphoma (FL) and CD5+ cyclin D1+ mantle cell lymphoma (MCL) may occur at extranodal sites (particularly the GI tract) but do so less commonly than MALT lymphoma. In both FL and MCL, the nodular infiltrates do not usually contain the reactive GCs often seen in MALT lymphoma. Lack of cyclin D1 expression is most useful in excluding MCL, since rare cases of MALT lymphoma may express partial/dim CD5. It should also be noted that other B-cell lymphomas, particularly FL, can also arise in association with chronic inflammatory states such as autoimmune conditions.

The dividing line between reactive inflammation (e.g., *Helicobacter pylori* gastritis or autoimmune sialoadenitis) and incipient MALT lymphoma is not precise particularly because multifocal, oligoclonal, or localized clonal B-cell proliferations may arise and regress over time. Findings that indicate lymphomatous transformation include sheet-like areas of monoclonal B cells, marginal zone colonization or infiltration of reactive GCs, and especially, destructive infiltrates with lymphoepithelial lesions [5]. A diagnosis of MALT lymphoma is also established if one of the characteristic chromosomal translocations or copy number aberrations is detected by cytogenetic analysis. The distinction between low-grade MALT lymphoma and large cell transformation can be difficult and is discussed below.

15.2.5. Etiology and Pathogenesis

MALT lymphomas are rare in organs with native lymphoid tissue such as the tonsil, Peyer's patches, and thymus, but instead arise at extranodal sites that normally lack organized lymphoid tissue. Chronic inflammation, secondary to bacterial infection or autoimmune disease, results in persistent expansion of B cells at these sites prior to the onset of lymphoma. In most cases, such clonal expansion of B cells appears to be driven by (and dependent on) prior expansion of helper T cells and the recruitment of immune accessory cells. This model has been best studied in gastric MALT lymphomas where T cells with T-cell receptor specificity for *H. pylori* antigens are found in chronic gastritis preceding a well-established lymphoma. This pathogenetic sequence is supported by the finding that eradication of bacterial infection in *H. pylori* gastritis by antibiotic therapy results in attenuation of the T-cell helper response and regression of many early-stage MALT lymphomas [4,10].

Autoimmune disease or bacterial infection are not the only factors implicated in the initiation of MALT lymphoma. The API2-MALT1 fusion protein produced by t(11;18)(q21;q21) [4], or the transcriptional upregulation of the BCL10 and MALT1 genes, by t(1;14)(p22;q32) and t(14;18)(q32;q21), respectively, all induce NF-kB activation which drives B-cell proliferation in early-stage MALT lymphomas in the absence of helper T cells. In nonneoplastic B cells, BCL10 and MALT1 bind together with BCR-activated CARMA in a cell surface "CBM" complex that links antigenic signaling to MALT1 activation of NF-kB [11]. MALT lymphomas with t(11;18), t(1:14) or t(14;18) bypass CBM regulation either by overexpressing BCL10 which triggers MALT1 oligomerization, or via the API2-MALT1 fusion which promotes oligomerization via the API2 moiety without requiring expression of BCL10.

The rare t(3;14)(p14;q32) translocation, most commonly seen in thyroid and skin MALT lymphomas [12], activates another growth regulator, FOXP1, [4] however, its exact oncogenic mechanism is not clear. The molecular genetics of MALT lymphomas without detectable chromosomal translocations remain poorly understood. It has been speculated that genomic amplification of certain chromosomal loci causes an increase in the transcript levels of NF-kB regulators such as TRAF2 or CARD9 (located at 9q34), RELA (located at 11q13), or MALT1 (located at 18q21-22), and leads to lymphomatous transformation in a manner similar to the translocation-driven cases.

15.2.6. Prognostic Factors and Treatment

The Ann Arbor system is routinely used for staging MALT lymphoma but can be problematic because low-level nodal or extranodal involvement may not be apparent by physical exam or radiologic studies. Additionally, involvement of multiple extranodal sites can be seen even in low-grade, indolent cases and usually does not indicate an aggressive course [7,13,14]. Combination computed tomography (CT)/positron emission tomography (PET) scans show promise in identifying active disease in nongastric MALT [15]. Staging bone marrow biopsy and aspirate with flow cytometry immunophenotyping is usually done, but may be omitted since the incidence of marrow involvement is so low.

Gastric MALT lymphoma associated with *H. pylori* is treated with three different antibiotics ("triple therapy") with subsequent assessment of therapeutic response by endoscopy every 3–6 months until the appearance of the stomach wall has normalized, and then annually for several years thereafter [13]. Response rates with antibiotics range from 60 to 90%, with a median interval to complete regression of 5 months [5]. Cases with t(11;18) or t(1;14) do not respond to antibiotic therapy [16] and more frequently present at an advanced stage [4]. For relapsed disease following *H. pylori* eradication or for *H. pylori*-negative cases, successful treatment involves a combination of surgery, radiation, or chemotherapy. Features associated with therapy resistance and recurrence in gastric MALT include invasion beyond the submucosa, spread of disease beyond the stomach, and the presence of increased large B cells in the infiltrate [5]. Considering all subtypes, the 5-year survival for gastric MALT is approximately 90% [5].

The course of MALT lymphoma outside of the stomach is usually extremely indolent. Most patients present with limited-stage disease and relapses are usually localized or occur at other MALT lymphoma sites (e.g., lung spread from a salivary gland MALT lymphoma). Asymptomatic patients with low tumor burden can be managed by a "watch-and-wait" approach or with localized radiotherapy [13]. Cases with presumed strong antigenic triggers, such as some ocular adnexal and cutaneous MALT lymphomas, may regress following antibiotic therapy [4]. Patients with advanced stage disease are typically treated similarly to other indolent lymphomas such as with single-agent rituximab or combination chemotherapeutic regimens [13]. Recurrences occurring after a prolonged disease-free interval are occasionally seen [7]. For nongastric MALT lymphoma, disease-associated mortality at 5 and 10 years is less than 10 and 20%, respectively [13], except in cases presenting with disseminated disease [17].

15.2.7. Patterns of Progression/Transformation

Like other subtypes of MZL, transformation to diffuse large B-cell lymphoma (DLBCL) occurs and is indicated by areas of the tumor with a sheet-like infiltrate of large cells (Fig. 15-5a). However, more commonly progression is manifested by gradual increases in the mix of large cells and more tissue destructive infiltrates (Fig. 15-5b). Spread of transformed MALT lymphomas into adjacent soft tissue is much more common than to a distant lymph node or bone marrow infiltration.

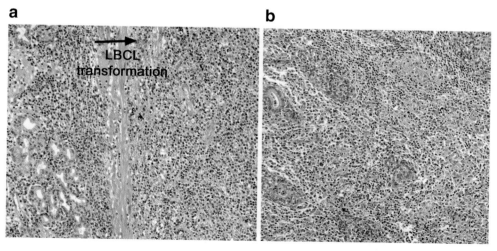

Fig. 15-5. *MALT lymphoma, progression patterns.* (**a**) Discrete large cell transformation (LBCL) of a gastric MALT lymphoma is seen associated with invasion into the muscularis. (**b**) Salivary gland MALT lymphoma with admixture of large cells, included among the lymphoepithelial lesions

Array comparative genomic hybridization (CGH) studies have identified partial or complete gains of chromosomes 3, 12, 18, and 22 as well as discrete chromosomal gains at 1p32, 9q33-34, 11q11-13, and 18q21-22 in translocation-negative cases of salivary gland or gastric MALT lymphoma [18,19]. Some genomic changes in ocular MALT lymphoma may be distinctive with losses at 6q23.3, 7q36.3, and 13q34 as well as the chromosomal gains described above [20]. As in other tumors, mutation and/or deletion of p53 and CDKN2A (p16) deletion have been implicated in initiating the genomic instability and cell cycle deregulation accompanying transformation [10].

15.3. Nodal Marginal Zone Lymphoma

15.3.1. Incidence and Clinical Features

NMZL is rare, comprising 1–2% of all lymphomas, usually occurs in adults with a median age of onset similar to that of MALT lymphoma (60 years), and affects males and females equally. Most patients are asymptomatic at diagnosis. Like other nodal small B-cell lymphomas, the disease tends to present in advanced stages with localized or generalized peripheral lymphadenopathy [13,21]. Bone marrow involvement at diagnosis has been reported in up to one-third of cases [13]. A distinct etiology remains unknown although an association with hepatitis C virus (HCV) has been reported in some series [21,22].

15.3.2. Diagnostic Features

In NMZL, lymph nodes typically show some degree of architectural preservation that includes reactive lymphoid follicles. Neoplastic lymphocytes surround and infiltrate these reactive follicles creating a "marginal zone" cuff around them (Fig. 15-6). Monocytoid B-cell lymphoma is a morphologic variant where all or most of the neoplastic lymphocytes have abundant pale cytoplasm imparting a pale nodular appearance (Fig. 15-7). Cases with prominent plasmacytic differentiation occur (Fig. 15-8) and raise the differential diagnosis lymphoplasmacytic lymphoma (LPL) which typically is associated with the presence of an IgM paraprotein.

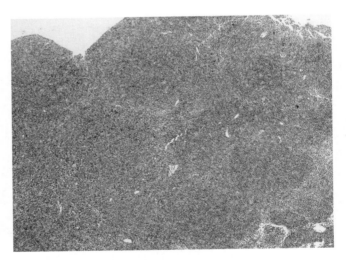

Fig. 15-6. *Nodal marginal zone lymphoma.* A nodular pattern is imparted by lymphomatous expansions of marginal zones and GC colonization

Fig. 15-7. *Nodal marginal zone lymphoma, monocytoid type.* Germinals centers are completely replaced by medium-sized lymphocytes with abdundant clear cytoplasm

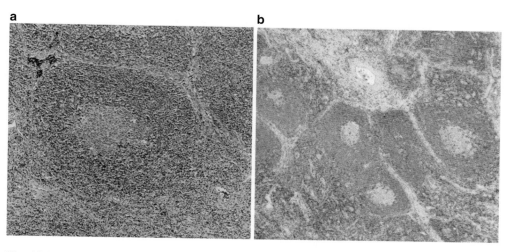

Fig. 15-8. *Nodal marginal zone lymphoma, plasmacytic type.* (**a**) Germinals centers are completely surrounded by mature-appearing plasma cells. (**b**) Immuoglobulin IHC shows strong monotypic cytoplasmic staining for kappa light chain

15.3.3. Laboratory Testing for Diagnosis

Immunohistochemistry or flow cytometric studies will identify a monoclonal B-cell population with an immunophenotype similar to that of MALT lymphoma. Monoclonal Ig gene rearrangements are also present. Trisomies of chromosomes 3, 7, 12, and 18 or deletions spanning chromosome region 6q21-25 have been detected by either conventional cytogenetic or FISH studies. The chromosomal translocations seen in MALT lymphomas are not detected [22]. Most, but not all, cases have mutated IGH variable regions with a usage bias toward VH3 and VH4 gene segments suggesting a post-GC origin [22].

15.3.4. Differential Diagnosis

The differential diagnosis of NMZL should always include primary extranodal MALT lymphoma since up to 30% of MALT cases can present with nodal involvement. SMZL is excluded if splenomegaly is not the predominant clinical finding. Prominent follicular colonization together with the nodular growth pattern may also raise the possibility of FL. The morphology and typical immunophenotype of NMZL (CD5, CD10, CD23, and cyclin D1 negative) are useful in excluding FL as well as other small B-cell lymphomas. Although LPL, which has a similar CD5- CD10- B-cell immunophenotype, may occasionally present with disease limited to the lymph node, it will be accompanied by an Ig paraprotein, usually of IgM type, and will show interstitial or diffuse bone marrow infiltration unlike NMZL.

`5.3.5. Etiology and Pathogenesis

The etiology and pathogenesis of NMZL are not well studied. This is largely due to the lack of characteristic phenotypic, molecular, and cytogenetic findings which make the reproducibility of this diagnosis difficult. HCV infection may play a role in the pathogenesis of some cases of NMZL which utilize the IGH VH1-69 segment, while in HCV-negative cases the VH3-34 segment is most frequently used [21,22].

15.3.6. Prognostic Factors and Treatment

The majority of patients with NMZL have an indolent clinical course. PET/CT is a useful tool for initial staging. The follicular lymphoma international prognostic index (FLIPI) may be used for prognostication and has been shown to identify patients with a significantly shorter survival [21]. A "watch-and-wait" approach may be appropriate for asymptomatic patients with low tumor burden whereas single-agent rituximab is often used for elderly patients or those with low-stage disease. Rituximab combined with CHOP chemotherapy is usually used for high-stage presentation [13]. Although frequent relapses are common in NMZL, 60–80% of patients survive longer than 5 years with a median survival approaching 10 years [13,21]. Overall, the prognosis appears to be less favorable than MALT lymphoma and SMZL, but similar to CLL/SLL [13].

15.3.7. Patterns of Progression/Transformation

The incidence of transformation to large cell lymphoma reported in the largest series was 16% (20 of 124 cases), occurring at a median time of 4.5 years from diagnosis [13]. Another study showed transformation occurring 10–76 months after diagnosis [22]. Progression may be largely independent of p53 or p16 inactivation [22] but more studies are needed.

15.4. Splenic B-cell Marginal Zone Lymphoma

15.4.1. Incidence and Clinical Features

SMZL is rare, comprising less than 2% of all lymphomas. The disease occurs in adults, affects males and females equally, and usually presents within the sixth decade of life. At presentation, patients typically have massive splenomegaly as well as low-level bone marrow and peripheral blood involvement [23]. The most common presenting symptom is abdominal discomfort due to massive splenomegaly. Patients also often have modest cytopenias primarily due to splenic sequestration as opposed to bone marrow infiltration [13]. The tumor nearly always involves the splenic hilar lymph nodes. Peripheral lymphadenopathy or involvement of extranodal sites is extremely rare. Like NMZL, an association with HCV has been reported in some series [23].

15.4.2. Diagnostic Features

In patients presenting with splenomegaly (and minimal lymphadenopathy), the diagnosis of SMZL is often accomplished by demonstration of low-level involvement of blood and/or bone marrow by a monoclonal CD5- CD10- B-cell lymphoma with compatible morphology.

In cases with unusual clinical features or equivocal immunophenotype, splenectomy is often done to clarify the diagnosis and demonstrates a micronodular gross appearance which corresponds histologically to both white and red pulp involvement. In SMZL, splenic white pulp nodules are expanded and characteristically have a central dark zone of admixed tumor lymphocytes and residual GC B cells, an attenuated or effaced mantle zone, and an expanded lighter-staining marginal zone composed of small to medium-sized cells with moderate amounts of pale cytoplasm (Fig. 15-9a) or complete expansion and effacement of the white pulp microarchitecture (Fig. 15-9b) [22,23]. Tumor cells also form small aggregates in the red pulp usually within the sinuses and cords [23].

Bone marrow involvement is almost always present and can be intrasinusoidal or nodular, sometimes with lymphoma surrounding and infiltrating reactive GCs (Fig. 15-10a). The infiltrate can sometimes be subtle, requiring immunohistochemical staining with a B-cell marker (e.g., CD20 or PAX5) for visualization (Fig. 15-10b) [22]. SMZL cells in blood are small to medium-sized with condensed chromatin, moderately abundant pale cytoplasm, and short polar villi (Fig. 15-11) [22,23]. Cases with a predominance of cells with such cytoplasmic processes have been named splenic lymphoma with villous lymphocytes and may have distinct clinical features.

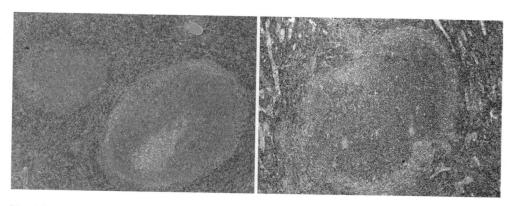

Fig. 15-9. *Splenic marginal zone lymphoma.* (**a**) White pulp is markedly expanded with preservation of a central reactive GC. (**b**) In the more common pattern, lymphoma replaces the white pulp GCs

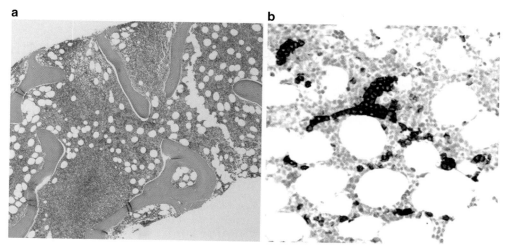

Fig. 15-10. *Splenic marginal zone lymphoma, bone marrow.* (**a**) Multiple interstitial lymphoid aggregates, including at least one created by colonization of a reactive GC. (**b**) Intrasinusoidal infiltration is characteristic in early/low-level marrow involvement (CD20 immunostain)

15.4.3. Laboratory Testing for Diagnosis

SMZL has an immunophenotype similar to that of MALT lymphoma, except that it is typically negative for CD43 and positive for IgD (Table 15-1) [22,23]. Allelic loss of chromosome 7q, specifically the 7q21-36 region centered on 7q32, is present in up to 50% of cases and is much more frequently seen in SMZL compared to other types of small B-cell lymphomas [22]. Gains of 3q (20–30% of cases), 4q, 5q, 9q, 12q (15–20%), 20q, and losses involving 6q, 7q, 14q, and 17p are also seen but are less specific [22–24]. Although these chromosomal deletions may be detected by conventional cytogenetic studies, FISH or array CGH are recommended for accurate detection. Overall, trisomy 3 is detected less frequently in cases of SMZL compared to other subtypes of MZL.

15.4.4. Differential Diagnosis with Hairy Cell Leukemia and Its Variants

The differential diagnosis of SMZL includes other low-grade B-cell lymphomas, particularly hairy cell leukemia (HCL), the ill-defined splenic B-cell lymphoma/leukemia, and hairy cell leukemia variant (HCL-v), since all three entities typically present with splenomegaly, bone marrow and peripheral blood involvement (Table 15-3). The morphology and typical immunophenotype (CD5, CD23, and cyclin D1 negative) of SMZL are useful in excluding

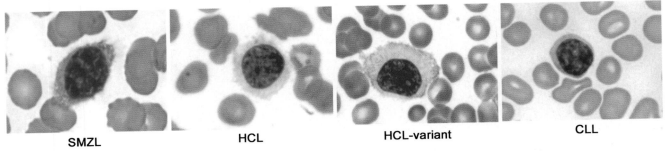

Fig. 15-11. *Low-grade B-cell lymproliferative disorders in peripheral blood.* Characteristic morphologies of splenic marginal zone lymphoma (**a**); hairy cell leukemia (**b**); hairy cell leukemia-variant (**c**); and chronic lymphocytic leukemia (**d**)

Table 15-3. Comparison of SMZL, HCL and HCL-v.

Type	Sites of involvement	Pattern of splenic involvement	Pattern of bone marrow involvement	Peripheral blood lymphocyte characteristics	Immunophenotype
SMZL	Spleen, splenic hilar lymph nodes, peripheral blood	Nodular white pulp and diffuse red pulp involvement	Nodular, interstitial, and intrasinusoidal pattern with preserved hematopoiesis	Small to medium in size, scanty basophilic cytoplasm with polar cytoplasmic projections	*Positive*: IgM and IgD *Variable*: CD11c, CD25, DBA.44 *Negative*: CD5, CD10, CD43, CD103, CD123
HCL	As above	Diffuse red pulp involvement and blood lake formation with obliteration of white pulp	Interstitial to diffuse often with suppression of hematopoiesis	Medium to large in size, more abundant cytoplasm with circumferential cytoplasmic projections, strong TRAP positivity	*Positive*: CD11c, bright CD25, CD103, CD123, FMC-7, annexin A1, DBA.44, bright IgM+ *Negative*: CD5, CD10
HCL-v	As above	Diffuse red pulp involvement and blood lake formation	Interstitial or nodular with preserved hematopoiesis	Similar to HCL but with a prominent single nucleolus and relatively condensed chromatin, TRAP weak to negative	As above for HCL except negative for CD25, annexin A1 and CD123 in most cases

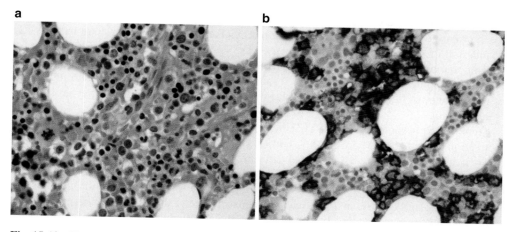

Fig. 15-12. *Hairy cell leukemia, bone marrow.* (**a**) Interstitial infiltration by this leukemia can be difficult to visualize on routine H&E staining. (**b**) CD20 immunostain highlights extensive involvement

CLL/SLL and MCL. The absence of CD43 expression, presence of IgD expression, and the anatomic site(s) of involvement are helpful features that can be used in the exclusion of NMZL and MALT lymphoma.

Patients with HCL generally have peripheral cytopenias and a characteristic monocytopenia. In contrast to SMZL, HCL typically presents with splenic white pulp atrophy and diffuse red pulp involvement with the formation of red blood cell lakes surrounded by neoplastic lymphocytes [25]. The morphologic appearance and pattern of bone marrow involvement by HCL is also much different from SMZL and typically shows an interstitial infiltrate composed of small lymphocytes with abundant cytoplasm and distinct cell borders giving rise to a "fried egg" appearance (Fig. 15-12a) [25]. These cells can be very difficult to visualize without immunohistochemistry (Fig. 15-12b).

Peripheral blood hairy cells, unlike the villous lymphocytes of SMZL, are medium to large-sized and have abundant pale cytoplasm with circumferential cytoplasmic projections in contrast to the polar projections seen in villous lymphocytes (Fig. 15-11). Hairy cells also show strong tartrate-resistant acid phosphatase (TRAP) cytochemical staining whereas villous lymphocytes in SMZL are weakly positive or negative [25]. The flow cytometric phenotype for HCL includes bright expression of surface immunoglobulin, with coexpression of CD11c, CD25, CD103, CD123, and FMC7. Annexin A1 is expressed in HCL but not in SMZL [23, 25].

HCL-v, a provisional entity in the 2008 WHO classification, describes cases that resemble classic HCL but shows variant cytological and immunophenotypic features as well as resistance to conventional HCL therapy [23]. Unlike HCL, HCL-v cases do not exhibit monocytopenia. Like HCL, circulating HCL-v lymphocytes are medium to large in size with more abundant often faintly basophilic cytoplasm and circumferential cytoplasmic projections; however, the nucleus resembles that of a prolymphocyte with a prominent single nucleolus and more condensed chromatin (Fig. 15-11). HCL-v is weakly positive or negative for TRAP and may lack CD25, CD123, and annexin A1 [26]. The relationship of HCL-v to cases previously described as CD5-negative atypical CLL, diffuse SMZL, or diffuse red pulp small B-cell lymphoma is still under study, leading the WHO committee to favor splenic B-cell lymphoma/leukemia, unclassifiable as an umbrella term for primary splenic low-grade B-cell lymphoproliferative disorders which are not typical for HCL or SMZL.

15.4.5. Etiology and Pathogenesis

Although its name implies a post-GC B-cell origin, the cell-of-origin of SMZL remains unclear. Absence of lymph node homing, along with surface expression of IgD and the presence of unmutated IGH in 50% of SMZL, [22,23] suggests an origin from B cells that have undergone extra-follicular maturation (i.e., outside of the GC). Such an alternate maturation pathway has been proposed for subsets of nonneoplastic marginal zone B cells, which share with SMZL, expression of some signaling molecules such as Notch2 [27]. Both chronic stimulation of splenic marginal zone B cells by HCV infection, which precedes SMZL in 20% of cases in some geographic areas, [22,23] and the frequent finding of productive IGH rearrangements utilizing one particular variable region (V1-2), [22] support a role for particular antigenic stimuli.

Genome expression studies of SMZL have shown an upregulation of mediators of NF-kB activation such as TRAF3, TRAF5, CD40, and LTB which may promote autonomous growth independent of a BCR signal as with translocation-driven MALT lymphomas. SMZL also expresses high levels of TCL1 which is typically a pre-GC marker that activates AKT kinase [22]. Finally, aberrant sonic hedgehog pathway signaling through loss of POT1 at 7q31 and/or SHH at 7q31 may be a consequence of the del(7q) [22,24]. Candidate transforming genes within the amplified areas of 3q23–q29 region have also been suggested [23].

15.4.6. Prognostic Factors and Treatment

The prognosis of SMZL is extremely favorable, with an overall median survival of at least 8–10 years. Adverse clinical prognostic factors include massive splenomegaly and poor performance status [22]. High beta-2 microglobulin concentrations, development of lymphadenopathy, involvement of nonhematopoietic sites, peripheral blood leukocytosis, and peripheral blood lymphocytosis have also been associated with shorter overall survival and progression free survival [22,23]. Complete response to initial treatment has been associated with longer survival and failure-free survival [22]. Molecular and cytogenetic factors associated with poor outcome include p53 alterations, unmutated Ig genes, and the presence of deletions at chromosome 7q [22,23]. Survival analyzes using cDNA microarray data identified shorter survival in cases with the expression of a subset of NF-kB pathway genes including TRAF5, REL, and PKC-alpha [22]. Overall survival was also shorter in cases with higher numbers of chromosomal losses identified by array CGH studies [22].

Approaches to treatment of SMZL vary at different centers [23]. Observation with followup exams and blood work every 6–12 months is widely used in asymptomatic individuals who have no adverse prognostic factors [13,22,23]. Splenectomy may be indicated for definitive diagnosis or as treatment for patients with cytopenias or massive splenomegaly [23]. Although not curative, splenectomy can provide symptomatic relief, long-term disease control and normalization of blood counts. Single-agent rituximab is highly active in SMZL, with an ORR of 100%, and a CR rate of 71% documented in a small Phase II study [13]. Chemotherapy with alkylating agents or purine analogs (fludarabine) alone or in combination with rituximab is typically reserved for patients with progression, and/or when splenectomy is contraindicated [13,22,23]. Successful therapy of SMZL with a-interferon and ribavirin in HCV-infected patients has also been reported [22,23].

15.4.7. Patterns of Progression and Transformation

Despite its indolent clinical course and response to splenectomy, the overall incidence of transformation to DLBCL in SMZL is 13–19% [13,22,28]. Cases with peripheral lymph node involvement at diagnosis, high tumor growth fraction, and del(7q) have been associated with higher rates of transformation [22,28]. The presence of large lymphoma cells in the bone marrow is an extremely adverse predictor whereas transformation detected in lymph nodes may respond well to chemotherapy [28]. Inactivation of p53 [28] has been implicated more commonly than p16 inactivation in transformation [22].

Suggested Readings

Du MQ. MALT lymphoma : recent advances in etiology and molecular genetics. J Clin Exp Hematop 2007;47:31–42.
- Thorough review of the etiologic roles of microbial pathogens and molecular genetic alterations in the different types of MALT lymphoma.

Kahl B, Yang D. Marginal zone lymphomas: management of nodal, splenic, and MALT NHL. Hematology Am Soc Hematol Educ Program 2008;2008:359–64.
- Succinct review of the different types of MZL lymphoma as well as the distinct clinical and therapeutic approaches currently employed for each entity.

Matutes E, Oscier D, Montalban C, et al. Splenic marginal zone lymphoma proposals for a revision of diagnostic, staging and therapeutic criteria. Leukemia 2008;22:487–95.
- Expert panel review and proposal of guidelines for diagnosis, differential diagnosis, staging, prognostic factors, treatment and response criteria for SMZL.

Mollejo M, Camacho FI, Algara P, Ruiz-Ballesteros E, Garcia JF, Piris MA. Nodal and splenic marginal zone B cell lymphomas. Hematol Oncol 2005;23:108–18
- Excellent review of NMZL and SMZL

References

1. Sagaert X, De Wolf-Peeters C, Noels H, Baens M. The pathogenesis of MALT lymphomas: where do we stand? Leukemia 2007;21:389–96.
2. Isaacson PG. Update on MALT lymphomas. Best Pract Res Clin Haematol 2005;18:57–68.
3. Wotherspoon AC, Ortiz-Hidalgo C, Falzon MR, Isaacson PG. *Helicobacter pylori*-associated gastritis and primary B-cell gastric lymphoma. Lancet 1991;338:1175–6.
4. Du MQ. MALT lymphoma: recent advances in aetiology and molecular genetics. J Clin Exp Hematop 2007;47:31–42.
5. Ferry JA. Extranodal lymphoma. Arch Pathol Lab Med 2008;132:565–78.
6. Thieblemont C, Berger F, Dumontet C, et al. Mucosa-associated lymphoid tissue lymphoma is a disseminated disease in one third of 158 patients analyzed. Blood 2000;95:802–6.
7. Raderer M, Streubel B, Woehrer S, et al. High relapse rate in patients with MALT lymphoma warrants lifelong follow-up. Clin Cancer Res 2005;11:3349–52.
8. Thieblemont C, Bastion Y, Berger F, et al. Mucosa-associated lymphoid tissue gastrointestinal and nongastrointestinal lymphoma behavior: analysis of 108 patients. J Clin Oncol 1997;15:1624–30.
9. Al-Saleem T, Al-Mondhiry H. Immunoproliferative small intestinal disease (IPSID): a model for mature B-cell neoplasms. Blood 2005;105:2274–80.
10. Isaacson PG. Gastric MALT lymphoma: from concept to cure. Ann Oncol 1999;10:637–45.
11. Rawlings DJ, Sommer K, Moreno-Garcia ME. The CARMA1 signalosome links the signalling machinery of adaptive and innate immunity in lymphocytes. Nat Rev Immunol 2006;6:799–812.
12. Remstein ED, Dogan A, Einerson RR, et al. The incidence and anatomic site specificity of chromosomal translocations in primary extranodal marginal zone B-cell lymphoma of mucosa-associated lymphoid tissue (MALT lymphoma) in North America. Am J Surg Pathol 2006;30:1546–53.
13. Kahl B, Yang D. Marginal zone lymphomas: management of nodal, splenic, and MALT NHL. Hematology Am Soc Hematol Educ Program 2008;2008:359–64.
14. A predictive model for aggressive non-Hodgkin's lymphoma. The international non-Hodgkin's lymphoma prognostic factors project. N Engl J Med 1993;329:987–94.
15. Perry C, Herishanu Y, Metzer U, et al. Diagnostic accuracy of PET/CT in patients with extranodal marginal zone MALT lymphoma. Eur J Haematol 2007;79:205–9.
16. Liu H, Ye H, RuskoneFourmestraux A, et al. T(11;18) is a marker for all stage gastric MALT lymphomas that will not respond to *H. pylori* eradication. Gastroenterology 2002;122:1286–94.
17. Talwalkar SS, Miranda RN, Valbuena JR, Routbort MJ, Martin AW, Medeiros LJ. Lymphomas involving the breast: a study of 106 cases comparing localized and disseminated neoplasms. Am J Surg Pathol 2008;32:1299–309.
18. Zhou Y, Ye H, Martin-Subero JI, et al. Distinct comparative genomic hybridisation profiles in gastric mucosa-associated lymphoid tissue lymphomas with and without t(11;18)(q21;q21). Br J Haematol 2006;133:35–42.

19. Zhou Y, Ye H, Martin-Subero JI, et al. The pattern of genomic gains in salivary gland MALT lymphomas. Haematologica 2007;92:921–7.
20. Kim WS, Honma K, Karnan S, et al. Genome-wide array-based comparative genomic hybridization of ocular marginal zone B cell lymphoma: comparison with pulmonary and nodal marginal zone B cell lymphoma. Genes Chromosomes Cancer 2007;46:776–83.
21. Arcaini L, Paulli M, Burcheri S, et al. Primary nodal marginal zone B-cell lymphoma: clinical features and prognostic assessment of a rare disease. Br J Haematol 2007;136:301–4.
22. Mollejo M, Camacho FI, Algara P, Ruiz-Ballesteros E, Garcia JF, Piris MA. Nodal and splenic marginal zone B cell lymphomas. Hematol Oncol 2005;23:108–18.
23. Matutes E, Oscier D, Montalban C, et al. Splenic marginal zone lymphoma proposals for a revision of diagnostic, staging and therapeutic criteria. Leukemia 2008;22:487–95.
24. Vega F, Cho-Vega JH, Lennon PA, et al. Splenic marginal zone lymphomas are characterized by loss of interstitial regions of chromosome 7q, 7q31.32 and 7q36.2 that include the protection of telomere 1 (POT1) and sonic hedgehog (SHH) genes. Br J Haematol 2008;142(2):216–26.
25. Sharpe RW, Bethel KJ. Hairy cell leukemia: diagnostic pathology. Hematol Oncol Clin North Am 2006;20:1023–49.
26. Matutes E, Wotherspoon A, Catovsky D. The variant form of hairy-cell leukaemia. Best Pract Res Clin Haematol 2003;16:41–56.
27. Troen G, Nygaard V, Jenssen TK, et al. Constitutive expression of the AP-1 transcription factors c-jun, junD, junB, and c-fos and the marginal zone B-cell transcription factor Notch2 in splenic marginal zone lymphoma. J Mol Diagn 2004;6:297–307.
28. Dungarwalla M, Appiah-Cubi S, Kulkarni S, et al. High-grade transformation in splenic marginal zone lymphoma with circulating villous lymphocytes: the site of transformation influences response to therapy and prognosis. Br J Haematol 2008;143:71–4.

Chapter 16

Follicular Lymphoma and Mantle Cell Lymphoma

Dan Jones

Abstract/Scope of Chapter This chapter covers the commonly-encountered follicular lymphoma and the more aggressive but rare mantle cell lymphoma. These two B-cell lymphomas are predominantly lymph node-based but show characteristic patterns of spread to the bone marrow and gastrointestinal tract. Both lymphomas progress through recognizable histologic stages that are characterized by increasing number of large tumor cells and accumulation of cell cycle genetic defects. Follicular lymphoma however shows a more clear requirement for stromal-derived cytokine signals and B-cell receptor pathway dysregulation for full transformation.

Keywords Follicular lymphoma (FL) · Follicular lymphoma · grading · Follicular lymphoma · FLIPI staging system · BCL2 · gene rearrangements · Follicular lymphoma · blastoid variant · Follicular lymphoma · diffuse · Pediatric follicular lymphoma · Follicular lymphoma · floral variant · Follicle lymphoma · BCL6 rearrangement · Follicular lymphoma · Castlemanoid variant · Follicular lymphoma · marginal zone pattern, Follicular lymphoma, in situ · Follicle center lymphoma · primary skin · NF-KB, REL amplification · Mantle cell lymphoma · Mantle cell lymphoma · blastoid · lymphomatous polyposis · Mantle cell lymphoma · Splenic variant · Cyclin D1 · Cyclin D3 · mantle cell lymphoma

16.1. Introduction

Follicular lymphoma and mantle cell lymphoma represent paradigms of the initiation-progression histogenetic model of lymphomagenesis discussed in Chap. 1. Although these tumors are defined based on their histologic and immunophenotype features, they both have characteristic initiating chromosomal translocations, t(14;18)/IGH-BCL2 and t(11;14)/CCND1-IGH, respectively. Later stages of lymphoma progression in both lymphomas involve the activation of common growth pathways and loss of tumor suppressors that largely determine the outcome.

16.2. Follicular Lymphoma

16.2.1. Incidence and Clinical Features

FL is the most common low-grade lymphoma, although there are marked geographic differences with a high incidence in the United States and Europe, and an extremely low incidence in parts of Asia [1,2]. The basis for these marked geographic variations is not yet known but may be related to population-based differences in genetic polymorphisms in immune

From: *Neoplastic Hematopathology*: Contemporary Hematology,
Edited by: D. Jones, DOI 10.1007/978-1-60761-384-8_16,
© Humana Press, a part of Springer Science+Business Media, LLC 2010

regulatory genes or in the age or prevalence in which common infections are acquired. In the United States, the median age at presentation for FL is 59 years, with roughly equal incidence in males and females. Rare cases presenting in childhood are thought to represent distinct variants with low rates of progression and frequent extranodal localization.

FL is almost always a systemic disease with multi-compartment lymphadenopathy. Bone marrow infiltration is detectable histologically in approximately 50% of cases, but low-level involvement can be detected using flow cytometric or molecular methods in 60–70%. Staging is done using the Ann Arbor classification, with risk stratification most commonly done using the FLIPI score.

As disease burden increases, extranodal spread is common, with FL often colonizing sites of chronic inflammation (e.g., folliculitis in skin) or involving body fluids. Transformation to diffuse large B-cell lymphoma can occur at a discrete nodal or extranodal site, which can sometimes be detected as an occult "hotspot" in nuclear medicine studies. A variant of FL largely restricted to the small bowel has an indolent course [3,4]. Conversely, a small cell blastoid variant that often shows high-level peripheral blood and bone marrow involvement has a worse outcome than typical small cleaved (grade 1) FL [5,6].

16.2.2. Diagnostic Features and Subcategories

FL has a characteristic nodular growth pattern in lymph node due to its displacement of reactive B cells within germinal centers (Fig. 16-1). Neoplastic follicles in FL tend to involve all areas of the node, extend into extracapsular areas, and include "cracking" or retraction artifact around the follicles in formalin-fixed sections. Partial or complete infarction of involved lymph nodes can be seen. Growth patterns are recorded as predominantly follicular (>75% of lymph node), mixed follicular and diffuse (25–75%) or predominantly diffuse (<25%), with worse outcome with increasing diffuse growth (Fig. 16-2) [7].

Histologic grading of follicular lymphoma (Fig. 16-3 and Table 16-1) has been traditionally done using the Mann-Berard criteria based on the number of noncleaved cells or centroblasts (Table 16-1), [9] with grades 1, 2, and 3 being correlated with progressively shorter survivals [10]. Grade 3 is often subdivided into type A (mixed centrocytes/centroblasts) and type B (only centroblasts), but the clinical significance of this distinction has not been convincingly demonstrated [7,11]. All FL grading schemes are somewhat subjective with poor inter-observer reproducibility [12]. FL usually shows a range of small, intermediate and large cells and a continuous spectrum of cleaved, polylobated, and "noncleaved" nuclear appearances, as well as spindle cell variants which are difficult to grade [13]. Grading based on cytologic preparations is equally problematic due to sampling issues (Fig. 16-4).

FL involving the spleen is usually confined to the white pulp [14]. FL involving fibrous tissue, such as in the groin, retroperitoneum, pleura or meninges, usually lacks nodular growth pattern, but instead infiltrates single-file or as nests between the fibrous bands. This sclerotic pattern encompasses most cases diagnosed as sclerosing or diffuse follicular lymphoma (Fig. 16-5),

Table 16-1. Cytological grading of follicular lymphoma.

	Morphology type	Mann–Berard criteria
Grade 1	Predominantly small cleaved (centrocytes)	0–5 centroblasts/HPF
Grade 2	Mixed	6-15 centroblasts/HPF
Grade 3		Greater than 15 centroblasts/HPF
3A	Large cleaved or mixed small and large	
3B	Large noncleaved (centroblasts) only	

Abbreviations: hpf: high-power field. Criteria for counting depending on field size are outlined in reference [8]

Fig. 16-1. *Follicular lymphoma.* (**a**) Lobulated gross appearance of an involved lymph node is shown. (**b**) Back-to-back neoplastic follicles are present throughout the entire lymph node

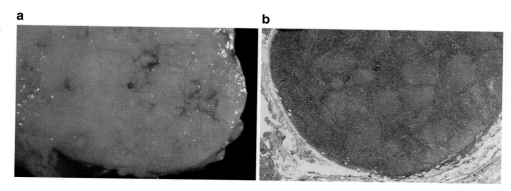

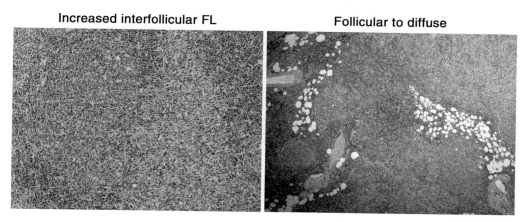

Increased interfollicular FL

Follicular to diffuse

Fig. 16-2. *Follicular lymphoma, progression patterns.* (**a**) Increased interfollicular tumor cells are present between two neoplastic follicles. (**b**) Nodular (*on left*) transitioning to a diffuse growth patterns (*on right*) is correlated with clinical disease progression

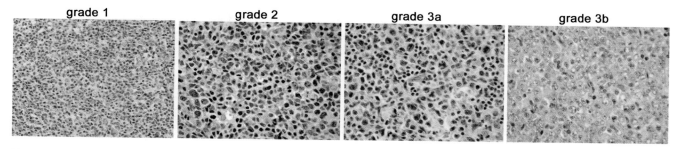

grade 1   grade 2   grade 3a   grade 3b

Fig. 16-3. *Follicular lymphoma, grading.* Illustrated are grade 1 (predominantly small cleaved cells), grade 2 (mixed large and small cleaved forms), grade 3A (increased large cells with both cleaved and noncleaved forms) and grade 3B (only large noncleaved forms present)

Fig. 16-4. *Follicular lymphoma, cytologic appearance.* (**a**) Grade 1 follicular lymphoma, with more irregular and cleaved nuclear contours in the lymphocytes, and numerous bare nuclei (H&E stained cytologic smear). (**b**) Reactive lymphadenitis showing polymorphous lymphoid infiltrate including nonneoplastic germinal center centrocytes (H&E stained cytologic smear)

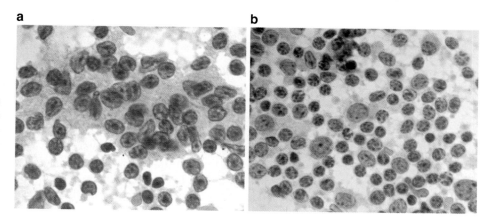

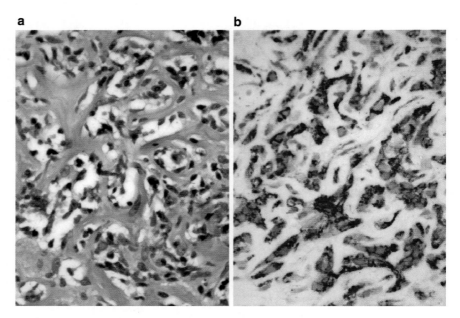

Fig. 16-5. *Follicular lymphoma, diffuse.* (**a**) Irregular lymphocytes infiltrating between sclerotic bands. (**b**) CD20 immunostain shows uniform positivity

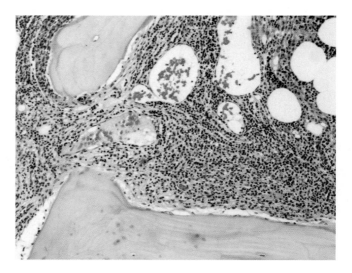

Fig. 16-6. Follicular lymphoma, bone marrow. Fibrotic paratrabecular aggregates are noted

which express BCL 2 and other FL-associated markers (e.g., BCL6, CD10) but can lack t(14;18) and instead have deletions involving chromosomal region (chr) 1p36 [15] consistent with a distinct entity. FL is the most common lymphoma type to involve body fluids, particularly pleural effusions and ascites, where it frequently shows large forms with bizarre or multilobate nuclei, even in low-grade cases.

Bone marrow involvement in FL is classically paratrabecular with lymphoid aggregates tightly opposed to bone trabeculae with associated reticulin deposition (Fig. 16-6). As a result of this fibrosis, FL tumor cells are poorly represented in marrow aspirates and are often missed by flow cytometry requiring immunostaining for confirmation. The presence of well-formed intertrabecular lymphoid follicles in the marrow should raise the diagnosis of marginal zone lymphoma (MZL) instead of FL. The leukemic blastoid variant of FL usually shows a diffuse pattern of marrow infiltration with a small to intermediate tumor cell size and nuclei with deep cleaves or furrows (known as "buttock" cells) [6]

16.2.3. Laboratory Testing for Diagnosis

Immunohistochemistry and flow cytometry remain the mainstays of diagnosis of FL. In paraffin sections, the demonstration of a CD10+BCL2+BCL6+B-cell infiltrate within follicles (Fig. 16-7) or infiltrating fibrous tissue is diagnostic. Flow cytometric studies will reveal a CD19+CD20+CD22+B-cell population that expresses CD10 and dim surface kappa or lambda monotypic immunoglobulin (Ig) light chain (Table 16-2). Except in rare transformed cases, FL lacks CD5 and CD43 expression, and shows variable CD11c, CD23, and CD38 expression. As the disease progresses, more prominent involvement of the interfollicular areas of the node is seen, and those tumor cells tend to downregulate CD10 and BCL6 expression.

Detection of the t(14;18)(q32;q21) is best performed using fusion FISH (separately labeled BCL2 and IGH probes that combine to give a two-color fusion signal) which will detect the translocation in 85–90% of cases. Approximately 7–10% of these false-negative results are due to alternate translocations, particularly involving the BCL6 locus at chromosome 3q27 (Table 16-3). Use of PCR to detect the t(14;18) translocation is complicated by the range of breakpoints involving the BCL2 gene on chromosome 18 which require multiple primer pairs for detection of all cases. The most frequently tested area is the 150 base pair major breakpoint region (MBR) which is involved in 65–70% of FL, followed by the minor cluster region (MCR) and intermediate cluster region (ICR) used in 5–10% and 2–3% of the cases, respectively.

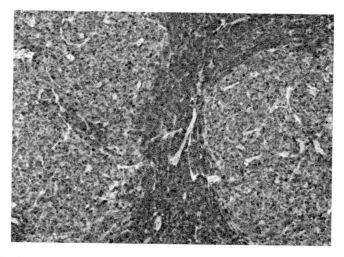

Fig. 16-7. *Follicular lymphoma, immunophenotype.* Neoplastic follicles are strongly and uniformly immunoreactive for BCL2 as are the small interfollicular T cells

Table 16-2. Differential diagnosis of B-cell lymphoma by flow cytometric markers.

	CD5	CD10	CD23	CD11c	CD43	CD20	Surface Ig
Follicular lymphoma	−	+	Var	Var	−	Var	Dim
Mantle cell lymphoma	+	−	−	−	+	Bright	Bright
Marginal zone lymphoma	−	−	Var	−	+	Bright	Bright
Small lymphocytic lymphoma	+	−	+	Subset	+	Often dim	Var
Lymphoplasmacytic lymphoma	−	−	Var	+	Var	+	+

Var: variable staining

Table 16-3. Variants of follicular lymphoma.

	Incidence, location	Morphology	Phenotypic features
Morphologic variants			
Marginal zone differentiation [16]	1–2%	Monocytoid or marginal zone differentiation in tumor cells around neoplastic follicles	Involvement of the BCL6 locus [17,18]
Floral variant [19]	<1%	Invasion of expanded reactive mantle B cells into follicles	May be CD5+ [20]
Castlemanoid	Pelvic and abdominal	Regressed Castlemanoid follicles	
In situ FL [21]	Rare	One to several neoplastic follicles in a background of reactive GCs	t(14;18) FISH useful to confirm, rebiopsy useful
Diffuse FL [15]	5–10% Inguinal, retroperitoneal	Low stage, grade 1–2	Often lack t(14;18), may show chr 1p36 deletions
Immunophenotype variants			
CD10- MUM1+ [22]	1–2%	More often diffuse, older patients, often grade 3	BCL6 translocation or amplification
Molecular variants			
Chromosome 3q27 alterations (BCL6) [23]	5%	Often grade 3B	BCL2– by IHC
BCL2 amplification [24]	1–2%	Often grade 3A or 3B	BCL2+ by IHC
Other genetic changes [25]		Often grade 3B	BCL2–/+ by IHC
Clinical variants			
Primary intestinal follicular lymphoma	Duodenum	Stage IE, IIE but otherwise identical to systemic FL	CD10+ BCL2+
Pediatric follicular lymphoma [26,27]	Testes, epididymis	Nodular, with large cell predominating	CD10+/– but no t(14;18) or BCL6 translocation
Cutaneous follicle center lymphoma [28]	Head and neck skin	Indolent but can show grade 3A morphology	CD10+HGAL+but no t(14;18) or BCL6 translocation

Abbreviations: FL: follicular lymphoma; FISH: fluorescence in situ hybridization; IHC: immunohistochemistry

Cytogenetic studies are often ineffective in early-stage FL due to failure to obtain metaphases. Progressed FL is much easier to karyotype but often has so many changes that interpretation is complex. A better method to catalog the large number of secondary genetic changes usually observed in progressed FL is array-based profiling using single nucleotide polymorphisms or comparative genomic hybridization (CGH), which can detect small genomic deletions and gains but not usually t(14;18) or other reciprocal translocations (Fig. 16-8).

16.2.4. Differential Diagnosis and Variants

The primary differential diagnoses of low-grade FL are with benign follicular hyperplasia and with marginal zone lymphoma. As summarized in Chap. 12, helpful features of FL in lymph node include loss of follicle polarity (no light–dark zones), back-to-back follicles replacing the entire node, and most importantly, expression of BCL 2 protein by the neoplastic B cells within the follicles. Flow cytometric studies are extremely helpful in demonstrating a clonal CD10+B-cell population; however, FL can have very dim surface CD10 and Ig light chain expression complicating diagnosis [29]. Marginal zone lymphomas of all types often show marked follicular colonization leading to the appearance of a purely nodular lymphoma [30]. In these cases, although BCL2+lymphoma B cells will be present in the follicles, they will be intermixed with reactive GC components. Other areas of lymph node will usually show marginal zone colonization or sheet-like areas of monocytoid B cells or plasmacytoid forms (see Chap. 15).

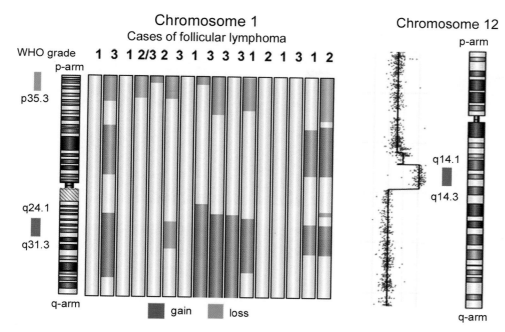

Fig. 16-8. *Follicular lymphoma, genomic analysis.* Array comparative genomic hybridization (CGH) reveals frequent chromosome 1 aberrations in follicular lymphoma which increase with tumor grade (*left panel*), as well as more localized gene-centric changes such as amplification at chromosome 12 q13-q14 encompassing the CDK2 and CDK4 loci (*right panel*)

Several patterns of nodal involvement by FL can present diagnostic difficulties (Table 16-3). The most common of these is sclerosing FL, which can resemble reactive fibrosis or inflammatory pseudotumor [31]. FL with marginal zone colonization has both nodular and marginal zone growth patterns (Fig. 16-9a, b) and often shows loss of CD10 and plasmacytoid differentiation in the marginal zone component but otherwise has a typical immunophenotype. Castlemanoid FL occurs in lymph nodes where the GCs are usually atretic, such as the groin and retroperitoneum, and is manifested by small, B-cell depleted follicles which may be overlooked (Fig. 16-9c). The floral variant of FL shows an inverted pattern with mantle zone B cells invading into neoplastic follicles (Fig. 16-9d) resembling nodular lymphocyte-predominant Hodgkin lymphoma or progressive transformation of GC; [19] a few of these lymphomas have been reported to express CD5 in addition to CD10 [20]. In all of these variants, demonstration of t(14;18)(q32;q21) by FISH can be helpful in unequivocally establishing the diagnosis of FL. In situ FL is focal infiltration of follicles by BCL2+ CD10+ monotypic B cells, including some cases in which only a single follicle is involved (Fig. 16-10). This variant which was initially believed to represent the earliest phase of FL development, more likely represents spread of FL from a more diffusely-involved site.

Finally, there are several nodular lymphomas that are closely related to classical FL. As discussed above, approximately 10% of morphologically and immunophenotypically typical FL will lack t(14;18)/IGH-BCL2 and instead have other initiating reciprocal translocations (Fig. 16-11). CD10-negative MUM1+ FL may represent a distinct entity, [22] but other cases are currently grouped with t(14;18)-containing cases (Table 16-3). *Pediatric follicle lymphoma,* a provisional subtype in the 2008 WHO classification, is distinguished based on particular presenting features, often in extranodal sites, and generally has a good prognosis despite its blastoid or large cell histologic appearance. *Follicle center lymphoma* refers to a nodular CD10+B-cell lymphoma that is restricted to skin. It is highly indolent and differs from FL, in that most show no or only minimal BCL2 protein expression in the follicular component (Fig. 16-12).

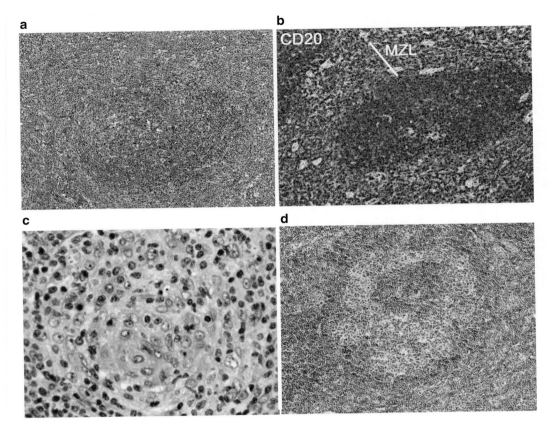

Fig. 16-9. *Follicular lymphoma, morphologic variants.* (**a**) Marginal zone differentiation in an otherwise typical t(14;18)-bearing follicular lymphoma is indicated by expanded marginal zone (MZL) cuffs around neoplastic follicles consisting of monotypic B cells. (**b**) CD20 is dimmer in the marginal zone component and CD10 was negative (not shown). (**c**) Castlemanoid grade 3B follicular lymphoma in a retroperitoneal lymph node. Small atretic follicles are replaced by large nucleolated B cells that were immunoreactive for BCL2 (not shown). (**d**) Floral variant of follicular lymphoma with small lymphocytes invading and disrupting neoplastic follicles

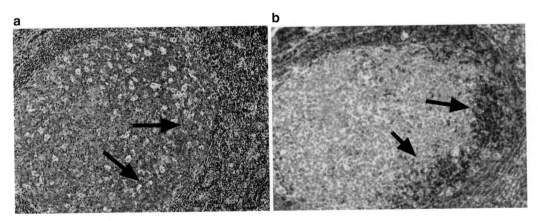

Fig. 16-10. *Follicular lymphoma, in situ.* A small focus of BCL2+B cells present in a reactive germinal centers. A biopsy performed six months later revealed typical grade 1 follicular lymphoma

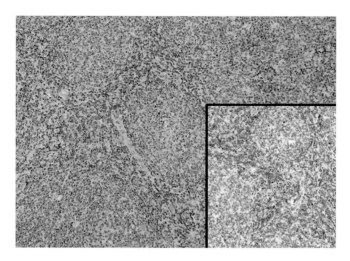

Fig. 16-11. *Follicular lymphoma, BCL2-negative.* CD10+nodular B-cell lymphoma with grade 3B histomorphology that is negative for BCL2 protein (inset). Cytogenetic analysis revealed t(3;14) (q27;q32) indicative of an IGH-BCL6 gene fusion

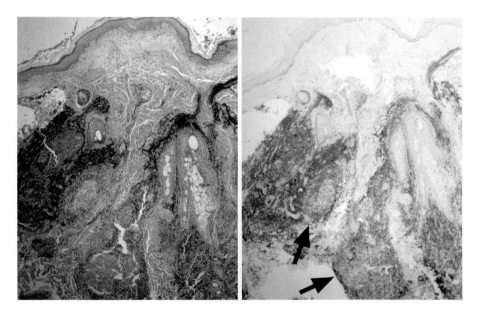

Fig. 16-12. *Follicle center lymphoma.* (**a**) Skin biopsy from the cheek shows superficial and deep nodular dermal lymphoid infiltrate composed of B-cell follicles surrounded by dense infiltrates of T cells. (**b**) BCL2 is negative within follicles (arrows), although CD10 and BCL6 were strongly expressed (not shown). Monoclonal IGH gene rearrangement was present

16.2.5. Etiology and Pathogenesis of Early Stage FL

The t(14;18)(q32;q21) translocation which initiates the pathogenesis of follicular lymphoma may arise from error-prone V–D–J recombination or from aberrant nonhomologous end-joining in the GC, [32] or at an earlier stage of B-cell development. If the latter occurs, t(14;18)-bearing naïve B cells would be expected to represent a first-step in oncogenesis requiring subsequent antigen selection and/or migration into the GC before overt FL could develop. This multi-step model of FL development is supported by the finding that transgenic overexpression of

Table 16-4. Markers in follicular lymphoma: the effects of BCL2 overexpression versus germinal center localization.

Gene or gene family	Gene function	Role in FL growth
GC B-cell markers also expressed in FL		
BCL6	Transcriptional factor	Drives GC transcriptional program
AICDA [39]	Activation-induced cytosine deaminase	Regulates somatic hypermutation
ID2 [37,40]	Transcription factor regulating AICDA	and class-switch recombination
MTA3 [41]	Transcriptional regulator (histone-dependent)	Epigenetic regulator for zinc finger transcriptional factors
LMO2 [42]	Transcriptional regulator	Epigenetic reprogramming
Centerin (SerpinA9) [43]	Serine proteinase inhibitor	
HGAL (GCET2) [44]	Cytokine-regulated kinase modulator	Cytokine receptor signal amplification
CBX7 [45]	Transcriptional repressor	
Overexpressed in FL relative to nonneoplastic GC B cells		
BCL2	Cell survival factor blocking apoptosis induction	BCR-independent survival in the GC microenvironment
Cell cycle regulators [36,37]	Increased CDK10, p120, altered CDKN1A (p21CIP1), CDKN2A (p16), BMI1 amplification	G1-S progression
TNFR/NF-kB pathway	CD27 (TNFRSF7), BAFF (TNFSF13B), TRAF and MALT1	BCR-independent growth signaling through admixed stromal elements
Cytokine signaling [37]	Increased IL2RG, IL4RA	As above
Adhesion molecules [37]	Increased CTNND1, CCR7	Linkage between FDC-GC adhesion, localization and growth signaling

Abbreviations: GC: germinal center; FL: follicular lymphoma; BCR: B-cell receptor; FDC: follicular dendritic cell

BCL2 in mouse models is not usually directly transforming, [33], that low levels of cells with t(14;18) translocations can be detected in individuals without lymphoma [34] and that nearly all t(14;18)-bearing lymphomas have GC-like gene signatures indicative of eventual GC localization. However, other models postulate that t(14;18) generation may occur at the GC stage by aberrant class-switch recombination with more rapid development of lymphoma [35].

BCL2 is a multifunctional mitochondrial and cytoplasmic protein that prevents apoptosis and is normally expressed in B cells up to the GC stage where it is transcriptionally downregulated by the GCB genetic program. BCL2 overexpression allows the FL precursors to evade BCR-mediated and TNFR death signals that normally control hyperproliferative B cells in the GC. Microarray studies clearly demonstrate that BCL2 upregulation induces a large number of genes including cytokine receptors, cell cycle regulators, [36,37] SOC3 [38] and other antiapoptotic genes (Table 16-4). Independent of BCL2 expression, GC localization also has a marked effect on gene expression in B cells mediated by the master transcriptional regulator BCL6 (Table 16-4). BCL2 overexpression in mice produces lymphoid hyperplasia, [46] with the development of lymphoma only in certain defined models, [38] suggesting that multiple other genetic events are required for FL transformation. These changes lead to hyper-responsiveness to BCR signaling in FL as compared to non-neoplastic GCB [47].

16.2.6. Patterns of Progression/Transformation

FL is one of the best studied models of tumor progression. The specific chromosomal loci which become deleted and amplified during the course of disease have been extensively studied by CGH, [48–52] and compared with those seen with other tumor types (summarized in Table 16-5). In some cases, these genomic changes can be directly correlated with effects on gene expression and morphology. For example, acquisition of MYC translocation accompanies blastic morphologic transformation [48,2,63]. The complex genomic changes associated with higher grade FL reflects acquisition of defects in DNA replication and repair (e.g., TP 53 deletion) and loss of cell cycle checkpoint control (e.g., deletions of CDK2NA) [49].

The shifts in gene expression with morphological progression in FL also reflect a shift from paracrine to autocrine signaling due to overexpression/hyperactivity of CD40 and other tumor necrosis factor receptors and resulting in ubiquitous activation of NF-kB signaling [48,64]. Upregulation of NF-kB activity through genomic amplification [52,65,66] or activating mutation [67] of RELA (at chr 2p15) is also seen with FL progression.

All of these studies highlight the importance of trophic signals from the stromal and nonneoplastic immune components in supporting the growth of early-stage FL [68]. The nodular character of FL implies that the GC microenvironment and its specialized follicular dendritic cells (FDC) and follicular helper T cells are all essential components in supporting lymphoma growth in its early stages (Fig. 16-13). Indeed, as FL progresses, there is a shift in the immunophenotype of lymphoma-associated stromal away from FDC markers [69] and shifts in the density of tumor-associated regulatory T cells [70] and macrophages [71]. Thus, genetic progression in FL can be conceived as of as stepwise shift from bidirectional supportive interactions between lymphoma and stroma to autonomous tumor cell growth [72].

Table 16-5. Comparison of secondary genetic alterations in follicular lymphoma and mantle cell lymphoma.[a]

	Follicular lymphoma		Mantle cell lymphoma	
	Incidence	*Effect*	*Incidence*	*Effect*
Cell cycle regulation				
CDK2, CDK4 amplification (chr 12q12-14 region)	30% [53]	Increased proliferation	25% [54]	nd
BMI1 amplification	Uncommon	nd	10–15% [55]	Increased proliferation
DNA repair/checkpoint				
TP53 mutation/deletion	6–30% [56, 57]	Increased grade, OS variable impact	26% [58]	Decreased OS
ATM mutation/deletion	10% [59]	Minimal impact on OS	56% [58]	Minimal impact on OS
Growth signaling				
REL genomic amplification	~25%[48, 60, 61]	Increased grade	Uncommon	nd

Abbreviations: nd: not determined; OS: overall survival
[a] Varies according to tumor grade. Studies covering FL not yet fully transformed to DLBCL

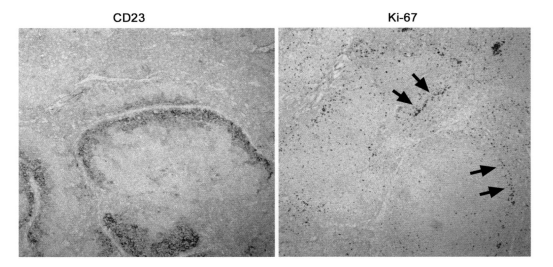

Fig. 16-13. *Follicular lymphoma, stromal interactions.* (**a**) CD23 immunostain is strongly reactive in the follicular dendritic cells (FDC) in only one area of the neoplastic follicles. (**b**) The proliferation marker Ki-67 is immunoreactive only in lymphoma cells in the area with fully differentiated CD23+ CD21+ FDC consistent with a supportive role for FDC in driving lymphoma proliferation

Table 16-6. Prognostic models for follicular lymphoma.

Marker(s)	Correlated with:	Reference(s)
Proliferation and apoptosis		
Increased proliferative index	Inferior OS	[76]
Increased apoptotic rate	Inferior OS in localized FL	[77]
Stromal-immune parameters		
T-cell GEP signature	Superior OS	[78]
FDC-like GEP profile	Inferior OS	
Tumor-associated sclerosis	Inferior OS	[79]
Increased CD68 + macrophages	Variable outcomes	[80,81]
Increased FOXP3 + T cells	Superior OS	[70,82,83]
Clinical predictors		
FLIPI	CR, TTP, OS	[84]

Abbreviations: OS: overall survival; FL: follicular lymphoma, CR: complete response; TTP: time to progression, GEP: gene expression profiling; FDC: follicular dendritic cells; FLIPI: follicular lymphoma international prognostic index

16.2.7. Prognostic Factors and Treatment Response

A number of large series have shown that clinical predictors reflected in the FLIPI score correlate both with outcome and the risk of large cell transformation, independent of therapy type [73,74]. Treatment strategies in FL are highly variable ranging from "watch-and-wait" to single agent rituximab or radiotherapy to aggressive CHOP (cyclophosphamide, doxorubicin, vincristine and prednisone)-type chemotherapy, autologous and nonmyeloablative stem cell transplantation (see Chap. 18). A national survey of treatment practice has indicated that treatment is usually based on FLIPI score, stage, and grade, with little use of radiotherapy [75].

As a result, there has been great interest in development of prognostic biomarkers to improve treatment stratification. This has included use of gene panels derived from microarray studies, or immunohistochemical markers of tumor proliferative capacity and stroma phenotype (Table 16-6) [85]. Recent studies have demonstrated that the number and type of immune accessory cells present within follicular and extrafollicular areas of the tumor have prognostic power, likely as a surrogate marker for tumor progression based on microenvironment-independent growth (i.e., a reflection of the paracrine to autocrine shift).

Regardless of the predictive model, analysis of blood or bone marrow during induction therapy using quantitative (q) PCR for the IGH-BCL2 rearrangements may be useful in more accurately assessing the level of residual disease following treatment [86,87]. However, the value of BCL2-IGH qPCR for monitoring levels of residual disease has been repeatedly questioned [88]. Similarly, the dim staining for surface Ig light chains has made MRD monitoring by flow cytometry more difficult than in other lymphoproliferative disorders. Therefore the optimal methods for monitoring response to treatment in FL remains to be determined.

16.3. Mantle Cell Lymphoma

16.3.1. Incidence and Clinical Features

MCL is rare representing less than 5% of all lymphomas although there are marked geographic differences with a higher incidence in the United States and Europe compared to Asia [1]. The median age of presentation is 63 years, with a threefold greater incidence in men than women. Presentations below 30 years old are extremely rare. The increased incidence and pattern of second malignancies is MCL suggests a role for germline genetic determinants of risk [89].

MCL is almost always a systemic disease with disseminated lymphadenopathy in 70–80%, splenic involvement in 50%, gastrointestinal (GI) tract involvement in 20–60%, and histologic evidence of bone marrow infiltration in 60–80%. Relapses in MCL often occur at extranodal sites, such as the GI tract, and may rarely involve skin or visceral organs. Several distinct clinical variants of MCL have been defined, including a GI tract-based form presenting as large mucosal nodules in the bowel and stomach known as *lymphomatous polyposis*. A variant with predominantly spleen, blood, and bone marrow involvement presenting with high serum beta-2 microglobulin is also recognized [90,91].

16.3.2. Diagnostic Features

MCL has several different growth patterns in lymph node, including colonization of the mantle zones (MZ) of primary or secondary follicles, infiltration of the GCs (nodular variants, Fig 16-14) and diffuse effacement (Fig. 16-15) [92,93]. The more indolent mantle zone variant is diagnosed when greater than 90% of the node shows preferential MZ colonization [94]. As disease progresses, there is a shift from mantle zone and nodular patterns to diffuse growth. The classical cytological features of MCL are that of an intermediate cell size with notched or indented nuclear contours and scant cytoplasm. A uniform admixture of epithelioid histiocytes is also common (Fig. 16-15). In contrast to FL, this is no standardized histologic grading scheme but blastoid and pleomorphic MCL are recognized higher-grade variants (Fig. 16-16) [95].

MCL in spleen show white pulp colonization with spill-over into the red pulp. GI tract involvement by MCL can be sparse infiltration of the lamina propria (on blind staging biopsies) or extensive diffuse infiltration invading into the muscularis in lymphomatous polyposis in 10–20% of patients (Fig. 16-17). Bone marrow involvement is typically nodular or interstitial (Fig. 16-18). The leukemic variant of MCL, seen in 5–10%, often has a prolymphocytoid or highly pleomorphic appearance in blood.

16.3.3. Laboratory Testing for Diagnosis

The demonstration of a CD5+CD23-B-cell infiltrate that strongly expresses cyclin D1 is diagnostic of MCL. Flow cytometric studies will reveal a CD19+CD20+CD22+B-cell population that expresses CD5 and moderate to bright surface monotypic Ig light chains, which is equally commonly lambda than kappa (Table 16-2). MCL are typically negative

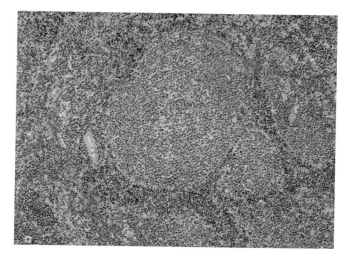

Fig. 16-14. *Mantle cell lymphoma, morphology.* Nodular growth within preexisting follicles, with spread into interfollicular areas

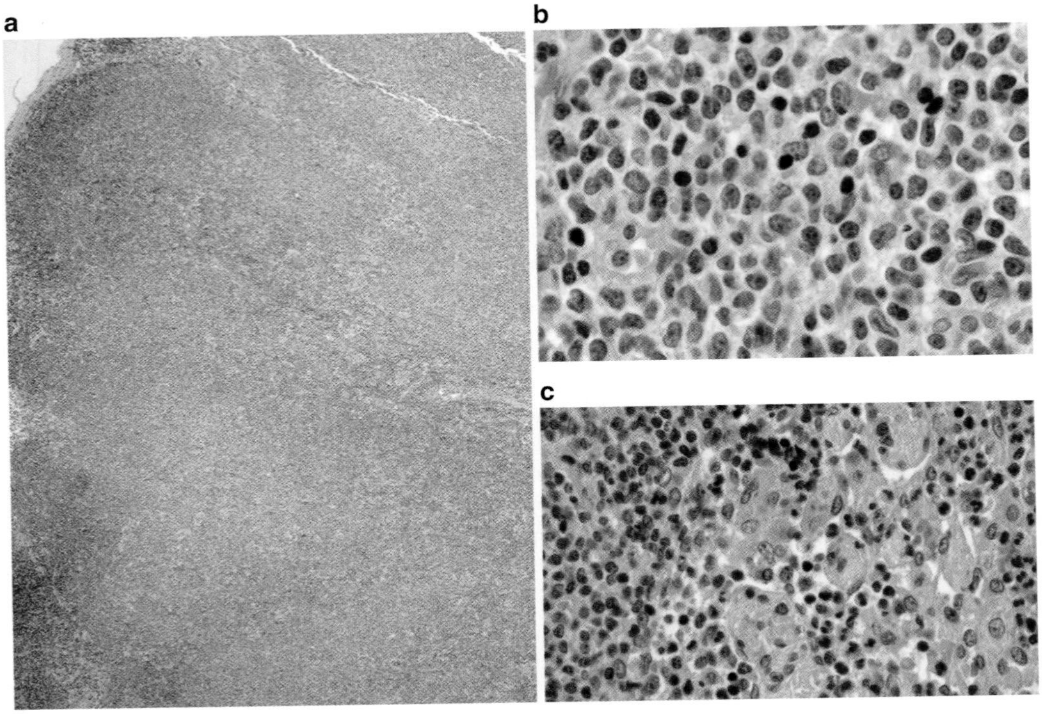

a

b

c

Fig. 16-15. *Mantle cell lymphoma, cytomorphologic features.* (**a**) Diffuse infiltrate of lymphoma cells; (**b**) Characteristic cytologic features of MCL include irregular to indented nuclear contours and scant cytoplasm. (**c**) Some cases show admixed pink epithelioid histiocytes/dendritic cells or loose granulomas, and eosinophils

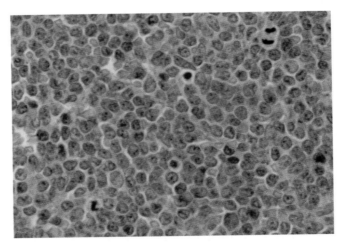

Fig. 16-16. *Mantle cell lymphoma, blastoid variant.* A combination of increased mitoses and fine, blastoid chromatin are noted

for CD23 and CD10, although partial expression may be rarely seen; [96–98] rare cases of transformed MCL may lack detectable CD5. Use of cyclin D1 immunostaining to detect focal involvement in GI tract and other extranodal sites is helpful.

Detection of the t(11;14)(q13;q32) is not required if cyclin D1 immunohistochemical expression is convincingly demonstrated but is best performed using fusion FISH which

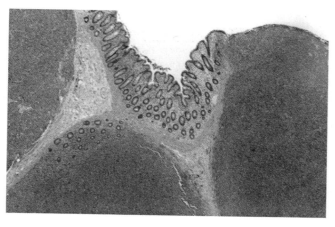

Fig. 16-17. *Lymphomatous polyposis.* Mantle cell lymphoma presenting as large mucosal nodules protruding into the bowel lumen

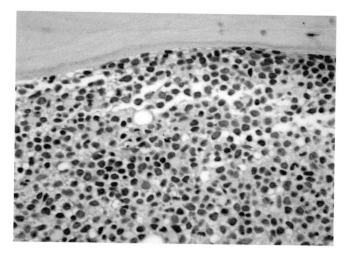

Fig. 16-18. *Mantle cell lymphoma, bone marrow.* Diffuse infiltrate of medium-sized lymphoma cells with sparse interspersed hematopoietic elements

will detect the translocation in 90% of cases. Use of PCR to detect the t(11;14) translocation is complicated by the wide range of breakpoints involving the CCND1 (cyclin D1) gene on chromosome 11. The most frequent translocation breakpoint around CCND1 is the ~100 base pair major translocation cluster (MTC) which is used in 30–35% of cases but the remainder of the breakpoints are widely scattered. Cytogenetic studies may miss the t(11;14) due to cryptic or complex translocations or because some MCL cases have highly unstable karyotypes. Approximately 5% of cases otherwise resembling classic MCL lack cyclin D1 rearrangement and may instead have translocations or transcriptional upregulation of other cyclins such as CCND3 [99].

16.3.4. Differential Diagnosis and Disease Variants

The primary differential diagnosis of MCL is with other CD5+B-cell lymphomas, particularly immunophenotypic variants of CLL/SLL. The identification of vaguely nodular proliferation centers in a CD5 + B-cell malignancy would indicate CLL/SLL, whereas GC colonization would favor MCL and should trigger cyclin D1 immunostaining. The classification of CD5 + CD23− B-cell lymphomas that resemble classical MCL but lack the t(11;14) translocation is somewhat controversial. Clinical and gene expression microarray studies in some of these cases, demonstrating an aggressive course and parallel dyregulation of cyclin D3, strongly favor grouping them with classical MCL.

The blastoid (or blastic) variant (BV) of MCL, defined as a tumor with fine nuclear chromatin reminiscent of lymphoblasts and an increased mitotic rate (greater than 20 mitotic figures per 10 high power microscope fields), likely represent a progression of classical MCL with higher cyclin D1 levels in part due to genomic amplification/aneuploidy [100]. Similarly, the pleomorphic variant of MCL likely represents a pattern of progression and not a distinct entity.

16.3.5. Etiology and Pathogenesis of Early-Stage MCL

MCL mostly have unmutated variable region Ig genes supporting emergence from pre-GC B cells. The predominance of lambda light chain expression in MCL (as opposed to kappa light chain preference for almost all other B-cell lymphomas) suggests a preferential or selective association with the B1 subset of naïve B cells. As with FL, transgenic mouse models of the CCND1-IGH translocation suggest that the t(11;14) is permissive for outgrowth of MCL but not fully transforming.

Because the progenitor cell of origin of MCL is not definitely known, which genes expressed in MCL are related to progression and which are related to the early phase of transformation (i.e., CCND1-related) is not yet clear. However, activation of the JAK-STAT pathway occurs in almost all cases [101]. Development of most sophisticated murine MCL models should begin to clarify which molecular changes are central to initial transformation [102].

16.3.6. Patterns of Progression/Transformation

The aggressive nature of MCL is accompanied in some patients by histologic progression to large cell (or blastoid) and pleomorphic forms [103]. In some cases, a particular chromosomal change can be linked to blastoid transformation, such as with the rare MYC translocation [104]. In general though, the genetic changes associated with blastoid or progressed MCL are more complex and are centered on cell cycle dysregulation (Table 16-5) [105,106] and chromosomal copy number changes due to centrosome defects [107,108]. Allelic loss or mutation in p53 occurs in more than 30% of MCL-BV, as does deletion/mutation of the DNA repair protein ATM. These changes, as with FL, lead to accumulation of many secondary chromosomal changes due to DNA replication in the face of unrepaired genetic damage. Altered sensitivity to apoptosis accompanies these cell cycle changes [109]. Proteomic analyses of aggressive FL and MCL reveals similar reprogramming of gene expression reflecting dysregulated p53 [110].

The rapid growth and therapy resistance of progressed MCL appear to result from overlapping changes in the G1-S mitotic checkpoint. Overexpression of cyclin dependent kinase 4 (CDK4), which is a cell cycle kinase that associates with cyclin D1, cooperates with overexpression of cdc28 protein kinase 1 (CKS1B) which assists in the degradation of the CDK inhibitor p27/Kip1 (Fig. 16-19) [106]. Loss of the CDK inhibitors CDKN1 (p21), CDKN2A (p16/INK4a) and CDKN2B (p15) also activates the cyclin D1 complex driving the hyperphosphorylation of RB1 and cell cycle progression. Other highly-expressed genes in MCL-BV that promote G1/S-checkpoint dysfunction

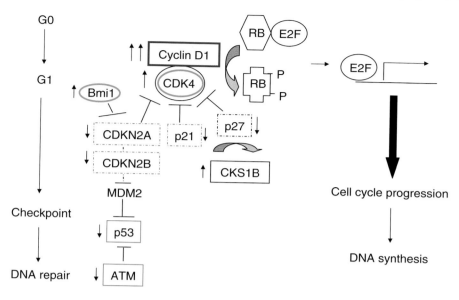

Gene amplification

Gene deletion, mutation, or methylation silencing

Transcriptional downregulation

Fig. 16-19. *Mantle cell lymphoma, multiple genetic aberrations at the G1-S checkpoint.* The CDKN2A gene at chr 9p21 encodes the p14/ARF and p16/IN4KA CDK inhibitors; CDKN2B also located at chr 9p21 encodes the p15/IN4KB CDK inhibitor

include the transcriptional regulator BMI1 (by gene amplification), the cyclin D1 activator MYBL (B-Myb) and the kinases PIM1, and PIM2.

One of the curious aspects of MCL progression is why so many identified genetic mechanisms that appear additive and redundant are required to dysregulate the G1-S transition. Many other tumor types, including FL, dysregulate similar components, but few neoplasms involve as many factors in the same G1-S complex. Part of the explanation may be that the initiating event, of MCL (overexpression of cyclin D1) is at the center of this regulatory loop. Therefore, different subpopulations of MCL may independently acquire changes that complement cyclin D1 dysregulation.

16.3.7. Prognostic Factors and Treatment

MCL is an aggressive malignancy which has poor outcomes with CHOP-type chemotherapy. The shift to use of more aggressive regimens such as hyper-CVAD with rituximab, especially when followed by allogeneic stem cell transplantation has improved outcomes [111]. Prognostic models for MCL are just beginning to be developed and have focused extensively on proliferation markers such as Ki-67, cyclin D1 transcript levels, or multigene predictors developed from microarray studies (Table 16-7). Unlike FL, there have been few studies that have focused on microenvironmental factors as prognostic markers.

Table 16-7. Prognostic models for mantle cell lymphoma.

Marker(s)	Correlated with	Reference(s)
Increased proliferation		
High Ki-67	FFS with R-HCVAD	[112,113]
	PFS	
High CCND1 levels	OS	[114,115]
GEP proliferation signature	OS	[114,115]
G1-S genetic alterations		
GEP MYC/MDM2 signature	OS	[114]
p53 mutation/deletion	OS	[58]
Stromal-immune parameters		
FDC phenotype in stroma	OS	[116]
Clinical predictors		
Older age, poor PS, Hgb < 12g/dl, PB involvement	OS	[117]
Older age, stage, and PB involvement	TTF	[118]

Abbreviations: OS: overall survival; FFS: failure-free survival; R-CVAD: rituximab plus fractionated cyclophosphamide, vincristine, doxorubicin, and dexamethasone; PFD: progression-free survival; GEP: gene expression profiling; FDC: follicular dendritic cells; TTF: time to treatment failure; PS: performance status; PB: peripheral blood

Suggested Readings

de Jong D. Molecular pathogenesis of follicular lymphoma: a cross talk of genetic and immunologic factors. J Clin Oncol 2005;23:6358–63.
   • A review highlighting the importance of bidirectional lymphoma–stroma interactions.

Jares P, Colomer D, Campo E. Genetic and molecular pathogenesis of mantle cell lymphoma: perspectives for new targeted therapeutics. Nat Rev Cancer 2007;7:750–62.
   • A review of the overlapping mechanisms of progression.

References

1. Anderson JR, Armitage JO, Weisenburger DD. Epidemiology of the non-Hodgkin's lymphomas: distributions of the major subtypes differ by geographic locations. Non-Hodgkin's Lymphoma Classification Project. Ann Oncol 1998;9:717–20.
2. Chang KC, Huang GC, Jones D, Tsao CJ, Lee JY, Su IJ. Distribution and prognosis of WHO lymphoma subtypes in Taiwan reveals a low incidence of germinal-center derived tumors. Leuk Lymphoma 2004;45:1375–84.
3. Bende RJ, Smit LA, Bossenbroek JG, et al. Primary follicular lymphoma of the small intestine: alpha4beta7 expression and immunoglobulin configuration suggest an origin from local antigen-experienced B cells. Am J Pathol 2003;162:105–13.
4. Sentani K, Maeshima AM, Nomoto J, et al. Follicular lymphoma of the duodenum: a clinicopathologic analysis of 26 cases. Jpn J Clin Oncol 2008;38:547–52.
5. Wang SA, Wang L, Hochberg EP, Muzikansky A, Harris NL, Hasserjian RP. Low histologic grade follicular lymphoma with high proliferation index: morphologic and clinical features. Am J Surg Pathol 2005;29:1490–6.
6. Melo JV, Robinson DS, De Oliveira MP, et al. Morphology and immunology of circulating cells in leukaemic phase of follicular lymphoma. J Clin Pathol 1988;41:951–9.
7. Hsi ED, Mirza I, Lozanski G, et al. A clinicopathologic evaluation of follicular lymphoma grade 3A versus grade 3B reveals no survival differences. Arch Pathol Lab Med 2004;128:863–8.
8. Swerdlow SH, Campo E, Harris NL, et al. WHO classification of tumours of haematopoietic and lymphoid tissues. Lyon: IARC Press, 2008.
9. Mann RB, Berard CW. Criteria for the cytologic subclassification of follicular lymphomas: a proposed alternative method. Hematol Oncol 1983;1:187–92.
10. Martin AR, Weisenburger DD, Chan WC, et al. Prognostic value of cellular proliferation and histologic grade in follicular lymphoma. Blood 1995;85:3671–8.

11. Hans CP, Weisenburger DD, Vose JM, et al. A significant diffuse component predicts for inferior survival in grade 3 follicular lymphoma, but cytologic subtypes do not predict survival. Blood 2003;101:2363–7.

12. Metter GE, Nathwani BN, Burke JS, et al. Morphological subclassification of follicular lymphoma: variability of diagnoses among hematopathologists, a collaborative study between the Repository Center and Pathology Panel for Lymphoma Clinical Studies. J Clin Oncol 1985;3:25–38.

13. Lim DG, Nga ME, Tan LH, et al. Primary nodal follicular lymphoma with spindle cell features: a potential diagnostic pitfall. Histopathology 2008;53:120–2.

14. Mollejo M, Rodriguez-Pinilla MS, Montes-Moreno S, et al. Splenic follicular lymphoma: clinico-pathologic characteristics of a series of 32 cases. Am J Surg Pathol 2009;33:730–8.

15. Katzenberger T, Kalla J, Leich E, et al. A distinctive subtype of t(14;18)-negative nodal follicular non-Hodgkin lymphoma characterized by a predominantly diffuse growth pattern and deletions in the chromosomal region 1p36. Blood 2009;113:1053–61.

16. Yegappan S, Schnitzer B, Hsi ED. Follicular lymphoma with marginal zone differentiation: micro-dissection demonstrates the t(14;18) in both the follicular and marginal zone components. Mod Pathol 2001;14:191–6.

17. Goodlad JR, Batstone PJ, Hamilton D, Hollowood K. Follicular lymphoma with marginal zone differentiation: cytogenetic findings in support of a high-risk variant of follicular lymphoma. Histopathology 2003;42:292–8.

18. Torlakovic EE, Aamot HV, Heim S. A marginal zone phenotype in follicular lymphoma with t(14;18) is associated with secondary cytogenetic aberrations typical of marginal zone lymphoma. J Pathol 2006;209:258–64.

19. Kojima M, Yamanaka S, Yoshida T, et al. Histological variety of floral variant of follicular lymphoma. APMIS 2006;114:626–32.

20. Tiesinga JJ, Wu CD, Inghirami G. CD5+ follicle center lymphoma. Immunophenotyping detects a unique subset of "floral" follicular lymphoma. Am J Clin Pathol 2000;114:912–21.

21. Sotomayor EA, Shah IM, Sanger WG, Mark HF. In situ follicular lymphoma with a 14;18 translocation diagnosed by a multimodal approach. Exp Mol Pathol 2007;83:254–8.

22. Karube K, Guo Y, Suzumiya J, et al. CD10-MUM1+ follicular lymphoma lacks BCL2 gene translocation and shows characteristic biologic and clinical features. Blood 2007;109:3076–9.

23. Bosga-Bouwer AG, Haralambieva E, Booman M, et al. BCL6 alternative translocation breakpoint cluster region associated with follicular lymphoma grade 3B. Genes Chromosomes Cancer 2005;44:301–4.

24. Guo Y, Karube K, Kawano R, et al. Low-grade follicular lymphoma with t(14;18) presents a homogeneous disease entity otherwise the rest comprises minor groups of heterogeneous disease entities with Bcl2 amplification, Bcl6 translocation or other gene aberrances. Leukemia 2005;19:1058–63.

25. Bosga-Bouwer AG, van Imhoff GW, Boonstra R, et al. Follicular lymphoma grade 3B includes 3 cytogenetically defined subgroups with primary t(14;18), 3q27, or other translocations: t(14;18) and 3q27 are mutually exclusive. Blood 2003;101:1149–54.

26. Bacon CM, Ye H, Diss TC, et al. Primary follicular lymphoma of the testis and epididymis in adults. Am J Surg Pathol 2007;31:1050–8.

27. Finn LS, Viswanatha DS, Belasco JB, et al. Primary follicular lymphoma of the testis in childhood. Cancer 1999;85:1626–35.

28. Xie X, Sundram U, Natkunam Y, et al. Expression of HGAL in primary cutaneous large B-cell lymphomas: evidence for germinal center derivation of primary cutaneous follicular lymphoma. Mod Pathol 2008;21:653–9.

29. Morice WG, Kurtin PJ, Hodnefield JM, et al. Predictive value of blood and bone marrow flow cytometry in B-cell lymphoma classification: comparative analysis of flow cytometry and tissue biopsy in 252 patients. Mayo Clin Proc 2008;83:776–85.

30. Naresh KN. Nodal marginal zone B-cell lymphoma with prominent follicular colonization – difficulties in diagnosis: a study of 15 cases. Histopathology 2008;52:331–9.

31. Kojima M, Matsumoto M, Miyazawa Y, Shimizu K, Itoh H, Masawa N. Follicular lymphoma with prominent sclerosis ("sclerosing variant of follicular lymphoma") exhibiting a mesenteric bulky mass resembling inflammatory pseudotumor. Report of three cases. Pathol Oncol Res 2007; 13:74–7.

32. Fenton JA, Vaandrager JW, Aarts WM, et al. Follicular lymphoma with a novel t(14;18) breakpoint involving the immunoglobulin heavy chain switch mu region indicates an origin from germinal center B cells. Blood 2002;99:716–8.

33. Bende RJ, Smit LA, van Noesel CJ. Molecular pathways in follicular lymphoma. Leukemia 2007;21:18–29.

34. Aster JC, Kobayashi Y, Shiota M, Mori S, Sklar J. Detection of the t(14;18) at similar frequencies in hyperplastic lymphoid tissues from American and Japanese patients. Am J Pathol 1992;141: 291–9.

35. Ruminy P, Jardin F, Picquenot JM, et al. S(mu) mutation patterns suggest different progression pathways in follicular lymphoma: early direct or late from FL progenitor cells. Blood 2008;112:1951–9.

36. Tracey L, Perez-Rosado A, Artiga MJ, et al. Expression of the NF-kappaB targets BCL2 and BIRC5/Survivin characterizes small B-cell and aggressive B-cell lymphomas, respectively. J Pathol 2005;206:123–34.

37. Husson H, Carideo EG, Neuberg D, et al. Gene expression profiling of follicular lymphoma and normal germinal center B cells using cDNA arrays. Blood 2002;99:282–9.

38. Vanasse GJ, Winn RK, Rodov S, et al. Bcl-2 overexpression leads to increases in suppressor of cytokine signaling-3 expression in B cells and de novo follicular lymphoma. Mol Cancer Res 2004;2:620–31.

39. Lossos IS, Levy R, Alizadeh AA. AID is expressed in germinal center B-cell-like and activated B-cell-like diffuse large-cell lymphomas and is not correlated with intraclonal heterogeneity. Leukemia 2004;18:1775–9.

40. Cattoretti G, Buttner M, Shaknovich R, Kremmer E, Alobeid B, Niedobitek G. Nuclear and cytoplasmic AID in extrafollicular and germinal center B cells. Blood 2006;107:3967–75.

41. Jaye DL, Iqbal J, Fujita N, et al. The BCL6-associated transcriptional co-repressor, MTA3, is selectively expressed by germinal centre B cells and lymphomas of putative germinal centre derivation. J Pathol 2007;213:106–15.

42. Natkunam Y, Zhao S, Mason DY, et al. The oncoprotein LMO2 is expressed in normal germinal-center B cells and in human B-cell lymphomas. Blood 2007;109:1636–42.

43. Montes-Moreno S, Roncador G, Maestre L, et al. Gcet1 (centerin), a highly restricted marker for a subset of germinal center-derived lymphomas. Blood 2008;111:351–8.

44. Natkunam Y, Lossos IS, Taidi B, et al. Expression of the human germinal center-associated lymphoma (HGAL) protein, a new marker of germinal center B-cell derivation. Blood 2005;105:3979–86.

45. Scott CL, Gil J, Hernando E, et al. Role of the chromobox protein CBX7 in lymphomagenesis. Proc Natl Acad Sci U S A 2007;104:5389–94.

46. McDonnell TJ, Nunez G, Platt FM, et al. Deregulated Bcl-2-immunoglobulin transgene expands a resting but responsive immunoglobulin M and D-expressing B-cell population. Mol Cell Biol 1990;10:1901–7.

47. Irish JM, Czerwinski DK, Nolan GP, Levy R. Altered B-cell receptor signaling kinetics distinguish human follicular lymphoma B cells from tumor-infiltrating nonmalignant B cells. Blood 2006;108:3135–42.

48. Davies AJ, Rosenwald A, Wright G, et al. Transformation of follicular lymphoma to diffuse large B-cell lymphoma proceeds by distinct oncogenic mechanisms. Br J Haematol 2007;136:286–93.

49. Fitzgibbon J, Iqbal S, Davies A, et al. Genome-wide detection of recurring sites of uniparental disomy in follicular and transformed follicular lymphoma. Leukemia 2007;21:1514–20.

50. Cheung KJ, Shah SP, Steidl C, et al. Genome-wide profiling of follicular lymphoma by array comparative genomic hybridization reveals prognostically significant DNA copy number imbalances. Blood 2009;113:137–48.

51. d'Amore F, Chan E, Iqbal J, et al. Clonal evolution in t(14;18)-positive follicular lymphoma, evidence for multiple common pathways, and frequent parallel clonal evolution. Clin Cancer Res 2008;14:7180–7.

52. Martinez-Climent JA, Alizadeh AA, Segraves R, et al. Transformation of follicular lymphoma to diffuse large cell lymphoma is associated with a heterogeneous set of DNA copy number and gene expression alterations. Blood 2003;101:3109–17.

53. Al-Assar O, Rees-Unwin KS, Menasce LP, et al. Transformed diffuse large B-cell lymphomas with gains of the discontinuous 12q12–14 amplicon display concurrent deregulation of CDK2, CDK4 and GADD153 genes. Br J Haematol 2006;133:612–21.

54. Allen JE, Hough RE, Goepel JR, et al. Identification of novel regions of amplification and deletion within mantle cell lymphoma DNA by comparative genomic hybridization. Br J Haematol 2002; 116:291–8.

55. Bea S, Tort F, Pinyol M, et al. BMI-1 gene amplification and overexpression in hematological malignancies occur mainly in mantle cell lymphomas. Cancer Res 2001;61:2409–12.

56. Davies AJ, Lee AM, Taylor C, et al. A limited role for TP53 mutation in the transformation of follicular lymphoma to diffuse large B-cell lymphoma. Leukemia 2005;19:1459–65.

57. O'Shea D, O'Riain C, Taylor C, et al. The presence of TP53 mutation at diagnosis of follicular lymphoma identifies a high-risk group of patients with shortened time to disease progression and poorer overall survival. Blood 2008;112:3126–9.

58. Greiner TC, Dasgupta C, Ho VV, et al. Mutation and genomic deletion status of ataxia telangiectasia mutated (ATM) and p53 confer specific gene expression profiles in mantle cell lymphoma. Proc Natl Acad Sci U S A 2006;103:2352–7.

59. Fang NY, Greiner TC, Weisenburger DD, et al. Oligonucleotide microarrays demonstrate the highest frequency of ATM mutations in the mantle cell subtype of lymphoma. Proc Natl Acad Sci U S A 2003;100:5372–7.

60. Ferreira BI, Garcia JF, Suela J, et al. Comparative genome profiling across subtypes of low-grade B-cell lymphoma identifies type-specific and common aberrations that target genes with a role in B-cell neoplasia. Haematologica 2008;93:670–9.

61. Goff LK, Neat MJ, Crawley CR, et al. The use of real-time quantitative polymerase chain reaction and comparative genomic hybridization to identify amplification of the REL gene in follicular lymphoma. Br J Haematol 2000;111:618–25.

62. Mohamed AN, Palutke M, Eisenberg L, Al-Katib A. Chromosomal analyses of 52 cases of follicular lymphoma with t(14;18), including blastic/blastoid variant. Cancer Genet Cytogenet 2001;126:45–51.

63. Knezevich S, Ludkovski O, Salski C, et al. Concurrent translocation of BCL2 and MYC with a single immunoglobulin locus in high-grade B-cell lymphomas. Leukemia 2005;19:659–63.

64. Sasaki Y, Derudder E, Hobeika E, et al. Canonical NF-kappaB activity, dispensable for B cell development, replaces BAFF-receptor signals and promotes B cell proliferation upon activation. Immunity 2006;24:729–39.

65. Fukuhara N, Tagawa H, Kameoka Y, et al. Characterization of target genes at the 2p15–16 amplicon in diffuse large B-cell lymphoma. Cancer Sci 2006;97:499–504.

66. Reader JC, Zhao XF, Butler MS, Rapoport AP, Ning Y. REL-positive double minute chromosomes in follicular lymphoma. Leukemia 2006;20:1624–6.

67. Starczynowski DT, Trautmann H, Pott C, et al. Mutation of an IKK phosphorylation site within the transactivation domain of REL in two patients with B-cell lymphoma enhances REL's in vitro transforming activity. Oncogene 2007;26:2685–94.

68. Ame-Thomas P, Maby-El Hajjami H, Monvoisin C, et al. Human mesenchymal stem cells isolated from bone marrow and lymphoid organs support tumor B-cell growth: role of stromal cells in follicular lymphoma pathogenesis. Blood 2007;109:693–702.

69. Chang KC, Huang X, Medeiros LJ, Jones D. Germinal centre-like versus undifferentiated stromal immunophenotypes in follicular lymphoma. J Pathol 2003;201:404–12.

70. Lee AM, Clear AJ, Calaminici M, et al. Number of CD4+ cells and location of forkhead box protein P3-positive cells in diagnostic follicular lymphoma tissue microarrays correlates with outcome. J Clin Oncol 2006;24:5052–9.

71. Glas AM, Knoops L, Delahaye L, et al. Gene-expression and immunohistochemical study of specific T-cell subsets and accessory cell types in the transformation and prognosis of follicular lymphoma. J Clin Oncol 2007;25:390–8.

72. de Jong D. Molecular pathogenesis of follicular lymphoma: a cross talk of genetic and immunologic factors. J Clin Oncol 2005;23:6358–63.

73. Salles GA. Clinical features, prognosis and treatment of follicular lymphoma. Hematology Am Soc Hematol Educ Program 2007;2007:216–25.

74. Montoto S, Davies AJ, Matthews J, et al. Risk and clinical implications of transformation of follicular lymphoma to diffuse large B-cell lymphoma. J Clin Oncol 2007;25:2426–33.

75. Friedberg JW, Taylor MD, Cerhan JR, et al. Follicular lymphoma in the United States: first report of the National Lymphocare Study. J Clin Oncol 2009;27:1202–8.

76. Koster A, Tromp HA, Raemaekers JM, et al. The prognostic significance of the intra-follicular tumor cell proliferative rate in follicular lymphoma. Haematologica 2007;92:184–90.

77. Logsdon MD, Meyn RE Jr, Besa PC, et al. Apoptosis and the Bcl-2 gene family – patterns of expression and prognostic value in stage I and II follicular center lymphoma. Int J Radiat Oncol Biol Phys 1999;44:19–29.

78. Leich E, Hartmann EM, Burek C, Ott G, Rosenwald A. Diagnostic and prognostic significance of gene expression profiling in lymphomas. APMIS 2007;115:1135–46.

79. Klapper W, Hoster E, Rolver L, et al. Tumor sclerosis but not cell proliferation or malignancy grade is a prognostic marker in advanced-stage follicular lymphoma: the German Low Grade Lymphoma Study Group. J Clin Oncol 2007;25:3330–6.

80. Farinha P, Masoudi H, Skinnider BF, et al. Analysis of multiple biomarkers shows that lymphoma-associated macrophage (LAM) content is an independent predictor of survival in follicular lymphoma (FL). Blood 2005;106:2169–74.

81. Canioni D, Salles G, Mounier N, et al. High numbers of tumor-associated macrophages have an adverse prognostic value that can be circumvented by rituximab in patients with follicular lymphoma enrolled onto the GELA-GOELAMS FL-2000 trial. J Clin Oncol 2008;26:440–6.

82. Carreras J, Lopez-Guillermo A, Fox BC, et al. High numbers of tumor-infiltrating FOXP3-positive regulatory T cells are associated with improved overall survival in follicular lymphoma. Blood 2006;108:2957–64.

83. Kelley T, Beck R, Absi A, Jin T, Pohlman B, Hsi E. Biologic predictors in follicular lymphoma: importance of markers of immune response. Leuk Lymphoma 2007;48:2403–11.

84. Marcus R, Imrie K, Solal-Celigny P, et al. Phase III study of R-CVP compared with cyclophosphamide, vincristine, and prednisone alone in patients with previously untreated advanced follicular lymphoma. J Clin Oncol 2008;26:4579–86.

85. Alvaro T, Lejeune M, Salvado MT, et al. Immunohistochemical patterns of reactive microenvironment are associated with clinicobiologic behavior in follicular lymphoma patients. J Clin Oncol 2006;24:5350–7.

86. Bowman A, Jones D, Medeiros LJ, Luthra R. Quantitative PCR detection of t(14;18) bcl-2/JH fusion sequences in follicular lymphoma patients: comparison of peripheral blood and bone marrow aspirate samples. J Mol Diagn 2004;6:396–400.

87. Mandigers CM, Meijerink JP, van't Veer MB, Mensink EJ, Raemaekers JM. Dynamics of circulating t(14;18)-positive cells during first-line and subsequent lines of treatment in follicular lymphoma. Ann Hematol 2003;82:743–9.

88. Paszkiewicz-Kozik E, Kulik J, Fabisiewicz A, et al. Presence of t(14;18) positive cells in blood and bone marrow does not predict outcome in follicular lymphoma. Med Oncol 2009;26:16–21.

89. Tort F, Camacho E, Bosch F, Harris NL, Montserrat E, Campo E. Familial lymphoid neoplasms in patients with mantle cell lymphoma. Haematologica 2004;89:314–9.

90. De Oliveira MS, Jaffe ES, Catovsky D. Leukaemic phase of mantle zone (intermediate) lymphoma: its characterisation in 11 cases. J Clin Pathol 1989;42:962–72.

91. Schlette E, Lai R, Onciu M, Doherty D, Bueso-Ramos C, Medeiros LJ. Leukemic mantle cell lymphoma: clinical and pathologic spectrum of twenty-three cases. Mod Pathol 2001;14:1133–40.

92. Weisenburger DD, Vose JM, Greiner TC, et al. Mantle cell lymphoma. A clinicopathologic study of 68 cases from the Nebraska Lymphoma Study Group. Am J Hematol 2000;64:190–6.

93. Weisenburger DD, Kim H, Rappaport H. Mantle-zone lymphoma: a follicular variant of intermediate lymphocytic lymphoma. Cancer 1982;49:1429–38.

94. Majlis A, Pugh WC, Rodriguez MA, Benedict WF, Cabanillas F. Mantle cell lymphoma: correlation of clinical outcome and biologic features with three histologic variants. J Clin Oncol 1997;15:1664–71.

95. Yatabe Y, Suzuki R, Matsuno Y, et al. Morphological spectrum of cyclin D1-positive mantle cell lymphoma: study of 168 cases. Pathol Int 2001;51:747–61.

96. Zanetto U, Dong H, Huang Y, et al. Mantle cell lymphoma with aberrant expression of CD10. Histopathology 2008;53:20–9.

97. Schlette E, Fu K, Medeiros LJ. CD23 expression in mantle cell lymphoma: clinicopathologic features of 18 cases. Am J Clin Pathol 2003;120:760–6.

98. Xu Y, McKenna RW, Kroft SH. Assessment of CD10 in the diagnosis of small B-cell lymphomas: a multiparameter flow cytometric study. Am J Clin Pathol 2002;117:291–300.

99. Wlodarska I, Dierickx D, Vanhentenrijk V, et al. Translocations targeting CCND2, CCND3, and MYCN do occur in t(11;14)-negative mantle cell lymphomas. Blood 2008;111:5683–90.

100. Ott G, Kalla J, Ott MM, et al. Blastoid variants of mantle cell lymphoma: frequent bcl-1 rearrangements at the major translocation cluster region and tetraploid chromosome clones. Blood 1997;89:1421–9.

101. Yared MA, Khoury JD, Medeiros LJ, Rassidakis GZ, Lai R. Activation status of the JAK/STAT3 pathway in mantle cell lymphoma. Arch Pathol Lab Med 2005;129:990–6.

102. Ford RJ, Shen L, Lin-Lee YC, et al. Development of a murine model for blastoid variant mantle-cell lymphoma. Blood 2007;109:4899–906.

103. Raty R, Franssila K, Jansson SE, Joensuu H, Wartiovaara-Kautto U, Elonen E. Predictive factors for blastoid transformation in the common variant of mantle cell lymphoma. Eur J Cancer 2003;39:321–9.

104. Hao S, Sanger W, Onciu M, Lai R, Schlette EJ, Medeiros LJ. Mantle cell lymphoma with 8q24 chromosomal abnormalities: a report of 5 cases with blastoid features. Mod Pathol 2002;15: 1266–72.

105. Izban KF, Alkan S, Singleton TP, Hsi ED. Multiparameter immunohistochemical analysis of the cell cycle proteins cyclin D1, Ki-67, p21WAF1, p27KIP1, and p53 in mantle cell lymphoma. Arch Pathol Lab Med 2000;124:1457–62.

106. de Vos S, Krug U, Hofmann WK, et al. Cell cycle alterations in the blastoid variant of mantle cell lymphoma (MCL-BV) as detected by gene expression profiling of mantle cell lymphoma (MCL) and MCL-BV. Diagn Mol Pathol 2003;12:35–43.

107. Ott G, Kalla J, Hanke A, et al. The cytomorphological spectrum of mantle cell lymphoma is reflected by distinct biological features. Leuk Lymphoma 1998;32:55–63.

108. Neben K, Ott G, Schweizer S, et al. Expression of centrosome-associated gene products is linked to tetraploidization in mantle cell lymphoma. Int J Cancer 2007;120:1669–77.

109. Rummel MJ, de Vos S, Hoelzer D, Koeffler HP, Hofmann WK. Altered apoptosis pathways in mantle cell lymphoma. Leuk Lymphoma 2004;45:49–54.

110. Weinkauf M, Christopeit M, Hiddemann W, Dreyling M. Proteome- and microarray-based expression analysis of lymphoma cell lines identifies a p53-centered cluster of differentially expressed proteins in mantle cell and follicular lymphoma. Electrophoresis 2007;28:4416–26.

111. Fayad L, Thomas D, Romaguera J. Update of the M.D. Anderson Cancer Center experience with hyper-CVAD and rituximab for the treatment of mantle cell and Burkitt-type lymphomas. Clin Lymphoma Myeloma 2007;8(Suppl 2):S57–62.

112. Garcia M, Romaguera JE, Inamdar KV, Rassidakis GZ, Medeiros LJ. Proliferation predicts failure-free survival in mantle cell lymphoma patients treated with rituximab plus hyperfractionated cyclophosphamide, vincristine, doxorubicin, and dexamethasone alternating with rituximab plus high-dose methotrexate and cytarabine. Cancer 2009;115:1041–8.

113. Raty R, Franssila K, Joensuu H, Teerenhovi L, Elonen E. Ki-67 expression level, histological subtype, and the International Prognostic Index as outcome predictors in mantle cell lymphoma. Eur J Haematol 2002;69:11–20.

114. Kienle D, Katzenberger T, Ott G, et al. Quantitative gene expression deregulation in mantle-cell lymphoma: correlation with clinical and biologic factors. J Clin Oncol 2007;25:2770–7.

115. Rosenwald A, Wright G, Wiestner A, et al. The proliferation gene expression signature is a quantitative integrator of oncogenic events that predicts survival in mantle cell lymphoma. Cancer Cell 2003;3:185–97.

116. Schrader C, Meusers P, Brittinger G, et al. Growth pattern and distribution of follicular dendritic cells in mantle cell lymphoma: a clinicopathological study of 96 patients. Virchows Arch 2006;448:151–9.

117. Samaha H, Dumontet C, Ketterer N, et al. Mantle cell lymphoma: a retrospective study of 121 cases. Leukemia 1998;12:1281–7.

118. Oinonen R, Franssila K, Teerenhovi L, Lappalainen K, Elonen E. Mantle cell lymphoma: clinical features, treatment and prognosis of 94 patients. Eur J Cancer 1998;34:329–36.

Chapter 17

Aggressive B-cell Lymphomas: Diffuse Large B-cell Lymphoma and Burkitt Lymphoma

Henry Y. Dong

Abstract/Scope of Chapter This chapter covers aggressive B-cell lymphomas, including diffuse large B-cell lymphoma and its recognized variants, as well as Burkitt lymphoma. Other types of aggressive B-cell tumors, namely acute B-lymphoblastic leukemia and mantle cell lymphoma, are covered in Chaps. 13 and 16, respectively.

Keywords Diffuse large B-cell lymphoma (DLBCL) • Burkitt lymphoma (BL) • Immunoblastic lymphoma • Plasmablastic lymphoma • MYC • Mediastinal large cell lymphoma (PMBL) • T-cell/histiocyte-rich large B-cell lymphoma (TCHRLBCL) • Diffuse large B-cell lymphoma, ALK+ • Diffuse large B-cell lymphoma, primary CNS • Diffuse large B-cell lymphoma, leg type • Intravascular DLBCL • Diffuse large B-cell lymphoma, Epstein-Barr virus • Human herpesvirus 8 • Primary effusion lymphoma • Multicentric Castleman disease • Lymphomatoid granulomatosis (LyG) • B-cell lymphoma, unclassifiable

17.1. General Features of Diffuse Large B-cell Lymphoma

17.1.1. The Current Approach to Classification

Diffuse large B-cell lymphoma (DLBCL) is an umbrella term for a variety of different intermediate- to high-grade lymphomas derived from mature B cells. All DLBCL cases share a diffuse growth pattern and predominant large tumor cell size, defined as being at least twice as large as a normal lymphocyte or with a nuclear size equal to or greater than that of a normal macrophage. Large cell lymphomas of T cell, natural killer cell, or unclear lineage are classified separately. Other terms used for DLBCL include *centroblastic* or *immunoblastic lymphoma, lymphosarcoma,* and *reticulosarcoma*. In the most recent WHO classification of hematopoietic malignancies, specific subtypes of DLBCL are defined based on the cell of origin, presumed pathogenesis (e.g., viral association), or their predominant site of involvement (Table 17-1), [1] whereas those that do not fit any of the individual entities are considered DLBCL, not otherwise specified (NOS). The recognized subtypes of DLBCL in the current WHO classification represent a fraction of the heterogeneity observed in this common tumor, so further changes in subclassification will likely occur in the coming years.

17.1.2. Incidence, Demographics, and Clinical Features

DLBCL is the most common subtype of adult lymphoma worldwide, comprising 30–40% of cases in Western countries and approximately 50% of lymphomas in China and many

From: *Neoplastic Hematopathology*: Contemporary Hematology,
Edited by: D. Jones, DOI 10.1007/978-1-60761-384-8_17,
© Humana Press, a part of Springer Science+Business Media, LLC 2010

Table 17-1. Subclassification of diffuse large B-cell lymphoma.

Categories in the 2008 WHO classification	Alternate methods of classification
DLBCL, NOS	*Morphologic variants*
DLBCL, specific histogenetic variants	Centroblastic
Primary mediastinal DLBCL	Immunoblastic
T-cell/histiocyte-rich DLBCL	Anaplastic
ALK+ DLBCL	Plasmablastic
DLBCL, distinctive extranodal variants	*Immunophenotypic variants*
Primary DLBCL of the CNS	GCB-like (CD10+)
Primary cutaneous DLBCL, leg type	Post-GCB (MUM1+)
Intravascular DLBCL	CD5+
DLBCL, primarily associated with viral infection	*Molecular subgroups*
EBV-associated DLBCL of the elderly	Lymphoma: GCB-like vs. ABC-like
Lymphomatoid granulomatosis	Stroma: Immune response vs.
DLBCL associated with chronic inflammation	angiogenic types
Plasmablastic lymphoma	
Primary effusion lymphoma	
Large B-cell lymphoma arising from HHV8+	
multicentric Castleman disease	
DLBCL, unclassifiable,	
intermediate between DLBCL and Burkitt lymphoma	
intermediate between DLBCL and classical Hodgkin	
lymphoma	

parts of Asia. DLBCL arises in all age groups, but occurs most commonly in the elderly, with approximately 25,000 new cases per year in the United States. Along with the Burkitt lymphoma (BL), DLBCL comprises the majority of all childhood B-cell lymphomas and is also the most common type of lymphoma associated with genetic and acquired immunodeficiency states. DLBCL can also arise rarely as a therapy-associated malignancy, most commonly following breast cancer or Hodgkin's lymphoma [2].

DLBCL can present with localized or generalized lymphadenopathy and is also the most common lymphoma type in nearly every extranodal site (see Chap. 27). Symptoms are highly dependent on the site(s) of presentation. Routine clinical evaluation requires anatomic staging, commonly using the Ann Arbor system, which is combined with laboratory data to derive the International Prognostic Index (IPI, Table 17-2) [3]. DLBCL is clinically aggressive, but potentially curable due to its high proliferation rate, especially in those tumors presenting at a low stage with a low IPI score. However, each DLBCL subtype has variable patterns of treatment response, relapse, and progression. Multiagent combination chemotherapy with cyclophosphamide, doxorubicin, vincristine, and prednisone (CHOP) is most commonly used for DLBCL and shows long-term remission rates in up to 40% of patients. The addition of the anti-CD20 antibody rituximab has improved overall survival by 10–15% (see Chap. 18). However, DLBCL still accounts for nearly 10,000 cancer deaths per year in the United States. Extensive molecular stratification and risk prediction modeling of DLBCL have been actively investigated in recent years in an attempt to predict therapy response and relapse as well as to better define mechanisms of transformation (see Chap. 32).

DLBCL may also arise as large cell transformation of a low-grade B-cell malignancy, such as follicular lymphoma (FL), marginal zone lymphoma (MZL), nodular lymphocyte predominant Hodgkin lymphoma (NLP-HL), classical Hodgkin lymphoma (CHL), or chronic lymphocytic leukemia/small lymphocytic lymphoma (CLL/SLL). Such transformed DLBCL shares many of the same genetic features as de novo DLBCL and is usually treated similarly. In some cases, the underlying low-grade lymphoproliferative neoplasm may be unrecognized at diagnosis, but can be suspected if cytogenetic studies reveal the genetic characteristics of a particular low-grade B-cell lymphoma.

Table 17-2. Clinical parameters affecting prognosis in lymphoma.

International Prognostic Index (IPI)
Unfavorable prognostic factors

- Age >60 yrs
- Poor performance status (ECOG>2)
- Extranodal involvement >2 sites
- High Ann Arbor stage (III or IV)
- High lactate dehydrogenase (LDH)

Risk group	Score (5 factors)	
	All patients	<60yrs
Low	0 or 1	0
Low-intermediate	2	1
High-intermediate	3	2
High	4 or 5	3-4

Eastern Cooperative Oncology Group (ECOG) performance status grading

0	Fully active without restriction
1	Restricted in physically strenuous activity
2	Ambulatory and capable of all self-care but unable to carry out any work activities.
3	Capable of only limited self-care, confined to bed or chair more than 50% of waking hours.
4	Completely disabled. Cannot carry on any self-care. Totally confined to bed or chair.

Ann Arbor staging system for lymphoma

I	Involvement of a single lymph node region or lymphoid structure (eg, spleen, thymus, Waldeyer's ring)
II	Involvement of two or more lymph node regions on the same side of the diaphragm
III	Involvement of lymph regions or structures on both sides of the diaphragm
IV	Involvement of extranodal site(s) beyond that designated E
	For all stages
A	No symptoms
B	Fever (>38°C), drenching sweats, weight loss (10% body weight over 6 months)
	For stages I to III
E	Involvement of a single, extranodal site contiguous or proximal to known nodal site.

Murphy staging system for high-grade lymphoma

I	A single tumor (extranodal) or single anatomic area (nodal) with the exclusion of mediastinum or abdomen
II	A single tumor (extranodal) with regional node involvement, or two or more nodal areas on the same side of the diaphragm, or two single (extranodal) tumors with or without regional node involvement on the same side of the diaphragm, or primary GI tract tumor, usually in the ileocecal area, with or without involvement of associated mesenteric nodes only
III	Two single tumors (extranodal) on opposite sides of the diaphragm or two or more nodal areas above and below the diaphragm, or primary intrathoracic tumors (mediastinal, pleural, thymic), or with extensive primary intra-abdominal disease, or paraspinal or epidural tumors regardless of other tumors site(s).
IV	Any of the above with initial CNS or bone marrow involvement.

17.1.3 Morphological Evaluation of DLBCL

In lymph node, DLBCL usually partially or completely effaces the architecture with frequent extracapsular extension and grows as either sheets or as individual cells dispersed in a dense background of nonneoplastic/inflammatory cells. Various degrees of sclerosis (in slower-growing tumors) and necrosis (in faster-growing tumors) are present. In extranodal tissue, DLBCL diffusely invades and replaces normal structures. In cytologic preparations, such as fine needle aspirate (FNA) smears and touch imprints, DLBCL can be readily recognized because of its large cell size, prominent nucleoli, and irregular nuclear contours with nose-like protrusions or indentations.

Although of limited prognostic utility, morphology subtyping of DLBCL can help in recognition of specific etiologic causes. *Centroblastic DLBCL*, the most common morphologic variant, resembles GC centroblasts with their round nuclei, vesicular, fine chromatin, and 2–4 distinct membrane-bound nucleoli, and discernible amphophilic cytoplasm (Fig. 17-1a). DLBCL with polylobate nuclei are often grouped with these cases are more common at certain extranodal sites, such as bone. *Immunoblastic DLBCL* are those where at least 90% of tumor cells resemble reactive immunoblasts with their prominent single, central nucleolus, and moderate amounts of amphophilic cytoplasm (Fig. 17-1b). *Plasmablastic DLBCL* has eccentric nuclei with prominent nucleoli, and abundant, often basophilic cytoplasm. *Anaplastic DLBCL* shows large polygonal, spindle- or bizarre-shaped tumor cells and often angulated or multilobated nuclei (Fig. 17-1c). Reed–Sternberg (RS)-like cells are common in this variant as well as atypical mitoses and frequently admixed inflammatory cells raising the differential diagnosis of CHL.

17.1.4. Use of Immunophenotyping in Diagnosis

Pan-B cell markers used for diagnosis of DLBCL by flow cytometry (FC) include CD19, CD20, CD22, and CD79a, whereas CD20, CD79a, and PAX5 are commonly used for immunohistochemistry (IHC) in fixed sections. Clonality can be confirmed by demontrating immunoglobulin (Ig) light chain restriction, defined as Igκ+cells greater than 4X the number of Igλ+cells, or Igλ+cells more than twice the number Igκλ+cells, using FC, or by in situ hybridization (ISH) or IHC in fixed sections in some cases. However, one should always be cautious when diagnosing or excluding DLBCL based only on FC alone. Review of a tissue section, cytologic cell block, or touch imprint is essential for avoiding errors due: to (1) frequent loss of fragile large lymphoma cells during FC sample processing; (2) absence of surface light chain on some tumor cells, particularly in mediastinal and plasmablastic DLBCL; (3) the presence of an obscuring predominant reactive lymphoid component, such as in T-cell-rich cases; and (4) a confusing immunophenotype such as CD5 and CD10 expression that is shared between DLBCLs and other B-cell lymphoproliferative disorders. In this regard, it is also important to note that judging cell size by the degree of FC forward light scatter may be misleading as some lymphomas (e.g., MZL) appear larger by FC than under the microscope.

Absence or dim expression of one or more pan-B antigens is a characteristic feature of some DLBCL subtypes at diagnosis or status-post treatment, particularly CD20 loss after

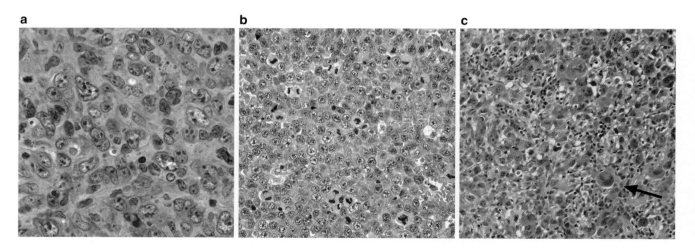

Fig. 17-1. Common morphologic variants of DLBCL include centroblastic (**a**), immunoblastic (**b**) and anaplastic (**c**) types with Reed–Sternberg-like cells (*arrow*)

use of rituximab. For these cases, other markers such as Ig heavy and/or light chains, CD22, CD79a, PAX5, and CD138 may help. CD138 is particularly useful in detecting plasmablastic/immunoblastic DLBCL (which often lack CD20) and these cases often also show cytoplasmic Ig light chain restriction detectable by IHC or ISH. Given its crisp nuclear staining pattern, the B-cell marker PAX5 can highlight tumor cases in cases with marked sclerosis or crush artifact, such as primary mediastinal B-cell lymphoma (PMBL) [4]. However, in DLBCL with extensive necrosis, CD20 immunostaining is usually retained, whereas nuclear markers, including PAX5, BCL1/cyclin D1, BCL6, MUM1, and Ki-67, will generally fail.

Many other markers that are routinely used in IHC are variably expressed in DLBCL. Strong CD30 expression is characteristic of DLBCL with a sinusoidal distribution, those associated with EBV, and cases with anaplastic morphology. About 10% of de novo DLBCL (i.e., unrelated to CLL or mantle cell lymphoma), are positive for CD5 and DLBCL may also aberrantly express T/NK cell antigens, such as CD2, CD7, CD8, and CD56. DLBCL associated with EBV may be identified by in situ hybridization for EBV-encoded RNAs (EBER), or expression of EBV latent membrane protein-1 (LMP1).

17.1.5. Use of Molecular Testing in Diagnosis

Molecular genetic assays may be useful in demonstrating B-cell clonality in difficult cases of DLBCL. However, although essentially all cases of DLBCL have clonally rearranged immunoglobulin genes, IGH polymerase chain reaction (PCR) assays can give a false-negative result in up to 15–20% of cases due to somatic mutations in the IGH primer binding sites which prevent amplification.

The monoclonal nature of DLBCL can also be established by detecting chromosomal translocations involving IGH and/or BCL6 genes that occur at high frequency in DLBCL. Translocations involving the BCL6 gene at chromosome 3q27 occur in about 30% of DLBCL, but they are not subtype specific since they occur in 5–10% of follicular lymphoma and rarely in T-cell lymphomas. About 30% of DLBCL have the t(14;18)(q32;q21) translocation producing the IGH/BCL2 fusion, which may or may not be related to transformation from an underlying follicular lymphoma. Finally, MYC translocations involving the immunoglobulin loci, while present in all cases of BL, also occur in 10–15% of DLBCLs or aggressive B-cell lymphomas with mixed features. Use of break-apart FISH probes which detect IGH, MYC, or BCL6 translocations irrespective of the partner genes (see Chap. 4) increases the detection frequency for these translocations and may be considered as an alternative clonality assay, especially when the IGH PCR fails to detect clonality.

17.1.6. Molecular and Immunophenotypic Subclassification

Gene expression profiles (GEP) established using large-scale gene expression arrays have led to recognition of several DLBCL subtypes with distinct clinical outcomes. The best studied are the GCB-like and the activated B cell (ABC)-like patterns [5]. The GCB and ABC signatures reflect fundamental differences in expression of hundreds of genes that largely match GCB and post-GC states of B-cell maturation. The GCB-like type highly expresses many genes that are also expressed in nonneoplastic GCB, and usually shows ongoing immunoglobulin gene somatic hypermutation, [6] whereas the ABC-like type shows expression of growth factor and signaling molecules seen in post-GC B cells where somatic hypermutation has ceased. DLBCL with plasmacytoid differentiation and most EBV-associated DLBCL have ABC-like features, whereas PMBL has a distinct GEP pattern. De novo CD5+ DLBCL may have an either GCB- or ABC-like GEP (Fig. 17-2).

As a group, the GCB-like DLBCL has a significantly better clinical outcome than the ABC-like type among patients treated with CHOP, with 5-year survival rates of 60 and 35%, respectively [5]. Some recent studies have shown that these outcome differences also apply to R-CHOP-treated patients [7,8]. In addition, GCB- and ABC-like DLBCL correlate with particular genomic changes reflective of distinct patterns of oncogenic progression For example, a subset of GCB cases show IGH/BCL2 rearrangements or amplification

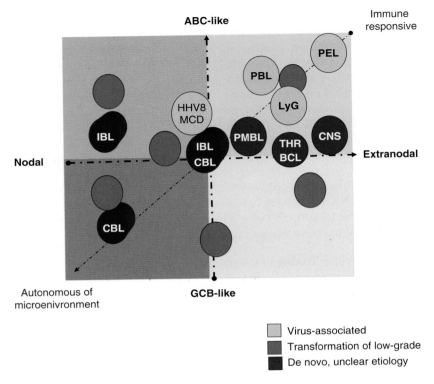

Fig. 17-2. *Intersection of maturation state, disease site, and genomic changes in diffuse large B-cell lymphoma.* The WHO DLBCL disease types can be mapped onto other pathogenetic features such as B-cell maturation stage of tumor cells (i.e., germinal center GC vs. post-GC types), sites of involvement, viral pathogenesis, or immunological responsiveness. DLBCL representing transformation of low-grade B-cell neoplasms are similarly heterogeneous. *Abbreviations*: ABC: activated B cell; PEL: primary effusion lymphoma; PBL: plasmablastic lymphoma; IBL: immunoblastic DLBCL; HHV8 MCD: DLBCL arising out of human herpesvirus 8+ multicentric Castleman disease; LyG: lymphomatoid granulomatosis; PMBL: primary mediastinal B-cell lymphoma; THRBCL: T-cell/histiocyte-rich large B-cell lymphoma; CNS: primary DLBCL of the central nervous system; CBL: centroblastic type of DLBCL; GCB: germinal center B cell

of the REL locus at chromosome 2q15, [5,9] features not seen in ABC-like DLBCL. In contrast, ABC-like cases display trisomy 3 and amplification of a small region on chromosome19, corresponding to upregulation of the ABC-associated genes FOXP1 and SPIB. These cases may also exhibit gains of chromosome 18q spanning the BCL2 and MALT1 loci, as well as deletions of chromosome 9p involving the CDKN2A (p16/INK4a) locus [9].

A number of studies have reported IHC-based correlates of the GCB vs. ABC molecular schema for DLBCL, most often using stains for CD10, BCL6, and MUM1 in the commonly used Hans scoring system [10]. GCB-like cases are positive for CD10 (with or without BCL6) and negative for MUM1, whereas ABC-like DLBCLs express MUM1 and lack CD10. Most studies agree that MUM1 (which is expressed in approximately 35% of DLBCL) is mutually exclusive with CD10 expression. BCL6 can be expressed in either GCB or ABC cases as a result of an activating promoter mutation or a chromosomal translocations and in those cases its expression will not reflect cell of origin. Likely for these reasons and due to differences in the quality and scoring criteria of the immunostains, IHC studies have not clearly shown differences in outcome stratification of DLBCL. Recent studies have added additional GCB-like markers such as HGAL [11] and LMO2, [12] and other ABC-like markers such as FOXP1, [13] which significantly improved outcome prediction in patients treated with either CHOP or R-CHOP. Nevertheless, there is not yet a consensus on the routine use of immunophenotyping for treatment stratification or on what markers would constitute the best routine IHC panel to determine prognosis and guide therapy selection.

GEP studies of DLBCL also identified distinct molecular signatures [7] related to tumor microenvironment that predict survival independently. Using cohorts of both CHOP and R-CHOP-treated patients, a "stroma-1" signature, enriched for genes responsible for increased host response, predicted a significantly better prognosis reminiscent of GCB-like DLBCL. It was also associated with histologic evidence of increased deposition of extracellular proteins and a prominent histiocytic infiltrate. A "stroma-2" signature rich in genes highly expressed in endothelial cells and in those encoding angiogenic factors and regulators predicted a poor prognosis and correlated with increased angiogenesis seen in the biopsies.

17.1.7. Prognostic Factors in DLBCL

In addition to an ABC-like GEP and IPI clinical factors, high-risk genetic changes in DLBCL include complex karyotype, MYC translocation, and TP53 loss (or p53 mutation). DLBCL with a MYC/IGH translocation do worse than those carrying a MYC translocation with other partner genes. Relapsed DLBCL frequently acquires additional genetic abnormalities and unstable karyotypes. Relapsed DLBCL that has been previously treated with rituximab may show a higher false-negative rate in nuclear medicine scans.

17.1.8. Differential Diagnosis

DLBCL with predominantly medium-sized cells, especially if cytoplasmic vacuoles are present on smears should be distinguished from BL, and cases with an anaplastic morphology may mimic CHL and/or ALCL. None of the commonly used pan-B markers are specific for B-cell tumors. CD20 and CD79a can be expressed in some T-cell lymphomas. Neuroendocrine carcinomas (Merkel cell carcinoma and small cell carcinoma) and CD19+ acute myeloid leukemias express PAX5. MUM1 is expressed in CHL and T-cell lymphoma, and CD138 is expressed in a number of nonhematopoietic neoplasms.

17.2. Histogenetic Variants of DLBCL

17.2.1. Primary Mediastinal Large B-cell Lymphoma (PMBL)

PMBL comprises 6–10% of DLBCL and it is twice as common in woman (median age, 35 years). PMBL is believed to arise from a specialized population of thymic B cells and warrants separate recognition because of its distinct clinical, morphologic, and genetic features. It often presents with shortness of breath due to a bulky anterior mediastinal mass, and commonly invades adjacent lung and spreads to adjacent lymph nodes. The rapid growth of PMBL may require urgent intervention due to superior vena cava syndrome or compression/invasion of lungs, pericardia, and pleura, a property that distinguishes it from mediastinal presentations of CHL. Lymphomas presenting with concurrent involvement of distant lymph nodes or bone marrow are excluded from this entity. PMBL also has a high rate of relapse in the kidney, adrenal, liver, and central nervous system (CNS). It usually responds well to initial treatment and has a relatively good prognosis, with approximately 50% of patients showing relapse and progression.

PMBL is composed of intermediate to large cells with frequently irregular or multilobate nuclear contours and moderate amounts of clear cytoplasm embedded in fibrosis with a reticulated or alveolar pattern (Fig. 17-3a). Sclerosis may be absent in rapidly growing tumors, whereas zonal necrosis is a common finding. Tissue crush artifact due to sclerosis

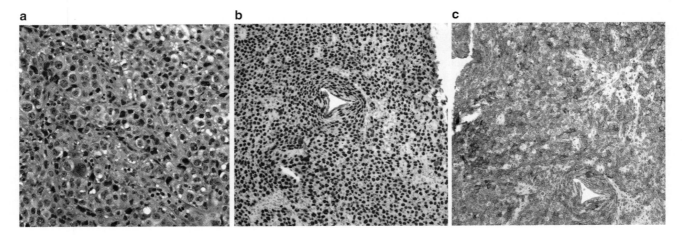

Fig. 17-3. *Mediastinal large B-cell lymphoma.* (**a**) Relatively monomorphic tumor lymphocytes infiltrate between fibrotic bands. (**b**) B-cell marker PAX5 is diffusely positive. (**c**) CD30 immunostain also shows diffuse membrane positivity

and the variable number of background reactive lymphocytes often make the diagnosis difficult on small biopsy samples. PMBL cells express CD20, PAX5 (Fig. 17-3b), and BCL6, with MUM1 positivity in up to 75% supporting an origin from post-GC activated B cells in most cases. More than 50% of cases show at least focal CD30 reactivity (Fig. 17-3c), but the staining is usually less uniform compared to CHL. Furthermore, the transcription factors BOB1 and OCT2 are positive, whereas they are usually negative or dim in CHL. MAL, TRAF1, and nuclear REL are positive in 62–75% of PMBL, but are uncommon in other types of DLBCL. CD10 and CD15 are usually negative, and EBER is always negative. FC has only limited diagnostic value because of the tissue sclerosis and the frequent absence of surface immunoglobulin on the tumor cells.

GEP of PMBL have shown an expression signature distinct from both GCB-like and ABC-like DLBCL, with some shared features with CHL such as upregulation of the NF-kB and JAK2 pathways [14]. This is correlated with amplification of the REL locus at chromosome 2p15 in 50%, and the JAK2 locus at chromosome 9q24 in 75%. Inactivating mutations in SOCS-1 are also seen. BCL2, BCL6, and MYC translocations are absent (Table 17-3).

17.2.2. T-cell/Histiocyte-Rich Large B-cell Lymphoma (TCHRLBCL)

TCHRLBCL is a DLBCL variety characterized by numerous nonneoplastic T cells and/or histiocytes. It comprises less than 10% of DLBCL and is most common in middle-aged men (median age, 49 years). It often involves deep lymph nodes in the retroperitoneum, as well as the liver, spleen, and bone marrow. Patients usually have high clinical stage at presentation, and tumors are largely refractory to CHOP-R chemotherapy.

In lymph node, TCHRLBCL shows diffuse effacement of the architecture, resulting in an abnormal appearance even on needle core biopsy. Whether in lymph node or extranodal sites, the neoplastic cells typically comprise less than 10% of the cellularity and are dispersed amid dense populations of small T cell and/or sheets of large epithelioid histiocytes. Small B cells, eosinophils, plasma cells, and neutrophils are usually completely absent. Tumor cell morphology is variable, sometime resembling Reed–Sternberg cells, with other cases having multilobate nuclei resembling the popcorn cells of NLPHL. Given the T-cell predominance, tumor cells may be missed by FC so IHC is recommended in all cases (Fig. 17-4). CD20 and BCL6 are uniformly positive, MUM1 is variable, and CD5, CD10, CD30, and BCL2 are expressed in only a minority of cases. The phenotype of the background T cells is variable with some cases showing a predominance of CD8+ cytotoxic cells; follicular T cells expressing PD-1 and/or CD57 are absent or rare.

Table 17-3. Molecular subgroups of DLBCL.

Variant	DLBCL-GCB	DLBCL-ABC	PMBL
Morphology	Often centroblastic, variable	Often immunoblastic, variable	Variable, with sclerosis
Phenotype	CD10±BCL6+MUM1- HGAL+LMO2+	CD10-BCL6±MUM1+ FOXP1+SPIB+BCL2+ Rarely IG/MYC	CD10-BCL6±MUM1± TRAF1+nREL+
Chromosomal translocations	t(14;18)/IGH-BCL2, 3q27/BCL6		
Commonly amplified chromosomal loci	2p15 (REL), 12q12 (CDK2/CDK4)	+3 (FOXP1), +18q(BCL2/MALT1),+19q(SPIB)	9q24 (JAK2), 2p15 (REL),
Commonly deleted chromosomal loci		9p (CDKN2A), 6q	16p13 (SOCSI)
IGH mutational status	Ongoing somatic hypermutation	Mutated	Mutated
Prognosis	Favorable	Unfavorable	Favorable
Median 5-yr survival	50–60%	15–30%	65%

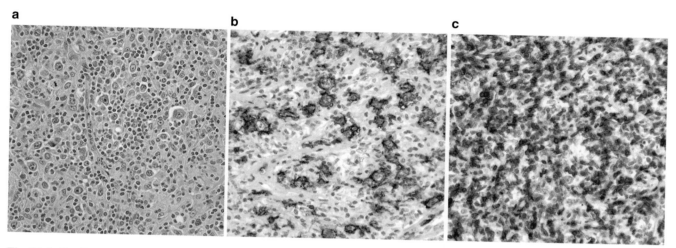

a   b   c

Fig. 17-4. *T-cell and histiocyte-rich large B-cell lymphoma.* (**a**) H&E section shows pleomorphic large cells in a histiocyte-rich background. (**b**) The large cells are exclusively B cells immunopositive for CD20; (**c**) small cells are exclusively CD3+ T cells

TCHRLBCL is likely a heterogeneous disorder, with some cases related to NLPHL. In particular, the "paragranuloma" variant of TCHRLBCL can develop as a transformation of preexisting NLPHL, [15] and the two tumors can even coexist in the same lymph node. Therefore, distinction of these two entities can be difficult whenever NLPHL acquires a diffuse growth pattern and has few associated small B cells. Table 17-4 lists some helpful distinctions. Spread of NLPHL outside of lymph nodes to liver or bone marrow is a sign of transformation to TCHRLBCL. Other subsets of DLBCL can show numerous nonneoplastic lymphocytes and histiocytes, such as EBV+tumors, and should not be diagnosed as TCHRLBCL [1].

17.2.3. DLBCL Expressing ALK

This is an extremely rare lymphoma comprising much less than 1% of DLBCL that has also been reported as ALK+plasmablastic lymphoma. It occurs in all age groups, but is most common in young to middle-aged men. Despite having been reported at extranodal sites, it is generally an aggressive nodal lymphoma and is insensitive to rituximab due to lack of CD20 expression. ALK+ DLBCL displays a sinusoidal distribution or forms large tumor nodules both grossly and microscopically mimicking carcinoma and melanoma. The lymphoma displays monotonous immunoblast-like cytology, but the cell size is much larger than regular immunoblasts. Like other lymphomas with sinusoidal localization, ALK+ DLBCL may have prominent membrane villous projections.

ALK+ DLBCL is negative for B-cell or T-cell markers, as well as CD30 (unlike ALK+ALCL) and CD45, but expresses granular cytoplasmic ALK and plasma cell antigens such as CD138, MUM1, and EMA [16]. The cells may also focally express cytoplasmic IgA (rarely IgG), CD4, CD43, and CD57. Unlike the t(2;5)/ALK-NPM1 translocation seen in ALK+ALCL, 60% of cases have t(2;17)(p23;q23) fusing clathrin (CLTC) and ALK; other cases may have cryptic insertion of 3'ALK sequences at chromosome 4q22-24.

17.3. Extranodal Variants of DLBCL

17.3.1. Primary DLBCL of the Central Nervous System (CNS)

DLBCLs may present in the CNS from systemic spread (often from PMBL), in immuno-suppressed patients (often HIV+), or in immunocompetent patients. The latter, known as primary DLBCL of the CNS, often present with neurological deficits, are mostly supraten-torial in location, may be multifocal, and are best detected by magnetic resonance imaging (MRI). Extracranial metastasis and bone marrow involvement are very rare. Biopsy usually shows perivascular parenchymal infiltration by clusters of tumor cells and subtle menin-geal spread, but the limited sampling afforded by brain biopsies will sometimes show only necrosis, foamy histiocytes, and rare CD20+ cells. Tumor cells are positive for BCL2, BCL6 (60–100%), MUM1 (~90%), and BCL6 (60–100%) with mutated IGH consistent with a post-GC origin [17]. Amplification of chromosomal region 18q21.31-33, including the BCL2 locus, and the deletion of chromosomal region 9q21 spanning CDKN2A are frequent findings; 30–40% of cases have BCL6 translocations, and BCL2 and MYC translocations are usually absent. High-dose intrathecal methotrexate therapy and involved field radiation are the primary treatment modalities.

17.3.2. Primary Cutaneous DLBCL, Leg Type

Most DLBCLs involving the skin are localized to the dermis (Stage IE), have an indolent course and can be easily treated with excision and/or radiotherapy. However, there is an aggressive variant of primary skin DLBCL typically presenting as bluish nodules on the lower extremities (in contrast to the trunk, head, and neck involvement seen more com-monly in indolent cases), which has been named "leg type". Such cases comprise about 20% of primary cutaneous B-cell lymphoma and commonly occur in elderly women having a 5-year survival of only 50%. The presence of multiple tumor nodules and rapid systemic spread are adverse risk factors. Both immunoblastic and centroblastic morphol-ogy are common, and epidermal or adnexal involvement is absent. Tumor cells display molecular signatures consistent with ABC-like DLBCL [18] and express BCL2, BCL6, MUM1, and FOXP1, but lack CD10 expression commonly seen in most of the cutaneous DLBCL of GCB origin. Deletions of chromosome 9p21 spanning the CDKN2A tumor suppressor are seen in 67% of cases. Translocations involving IGH, BCL6, and MYC may be seen.

17.3.3. Intravascular DLBCL

This is an exceedingly rare type of extranodal DLBCL with a characteristic intravascular pattern of growth that can be diagnosed incidentally during biopsy for other reasons. It often presents with symptoms related to vasculitis and thrombosis in various organs such as brain (stroke and infarct), lung (pneumonia and pulmonary embolism), kidney (infarction or renal insufficiency), adrenal (endocrine disorders), or skin. Although there is often preferential involvement of some organs, it is a systemic disease with bone marrow involvement in nearly all cases that can be demonstrated by immunostaining. Delays in diagnosis due to the subtlety and focal nature of the intravascular infiltrates often lead to a terminal disease

Table 17-4. Helpful features for differential diagnoses between TCHRLBCL, NLP-HL and CHL.

Features	T-cell and histiocyte-rich large B-cell lymphoma	Nodular lymphocyte predominant Hodgkin lymphoma	Classical Hodgkin lymphoma(i.e., follicular and lymphocyte-rich types)
Patient	Mid-age man (median 49 years)	Mid-age man (30–50 years)	Bimodal
Locations	LN (retroperitoneal, etc.), spleen, BM	LN (axillary, neck, inguinal)	LN, mediastinal, extranodal
Ann Arbor stage/IPI	Intermediate to high	Low	Variable
Prognosis	Poor	Good	Generally good
Growth, morphology	Diffuse, variable cytology	Nodular, L&H cells	Nodular or diffuse. RS-/Lacunar cells
Tumor-associated reactive B cells	Absent	Numerous in a nodular pattern	Variable
Tumor-associated reactive T cells	CD8+CD57-PD1-, with minimal resetting of tumor cells	CD4+CD57+PD1+, with prominent resetting of tumor cells	CD4+CD57±PD1±, with focal rosetting of tumor cells
Histiocytes	Numerous, sheets/aggregates	Uncommon	Many
Inflammatory cells	Absent	Absent	Common (eosinophils, neutrophils)
FDC meshwork	Absent	Expended	Variable
Immunophenotype	CD20+BCL6+MUM1±IgD-CD45+EBER-	CD20+BCL6+MUM1±IgD±CD45+EBER-	CD20±BCL6±MUM1+ IgD-CD15+CD30+CD45-EBER±

LN: lymph node; *BM:* bone marrow; *FDC:* follicular dendritic cell

with death before chemotherapy is initiated. Most cases have an immunoblastic or anaplastic appearance and express BCL2 and MUM1, consistent with a post-GC/ABC-like origin. Rare lymphomas of NK/T-cell origin with similar presentation have also been reported.

17.4. Variants of DLBCL Associated with Viral Infections

17.4.1. The Role of Herpesviruses in DLBLC

Viral-associated DLBCL are the most common malignancies in patients with an underlying immunodeficiency, whether it is related to primary immunodeficiencies, chronic iatrogenic immunosuppression, human immunodeficiency virus (HIV) infection and other chronic infections, transplantation, or age-related declines in immune function. The two primary viral agents involved in lymphomagenesis are the gamma herpesviruses, EBV and human herpesvirus (HHV)8. EBV is endemic among all populations worldwide, with seropositivity rates of over 90% in adults in the United States. However, geographic differences in genetic strains of the virus, age of primary infection, and patient socioeconomic status lead to differences in the profile of EBV-associated malignancies in different countries. HHV8 infects up to 5% of the population in the United States, with higher percentages in Europe, and up to 40–70% seropositivity rates in some parts of Africa. HHV8-associated malignancies are rare in Western countries, except in the context of severe immunodeficiency.

Nearly all EBV- and HHV8-associated DLBCLs are MUM1+ and CD10-, consistent with a post-GC/ABC-like origin. Plasma cell differentiation is also very common. Most of these lymphomas are clinically aggressive with median survivals of only months to 1–2 years. EBER detected by ISH is the most useful marker to demonstrate EBV infection in the tumor cells, and latency associated nuclear antigen (LANA)-1 detected by IHC is the most useful marker of HHV8 infection. Detection of LMP1 by IHC in EBV+lymphomas is typically associated with reactivation of EBV replication. The comparisons between variants of viral-associated DLBCL are listed in Table 17-5.

17.4.2. Acquired Immunodeficiency Syndrome (AIDS)-Associated DLBCL

Prior to the advent of highly active anti-retroviral therapy, there was a 110- to 200-fold increase in the incidence of lymphoma in HIV-infected patients, the majority of which were

Table 17-5. Diffuse large B-cell lymphomas associated with herpesvirus infection.

Variant	EBV	HHV8	Body Sites	Morphology	Immunophenotype	Risk factors	Prognosis
EBV+DLBCL of the elderly	EBER+ LMP1+	–	Lymph node, extranodal	Pleomorphic, plasmacytoid	CD45+CD20+PAX+ MUM1+CD30±	Elderly population	Usually poor
DLBCL associated with chronic inflammation	EBER+ LMP1+	–	Joint capsule and cavity walls	Variable	CD45+CD20+PAX+ MUM1+CD30+	Surgical prostheses or foreign body-related inflammation	Usually poor
Lymphomatoid granulomatosis	EBER+ LMP1+	–	Lung, skin, brain	Pleomorphic, angiocentric	CD45+CD20+PAX+ MUM1+CD30+	Geographic variations, related to EBV type?	Variable, dependent on grading
Plasmablastic lymphoma	EBER+ LMP1-	–	Oral cavity, GI tract, soft tissue	Immunoblastic, plasmablastic	CD45+MUM1+ CD138+CD20- PAX5-CD30±,cIg±	Immunodeficient young males, elderly	Poor
Primary effusion lymphoma	EBER+ LMP1-	+	Body cavity	Immunoblastic, anaplastic	CD45+ MUM1+ CD138+CD20- PAX5-CD30±,cIg±	Immunodeficient young males, elderly in HHV8 endemic areas	Poor
LBCL arising in HHV8-associated multicentric Castleman disease	–	+	Lymph node, spleen	Immunoblastic, plasmablastic	CD45+ MUM1+ CD138- CD20+ PAX5-CD30-cIgM/ Igλ+IgD-	Immunodeficient young males, elderly in HHV8 endemic areas	Poor

EBV-associated DLBCL and BL. Currently, in the United States, there has been a marked reduction in the incidence of AIDS-associated lymphomas, which are now limited to patients who are refractory to, or noncompliant with, therapy. Involvement of various extranodal sites is frequently seen, and tumor cell morphology ranges from polymorphous B-cell infiltrates with oligoclonal IGH gene rearrangements to monomorphous high-grade immunoblastic DBLCL similar to the range of features seen in posttransplant tumors (see Chap. 30).

17.4.3. Lymphomatoid Granulomatosis (LyG)

LyG is an extranodal EBV+B-cell lymphoproliferative disorder that characteristically presents with multifocal angiocentric lesions, most commonly involving lung (bilateral pulmonary nodules in middle and lower lobes), skin (multiple nodules or ulcers), CNS, and less commonly kidney and liver. Although most common in middle-aged men, it affects a wide age range and is associated with an immunocompromised state in many patients. The EBV+large cells typically have a perivascular distribution with vascular invasion, and are regularly positive for CD30 as well as both EBER and LMP1. Prognosis of LyG depends on histological grade (Table 17-6), with disease progression manifested by an increased number of EBV+tumor cells and a decreased number of reactive CD4+ T cells.

17.4.4. DLBCL Associated with Chronic Inflammation

The outgrowth of an EBV+DLBCL in response to unremitting chronic suppurative inflammation was first recognized in Japan in patients who had a history of pyothorax. Such pyothorax-associated lymphoma (PAL) typically occurred after 10–20 years of persistent inflammation. Similar lymphomas have now been reported following chronic osteomyelitis, chronic skin ulcers, and around protheses and metallic implants. The tumor infiltrates dense fibrotic linings or capsule of cavities and joint spaces and can show just focal nests of EBER+and LMP1+ large B cells. Surgical debulking with complete tumor resection has been reported to improve survival, but the overall prognosis is poor, possibly due to delays in diagnosis. Patients with rheumatoid arthritis may also develop DLBCL near inflamed joints, but these neoplasms are usually negative for EBV.

Table 17-6. Histological grading of lymphomatoid granulomatosis.

Features	Grade 1	Grade 2	Grade 3
Polymorphic background	Dominant	Significant	Focal
Necrosis	Focal	Frequent	Extensive
Tumor cells	Rare (need IHC)	Occasional, may be in clusters	Frequent, may be in aggregates
	<5/hpf	5–20/hpf, may be up to 50/hpf	>50/hpf
Outcome	Wax & wane, may regress	May have durable response to therapy	Same as EBV+DLBCL

17.4.5. Plasmablastic Lymphoma

Plasmablastic lymphoma is typically an EBV+extranodal, extramedullary lymphoma with immunoblastic or plasmablastic morphology that is negative for pan-B-cell antigens (Fig. 17-5). Although initially reported to be restricted to the oropharynx in patients with AIDS, [19] it also occurs at other sites such as the gastrointestinal tract, bone, and soft tissues, and in patients without HIV infection [20]. Some patients may have a low-level serum paraprotein (usually IgG kappa or lambda), but the tumor cells only infrequently exhibit cytoplasmic immunoglobulin expression by IHC. Nodal involvement is very rare and tends to be found in elderly patients without an identifiable immunodeficiency state. Plasmablastic lymphoma should be distinguished from plasmablastic transformation of myeloma, as the latter usually has the characteristic triad of lytic bone lesions, plasmacytosis, and prominent monoclonal gammopathy, as well as expression of cytoplasmic immunoglobulin, and is typically negative for EBV. Occasional cases of high-grade lymphoma that have typical plasmablastic morphology and immunophenotype but lack evidence of EBV infection may be encountered.

17.4.6. Primary Effusion Lymphoma (PEL)

PEL, also known as body-cavity lymphoma, is a highly aggressive extranodal tumor invariably associated with HHV8 infection (Fig. 17-6). A vast majority of cases are also positive for EBV. PEL presents with massive serous effusions in one or more of the large body cavities (i.e., pleura space, pericardium, or peritoneum) without localized masses, adenopathy, or organomegaly [21]. PEL cells exhibit immunoblastic or anaplastic morphology and are often extremely pleomorphic. They lack most pan-B-cell markers, but express CD45, MUM1, and CD138. CD30, EMA, and CD79a are variably expressed. Similar appearing tumors arising as a tissue-based lymphoma have been described as extra-cavitary PEL.

17.4.7. EBV+DLBCL of the Elderly

There is an increasing recognition that age-related declines in T-cell surveillance can lead to emergence of nodal and extranodal systemic EBV+DLBCL in elderly patients, and are termed senile EBV-associated lymphoproliferative disorders [22]. While this entity is defined in the 2008 WHO classification as a disease of patients >65 year-old, it does occasionally occur in younger patients. The boundaries of this EBV-associated DLBCL are currently under investigation, but the diagnosis should only be made when a tumor does not fit other entities. This lymphoma should be suspected whenever a DLBCL has areas containing Reed-Sternberg-like cells, polymorphic infiltrates with plasmacytoid features, and zonal necrosis. There is usually variable expression of CD30, and cytoplasmic light chain restriction is commonly identifiable, especially when sheets of immunoblasts or plasmablasts are present.

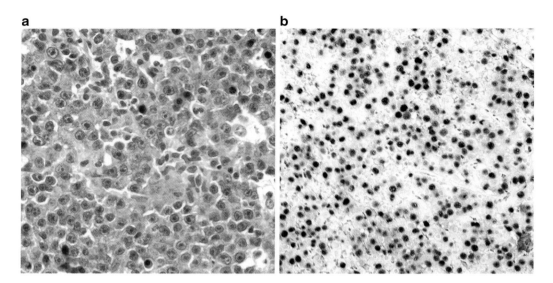

Fig. 17-5. *Plasmablastic lymphoma.* (**a**) Tumor cells have immunoblastic to plasmablastic morphology. (**b**) EBV is present in all tumor cells as seen by EBER ISH

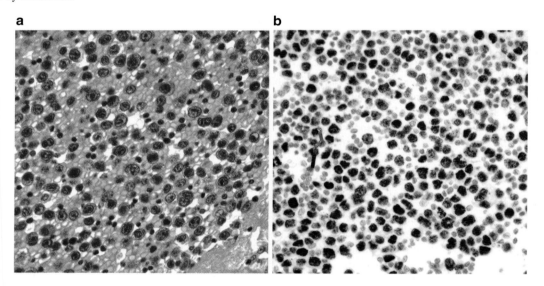

Fig. 17-6. *Primary effusion lymphoma.* (**a**) Cell block preparation shows large pleomorphic tumor cells. (**b**) HHV8 infection is detected by LANA-1 immunostain

17.4.8. Large B-cell Lymphoma Arising from HHV8+ Multicentric Castleman Disease (MCD)

This is primarily a nodal IgM plasmablastic lymphoma arising from MCD and is the only known lymphoma subtype exclusively associated with HHV8 without EBV coinfection. In a minority of patients, it may disseminate to the GI tract, liver, lungs, or evolve into a leukemic phase. The early lesions manifest as monotypic IgM + Igλ + plasmablastic proliferations localized to the mantle zones of MCD follicles, [23] which then evolve into microscopic aggregates (*micro-lymphoma*) and eventually frank lymphoma with confluent sheets of tumor cells (Fig. 17-7). Unlike EBV + extranodal plasmablastic lymphoma, HHV8+ plasmablastic lymphoma arising from MCD exhibit intense cytoplasmic expression of IgM and lambda light chain (rarely kappa). The tumor cells express CD20 (weak) and MUM1, but

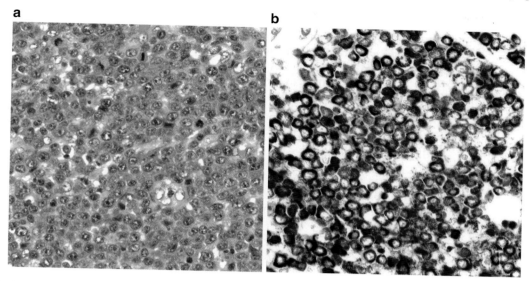

Fig. 17-7. *HHV8+ plasmablastic lymphoma arising in multicentric Castleman's disease.* (**a**) Diffuse infiltrate of tumor cells with plasmablastic differentiation. (**b**) Cytoplasmic IgM expression is demonstrated by immunostain

lack PAX5 and CD138. A distinct and much more indolent germinotropic lymphoproliferative disorder that expresses both EBV and HHV8 can arise in lymph nodes of immunocompetent patients and should be regarded as a different disease.

17.5. Burkitt Lymphoma and Its Variants

17.5.1. Introduction

Burkitt lymphoma (BL), previously known as small noncleaved cell or undifferentiated lymphoma, is an aggressive, but often curable B-cell lymphoma of medium-sized tumor cells with high mitotic rate. Cases with bone marrow involvement were formerly diagnosed as ALL-L3 subtype. The initiating factor in BL is a chromosomal translocation that drives expression of the MYC oncogene by juxtaposition to the transcriptional enhancer of the immunoglobulin genes, usually IGH. Based on GEP studies, IGH somatic mutation status, and immunophenotype, BL is classified as a GCB-derived lymphoma. The MYC-IGH translocations may thus arise following aberrant receptor-editing, somatic hypermutation, or class switch recombination in the germinal center.

17.5.2. Incidence, Demographics, and Clinical Features

BL consists of three clinical variants that share similar morphologic and immunophenotypic features but differ in their geographic distribution, sites of involvement, and frequency of association with EBV. First recognized by Dennis Burkitt in1958, endemic BL occurs with a high incidence in equatorial Africa, with a peak incidence between 4 and 7 years old and a male-to-female ratio of 2:1. More than 50% of patients present with facial/jaw masses and often systemic disease involving terminal ileum/cecum, kidney, gonads, salivary glands, breasts, and bone marrow. Nearly all cases of endemic BL are positive for EBV. Sporadic BL mostly occurs in young adults representing 1–3% of lymphoma in this age cohort (M:F ratio of 2–3:1) and usually presents as an abdominal mass in the ileocecal region, but can also involve lymph node, kidney, gonads, or the breasts. Only 20–40% of cases are positive for EBV. Immunodeficiency-associated BL is primarily associated with HIV infection, has a high association with EBV, and typically involves lymph nodes and bone marrow.

BL presents as a rapidly-enlarging lymph node or extranodal mass, or an acute leuke-mia. Many patients present at high stage, with frequent bone marrow (30–40%) and CNS (15–20%) involvement. The modified Murphy system is used for staging (Table 17-2) [1]. When treated with intensive chemotherapy including cytarabine and intrathecal methotrex-ate, BL is curable in up to 90% of patients with low-stage disease and 60–80% of patients with advanced disease. Tumor lysis syndrome may occur during induction therapy. Children tend to have a better prognosis than adults who may have difficulties tolerating intensive chemotherapy. Prognosis is mainly related to the IPI score and/or Murphy stage.

17.5.3. Morphologic Evaluation of Burkitt Lymphoma

BL is composed of monotonous, medium-sized cells with high mitotic rate diffusely displac-ing normal architecture in extranodal tissue or lymph node. Confluent tumor cell necrosis may be prominent, especially in extranodal cases, and reactive lymphocytes are rare. Admixed in the monotonous tumor cells are benign tingible-body macrophages with engulfed cell debris in the expanded pale cytoplasm known as the "starry-sky" pattern (Fig. 17-8). BL cells have round nuclei, clumped fine chromatin, a few distinct small nucleoli, and discern-ible basophilic cytoplasm with frequently "squared-off" cell borders between neoplastic cells. On a touch imprint or cytospin slide, BL cells show numerous cytoplasmic vacuoles. The proliferation fraction is very high, approaching 100% by Ki-67 immunostains. Cells in immunodeficiency-associated BL and some cases of sporadic BL may have eccentric nuclei, somewhat more conspicuous nucleoli, and appreciable variation in cell size.

17.5.4. Use of Immunophenotyping in Diagnosis

BL expresses pan-B markers (CD19, CD20, and CD22) as well as CD10, CD38 (bright), CD43, BCL6, and surface IgM and Ig light chain, but is negative for BCL2 and TdT (Fig. 17-8). Nearly all endemic BL cases harbor the EBV genome and are thus positive for EBER by ISH or EBNA1 by IHC. Approximately 30% of sporadic BL and immunodeficiency-associ-ated BL are also positive for EBER. EBV LMP1 is not expressed. Rare cases of BL may be weakly positive for BCL2 protein, which is unrelated to BCL2 translocations [24].

17.5.5. Use of Molecular Cytogenetic Testing in Diagnosis

All cases of BL should demonstrate chromosomal translocation between MYC (chr 8q22) and the either the IGH gene (chr 14q32) or less commonly the immunoglobulin light chain genes (IGK at chr 2q12, and IGL at chr 22q11). Such deregulated, constitutive MYC expression driven by the Ig enhancer is the transforming event in BL. In contrast, levels

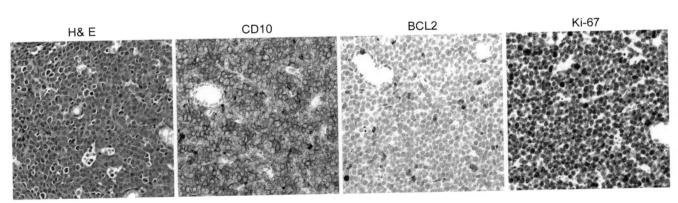

Fig. 17-8. *Burkitt lymphoma.* A monomorphic proliferation of blastoid lymphocytes with starry-sky appearance is noted on H&E. Tumor is immunoreactive for CD10, but BCL2 immunostain is negative. The proliferative marker Ki-67 is immunoreactive in all tumor cells

of MYC transcript or protein may not be discernibly higher in BL than in other lymphomas. Translocations are best detected by breakapart FISH using probes that span the MYC breakpoint, though FISH detecting the MYC/IGH fusion is more specific for BL. G-banding karyotype will show the MYC translocation and other gross chromosomal abnormalities, if any. The breakpoints in the MYC gene are widely scattered, Long-range PCR and Southern blot can be used for detection of MYC/IGH, though they have been largely replaced by FISH analysis.

In the endemic variant of BL, the translocation breakpoints are usually in the 5'-untranslated region of MYC and the joining region of IGH driving transcription from the endogenous MYC promoter, whereas in sporadic cases they are often downstream of MYC exon 1 and in the IGH switch regions utilizing the 3' enhancer of IGH. These differences may result from the mechanism of transformation. Rare cases of MYC translocation-negative BL have also been reported, in which deregulated MYC expression appears to be closely correlated with downregulation of the regulatory microRNA mir-34b [25].

GEP studies have identified a unique BL molecular signature that is different from DLBCL in nearly all cases of classical BL. However, up to 17% of high-grade lymphomas that do not completely fit all criteria for classical BL can show similar GEP and up to 27% of other high-grade B-cell lymphomas can display GEP features intermediate between BL and DLBCL [26,27]. These findings support the establishment of an entity, as in 2008 WHO schema, of B-cell lymphoma with features intermediate between DLBCL and BL. These cases nearly always present diagnostic and clinical difficulties, as discussed below.

17.6. B-cell Lymphoma, Unclassifiable, with Features Intermediate Between DLBCL and BL

This category comprises aggressive B-cell lymphomas that are difficult to classify. They display features closely resembling BL but vary to differing degrees in their morphology, immunophenotype and genetics (Fig. 17-9). For example, a BL-like lymphoma may show more variable cytomorphology, such as increased number of large cells and more irregular nuclear contours. Cases with morphology typical of BL may have strong BCL2 expression and harbor both t(14;18) and t(8;14), that may be either de novo or represent transformation of follicular lymphoma (Fig. 17-10). Indeed, when routine FISH analysis is performed, up to 2.5% of DLBCL may have both t(8;14) and t(14;18), and such "double-hit" cases have very poor outcome. Rare B-ALL/BL hybrid cases may have MYC translocation and classical BL morphology, but display a mixed phenotype (e.g. surface Ig+ and CD10+ but with TdT expression). Cases with typical BL morphology and immunophenotype but no identifiable MYC translocation may be diagnostically challenging, though they might be best considered as BL, especially in young patients who might be expected to benefit from the intensive chemotherapy given for BL.

17.7. B-cell Lymphoma, Unclassifiable, with Features Intermediate Between DLBCL and CHL

This category covers so-called gray-zone lymphoma and large B-cell lymphoma with Hodgkin-like features. It mostly reflects the diagnostic overlaps between PMBL and CHL in young adults presenting with a mediastinal mass though similar lymphomas have been reported at other sites as well. The classification difficulties arise when there is a sheet-like proliferation of large lymphocytes that show a CHL-like immunophenotype (CD20–, CD15+), or conversely the histologic appearance of nodular sclerosis CHL but with tumor cells positive for CD20, CD79a, and/or CD45, and negative for CD15. In most cases, the tumor cells will be larger and more pleomorphic than is typical for PMBL but lack a classical Reed-Sternberg appearance, and may strongly express the B-cell transcription factors PAX5,

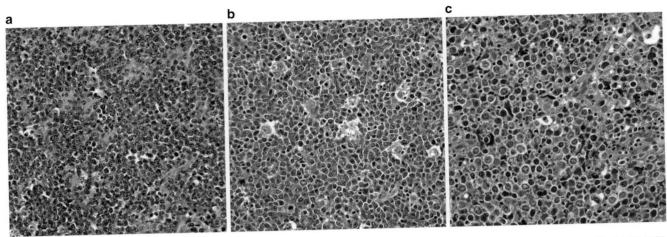

Fig. 17-9. *High-grade lymphomas with unusual features.* (**a**) Burkitt lymphoma with some pleomorphic and large tumor cells.(**b**) DLBCL with high mitotic rate and smaller tumor cell size. MYC translocation was not detected. (**c**) DLBCL with MYC-IGH translocation detected by FISH

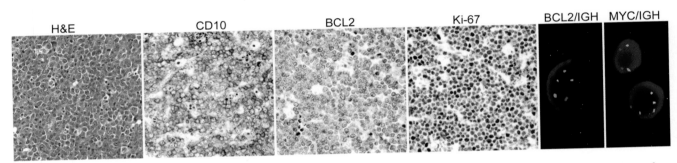

Fig. 17-10. *Burkitt-transformation of follicular lymphoma.* Tumor cells have high-grade cytologic features on H&E stain, but more pleomorphism is present than is typical of BL. CD10 immunostain is diffusely positive, but unlike BL, BCL2 is strongly immunoreactive. Ki-67 immunostain highlights nearly 100% of tumor cells. Dual t(14;18) and t(8;14) is detected by FISH using dual color, dual fusion probes. Left side of panel is BCL2/IGH probe pattern in tumor cells (two yellow fusion signals, 1 normal green and an extra green signal due to an additional IGH translocation, 1 normal red); right panel is MYC/IGH probe with a tumor cell at the bottom (with two fusion signals) and a nonneoplastic cell at the top (two normal red and green signals)

Table 17-7. Helpful features for differential diagnosis of Burkitt lymphoma and diffuse large B-cell lymphomas.

Features	Burkitt lymphoma	Intermediate BL/ DLBCL	Diffuse large B-cell lymphomas
Morphology	Medium-sized cells, monotonous	Medium-sized cells heterogeneous	Large cells ± medium-sized cells, variable
Proliferation (Ki67)	>95%, homogeneous	Often >90% often heterogeneous	<90% or >90%, heterogeneous
BCL2 (IHC)	Negative, rarely positive (weak)	Negative or positive	Positive or negative
Karyotype	Simple	Simple or complex	Complex or simple
MYC translocation	MYC/IG	MYC/IG, MYC/ non-IG; 30–50%	MYC/non-IG, MYC/IG; 10%
Other translocations	None	BCL2, BCL6, complex	BCL2, BCL6, complex

BOB1, and OCT2 (like PMBL) along with CD30. In some cases that have separate areas resembling CHL and DLBCL, the tumor may be better classified as composite lymphoma. These borderline cases probably reflect a shared biology, since microarray studies have shown overlap in the molecular signature between CHL and PMBL [28].

Suggested Readings

Staudt LM and Dave S. The biology of human lymphoid malignancies revealed by gene expression profiling. Adv Immunol 2005;87:163–208
- A comprehensive review of studies on the molecular characterization of DLBCL.

Harris NL and Horning SJ. Burkitt's lymphoma – the message from microarrays. N Engl J Med 2006;354:2495–8.
- An updated discussion on gene expression of DLBCL and borderline diseases.

References

1. Swerdlow SH, Campo E, Harris NL, et al. WHO classification of tumors of hematopoietic and lymphoid tissues. Lyon: IARC Press, 2008.
2. Rueffer U, Josting A, Franklin J, et al. Non-Hodgkin's lymphoma after primary Hodgkin's disease in the German Hodgkin's Lymphoma Study Group: incidence, treatment, and prognosis. J Clin Oncol 2001;19:2026–32.
3. Armitage JO. Staging non-Hodgkin lymphoma. CA Cancer J Clin 2005;55:368–76.
4. Dong HY, Browne P, Liu Z, Gangi M. PAX-5 is invariably expressed in B-cell lymphomas without plasma cell differentiation. Histopathology 2008;53:278–87.
5. Rosenwald A, Wright G, Chan WC, et al. The use of molecular profiling to predict survival after chemotherapy for diffuse large-B-cell lymphoma. N Engl J Med 2002;346:1937–47.
6. Lossos IS, Alizadeh AA, Eisen MB, et al. Ongoing immunoglobulin somatic mutation in germinal center B cell-like but not in activated B cell-like diffuse large cell lymphomas. Proc Natl Acad Sci U S A 2000;97:10209–13.
7. Lenz G, Wright G, Dave SS, et al. Stromal gene signatures in large-B-cell lymphomas. N Engl J Med 2008;359:2313–23.
8. Fu K, Weisenburger DD, Choi WW, et al. Addition of rituximab to standard chemotherapy improves the survival of both the germinal center B-cell-like and non-germinal center B-cell-like subtypes of diffuse large B-cell lymphoma. J Clin Oncol 2008;26:4587–94.
9. Lenz G, Wright GW, Emre NC, et al. Molecular subtypes of diffuse large B-cell lymphoma arise by distinct genetic pathways. Proc Natl Acad Sci U S A 2008;105:13520–5.
10. Hans CP, Weisenburger DD, Greiner TC, et al. Confirmation of the molecular classification of diffuse large B-cell lymphoma by immunohistochemistry using a tissue microarray. Blood 2004;103:275–82.
11. Lossos IS, Alizadeh AA, Rajapaksa R, Tibshirani R, Levy R. HGAL is a novel interleukin-4-inducible gene that strongly predicts survival in diffuse large B-cell lymphoma. Blood 2003;101:433–40.
12. Natkunam Y, Farinha P, Hsi ED, et al. LMO2 protein expression predicts survival in patients with diffuse large B-cell lymphoma treated with anthracycline-based chemotherapy with and without rituximab. J Clin Oncol 2008;26:447–54.
13. Banham AH, Connors JM, Brown PJ, et al. Expression of the FOXP1 transcription factor is strongly associated with inferior survival in patients with diffuse large B-cell lymphoma. Clin Cancer Res 2005;11:1065–72.
14. Savage KJ, Monti S, Kutok JL, et al. The molecular signature of mediastinal large B-cell lymphoma differs from that of other diffuse large B-cell lymphomas and shares features with classical Hodgkin lymphoma. Blood 2003;102:3871–9.
15. Boudova L, Torlakovic E, Delabie J, et al. Nodular lymphocyte-predominant Hodgkin lymphoma with nodules resembling T-cell/histiocyte-rich B-cell lymphoma: differential diagnosis between nodular lymphocyte-predominant Hodgkin lymphoma and T-cell/histiocyte-rich B-cell lymphoma. Blood 2003;102:3753–8.
16. Delsol G, Lamant L, Mariame B, et al. A new subtype of large B-cell lymphoma expressing the ALK kinase and lacking the 2; 5 translocation. Blood 1997;89:1483–90.

17. Montesinos-Rongen M, Siebert R, Deckert M. Primary lymphoma of the central nervous system: just DLBCL or not? Blood 2009;113:7–10.

18. Hoefnagel JJ, Dijkman R, Basso K, et al. Distinct types of primary cutaneous large B-cell lymphoma identified by gene expression profiling. Blood 2005;105:3671–8.

19. Delecluse HJ, Anagnostopoulos I, Dallenbach F, et al. Plasmablastic lymphomas of the oral cavity: a new entity associated with the human immunodeficiency virus infection. Blood 1997;89:1413–20.

20. Dong HY, Scadden DT, de Leval L, Tang Z, Isaacson PG, Harris NL. Plasmablastic lymphoma in HIV-positive patients: an aggressive Epstein–Barr virus-associated extramedullary plasmacytic neoplasm. Am J Surg Pathol 2005;29:1633–41.

21. Nador RG, Cesarman E, Chadburn A, et al. Primary effusion lymphoma: a distinct clinicopathologic entity associated with the Kaposi's sarcoma-associated herpes virus. Blood 1996;88:645–56.

22. Oyama T, Ichimura K, Suzuki R, et al. Senile EBV + B-cell lymphoproliferative disorders: a clinicopathologic study of 22 patients. Am J Surg Pathol 2003;27:16–26.

23. Du MQ, Liu H, Diss TC, et al. Kaposi sarcoma-associated herpesvirus infects monotypic (IgM lambda) but polyclonal naive B cells in Castleman disease and associated lymphoproliferative disorders. Blood 2001;97:2130–6.

24. Lin P, Medeiros LJ. High-grade B-cell lymphoma/leukemia associated with t(14;18) and 8q24/MYC rearrangement: a neoplasm of germinal center immunophenotype with poor prognosis. Haematologica 2007;92:1297–301.

25. Leucci E, Cocco M, Onnis A, et al. MYC translocation-negative classical Burkitt lymphoma cases: an alternative pathogenetic mechanism involving miRNA deregulation. J Pathol 2008;216:440–50.

26. Dave SS, Fu K, Wright GW, et al. Molecular diagnosis of Burkitt's lymphoma. N Engl J Med 2006;354:2431–42.

27. Hummel M, Bentink S, Berger H, et al. A biologic definition of Burkitt's lymphoma from transcriptional and genomic profiling. N Engl J Med 2006;354:2419–30.

28. Traverse-Glehen A, Pittaluga S, Gaulard P, et al. Mediastinal gray zone lymphoma: the missing link between classic Hodgkin's lymphoma and mediastinal large B-cell lymphoma. Am J Surg Pathol 2005;29:1411–21.

Chapter 18

Therapy of B-cell Lymphoproliferative Disorders

Nathan Fowler, Sandra Horowitz, and Peter McLaughlin

Abstract/Scope of Chapter The majority (>80%) of both aggressive and indolent variants of NHL are of B-cell origin, and their treatment is discussed in this chapter. Therapeutic options range from close observation with intervention only with disease progression to treatment at diagnosis with intensive multiagent regimens. With the development of new chemotherapeutic regimens and advances in supportive care, improved outcomes are becoming apparent. The introduction of antibody immunotherapy, immunomodulatory agents, and small molecules that target lymphoma signaling pathways are leading to further customized therapies.

Keywords Lymphoma, B-cell, therapy • CHOP chemotherapy • Targeted therapy • B-cell lymphomas • Immunotherapy • antibody use in lymphoma • Pharmacogenetics • B-cell lymphoma

18.1. Introduction

Non-Hodgkin's lymphoma (NHL) is expected to be diagnosed in over 60,000 new patients in 2009 in the United States [1]. The vast majority (>80%) of both aggressive and indolent variants of NHLs are of B-cell origin (Fig. 18-1)[2] and are discussed in this chapter. The treatment of Hodgkin lymphoma and T-cell neoplasms are discussed in Chaps. 21 and 23, respectively.

Although some patients will attain prolonged progression-free survival with standard therapeutic regimens, many others will ultimately relapse and die of their disease. Despite the development of new chemotherapeutic agents and advances in supportive care that have improved responses and overall survival, improvements in therapy are needed [3, 4]. Here, we summarize the standard cytotoxic chemotherapeutic regimens and their variants, but also explore the more recent introduction of antibody immunotherapy and targeted agents into both frontline and salvage regimens.

18.2. Clinical Workup and Staging

The initial workup of patients with newly diagnosed NHL includes a complete physical exam with a focus on common nodal sites such as the neck, axilla, and groin, as well as attention to the size of the spleen and liver. An excisional biopsy of a lymph node or involved extranodal site is almost always required for definitive diagnosis and subclassification of lymphoma and should be obtained whenever possible [5]. A fine needle aspirate (FNA) is generally not

From: *Neoplastic Hematopathology*: Contemporary Hematology,
Edited by: D. Jones, DOI 10.1007/978-1-60761-384-8_18,
© Humana Press, a part of Springer Science+Business Media, LLC 2010

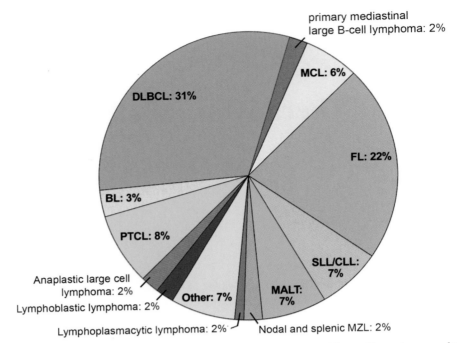

Fig. 18-1. Incidence of non-Hodgkin lymphoma subtypes in the United States. Percentages are derived from the 2001 WHO classification of Tumors of the Hematopoietic and Lymphoid Tissues (IARC Press). Lymphoblastic leukemia is not included. However, there is considerable geographic and age-related variation in the incidence of different lymphoma types. Abbreviations are as in Table 18-1

Table 18-1. Staging procedures for common non-Hodgkin lymphoma (NHL) types.

Subtype	Physical exam, focus on nodal sites, spleen	CT neck, chest, abdomen, pelvis	PET/CT scan	BM aspirate and biopsy	Upper and lower endoscopy	Lumbar puncture
DLBCL	+	+	+	+	−	+, if HIV+, testicular or epidural involvement, >2 extranodal sites
BL	+	+	+	+	−	+
FL	+	+	+/−	+	−	−
MZL (MALT)	+	+	+/−	+	+	−
MCL	+	+	+	+	+	+, if blastoid variant or neurologic symptoms
SLL/CLL	+	+	+/−	+	−	−

DLBCL diffuse large B-cell lymphoma, *BL* Burkitt lymphoma, *FL* follicular lymphoma, *MZL* marginal zone lymphoma of mucosal-associated lymphoid tissue (MALT) type, *MCL* mantle cell lymphoma, *SLL* small lymphocytic lymphoma, *CLL* chronic lymphocytic leukemia, +/− testing optional, −testing not required

acceptable for diagnosis, but with the addition of a large caliber needle biopsy can sometimes be adequate. For the majority of lymphoma subtypes, baseline CT and PET scans should be performed (Table 18-1). [6, 7] Sampling of the cerebrospinal fluid (CSF) should also be obtained in lymphomas with high-grade cytomorphology, testicular primaries, and those arising in patients with human immunodeficiency virus (HIV) infection. Bone marrow aspirate and biopsy should be performed on all patients, with flow cytometry performed on aspirate samples. Cytogenetic analysis is useful in suspected high-grade malignancies to distinguish

Table 18-2. Ann Arbor staging system [6].

Stage	Distribution of Disease
I	Involvement of a single lymph node region (I) or involvement of a single extralymphatic site or organ (I-E)
II	Involvement of two or more lymph node regions on the same side of the diaphragm (II) or with involvement of limited contiguous extralymphatic organ or tissue (II-E)
III	Involvement of lymph node regions on both sides of the diaphragm (III), which may include the spleen (IIIs) and or limited contiguous extralymphatic organ or site (III-E).
IV	Multiple or disseminated foci of involvement of one or more extralymphatic organs or tissues with or without lymphatic involvement.

Burkitt lymphoma, and diffuse large B-cell lymphoma from other aggressive hematopoietic tumors.

The most widely accepted lymphoma staging systems utilize an anatomic schema such as the Ann Arbor classification (Table 18-2). [6] Other staging approaches for aggressive lymphoma, such as the Murphy score often utilized for Burkitt lymphoma (BL) in children, are discussed in Chap. 17. Risk stratification scores have been developed for common lymphomas types, including the international prognostic index (IPI) in diffuse large B-cell lymphoma (DLBCL, Chap. 17), and the follicular lymphoma IPI (FLIPI, Chap. 16). These scores are useful in identifying patients with high risk of relapse and/or disease progression and may guide the use of additional diagnostic and disease monitoring as well as timing of treatment.

18.3. Therapy

18.3.1. Treatment Versus Observation

There are various management options for patients with newly-diagnosed B cell lymphoma, and the clinician's decision is often influenced by the presentation, stage, and classification of disease. While patients with indolent NHL can often be observed for prolonged periods without treatment, patients with intermediate or aggressive disease require prompt combination therapy. In cases of localized (stage I and II) disease, there can also be a role for radiation therapy, frequently in conjunction with chemotherapy.

18.3.2. Combination Cytotoxic Chemotherapy

The treatment of NHL underwent a major advance with the development of combination chemotherapy regimens utilizing agents with different mechanisms of action and toxicity profiles (Table 18-3). By combining cytotoxic agents of differing classes, there is a potential to overcome resistance while minimizing side effects. In addition, preclinical studies have demonstrated increased apoptosis rates as well as a synergistic effect between several classes of anti-neoplastic agents such as alkylating agents and anthracyclines (Table 18-4). Although current intensive chemotherapy approaches are designed to be preferentially toxic to the malignancy due to its intrinsic growth and apoptotic properties, all regimens also carry risks of toxicity to, and mutagenesis of, nonneoplastic cells.

There are a large variety of commonly-used multiagent chemotherapeutic regimens in the treatment of NHL (See Tables 18-4 and 18-5 for a listing of drugs in various combinations). Although CHOP, with the addition of anti-CD20 immunotherapy (rituximab/Rituxan), is the most commonly-used therapy for DLBCL, different combinations may be employed for other NHL subtypes. For example, the more intensive hyper-CVAD regimen is now commonly used for mantle cell lymphoma, lymphoblastic lymphoma, BL, and aggressive variants of DLBCL. CLL/SLL and other low-grade NHLs may be effectively treated by 3-drug

Table 18-3. Mechanisms of action of common chemotherapy classes.

Drug Class	Mechanism of Action	Examples
Alkylating agents	Active metabolites alkylate DNA through the formation of reactive intermediates which form covalent linkages with various nucleophilic groups (e.g., phosphate, amino, sulfhydryl, hydroxyl groups). Inhibition of DNA synthesis and function.	Cyclophosphamide, Ifosfamide
Antimetabolites: Folate antagonists	Inhibition of dihydrofolate reductase enzyme leads to the depletion of critical reduced folate and a resultant inhibition of DNA, RNA, thymidylate and purine synthesis.	Methotrexate
Deoxycytidine analogs	Active metabolites are incorporated into DNA during replication and result in strand termination and inhibition of DNA synthesis and function. Additionally, DNA polymerases are inhibited; leading to disruption of DNA chain elongation, synthesis and repair.	Cytarabine (Ara-C); Gemcitabine
Purine analogs	Active metabolites are incorporated into DNA, inhibiting DNA chain extension. DNA synthesis is inhibited via the inhibition of ribonucleotide reductase and DNA polymerases.	Fludarabine Pentostatin
Anthracyclines	Bind to DNA by intercalation between DNA strands inhibiting DNA synthesis and function. Inhibit topoisomerase II and DNA-dependent RNA polymerase leading to DNA breaks and faulty DNA replication and transcription. Form iron-doxorubicin complexes via iron chelation which bind to DNA and produce free radicals that cleave DNA strands.	Doxorubicin Mitoxantrone
Vinca alkaloids	Disrupt the assembly of microtubules by inhibiting tubulin polymerization. This results in mitotic arrest in metaphase, ultimately leading to cell death.	Vincristine
Epipodophyllotoxins	Inhibit topoisomerase II by stabilizing topoisomerase II-DNA complexes. Prevents DNA unwinding and results in the inhibition of DNA synthesis.	Etoposide
Corticosteroids	Directly toxic to lymphocytes	Dexamethasone
Platinum analogs	Covalently bind to DNA, forming intra- and interstrand DNA cross-links. Leads to DNA breakage and inhibition of DNA synthesis.	Cisplatin; Carboplatin
Taxanes	Promote microtubule assembly and stability and prevent microtubule disassembly. Interfere with mitosis; inhibiting cell replication and inducing apoptosis in dividing cells.	Paclitaxel; Docetaxel

combinations such as CVP, FND, or FCR. There are also considerable variations in dosing and drug combinations (Table 18-5) and in the number of cycles of chemotherapy given.

18.3.3. Targeted Therapy of Lymphoproliferative Disorders with Monoclonal Antibodies

The development of targeted antibody therapies directed against surface B-cell antigens on the malignant lymphoma cell has revolutionized the treatment of NHL (Fig. 18-2). The widespread application of monoclonal antibody therapy was made possible with the development of hybridomas and recombinant engineering technology allowing the production of large quantities of both chimeric and native antibodies [8]. Antibody reagents may be used alone or conjugated to radionuclide or toxins, and produce their effects through antibody-dependent cytotoxicity, complement-mediated cytotoxicity, or direct apoptotic effects due to antagonist or agonist action (Table 18-6). In lymphoma therapy, this is most prominently represented by the use of antibody reagents directed against the pan-B-cell marker CD20 (such as rituximab and ibritumomab tiuxetan/Zevalin), but other antigens such as CD19, CD22, CD25, and CD30 have also been effectively targeted. The majority of antibodies in

Table 18-4. Combination chemotherapy regimens.

Acronym	Agents	Typical disease utilization	Frontline or salvage
COP/CVP [16]	Cyclophosphamide, vincristine, prednisone	Indolent B-NHL, CLL	Both
FCR	Fludarabine, cyclophosphamide, rituximab	CLL	Mainly frontline
CHOP [17] +/− rituximab	COP agents, plus: doxorubicin	DLBCL; indolent B-NHL	Both
EPOCH [18]	CHOP agents, plus: etoposide	HIV-related lymphoma; MCL, DLBCL	Mainly frontline
Hyper-CVAD [18] +/− rituximab	CHOP agents with dexamethasone (instead of prednisone), alternating with methotrexate and cytarabine	MCL, BL, lymphoblastic lymphoma, and other aggressive lymphomas	Both
CODOX-M/IVAC [19]	CHOP agents, minus: prednisone; plus: mid-cycle high dose methotrexate alternating with ifosfamide, mesna, etoposide, cytarabine (IVAC)	BL	Frontline
ACVBP [3]	CHOP agents; with bleomycin and vindesine[a] (instead of vincristine)	DLBCL	Frontline
FND [20]	Fludarabine, mitoxantrone, dexamethasone	Indolent B-NHL or MCL	Both
DHAP [18]	Dexamethasone, cytarabine, cisplatin	DLBCL	Salvage
ICE [18]	Ifosfamide, mesna, carboplatin, etoposide	DLBCL	Salvage
MINE [21]	Mesna, ifosfamide, mitoxantrone, etoposide	Indolent B-NHL or DLBCL	Salvage
R-GemOx[b] [18]	Rituximab, gemcitabine, oxaliplatin	DLBCL	Salvage
TTR[b] [18]	Topotecan, paclitaxel, rituximab	DLBCL	Salvage

Lymphoma abbreviations are as in Table 18-1

[a] Vindesine not available in the United States

[b] Some regimens developed mainly or only in the rituximab era; virtually all others can be given in conjunction with rituximab, e.g., the R-CHOP regimen

Table 18-5. Variants of chemotherapy regimens.

Basic regimen[a]	Variant acronym	Notable differences
CHOP	CHOP-14 [18]	CHOP regimen given every 14 days instead the standard 21 day cycle.
	m-BACOD [17]	Low dose methotrexate, bleomycin added, dexamethasone instead of prednisone
	MACOP-B [17]	Methotrexate, bleomycin added
DHAP	ESHAP [18]	Etoposide added, methylprednisolone (instead of dexamethasone)
	ASHAP [18]	Doxorubicin added, methylprednisolone (instead of dexamethasone)
FND	FN [20]	Dexamethasone deleted
	FC [20]	Cyclophosphamide added; mitoxantrone and dexamethasone deleted
	PCR [22]	Pentostatin (instead of fludarabine), cyclophosphamide, rituximab; mitoxantrone and dexamethasone deleted
	R-FCM [20]	Rituximab and cyclophosphamide added; dexamethasone deleted

[a] See Table 18-4 for comparison

use therapeutically target markers that are expressed on most normal B cells as well as lymphoma cells, but more recent reagents have targeted the activation and signaling molecules that tend to be preferentially upregulated in lymphoma.

Problems with antibody-based immunotherapy can include antigen shedding or modulation (e.g., CD20 loss on lymphoma cells at relapse following rituximab) and the development of neutralizing antibodies due to an immune reaction against the antibody itself. These difficulties have been progressively overcome with the identification of the most stably-expressed antigenic targets, modulation of the dose and duration of immunotherapy, and reengineering of therapeutic antibodies to be fully humanized or defucosylated. As a result, monoclonal antibody therapy has now become integrated into the majority of newly-diagnosed and relapsed treatment regimens for lymphoma [8]. Although the addition of antibody immunotherapy (particularly rituximab) has improved outcomes for both indolent B-cell NHL and DLBCL, recurrent disease may lack the antigen target requiring the use of a different therapeutic antibody in the relapse setting.

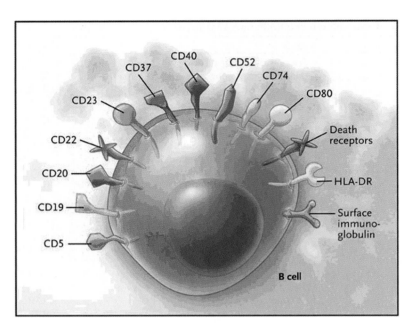

Fig. 18-2. Antigen targets on the surface of a B cell. Image reprinted with permission from: Cheson B, Leonard J. N Engl J Med 2008;359:613–26

Table 18-6. Monoclonal antibodies used as immunotherapeutics [8].

Antibody Target	Antibody Construct	Example(s)
CD20	Naked antibody	Rituximab
	Radioimmunotherapy	Tositumomab, ibritumomab tiuxetan
CD22	Naked antibody	Epratuzumab
	Immunotoxin	CMC-544[a]
CD52	Naked antibody	Alemtuzumab
CD25	Immunotoxin	Denileukin diftitox
CD80	Naked antibody	Galiximab[a]
CD40	Naked antibody	SGN-40[a]

[a]Investigational agent

18.3.4. Toxicities of Common Lymphoma Therapies

Chemotherapy regimens used to treat lymphoma are associated with a unique set of toxicities as well as common side effects such as myelosuppression, alopecia, mucositis, nausea, and vomiting. Secondary immunosuppression due to chemotherapy effects on normal immune cells can lead to the reactivation of latent infections, such as herpesviruses and hepatitis B and C, or put patients at risk for infection from opportunistic organisms. Some agents, such as doxorubicin and vincristine, can cause significant local damage with direct tissue exposure (e.g., infiltration of intravenous catheters).

Tumor lysis syndrome (TLS) is a rare but dramatic "toxicity" which is occasionally seen with initial treatment of aggressive lymphomas. The release of intracellular potassium, phosphate, uric acid, and cellular debris can overwhelm the kidneys' capacity to maintain homeostasis, leading to electrolyte abnormalities, acute renal failure and in rare cases, multiorgan failure. Careful monitoring as well as prophylaxis with hydration, allopurinol, alkalinization of the urine, or rasburicase can prevent the majority of severe presentations and their sequelae (Table 18-7).

Excellent countermeasures exist for many of the above mentioned toxicities. For example, the National Comprehensive Cancer Network (NCCN) and the American Society of Clinical Oncology (ASCO) have developed supportive care guidelines for the use of antiemetics and

Table 18-7. Common drug-related toxicities and countermeasures [23].

Drug	Toxicity	Prophylaxis/countermeasure
Bortezomib	Peripheral neuropathy	• Discontinue/decrease dose if symptoms persist/worsen
Cisplatin	Nephrotoxicity and associated magnesium wasting Neuropathy	• Aggressive hydration • Monitor serum creatinine and magnesium levels • Neurologic monitoring • Dose discontinuation/adjustment
Cytarabine	Rash, fever, myalgias	• Premedication with corticosteroids
Doxorubicin Mitoxantrone	Cardiomyopathy	• Administer as continuous infusion vs bolus • Do not exceed lifetime dose of approx. 450 mg/m^2 • Monitor cardiac function
Ifosfamide Cyclophosphamide	Hemorrhagic cystitis	• Aggressive hydration with concurrent use of mesna
Methotrexate	Nephrotoxicity Hepatotoxicity, mucositis, bone marrow suppression	• Aggressive hydration with alkalinization of urine • Timed leucovorin rescue
Vincristine Vinblastine	Peripheral neuropathy	• Max dose of vincristine 2 mg/cycle • Discontinue/decrease dose if symptoms persist/worsen
Rituximab other monoclonal antibodies	Infusion related hypersensitivity: fever, chills (typically first-dose effect)	• Interrupt/decrease rate of infusion • Premedicate with acetaminophen/diphenhydramine

growth factors in the management of nausea and vomiting, and myelosuppression, respectively [9]. Guidelines for the prevention and management of TLS have also been proposed [10].

18.3.5. Drug Interactions

Oncology patients are at high risk for drug-drug interactions due to the multiple medications they receive (e.g., chemotherapeutics, antiemetics, over the counter medications, pain medications). Given the toxic nature and narrow therapeutic index of chemotherapeutic agents, an awareness of potential drug-drug interactions is essential in minimizing drug toxicity and maximizing efficacy. Drug-drug interactions may be classified as pharmaceutical, pharmacokinetic, or pharmacodynamic. Pharmaceutical interactions occur when two or more compounds interact due to physical and/or chemical incompatibilities (e.g., the precipitation of ondansetron when it is combined with bicarbonate). Pharmacokinetic interactions arise when one drug interferes with the absorption, distribution, metabolism, or elimination of another drug (e.g., drug interactions involving the metabolizing cytochrome P450 system), such as the concurrent use of voriconazole and vincristine. Pharmacodynamic interactions occur with two or more drugs that influence the same physiologic outcome. Pharmacodynamic effects can be broadly classified as antagonistic, additive, or synergistic. The favorable pharmacodynamic drug-drug interactions form the basis for many combination chemotherapy regimens.

It has long been recognized that patients respond differently to chemotherapy, both in terms of response and toxicity. The study of pharmacogenomics has emerged to study the specific genetic polymorphisms in drug targets, drug transporters and metabolizing enzymes. By identifying individual polymorphisms, we may hope to be able to predict the safety and efficacy of a particular drug in individual patients and therefore ultimately develop a more individualized approach to lymphoma treatment.

18.4. Assessment of Response to Therapy

Response to initial therapy is usually assessed after 2–3 cycles of systemic treatment and at the end of treatment, unless early progression is suspected. CT imaging of the neck, chest, abdomen, and pelvis is recommended with attention to known sites of disease and major lymphoid organs. PET scanning is also increasingly being used for response assessment in some lymphomas, notably DLBCL [11]. While PET scanning can potentially identify sites of residual disease, there is little evidence to support a change in therapy based upon PET findings alone [11]. Bone marrow aspiration and biopsy are recommended at the completion of therapy in patients with known marrow involvement at diagnosis.

18.5. Treatment of Relapsed Lymphoma

Histologic confirmation is essential to distinguish relapsed lymphoma from a second malignancy or a nonneoplastic process and to detect transformation to a more aggressive form. When relapse is confirmed, staging, methods are similar to those used at diagnosis. Because of the potential risk of additive cardiotoxicity, patients with prior anthracycline use should also have repeat cardiac function testing.

The options for treatment in patients with relapsed disease are varied. When deciding on a course of treatment, several factors should be weighed carefully. Examples include the performance status of the patient, the amount, type, and response to prior therapy, the location of relapse, and the goals of treatment (curative vs. palliative). If a patient experiences a relapse soon after initial therapy, the choice of systemic therapy is often made with a search for non-cross resistant or differing classes of chemotherapeutics.

The role of high-dose chemotherapy followed by hematopoietic stem cell transplant for patients with relapsed or refractory disease is evolving. Ample literature demonstrates a benefit in the long-term outcomes in patients with aggressive NHL treated with autologous stem cell transplant (ASCT) in the second remission following systemic therapy [12]. With relapsed indolent lymphomas, there may be a benefit from allogeneic transplantation in young patients with good performance status [13]. Clinical trials are underway to further define the ideal role of hematopoietic stem cell transplant in the setting of relapsed and/or refractory indolent NHL. In light of the impact of ASCT in the setting of relapse, studies have also explored the use of front-line ASCT as a consolidation approach for high-risk patients. This approach has gained acceptance in only a few settings (e.g., mantle cell lymphoma) [14].

18.6. Investigational Agents in Lymphoma: Targeting Growth and Death Pathways

Newer therapies are often directed at mechanisms that are known to be dysregulated in a significant number of lymphomas, such as cell cycle and growth regulatory pathways, programmed cell death, and intracellular protein assembly/degradation. Reactivation of tumor suppressor genes through epigenetic approaches (e.g., hypomethylating agents and histone deacetylase inhibitors) and targeting the microenvironment through the use of immunomodulatory drugs (IMiDs) are both areas of active research [15].

One example of a new approach to therapy is targeting the nuclear factor kappa (NF-k) B pathway through proteasome inhibition. The 26S proteasome is an intracellular protein degradation structure. Among its many protein substrates is phosphorylated IkB, which normally complexes with NF-kB. The proteasomal degradation of IkB, an inhibitor of NF-kB, permits free NF-kB to move from the cytoplasm into the nucleus, where it can activate proliferation and/or anti-apoptotic genes; an action which is opposed by proteasome inhibitors. NF-kB family genes are dysregulated in many B-cell malignancies, ranging from myeloma to some subtypes of DLBCL. Therapy with proteasome inhibitors can lead to sequestration in the cytoplasm of the NF-kB-IkB complex, thereby preventing the nuclear signaling of free NF-kB [15].

Table 18-8 lists several other examples of biological pathways for which targeted therapeutic approaches are under development. It is clear that advances in our understanding of lymphoma biology are leading to new therapies. Examples include dysregulation of

Table 18-8. Promising targets for therapy in lymphoma [24].

Target	Signaling pathway impacted	Agent	Candidate lymphoma subtypes
Mammalian target of rapamycin (mTOR)	PI3K/Akt	Temsirolimus	MCL; other NHL
26S proteasome	NF-kB; others	Bortezomib	MCL; other NHL
Cyclin-dependent kinases (CDK)	G1-S cell cycle progression	Flavopiridol, roscovitine	MCL; other NHL
SYK kinase	B-cell receptor (BCR)	Fostamatinib disodium	CLL; DLBCL
Protein kinase C (PKC)	BCR and PI3K/Akt	Enzastaurin	DLBCL; other NHL
Bcl-6	Germinal center B cell transcriptional program	B peptide inhibitor	DLBCL
Immunomodulatory drugs (IMiDs)	T-cell activation, tumor-associated microenvironment	Lenalidomide, thalidomide	MCL; other NHL
Bcl-2 and related anti-apoptotic factors	Intrinsic and extrinsic apoptotic pathways	Oblimersen	FL, other NHL

Abbreviations as in Table 18-1

the anti-apoptotic protein Bcl-2 in follicular lymphoma, the cell cycle regulatory cyclin D1 pathway in MCL, and the B-cell receptor signaling abnormalities in some cases of DLBCL. It is also clear that we have much to learn since agents developed against a specific target are often found to have off-target effects. Therefore, careful clinical research needs to be linked with the laboratory advances.

References

1. Jemal A, Siegel R, Ward E, et al. Cancer statistics, 2008. Ca Cancer J Clin 2008;58:71–96.
2. Swerdlow S, Campo E, Harris N, eds. World health organization classification of tumours of haematopoietic and lymphoid tissues. IARC Press: Lyon, 2008.
3. Coiffier B. State-of-the-art therapeutics: diffuse large B-cell lymphoma. J Clin Oncol 2005;23:6387–93.
4. Swenson W, Wooldridge J, Lynch C, Forman-Hoffman V, Chrischilles E, Link B. Improved survival of follicular lymphoma patients in the united states. J Clin Oncol 2005;23:5019–26.
5. Gascoyne R. Establishing the diagnosis of lymphoma: from initial biopsy to clinical staging. Oncology 1998;10:11–6.
6. Lister TA, Crowther D, Sutcliffe SB. et al "Report of a committee convened to discuss the evaluation and staging of patients with Hodgkin's disease: Cotswolds meeting". J Clin Oncol 1989;11:1630–6.
7. Cheson B, Pfistner B, Juweid M, et al. Revised Response Criteria for Malignant Lymphoma. J Clin Oncol 2007;25:579–86.
8. Cheson B, Leonard J. Monoclonal antibody therapy for B-cell non-Hodgkin's lymphoma. N Engl J Med 2008;359:613–26.
9. 2008/2009 National Comprehensive Cancer Center Guidelines. (Accessed March 12, 2009, at: http://www.nccn.org/professionals/physician_gls/f_guidelines.asp)
10. Coiffier B, Altman A, Pui C, Younes A, Cairo M. Guidelines for the Management of Pediatric and Adult Tumor Lysis Syndrome: An Evidence-Based Review. J Clin Oncol 2008;16:2767–78.
11. Juweid M, Stroobants S, Hoekstra O, et al. Use of Positron Emission Tomography for Response Assessment of Lymphoma: Consensus of the Imaging Subcommittee of International Harmonization Project in Lymphoma. J Clin Oncol 2007;25:571–8.
12. Philip T, Guglielmi C, Hagenbeek A, et al. Autologous bone marrow transplantation as compared with salvage chemotherapy in relapses of chemotherapy-sensitive non-Hodgkin's lymphoma. N Engl J Med 1995;333:1540–5.
13. Khouri I, Saliba R, Hosing C, et al Autologous stem cell vs nonmyeloablative allogeneic transplantation after high-dose rituximab-containing conditioning regimens for relapsed chemosensitive follicular lymphoma. Blood 2005; 106:19a, (abstr 48).
14. Dreyling M, Lenz G, Hoster E, et al. Early consolidation by myeloablative radiochemotherapy followed by autologous stem cell transplantation in first remission significantly prolongs progression-free survival in mantle-cell lymphoma: Results of a prospective randomized trial of the European MCL Network. Blood 2005;105:2677–84.

15. Johnson P. New targets for lymphoma treatment. Ann Oncol 2008;19 Suppl 4;56-9.

16. Marcus R, Imrie K, Belch A, et al. CVP chemotherapy plus rituximab compared with CVP as first-line treatment for advanced follicular lymphoma. Blood 2005;105:1417-1423.

17. Fisher RI, Gaynor ER, Dahlberg S, et al. Comparison of a standard regimen (CHOP) with three intensive chemotherapy regimens for advanced non-Hodgkin's lymphoma. N Engl J Med 1993;328:1002–6.

18. Gisselbrecht C. Use of rituximab in diffuse large B-cell lymphoma in the salvage setting. Br J Hemae 2008;143:607–21.

19. Perkins A, Friedberg J. Burkitt lymphoma in adults. Hematology 2008;1:341–8.

20. Anderson V, Perry C. Fludarabine: A review of its use in non-Hodgkin's lymphoma. Drugs. 2007;67:1633–55.

21. Rodriguez MA, Cabanillas FC, Hagemeister FB, et al. A phase II trial of mesna/ifosfamide, mitoxantrone and etoposide for refractory lymphomas. Ann Oncol 1995;6:609–11.

22. Samaniego F, Fanale M, et al. Pentostatin, Cyclophosphamide, and Rituximab (PCR) Achieve High Response Rates in Indolent B-Cell Lymphoma without Prolonged Myelosuppression. Blood 2008;112:835.

23. Zinzani P. Salvage Chemotherapy in Follicular Non-Hodgkin's Lymphoma: Focus on Tolerability. Clin Lymph & Myeloma 2006;7:115–24.

24. Abramson J, Shipp M. Advances in the biology and therapy of diffuse large B-cell lymphoma: moving toward a molecularly targeted approach. Blood 2005;106:1164–74.

Chapter 19

Plasma Cell Myeloma and Other Plasma Cell Dyscrasias

Marwan A. Yared

Scope of Chapter/Abstract This chapter covers plasma cell neoplasms, including plasma cell myeloma and lymphoplasmacytic lymphoma (LPL)/ Waldenström macroglobulinemia (WM) involving the bone marrow. LPL involving extramedullary sites is discussed in Chap. 15.

Keywords Plasma cell myeloma • Multiple myeloma • Myeloma, smoldering • Myeloma, non-secretory • Plasma cell leukemia • Plasmacytoma • Amyloidosis, primary • Paraprotein • Myeloma, gene expression profiling • Myeloma, minimal residual disease • Myeloma, IGH translocations • Myeloma, staging systems, lymphoplasmacytic lymphoma • Waldenström macroglobulinemia • M-protein • Flow cytometry, DNA content/ploidy analysis • Cyclin D1, myeloma • Plasma cell myeloma, cyclin group • Plasma cell myeloma, MAF group • Plasma cell myeloma, anueploidy

19.1. Overview of Plasma Cell Neoplasms

Plasma cell neoplasms encompass a group of diseases with varying clinical manifestations but with at least one common feature, the production by neoplastic plasma cells with a monoclonal immunoglobulin protein (M-protein, or paraprotein). These diseases include plasma cell myeloma (PCM) (and its clinical variants), solitary plasmacytoma of bone, extraosseous plasmacytoma, and the monoclonal immunoglobulin deposition diseases (primary amyloidosis and monoclonal light and heavy chain deposition diseases) (Fig. 19-1). The clinical variants of PCM now recognized by the World Health Organization (WHO) are symptomatic PCM, asymptomatic PCM (also known as smoldering PCM), nonsecretory myeloma, and plasma cell leukemia (PCL).

PCM will be the primary focus of this chapter, but other plasma cell neoplasms enter into the differential diagnosis. Solitary plasmacytoma of bone lacks evidence of systemic dissemination or diagnostic features of PCM, but can undergo progression to myeloma. Extraosseous plasmacytoma is restricted to extramedullary tissues, most frequently the upper respiratory tract, usually only produces symptoms related to its mass effect, and rarely progresses to PCM. Primary amyloidosis is the deposition of immunoglobulin light chain aggregates that show apple-green birefringence on a Congo red stain (i.e., AL amyloid) and usually sparse clonal plasma cell proliferations. Clinical manifestations of the effects of amyloid on producing organ or tissue dysfunction include nephrotic syndrome, heart failure, malabsorption, peripheral neuropathy, and bleeding disorders. The related light and heavy chain deposition diseases are due to deposition of non-birefrigent immunoglobulin and produce a similar range of effects although their ultrastructural appearance is different than amyloid. These include the immunoglobulin "heavy chain deposition" disorders which

From: *Neoplastic Hematopathology*: Contemporary Hematology,
Edited by: D. Jones, DOI 10.1007/978-1-60761-384-8_19,
© Humana Press, a part of Springer Science+Business Media, LLC 2010

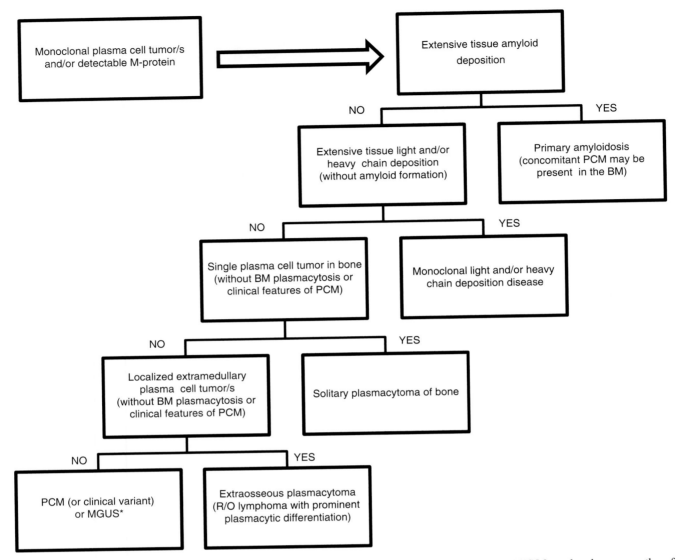

Fig. 19-1. An algorithmic approach to the diagnosis of plasma cell neoplasms. *BM* Bone marrow, *MGUS* Monoclonal gammopathy of undetermined significance, *PCM* Plasma cell myeloma, *R/O* Rule out.*See Fig. 19-2 for diagnostic algorithm of PCM, its clinical variants, and MGUS

are different from "heavy chain disease," which is a variant of intestinal marginal zone lymphoma of MALT type that has plasmacytic differentiation (see Chap. 15).

Although considered to be a plasma cell dyscrasia because neoplastic plasma cells are part of the disease, lymphoplasmacytic lymphoma (LPL) is spectrum neoplasm composed of variable numbers of B cells with plasmacytoid differentiation and plasma cells, which often but do not always produce an IgM paraprotein. Waldenström macroglobulinemia (WM) is defined as an IgM monoclonal gammopathy of any concentration associated with LPL involving the bone marrow (BM) [1].

Finally, monoclonal gammopathy of undetermined significance (MGUS) is considered to be a precursor lesion that may progress to a plasma cell neoplasm or LPL depending on the nature of the monoclonal protein produced.

The discussion in this chapter will focus on PCM and its clinical variants, and LPL/ WM involving the BM. Chapter 15 discusses the differential of LPL in the lymph node with marginal zone lymphoma.

19.2. Plasma Cell Myeloma

19.2.1. Definition, Incidence, Demographics, and Clinical Features

Plasma cell myeloma is a neoplasm of terminally-differentiated B cells which involves the BM in a multifocal fashion. Extramedullary disease can occur and is usually a sign of advanced disease. An M-protein is found in the serum and/or in the urine of most patients. With an estimated yearly incidence of 20,000, PCM represents 1% of all malignancies. It is more frequent in older males with a median age of 50 years and a male to female ratio of 1.4:1 and occurs twice as frequently in African Americans as in Caucasians.

The clinical features of PCM are mainly due to the accumulation of neoplastic plasma cells and/or deposition of the M-protein they produce, ultimately causing organ failure. They include the CRAB complex (signifying hypercalcemia, renal insufficiency, anemia, and bone lesions), recurring infections, polyclonal hypogammaglobulinemia, and hypoalbuminemia. Bone lesions are typically lytic, and involve the areas of the BM with the most active hematopoiesis (vertebrae, ribs, skull, pelvis, femur, clavicle, and scapula, in descending order of frequency of involvement) [2, 3].

19.2.2. Diagnostic Categories

The major and minor diagnostic criteria for PCM and its clinical variants described in the 2001 WHO classification of tumors of hematopoietic and lymphoid tissues have been modified in the 2008 WHO classification (Fig. 19-2) [2,3]. As a result, indolent myeloma,

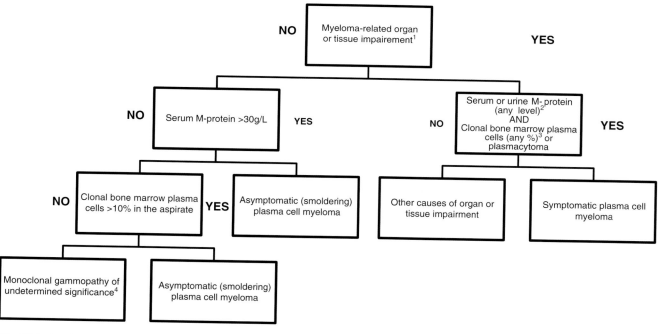

Fig. 19-2. An algorithmic approach to the diagnosis of plasma cell myeloma and its clinical variants and to MGUS, focusing on 3 primary diagnostic elements. 1. Organ and tissue impairment: CRAB (hypercalcemia, renal insufficiency, anemia, bone lesions), hyperviscosity, amyloidosis, or recurrent infections. 2. Paraprotein levels: most cases have >30 g/L of IgG or >25 g/L of IgA in the serum, or >1 g/24 h of light chain in the urine. 3. Marrow plasma cells: usually >10% of nucleated cells in the BM aspirate. 4. Low-level of plasma cells with a serum M-protein level <30 g/L

a previously recognized clinical variant of PCM, is no longer separately recognized. Retained are the categories of smoldering myeloma (now also referred to as asymptomatic PCM), non-secretory myeloma, and PCL.

The diagnosis of PCM (also referred to as symptomatic PCM) now requires the presence of manifestations of myeloma-related end organ damage, a serum or urine M-protein, and monoclonal plasma cells in the BM or plasmacytoma. Manifestations of myeloma-related end organ damage include the CRAB complex, hyperviscosity, amyloidosis, or recurrent infections. Minimum levels of serum or urine M-protein are no longer required for diagnosis. However, WHO recognizes that most cases will have >30 g/L of IgG or >25 g/L of IgA in the serum, or >1 g/24 h of urine light chain. Similarly, minimum levels of marrow involvement with clonal plasma cells are no longer required for diagnosis. Still, the WHO recognizes that most cases will have monoclonal plasma cells exceeding 10% of nucleated cells in the marrow.

The diagnosis of asymptomatic (smoldering) myeloma now requires the absence of manifestations of myeloma-related end organ damage. In addition, a serum M-protein level of >30 g/L and/or clonal plasma cells comprising 10% or more of nucleated marrow cells are required.

Non-secretory myeloma is defined as PCM without a detectable M-protein on immunofixation electrophoresis. Most such cases will however have cytoplasmic M-protein demonstrable by immunohistochemistry.

The diagnosis of PCL requires the presence of clonal plasma cells in the peripheral blood comprising 20% or more of leukocytes or exceeding 2×10^9/L. Primary PCL is present at the time of diagnosis of PCM. Secondary PCL develops at a later stage after the diagnosis of PCM is established.

19.2.3. Pathologic Features

While typically a disease of the BM, PCM can also involve extramedullary sites. Regardless of location, PCM is characterized by a proliferation of plasma cells that may or may not displace the normal architecture, depending on the pattern of involvement. BM involvement is typically multifocal and the pattern of involvement can be interstitial, nodular, paratrabecular, diffuse, or a combination of these patterns (Fig. 19-3) [4]. The plasma cell morphology is variable. Some cases show mature plasma cells with a morphology that is very similar or even identical to that of benign plasma cells with an eccentric nucleus, condensed "clock-face"

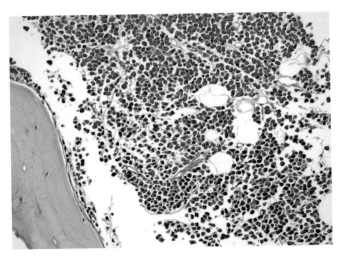

Fig. 19-3. Plasma cell myeloma, BM biopsy. An example of diffuse involvement, with sheets of plasma cells displacing normal marrow elements

chromatin, ample basophilic cytoplasm, a perinuclear clearing or hof, and no visible nucleoli. Other cases show atypical plasma cells. Features of atypical morphology may include large size, multinuclearity, irregular nuclear contour, prominent nucleoli, or frank anaplastic cyto-morphology with large bizarre nuclei (Fig. 19-4). Rarely, some cases show plasma cells with a small lymphocyte-like morphology, including small size, very high nuclear/cytoplasmic ratio with scant cytoplasm and no visible perinuclear hof, dark chromatin, and inconspicuous or absent nucleoli. Other cases show immature plasmablasts with a high nuclear/cytoplasmic ratio, scant cytoplasm with or without a perinuclear hof, non-condensed chromatin, and a central prominent nucleolus (Fig. 19-5). As discussed previously, there is no minimum levels of involvement of the BM required for the diagnosis of PCM, but most cases of symptomatic PCM have plasma cells comprising >10% of nucleated cells. Moreover, large plasma cell aggregates or sheets that displace the normal marrow elements are also indicative of involvement by PCM.

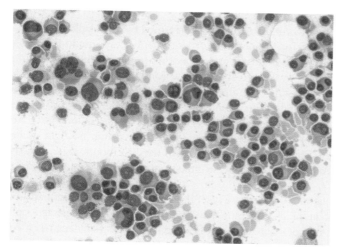

Fig. 19-4. Plasma cell myeloma, BM aspirate smear. Atypical plasma cells with irregular nuclear con-tour, multinuclearity, or bizarre nuclei. Interspersed are more mature plasma cells showing a smaller size, an eccentric nucleus with a perinuclear hof, darker chromatin, and absent nucleoli

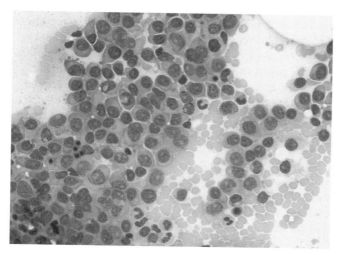

Fig. 19-5. Plasma cell myeloma, plasmablastic type, BM aspirate smear. Plasmablasts have an open chromatin, scant cytoplasm, and a prominent central nucleolus

19.2.4. Laboratory Testing for Diagnosis

The gold standard laboratory techniques for the diagnosis of PCM remain the morphologic examination of routinely-stained BM aspirate smears and biopsy sections, and analysis of the M-protein by electrophoresis, and immunofixation. In addition to these time-honored methods, relatively newer tests are available which arguably provide more accurate and sensitive methods of diagnosis, albeit at a higher cost. Some of these newer tests also allow for better characterization of the disease and include the free light chain assay, immunohisto-chemistry/in-situ hybridization, flow cytometry, conventional cytogenetics, and fluorescent in-situ hybridization (FISH).

Morphologic examination is usually performed on BM aspirate smears stained with Romanowsky's stain, and/or BM biopsy sections stained with hematoxylin and eosin (H&E). An alternative to the H&E is the periodic acid Schiff (PAS) stain. We prefer using the PAS stain since it does not stain erythrocytes thus resulting in a cleaner background, with a dark gray–violet hue to the cytoplasm making the plasma cells stand out better against myeloid precursors, which stain pink or red.

Serum and urine M-protein analysis is performed by electrophoresis and immunofixation. These methods allow for the detection, identification, and quantification of the M-protein and provide information about the polyclonal immunoglobulin and albumin content of the specimen. In addition to these tests, we now routinely perform the free light chain assay. This is an immunoassay that can detect free light chains at a much lower level (2–4 mg/L) when compared with immunofixation which can only detect light chains at a minimum level of 100–150 mg/L. This improved sensitivity allows for the detection of free light chains in cases of non-secretory myeloma and amyloidosis in which no light chains were detected by other methods. Finally, these tests are also used to monitor the post-therapy M-protein levels, which remains one of the most important markers used to monitor the course of the disease [5–7].

Immunohistochemical stains are useful in challenging or minimally-involved cases to highlight rare or atypical-appearing plasma cells not readily detected on routine staining, and to prove the monoclonal status of these cells. CD138 (syndecan-1, a collagen-1 binding proteoglycan) is strongly expressed by plasma cells and not by other cells within the BM. Immunohistochemical stains for kappa and lambda light chains allow for the relative enumeration of kappa- and lambda-expressing cells. A kappa/lambda ratio of >10 or <0.1 is considered proof of monoclonality, although several other cutoff values have been reported [8–10]. However, immunohistochemical stains for light chains, especially kappa, can produce strong, non-specific background staining. We find that in situ hybridization studies for light chains are easier to interpret with less background staining and are thus preferred for assessing the monoclonality of plasma cells in paraffin-embedded tissues.

Flow cytometric (FC) analysis of the BM aspirate should also be part of the initial diagnostic and follow-up workup of patients with PCM. FC allows for phenotyping the disease cells, as well as assessing monoclonality by analysis of their cytoplasmic immunoglobulin content. Moreover, FC allows for analyzing DNA ploidy and proliferative activity of the disease cells [8].

The phenotype of neoplastic plasma cells is somewhat different from that of normal plasma cells. Both strongly express the activation marker CD38, which is found on many other hematopoietic cells but is not as brightly expressed as it is on plasma cells, CD138, which is not expressed by other hematopoietic elements, and the B-cell marker CD79a. Plasma cells are mostly negative for the leukocyte common antigen CD45. Unlike normal plasma cells, neoplastic plasma cells are usually negative for the B-cell marker CD19 and most express the adhesion molecule CD56 (except in PCL cases which can be negative for CD56). Other markers that might be aberrantly expressed by neoplastic plasma cells are CD117, CD20, CD45, CD52, CD33, CD28, and CD10 [11–14].

DNA ploidy, measured by FC is expressed as a DNA index, obtained by dividing the DNA content of the neoplastic cells by that of the normal cells present in the same sample, with diploid cells having a DNA index of 1. Aneuploidy is further divided into the following categories: hypodiploidy when the DNA index is <0.95, corresponding to a chromosome number of up to 44–45; pseudodiploidy, when the DNA index is 0.95–1.05, corresponding to a chromosome number of 44/45 to 46/47; hyperdiploidy, with a DNA index of >1.05 and a chromosome number greater than 46/47 but ≤75; and near-tetraploidy, with a DNA index of >1.75 and a chromosome number of >75 (Table 19-1). The reported incidence of aneuploidy in PCM varies widely. In one study of more than 800 untreated cases, 54% were aneuploid. Of these, 83% were hyperdiploid, 15% were biclonal with each population showing a different ploidy, and the remaining 2% were hypodiploid [5]. The proliferative activity of plasma cells, also known as the plasma cell labeling index (PCLI), is a measure of the percentage of tumor cells in the synthetic cell cycle phase (S-phase). Measured by staining plasma cells with propidium iodide, PCLI>3% correlates with poor outcome [5,15].

Conventional cytogenetics remains the main method utilized for the detection of chromosomal abnormalities in PCM, despite the technical limitations due to the low proliferative fraction of many plasma cells. Using this technique, abnormalities are detected in <50% of cases [16]. Detection of chromosomal abnormalities using FISH, on the other hand, increases the yield significantly, and it is now accepted that almost all cases of PCM have chromosomal abnormalities [17,18]. Another advantage of FISH is the ability to perform the test on paraffin-embedded tissues, obviating the need for fresh tissue. Regardless of the method used, the cytogenetic abnormalities detected in PCM include both numerical and structural ones, and cases frequently show complex abnormalities. About 60% of cases show numerical abnormalities which are usually gains of odd-numbered chromosomes, including 3, 5, 7, 9, 11, 15, 19, and 21. These cases are mostly hyperdiploid and only rarely have structural chromosomal abnormalities.

The other 40% of PCM are non-hyperdiploid and most have one of five recurring translocations involving the immunoglobulin heavy chain gene (IGH) at chromosomal location (chr) 14q32 and a partner oncogene. The partner oncogenes in these translocations are, in order of frequency, CCND1 (cyclin D1) at chr 11q13, FGFR3 and WHSC1 (MMSET) at chr 4p16, MAF at chr 16q23, CCND3 (cyclin D3) at chr 6p21, and MAFB at chr 20q12. These translocations lead to upregulation of these oncogenes with a possible more favorable prognosis in cases with t(11;14)/CCND1-IGH and an adverse effect on prognosis in cases with t(4;14)/IGH-FGFR3 or t(14;16)/IGH-MAF (Table 19-2). Monosomies, also commonly seen in PCM, most frequently affect chromosomes 13, 14, 16, and 22, with monosomy 13

Table 19-1. Categories of DNA aneuploidy in PCM.

Aneuploid category	Number of chromosomes	Corresponding DNA index
Hypodiploid	< 44–45	< 0.95
Pseudodiploid	44/45–46/47	0.95–1.05
Hyperdiploid	> 46/47 and ≤75	> 1.05
Near tetraploid	> 75	As close to 2.0 (usually > 1.75)

Table 19-2. Recurring translocations involving IGH in PCM.

Abnormality	Prevalence in PCM (%)	Up-regulated oncogene/s	Effect on prognosis
t(11:14)(q13;q32)	16	CCND1 (cyclin D1)	? Favorable
t(4:14)(p16;q32)	15	FGFR3 and/or MMSET	Adverse
t(14:16)(q32;q23)	5	MAF	Adverse
t(6:14)(p21;q32)	3	CCND3 (cyclin D3)	Unknown
t(14:20)(q32;q12)	2	MAFB	Unknown

Data derived from reference [15]

Table 19-3. Chromosomal abnormalities in hyperdiploid and non-hyperdiploid PCM.

	Number of chromosomes	Trisomies of odd-numbered chromosomes	Translocations involving IgH	Monosomy 13	Overall prognosis
Hyperdiploid PCM	48–75	Yes	In <30% of cases	Less common	Better
Non-hyperdiploid PCM	<48 or >75	No	In >85% of cases	More common	Worse

Table 19-4. Comparison of clinical and pathological features of plasma cell myeloma and lymphoplasmacytic lymphoma.

	Neoplastic population/s	Sites of involvement	Clinical presentation	Lytic bone lesions	M-protein	Ploidy	Cytogenetic abnormalities
Plasma cell myeloma	Plasma cells	BM/PB (Extramedullary involvement is rare)	End-organ damage (CRAB)	Yes	IgG IgA	Frequently aneuploid	Complex
Lymphoplasmacytic lymphoma	Lymphocytes Plasmacytoid lymphocytes Plasma cells	BM/PB LN Spleen	Symptoms of anemia WM	No	IgM	Diploid	Rare

BM Bone marrow, *CRAB* Hypercalcemia, renal insufficiency, anemia, bone lesions, *LN* Lymph nodes, *PB* Peripheral blood, *WM* Waldenström macroglobulinemia

more commonly found in non-hyperdiploid PCM (Table 19-3). Chromosome 13 abnormalities (monosomy or partial deletion) are detected in 10%–20% of all PCM patients and are associated with lower response rates to therapy and shorter survival. Other less common recurring genetic abnormalities detectable by FISH or other molecular methods include RAS mutations, inactivation of p53, inactivation of tumor suppressors at the G1-S cell cycle transition, PTEN mutations, and rarely, complex karyotypic abnormalities involving the MYC locus at chr 8q24 [15,18]. The interactions between aneuploidy and other molecular findings are summarized in Table 19-3.

19.2.5. Differential Diagnosis

In the BM, the differential diagnosis of PCM includes reactive plasmacytosis and LPL. Reactive BM plasma cells usually have a mature morphology and reside around blood vessels, individually or in small clusters and do not displace other marrow elements. Neoplastic plasma cells may have mature morphology, but will show some atypical cytologic features and involve the BM in a pattern different from reactive plasma cells. In the interstitial pattern of PCM, plasma cells are not necessarily displacing other elements, but are found widely distributed throughout the medually space and are not restricted to perivascular areas. In the nodular and diffuse patterns, plasma cells are present in large aggregates or sheets that displace other marrow elements. Even with these differences between reactive and neoplastic plasmacytoses, some cases are challenging, especially those with a minimal initial involvement at diagnosis, and cases with MRD after therapy. In such cases, ancillary studies like immunohistochemical or in-situ hybridization studies for light chains can be helpful in determining if a plasma cell population is reactive or neoplastic.

Lymphoplasmacytic lymphoma involving the BM typically shows a mixed population of cells with a predominant lymphocytic component and variable numbers of plasmacytoid lymphocytes and plasma cells. In addition, increased mast cells and Dutcher bodies are typically seen. However, rare cases of LPL with an extensive plasma cell component can be mistaken for PCM purely on a morphologic basis. Fortunately, the clinical and laboratory disease characteristics are usually typical of LPL and make the distinction straightforward. These include production of an IgM paraprotein and resultant clinical WM, absence of lytic bone lesions, normal cytogenetics, and diploidy, features not usually seen in PCM (Table 19-4).

In extramedullary sites, reactive plasmacytosis and LPL remain on the differential diagnosis list for PCM. In addition, other B-cell lymphomas with extensive plasmacytoid differentiation should be ruled out. Reactive plasmacytosis is known to occur in the gastro intestinal tract. In the oral cavity, the mucous membrane can be involved by extensive sheets of plasma cells mimicking the involvement by extramedullary PCM. This has also been described in the mucosa at other sites and has been designated by different names like plasma cell mucositis and mucous membrane plasmacytosis [19–21]. Lymphoplasmacytic lymphoma and other B-cell lymphomas with extensive plasmacytic differentiation involving extramedullary sites are discussed in Chap. 15.

19.2.6. Prognosis, Predictive Factors, and Patterns of Progression

Despite the advent of modern therapeutic modalities, the median survival in PCM patients is relatively short (3–4 years) with a very wide range (few months to >10 years) reflecting the heterogeneity of the disease and factors influencing outcome [22]. At the time of diagnosis, demographic and clinical factors and the type of initiating genetic change(s) are the major determinants of outcome. As the disease progresses, the type of acquired cytogenetic and molecular changes are the main determinants of outcome. Favorable prognostic factors include a good performance status, age <70 years, African American ethnicity, and a competent immune surveillance system as reflected by a peripheral blood CD4+ T-cell count of >700×10⁶/mL. Among initiating genetic changes, t(11;14)(q13;q32) and hyperdiploidy are associated with a better outcome (Tables 19-2 and 19-3). Deletion of 13q14 and monosomy 13 impart an adverse prognosis. Other adverse acquired genetic changes include deletions of 17p13 (TP53 loss), activating KRAS, NRAS, or FGFR3 mutations, and chromosome 1q21 abnormalities producing amplification and/or overexpression of CKS1B. Secondary chromosomal translocations that dysregulate MYC through the immunoglobulin gene(s) can occur early or late in the disease process and have an adverse effect on outcome.

Other prognostic markers not necessarily related to specific disease evolutionary stages include tumor burden, biochemical markers (serum β2-microglobulin, lactate dehydrogenase (LDH), C-reactive protein (CRP), albumin, and others), cytomorphologic and phenotypic characteristics of the neoplastic plasma cells, and the tumor proliferative activity. The Durie-Salmon staging system (Table 19-5) uses the M-protein level, extent of bone lesions, hemoglobin

Table 19-5. Durie and Salmon staging system for multiple myeloma.

Stage	Criteria	Tumor burden (cells×10¹²/m²)
I	Normal hemoglobin and serum calcium No or solitary bone lesion on X-ray Low M-protein levels: IgG <50 g/L IgA <30 g/L Urine light chain <4g/24 h	Low (<0.6)
II	Fitting neither Stage I nor Stage III	Intermediate (0.6–1.2)
III	Hemoglobin <8.5 g/dL, serum calcium >12 mg/dL Advanced lytic bone lesions on X-ray High M-protein levels: IgG >70 g/L IgA >50 g/L Urine light chain >12 g/24 h	High (>1.2)

Stages are further subclassified based on renal function into: A. Serum creatinine <2 mg/dL or B. Serum creatinine ≥2 mg/dL. Definitions as in reference [23]

Table 19-6. International Staging System for multiple myeloma.

Stage	Criteria	Median Survival (months)
I	Serum β_2-microglobulin <3.5 mg/L Serum albumin ≥3.5 g/dL	62
II	Not stage I or III*	44
III	Serum β_2-microglobulin ≥5.5 mg/L	29

*There are two categories for stage II: serum β_2-microglobulin <3.5 mg/L but serum albumin <3.5 g/dL; or serum β_2-microglobulin 3.5 to <5.5 mg/L irrespective of serum albumin level. Criteria derived from reference [22]

level, and serum calcium to predict the tumor burden and classify cases accordingly into one of three stages with different median survivals. Each stage is further subclassified into a lower or higher risk category based on renal function [23]. The more recent International Staging System for multiple myeloma (Table 19-6) uses serum β2-microglobulin and albumin levels to classify cases into one of three stages with different median survivals [22]. Bartle described 6 cytomorphologic types of plasma cells that classify cases into one of three grades with different median survivals. Not surprisingly, the plasmablastic type, which is now widely considered to have a worse outcome, corresponds to the highest Bartl grade with the worse median survival [4]. The immunophenotype of neoplastic plasma cells is also considered to have prognostic value. Lack of CD45 expression has been associated with an adverse prognosis as has upregulation of CD56. Other findings associated with an adverse prognosis are lack of expression of CD19 or CD28. Expression of CD117 is associated with a favorable prognosis. A high tumor proliferative activity, corresponding to PCLI >3%, portends an unfavorable prognosis.

The different stages of progression of PCM are correlated with acquisition of specific genetic changes. IGH translocations arise early, likely due to an aberrant recombination in a germinal center B cell, with stepwise progression from MGUS to asymptomatic (smoldering) myeloma, classical myeloma, and perhaps to extramedullary dissemination or PCL. Occurrence of secondary genetic events (e.g., activating RAS mutations) occur commonly at the transition from the MGUS into PCM. Other secondary genetic events occur as the disease progresses (e.g., FGFR3 mutations) may facilitate PCM independence from BM stromal trophic signals with MYC BM dysregulation, methylation and inactivation of the tumor suppressor genes such as p15 and p16 driving genetic instability. TP53 inactivation is a late event often accompanying the extramedullary dissemination [18, 24–29].

Regardless of the particular initiating genetic event (i.e. hyperdiploid versus non-hyperdiploid with IgH translocations), most cases of PCM show dysregulation and overexpression of one or more cyclin D gene(s) which leads to phosphorylation of the retinoblastoma protein (Rb) and its dissociation from E2F transcription factor which then drives the cell cycle from G1 to S. The cyclin genes that are dysregulated by one or more of the early genetic events in PCM include cyclins D1, D2, and D3. Cyclin D1 is dysregulated by t(11;14)(q13;q32) or its overexpression due to gene dosage in hyperdiploid cases. Cyclin D2 is dysregulated by t(4;14)(p16;q32) but also by activation of the MAF and MAFB transcription factors as a result of t(14;16)(q32;q23) and t(14;20)(q32;q12), respectively. Cyclin D3 is dysregulated by t(6;14)(p21;q32) [18,30].

Because of these changes, gene expression profiling can now identify cases with any one of the five recurring primary IgH translocations or specific trisomies, and cases with overexpression of particular cyclin D genes. Using this information, PCM cases can be grouped into 8 different translocation/cyclin D (TC) groups that not only have different gene expression profiles but also show differing clinical characteristics (Table 19-7). Groups containing cases with recurring translocations are designated by the partner gene translocated next to

Table 19-7. Genetic events and clinical features of translocation/cyclin D groups of plasma cell myeloma.

Group	Genetic event	Gene at breakpoint	Overexpressed cyclin D	Proliferation index	Lytic bone disease (% positive MRI)	Extramedullary disease	Prognosis
Chr 6p21	t(6:14)(p21;q32)	CCND3	D3	Average	100		? Good
Chr 11q13	t(11:14)(q13;q32)	CCND1	D1	Average	94		Good
Chr 4p16	t(4:14)(p16;q32)	FGFR3/MMSET	D2	Average	57	+	Poor
MAF genes	t(14:16)(q32;q23)	MAF	D2	High	55	+	Poor
	t(14:20)(q32;q12)	MAFB					
Cyclin D1	Hyperdiploid	None	D1	Low	86		Good
Cyclin D1+D2	Hyperdiploid	None	D1 and D2	High	100		? Poor
Cyclin D2	Hyperdiploid	None	D2	Average	67		?
None	None	None	None	Average	100		? Good

Data are derived from references [18,30]

Table 19-8. Different methods used to detect minimal residual disease in plasma cell myeloma.

	BM Morphologic Examination	Flow Cytometry	FISH	Fluorescent IgH PCR	Clone-specific IgH PCR
Sensitivity	10^{-2}	10^{-2}–10^{-4}	10^{-2}–10^{-3}	10^{-3}–10^{-4}	10^{-6}
Quantitation of malignant plasma cells	Manual count	Semi-quantitative	No	Semi-quantitative	Quantitative

Sensitivity is derived from the ratio of number of malignant cells detected divided by number of normal cells in the specimen

IGH or its original locus. These categories include the 6p21 group of tumors which express cyclin D3, the 11q13 group of tumors which express cyclin D1, and the MAF- and MAFB-translocated cases and the chr 4p16 group which overexpress cyclin D2. Cases containing hyperdiploidy are designated by their dysregulated cyclin D gene(s). These include the D1 group of tumors which express increased cyclin D1, the D1+D2 group of tumors which express increased cyclin D1 and cyclin D2, the D2 group of tumors which express increased cyclin D2, and a group of tumors that do not show increased levels of cyclins D1, D2, or D3. Clinical differences among these groups include a higher percentage of lytic bone lesions, detected by MRI, in the 11q13, D1, and D1+D2 groups, a higher proliferation index in the D1+D2 and MAF groups, an overall good prognosis in the 11q13 and D1 groups, and an overall poor prognosis in the 4p16 and MAF groups. Of interest, the 4p16 and MAF groups are also known to be associated with extramedullary disease and, not surprisingly, the lowest incidence of lytic bone lesions seen by MRI [30].

19.2.7. Monitoring After Treatment

No matter what method or test is used, the goal of disease monitoring after treatment is to assess the initial response to the administered therapy and to predict early relapse and direct further management accordingly. A major part of monitoring patients with PCM after therapy remains the serial assessment of the M-protein level, which provides an assessment of tumor burden, using the standard protein analysis methods or the more sensitive serum free light chain assay. In addition, detection of MRD is done using one or more of several plasma cell enumeration methods, each with its own level of sensitivity, advantages, and disadvantages. These methods include morphologic BM examination, FISH, flow cytometry, and polymerase chain reaction (PCR) (Table 19-8).

Morphologic BM examination, including the use of immunohistochemical stains, is routinely done for disease monitoring and can achieve a sensitivity of 10^{-2} (one myeloma cell in 100 normal cells). Multiparameter flow cytometry can be used to detect residual neoplastic plasma cells showing an aberrant phenotype with loss of CD19 and/or expression of CD56, CD28, or CD117, and can achieve a sensitivity of 10^{-2}–10^{-4}. A semiquantitative measurement of residual malignant plasma cells can also be performed by flow cytometry. Interphase FISH can be used to detect deletion 13q14, deletion 17p13, 11q abnormalities, hyperdiploidy, and many other cytogenetic abnormalities commonly seen in the PCM. It can achieve a sensitivity of 10^{-2}. The newer target FISH method is reported to have a sensitivity of 10^{-3}. However, quantitative measurement of malignant plasma cells is currently not routinely performed by FISH. Several PCR techniques are utilized for MRD detection in PCM. Standard IgH PCR has a sensitivity of 10^{-3} to 10^{-4}, but can only provide a semiquantitative measurement of malignant plasma cells. Clone-specific PCR techniques, both quantitative and qualitative, can achieve sensitivity of 10^{-6} and accurately quantify the clonal plasma cells in the specimen. However, being highly specific for the disease clone, they are not universally applicable to all patients as clone-specific primers must be designed (see Chap. 4) [24,31–33].

19.3. Lymphoplasmacytic Lymphoma Involving the Bone Marrow

19.3.1. Definition, Incidence, Demographics, and Clinical Features

Lymphoplasmacytic lymphoma (LPL) is a disease of small B cells, plasmacytoid lymphocytes, and plasma cells, which is often but not always characterized by production of an IgM paraprotein. While usually involving the BM, LPL can also affect the extramedullary locations like lymph nodes and spleen. Waldenström macroglobulinemia (WM) was previously considered to be a clinical syndrome occurring in any disease resulting in secretion of IgM, whether LPL or other. Now, WM is defined as an IgM monoclonal gammopathy of any concentration, in the background of LPL involving the BM [1]. LPL is a disease of adults with a median age of 65 years and a slight male predominance. It is a relatively rare disease constituting <5% of non-Hodgkin lymphomas [34]. Patients usually present with symptoms attributable to tumor infiltration and/or the presence of an IgM M-protein. The former include anemia mainly, and other symptoms depending on the infiltrated organ. Of note, unlike PCM, LPL does not cause lytic bone lesions (Table 19-4). Symptoms attributable to the presence of an IgM M-protein can be divided into those caused by circulating IgM, IgM deposition in tissues, and the autoantibody activity of IgM. Since it is a large pentameric molecule, circulating IgM causes serum hyperviscosity in about 30% of patients with WM with resultant cardiovascular, neurologic, and ocular manifestations. IgM is also known to interact with coagulation factors, potentially causing bleeding and clotting abnormalities. Circulating IgM can also cause cryoglobulinemia. IgM deposition in tissues occurs mainly in the kidneys, gastrointestinal tract, and skin, and causes proteinuria (but not usually renal insufficiency or cast nephropathy), as well as diarrhea, and cutaneous papules and nodules. Finally, the autoantibody activity of IgM can potentially cause a variety of autoimmune phenomena like immune hemolytic anemia and neuropathies in about 20% of patients [35,36].

19.3.2. Pathologic Features

LPL usually involves the BM. Less frequently, extramedullary sites are also involved, usually lymph nodes and spleen. In the BM, the pattern of involvement can be interstitial, nodular, or diffuse (Figs. 19-6 and 19-7). The lesion is usually predominantly comprised of small lymphocytes with a variable number of larger plasmacytoid lymphocytes and plasma cells. Dutcher bodies (cytoplasmic immunoglobulin inclusions in lymphocytes) and admixed mast cells are common features (Fig. 19-8). Morphologic variants of LPL have been described, including lymphoplasmacytoid (where mature lymphocytes predominate),

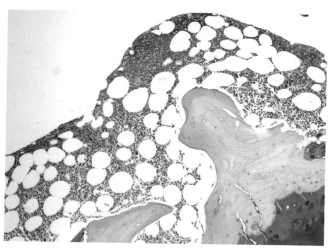

Fig. 19-6. Lymphoplasmacytic lymphoma in BM biopsy. A small lymphoplasmacytic aggregate is visible in the upper middle of the biopsy

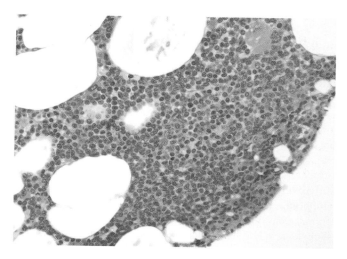

Fig. 19-7. Lymphoplasmacytic lymphoma in BM biopsy. The same lymphoplasmacytic aggregate as in Fig. 19-6 shows mostly lymphoplasmacytoid lymphocytes and scattered mast cells

lymphoplasmacytic (where transitional plasmacytic forms are common), and polymorphous (where cytologic atypia is pronounced), with the latter type having a worse outcome [37].

19.3.3. Laboratory Testing for Diagnosis

In our institution, laboratory testing for LPL is similar to that for PCM except for the inclusion of markers of mature B-lymphomas during FC immunophenotyping, including analysis of surface immunoglobulins, and CD5 and CD10. Analysis of the genetic makeup of the cells is also done in a fashion similar to PCM, however no specific oncogene or cytogenetic abnormalities are usually identified in LPL. The most frequently reported structural chromosome abnormality in LPL/WM is usually deletion of chromosome region 6q. The most frequently reported numerical chromosome abnormalities are trisomy 4, trisomy 5, and monosomy 8 [38,39].

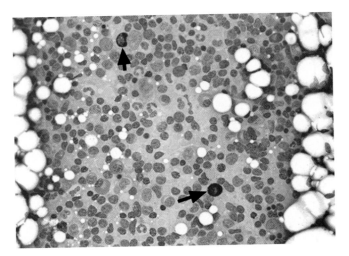

Fig. 19-8. Lymphoplasmacytic lymphoma in BM aspirate. The typical cellular composition of LPL includes small lymphocytes, plasmacytoid lymphocytes, and plasma cells. Rare mast cells are also present (arrows)

19.3.4. Differential Diagnosis

As previously discussed, PCM is the most important differential diagnosis in BM involved by LPL with a prominent plasmacytoid component. Another important diagnostic consideration is involvement by a marginal zone lymphoma with prominent plasmacytoid differentiation. Secretion of an IgM paraprotein, while supportive of a diagnosis of LPL, can rarely occur in marginal zone lymphoma. Immunophenotypic analysis is also not helpful in this distinction since both marginal zone lymphoma and LPL have a virtually identical phenotypic profile, with commonly-used markers. In such cases, the clinical profile is of paramount importance in determining the nature of the disease. Any evidence of concurrent or previous involvement by lymphoma of tissues or organs considered usual sites of marginal zone lymphoma, like the gastrointestinal tract or salivary glands, would favor the diagnosis of marginal zone lymphoma.

Reactive lymphocytosis is another important consideration in a BM with a lymphoplasmacytic infiltrate. Phenotypic analysis by immunohistochemical stains might not be conclusive in determining if a lymphoid infiltrate present in the BM represents involvement by LPL or is reactive, partly due to the CD5- and CD10-negative phenotype of LPL lymphocytes [37]. FC with analysis of surface immunoglobulin expression is usually helpful in determining the clonal nature of the lymphoid population present in the specimen. Additionally, evidence of monoclonal plasma cells by FC or DNA content alterations in the plasma cell component can be supportive of involvement by LPL.

19.3.5. Prognosis, Predictive Factors, and Patterns of Progression

LPL is usually an indolent disease with a median survival of 5–10 years. Significant outcome predictive factors are age, hemoglobin concentration, β_2-microglobulin, and serum albumin. Similarly to the absence of characteristic findings by cytogenetic analysis, gene expression profiling studies have not yet identified distinct genetic subgroups of LPL, even among del6q cases [40]. Indeed, LPL/WM cases show more overlap in their expression profiles with chronic lymphocytic leukemia (and even non-neoplastic B cells) than they do with PCM. Some differentially-expressed genes include components of the MAP kinase and cytokine signaling pathways, including IL-6, which thus represents a potential target for therapy [40].

19.3.6. Monitoring After Treatment

Similarly to PCM, serial determination of M-protein levels is an important part of disease monitoring in patients with LPL. FC analysis is also an important tool for the detection of MRD. However, due to the lack of characteristic cytogenetic abnormalities in LPL, ancillary tests like FISH and PCR currently play a less important role in MRD detection.

Selected Reviews

- Ho PJ, Campbell LJ, Gibson J, Brown R, Joshua D. The biology and cytogenetics of multiple myeloma. Rev Clin Exp Hematol 2002;6:276–300. (An in-depth review of normal and abnormal plasma cell development)
- San Miguel JF, Gutierrez NC, Mateo G, Orfao A. Conventional diagnostics in multiple myeloma. Eur J Cancer 2006;42:1510–9. (An in-depth review of diagnostic methods in plasma cell myeloma)
- Fonseca R, Barlogie B, Bataille R, et al. Genetics and cytogenetics of multiple myeloma: A workshop Report. Cancer Res 2004;64:1546–58. (An in-depth review of genetic abnormalities of plasma cell myeloma).

References

1. Owen RG, Treon SP, Al-Katib A, et al. Clinicopathological definition of Waldenstrom's macroglobulinemia: consensus panel recommendations from the Second International Workshop on Waldenstrom's Macroglobulinemia. Semin Oncol 2003;30:110–5.
2. Jaffe ES, Harris NL, Stein H, Vardiman JW, eds. World Health Organization classification of tumours. Pathology and genetics of tumours of haematopoietic and lymphoid tissues. Lyon: IARC Press, 2001.
3. Swerdlow SH, Campo E, Harris NL, et al., eds. WHO classification of tumours of haematopoietic and lymphoid tissues. IARC: Lyon, 2008.
4. Bartl R, Frisch B, Fateh-Moghadam A, Kettner G, Jaeher K, Sommerfeld W. Histologic classification and Staging of multiple myeloma: A retrospective and prospective study of 674 cases. Am J Clin Pathol 1987;87:342–55.
5. San Miguel JF, Gutierrez NC, Mateo G, Orfao A. Conventional diagnostics in multiple myeloma. Eur J Cancer 2006;42:1510–9.
6. Pratt G. The evolving use of serum free light chain assays in haematology. Br J Haematol 2008;141:413–22.
7. Kang SY, Suh JT, Lee HJ, Yoon HJ, Lee WI. Clinical usefulness of free light chain concentration as a tumor marker in multiple myeloma. Ann Hematol 2005;84:588–93.
8. Peterson LC, Brown BA, Crosson JT, Mladenovic J. Application of the immunoperoxidase technique to bone marrow trephine biopsies in the classification of patients with monoclonal gammopathies. Am J Clin pathol 1986;85:688–93.
9. Eckert F, Schmid I, Kradolfer D, Schmid U. Bone marrow plasmacytosis – an immunohistological study. Blut 1986;53:11–9.
10. Majumdar G, Grace RJ, Singh AK, Slater NG. The value of the bone marrow plasma cell cytoplasmic light chain ratio in differentiating between multiple myeloma and monoclonal gammopathy of undetermined significance. Leuk Lymphoma 1992;8:491–3.
11. Lin P, Owens R, Tricot G, Wilson CS. Flow cytometric immunophenotypic analysis of 306 cases of multiple myeloma. Am J Clin Pathol 2004;121:482–8.
12. Mateo G, Castellanos M, Rasillo A, et al. Genetic abnormalities and patterns of antigenic expression in multiple myeloma. Clin Cancer Res 2005;11:3661–7.
13. Almeida J, Orfao A, Mateo G, et al. Immunophenotypic and DNA content characteristics of plasma cells in multiple myeloma and monoclonal gammopathy of undetermined significance. Pathol Biol 1999;47:119–27.
14. Pellat-Deceunynck C, Bataille R, Robillard N, et al. Expression of CD28 and CD40 in human myeloma cells: a comparative study with normal plasma cells. Blood 1994;84:2597–603.
15. Fonseca R, Barlogie B, Bataille R, et al. Genetics and cytogenetics of multiple myeloma: A workshop Report. Cancer Res 2004;64:1546–58.

16. Ho PJ, Campbell LJ, Gibson J, Brown R, Joshua D. The biology and cytogenetics of multiple myeloma. Rev Clin Exp Hematol 2002;6:276–300.

17. Avet-Loiseau H, Attal M, Moreau P, et al. Genetic abnormalities and survival in multiple myeloma: the experience of the Intergroupe Francophone du Myelome. Blood 2007;109:3489–95.

18. Bergsagel PL, Kuehl WM. Molecular pathogenesis and a consequent classification of multiple myeloma. J Clin Oncol 2005;23:6333–8.

19. Keren DF. Intestinal mucosal immune defense mechanisms. Am J Surg Pathol 1988; 12:100-5.

20. Bharti R, Smith D. Mucous membrane plasmacytosis: A case report and review of the literature. Dermatol Online J 2003;9:15.

21. Solomon LW, Wein RO, Rosenwald I, Laver N. Plasma cell mucositis of the oral cavity: a report of a case and review of the literature. Oral Surg Oral Med Oral Pathol Oral Radiol Endod 2008;106:853–60.

22. Greipp PR, San Miguel J, Durie BG, et al. International staging system for multiple myeloma. J Clin Oncol 2005;23:3412–20.

23. Durie BG, Samlon SE. A clinical staging system for multiple myeloma. Correlation of measured myeloma cell mass with presenting clinical features, response to treatment, and survival. Cancer 1975;36:842–54.

24. Fonseca R, San Miguel J. Prognostic factors and staging in multiple myeloma. Hematol Oncol Clin N Am 2007;21:1115–40.

25. Shaughnessy J. Amplification and overexpression of CKS1B at chromosome band 1q21 is associated with reduced levels of p27^{Kip1} and an aggressive clinical course in multiple myeloma. Hematology 2005;10:117–26.

26. Bergsagel PL, Kuehl WM. Chromosome translocations in multiple myeloma. Oncogene 2001;20: 5611–22.

27. Chesi M, Nardini E, Brents L, et al. Frequent translocation t(4;14)(p16.3;q32.3) in multiple myeloma is associated with increased expression and activating mutations of fibroblast growth factor receptor 3. Nat Genet 1997;16:260–4.

28. Liu P, Leong T, Quam L, et al. Activating mutations of N- and K-ras in multiple myeloma show different clinical associations: analysis of the Eastern Cooperative Oncology Group Phase III trial. Blood 1996;88:2699–706.

29. Gutierrez NC, Garcia-Sanz R, San Miguel JF. Molecular biology of myeloma. Clin Transl Oncol 2007;9:618–24.

30. Bergsagel PL, Kuehl WM, Zhan F, Sawyer J, Barlogie B, Shaughnessy J. Cyclin D dysregulation: an early and unifying pathogenic event in multiple myeloma. Blood 2005;106:296–303.

31. Fenk R, Haas R, Kronenwett R. Molecular monitoring of minimal residual disease in patients with multiple myeloma. Hematology 2004;9:17–33.

32. Davies FE, Rawstron AC, Owen RG, Morgan GJ. Minimal residual disease monitoring in multiple myeloma. Best Pract Res Clin Hematol 2002;15:197–222.

33. Slovak ML, Bedell V, Pagel K, Chang KL, Smith D, Somlo G. Targeting plasma cells improves detection of cytogenetic aberrations in multiple myeloma: phenotype/genotype fluorescence in situ hybridization. Cancer Genet Cytogenet 2005;158:99–109.

34. Vitolo U, Ferreri AJ, Montoto S. Lymphoplasmacytic lymphoma-Waldenstrom macroglobulinemia. Crit Rev Oncol Hematol. 2008;67:172–85.

35. Vijay A, Gertz MA. Waldenstrom macroglobulinemia. Blood 2007;109:5096–103.

36. Dimopoulos MA, Kyle RA, Anagnostopoulos A, Treon SP. Diagnosis and management of Waldenstrom's macroglobulinemia. J Clin Oncol 2005;23:1564–77.

37. Konoplev S, Medeiros LJ, Bueso-Ramos CE, Jorgensen JL, Lin P. Immunophenotypic profile of lymphoplasmacytic lymphoma/ Waldenstrom macroglobulinemia. Am J Clin Pathol 2005;124:414–20.

38. Terre C, Nguyen-Khac F, Barin C, et al. Trisomy 4, a new chromosomal abnormality in Waldenstrom's macroglobulinemia: a study of 39 cases. Leukemia 2006;20:1634–6.

39. Mansoor A, Medeiros LJ, Weber D, et al. Cytogenetic findings in lymphoplasmacytic lymphoma/ Waldenstrom macroglobulinemia. Am J Clin pathol 2001;116:543–9.

40. Chng WJ, Schop RF, Price-Troska T, et al. Gene-expression profiling of Waldenstrom macroglobulinemia reveals a phenotype more similar to chronic lymphocytic leukemia than multiple myeloma. Blood 2006;108:2755–63.

Chapter 20

Hodgkin Lymphoma

Robert Lin, Dan Jones, and Sherif Ibrahim

Abstract/Scope of Chapter This chapter covers the clinical features, classification, differential diagnosis, and pathogenesis of Hodgkin lymphoma. Differences between the histogenesis and appearance of classical subtypes (nodular sclerosis, mixed cellularity, lymphocyte-rich, and lymphocyte-depleted) and the nodular lymphocyte predominant type are covered.

Keywords Hodgkin lymphoma • Reed-Sternberg (R-S) cell • Hodgkin lymphoma, L&H (lymphocytic/histiocytic) cell • Nodular lymphocyte predominant Hodgkin lymphoma (NL-PHL) • Hodgkin lymphoma, classical type (CHL) • Hodgkin lymphoma, nodular sclerosis type (NSCHL) • Hodgkin lymphoma, mixed cellularity (MCCHL) • Hodgkin lymphoma, lymphocyte rich (LRHL) • Hodgkin lymphoma, lymphocyte depleted (LDHL) • Epstein-Barr Virus (EBV), Hodgkin lymphoma, CD15 • Hodgkin lymphoma, CD30 • Hodgkin lymphoma, progressive transformation of germinal centers (PTGC) • T-cell/histiocyte-rich B-cell lymphoma (TCHRBCL), differential with Hodgkin lymphoma • Anaplastic large cell lymphoma (ALCL), differential with Hodgkin lymphoma • Primary mediastinal large B-cell lymphoma (PMLBCL), differential with Hodgkin lymphoma • Grey zone lymphoma

20.1. Pathogenesis and Historical Perspective

Hodgkin lymphoma (HL) is now understood to comprise several related neoplasms that arise from germinal center (GC) B cells. The characteristic histologic feature of HL, namely sparse large neoplastic cells embedded within dense infiltrates of nonneoplastic inflammatory cells, is a function of the secretion of abundant chemotactic chemokines and cytokines by the tumor cells [1]. In nodular lymphocyte predominant (NLP)HL, the predominant reactive cells are small lymphocytes, whereas in classical (C)HL, the inflammatory cells include eosinophils, histiocytes, and neutrophils as well as small lymphocytes. CHL is further subdivided into nodular sclerosis, mixed cellularity (MC), lymphocyte-depleted, and lymphocyte-rich (LR) subtypes based on the inciting agents [Epstein-Barr virus (EBV) in most MCCHL], histologic pattern, and density of tumor cells (Table 20-1) [2].

The classification of HL has a fascinating 150-year history characterized by a lively debate concerning the origin of the neoplastic cells, and initially, if the entity was a neoplasm at all. Not until recently was the designation changed from "Hodgkin disease" to "Hodgkin lymphoma". Thomas Hodgkin first described a series of cases based on the distinctive gross autopsy findings

From: *Neoplastic Hematopathology*: Contemporary Hematology,
Edited by: D. Jones, DOI 10.1007/978-1-60761-384-8_20,
© Humana Press, a part of Springer Science+Business Media, LLC 2010

in 1832, and he was recognized for this discovery when Wilks performed a similar study in 1856. Interestingly, retrospective review of Hodgkin's original autopsy material concluded that half of the cases actually represented infectious processes, including tuberculosis, syphilis, or infectious mononucleosis. Dorothy Reed and Carl Sternberg gave their names to the distinctive appearance of the CHL tumor cell, based on their drawings done around 1900 [3].

Classification schemes for HL were among the first in tumor biology to be based on both clinical behavior and histomorphology. Most of the currently known HL categories were recognized as distinct by Jackson and Parker in 1944, and Lukes and Butler in 1966. The next major advance in understanding came in the mid-1990s with the demonstration through single-cell PCR analysis that nearly all cases of CHL represent clonal B-cell malignancies that have crippling (non-functional) mutation in their immunoglobulin genes leading to partial loss of their B-cell phenotype [4·5]. These studies and similar studies in NLPHL convincingly demonstrated a GC B-cell origin and provided a mechanistic explanation for the absence of expression of many B-cell markers in HL (Fig. 20-1) [6,7]. As a result, the term

Table 20-1. Historical developments in the recognition of Hodgkin lymphoma.

1832	Thomas Hodgkin publishes initial series
1856	Wilks names entity after Hodgkin
1872–1878	Langhans and Greenfield describe histology of entity
1898–1902	Sternberg and Reed define characteristic neoplastic cell
1947	Jackson and Parker sub-classify by histology as Hodgkin granuloma, sarcoma, and paragranuloma
1966	Lukes and Butler propose classification of nodular sclerosing, mixed-cellularity, and lymphocyte depleted
1994	REAL classification recognizes nodular lymphocyte predominant Hodgkin lymphoma
2001	WHO recognizes Hodgkin's disease as a lymphoma and lymphocyte-rich classical Hodgkin as a subtype
2008	Growing body of evidence supports a germinal center origin for Hodgkin lymphoma

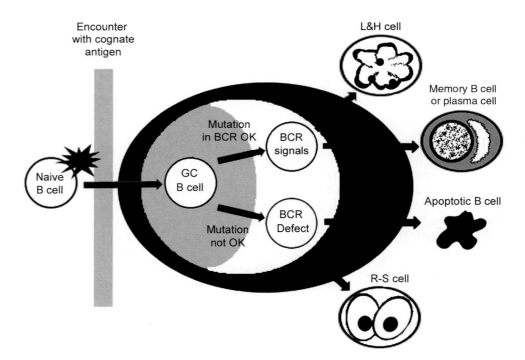

Fig. 20-1. Proposed origin of NLPHL (LP/L&H cell) and CHL (R-S cell) from germinal center B cells without or with crippling mutations in the B-cell receptor (BCR)

"non-Hodgkin's lymphoma" could be a considered a historical remnant as the category of B-cell lymphomas has expanded to include CHL and NLPHL as special subtypes.

20.2. Epidemiology

HL comprises ~30% of lymphomas in Western countries, presenting with a bimodal age distribution with incidence peaks at 15–35 years and at 70–80 years. Worldwide, there are dramatic differences in the overall HL incidence, subtype, and age distributions likely due to differences in each country's socioeconomic status that influence the average age at which primary EBV infection is acquired [8]. Incidence is lowest in Asia, [9] and statistical studies in Europe and North America from 1993 to 1997 show a slight male predominance for HL, with an annual incidence of 1.3–4.0 per 100,000 in males and 0.9–3.1 per 100,000 in females [10].

In the United States, the M:F ratio is 1.2:1, with the highest incidence in whites of non-Hispanic origin. NSCHL accounts for ~70% of CHL cases in Western countries, but it is less common in developing countries where the proportion of EBV+ HL is higher. The bimodal age distribution (Fig. 20-2) is produced by subsets of NSCHL occurring mostly in younger, white populations and then subsequently MCCHL cases occurring preferentially in older, white males.

20.3. Nodular Lymphocyte-Predominant Hodgkin Lymphoma (NLPHL)

20.3.1. Clinical Features

NLPHL is most commonly seen in young men who present with a single enlarged lymph node in the axillae, neck, or groin, and have few, if any, other signs or symptoms [11]. Evidence of systemic disease is almost always absent by clinical exam, radiology scans, or laboratory tests with a normal serum lactate dehydrogenase (LDH) level and erythrocyte

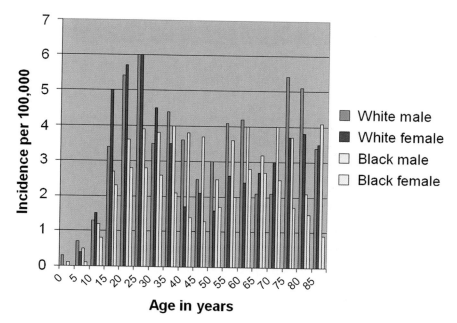

Fig. 20-2. Bimodal age distribution of presentation of Hodgkin lymphoma in the United States (1973–1997). Peaks are noted for patients between 15–35 years of age (mostly nodular sclerosis type), and 70–80 years of age (increased mixed cellularity cases). Data drawn from the Surveillance Epidemiology and End Results (SEER) registry, as summarized in reference [43]

sedimentation rate (ESR). Current therapies are conservative, including localized radio-therapy and multiagent chemotherapy if bulky disease or adverse predictors are present (See Chap. 21). Relapses, which occur in 10%–20% of patients, are usually localized to the initial site(s), and can occur many years after presentation. Spread to multiple lymph node groups, to extranodal sites (commonly liver and lung), or to bone marrow, is almost always indicative of the transformation to diffuse large B-cell lymphoma (DLBCL).

20.3.2. Morphologic and Immunophenotypic Features

The involved lymph node in NLPHL is usually moderately enlarged by an expansile, nodular proliferation of small, mature lymphocytes with scattered large tumor cells (Fig. 20-3). Known as lymphocytic and histiocytic (L&H), LP, or popcorn cells, these neoplastic cells have folded or multilobated vesicular nuclei with multiple, basophilic, small nucleoli (Fig. 20-4), although more typical HL tumor cells can also be seen. The nodules in NLPHL represent follicles with a CD21+ follicular dendritic cell meshwork that have been markedly expanded by recruitment of nonneoplastic mantle zone B cells, epithelioid histiocytes/dendritic cells, [12]

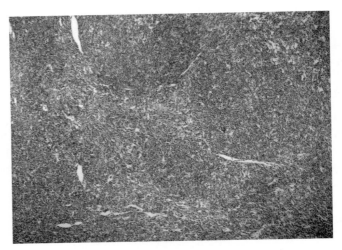

Fig. 20-3. Nodular lymphocyte predominant Hodgkin lymphoma. Lymph node effaced by multiple nodules (*right*) in a background of progressive transformation of germinal centers

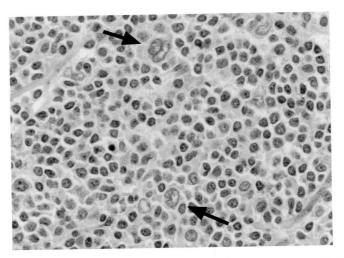

Fig. 20-4. L&H cells in nodular lymphocyte predominant Hodgkin lymphoma. Lobulated L&H or "popcorn" cell with multiple, small nucleoli (arrows)

and follicular-type CD57+ BCL6+ CD134+ T cells that sometimes rosette around the L&H cells (Fig. 20-5a) [13]. Unlike CHL, few neutrophils or eosinophils are noted and sclerotic bands surrounding the nodules are absent.

In almost all cases, the L&H cells are positive for CD45/leukocyte common antigen (LCA) and pan-B-cell markers [CD20 (Fig. 20-5b), CD79a, PAX5] as well as the transcription factors expressed in GC B cells, including BCL6, Bob-1/ POU2AF1, and Oct-2/POU2F2 [6]. They are negative for CD15 and EBV. Occasionally, L&H cells are positive for CD30 but lack the uniform, strong positivity seen in CHL.

In some NLPHL cases, tumor cells extend between the nodules in a serpiginous pattern, or have focal diffuse areas (Fig. 20-6) admixed with more typical nodules [14]. These changes

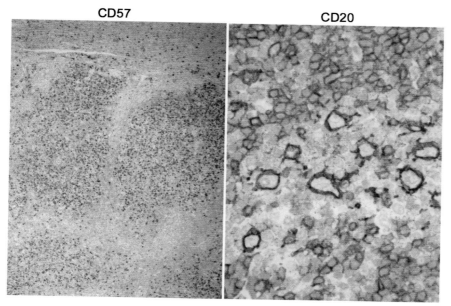

Fig. 20-5. Nodular lymphocyte predominant Hodgkin lymphoma (**a**) Tumor nodules are expanded follicles with increased numbers of follicular-type T cells (CD57 immunostain). (**b**) CD20 immunostain highlights both the L&H tumor cells and the nonneoplastic mantle zone B cells

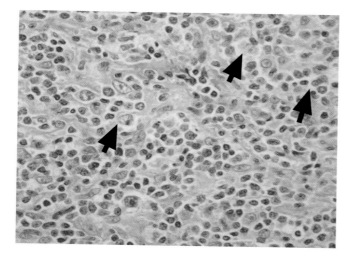

Fig. 20-6. Lymphocyte predominant Hodgkin lymphoma, diffuse growth pattern. Extrafollicular small lymphocytes and L&H-type tumor cells (*arrows*). Other areas of the lymph node showed typical NLPHL nodules

may represent tumor progression, as these variants typically showed increased numbers of T cells and lack small lymphocytes. Diffuse LPHL growth raises the possibility of transformation to T-cell/histiocyte-rich B-cell lymphoma (TCHRBCL), which occurs in 3–5% of patients, especially those with multiple recurrences.

20.3.3. Pathogenesis

Given the immunophenotype, follicular localization, and tight association of L&H cells with follicular T cells, it is clear that NLPHL is a neoplasm of GC B cells. This has been confirmed by single-cell microdissection studies that have shown identical clonal IGH rearrangements in tumor cells within a nodule, and mutated IGH variable regions in a pattern consistent with ongoing somatic mutation [6]. However, the extremely indolent nature of most NLPHL cases suggests that the proliferative capacity of L&H cells is limited, and their ability to spread outside of the GC microenvironment is minimal.

L&H cells transform the GC into an expansile follicle nearly identical to those seen in progressive transformation of germinal centers (PTGC), which is a reaction pattern observed in persistent follicular hyperplasia. Based on an analysis of the activation state of the follicular homing T cells, PTGC appears to represent an abnormal termination pattern of the GC reaction, whereby follicular homing T cells continue to be generated in the paracortex and seed the GC [15]. L&H cells in NLPHL appear to mimic this state producing a similar mix of mantle zone B cells and follicular T cells. However, the expansile nodules in NLPHL are typically larger and more uniform than those seen in PTGC, and show the presence of L&H tumor cells. Intriguingly, a proportion of patients with NLPHL will show persistent and marked PTGC on followup lymph node biopsies that are negative for tumor suggesting that the expansion of follicular T cells underling PTGC may, in fact, be a predisposing factor for NLPHL outgrowth or persistence.

20.3.4   Differential Diagnosis

The primary diagnostic considerations are between NLPHL and PTGC on the benign end (as discussed above), and between NLPHL and TCHRBCL. Since the expansile follicles can be identical in NLPHL and PTGC, distinction relies on finding the L&H tumor cells, which can often be quite sparse and may be highlighted only with CD20 immunostains. The nodules in NLPHL tend to be larger and transform the entire lymph node, whereas PTGC follicles will usually always show adjacent hyperplastic and/or regressed GCs (Fig. 20-7).

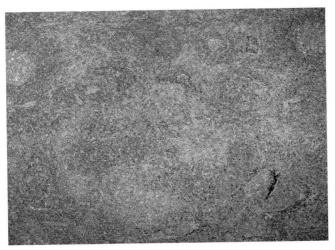

Fig. 20-7. Progressive transformation of germinal centers. A large disrupted transformed follicle in the center of the figure is surrounded by multiple hyperplastic and regressed germinal centers

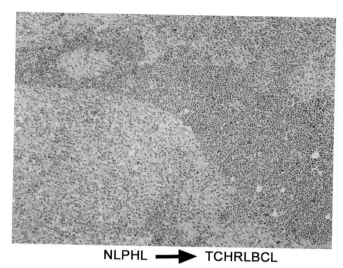

NLPHL ➤ TCHRLBCL

Fig. 20-8. Large cell lymphoma transformation in lymphocyte predominant Hodgkin lymphoma. Lymph node with NLPHL nodules (with a more fibrotic appearance than is typically seen) are associated with diffuse extrafollicular proliferations of small lymphocytes and large nucleolated tumor cells, consistent with transformation to T-cell/histiocyte-rich large B-cell lymphoma (TCHRLBCL). Spread of this lymphoma to bone marrow and liver was also noted

The paragranuloma variant of TCHRBCL shows vague nodular growth and clustering of tumor B cells will be evident on B-cell immunostains [16]. However unlike NLPHL, the infiltrate in TCHRBCL is not folliculocentric and CD57+ BCL6+ T-cell rosettes are absent. More problematic is the distinction between diffuse growth in LPHL (Fig. 20-6) and transformation to DLBCL. Unequivocal evidence of large cell transformation of NLPHL is heralded by sheet-like growth of large B cells outside of nodules (Fig. 20-8) and a shift in the lymphocyte background from predominantly B cells to predominantly T cells, often with a persistent activation (CD38+) immunophenotype (Fig. 20-9) [13]. Systemic spread of NLPHL to the liver or bone marrow almost certainly indicates a shift to TCHRBCL (Fig. 20-9), [17] since this indicates that the tumor no longer requires the lymph node microenvironment for growth.

Another important differential is with the follicular variant of LRCHL which is also frequently folliculocentric. In one study, nearly 21% of cases of NLPHL diagnosed by morphology alone had an immunophenotype consistent with LRCHL [18]. LRCHL may be distinguished morphologically from NLPHL by the presence of the RS-like neoplastic cells in the mildly expanded mantle zone cells, eccentrically surrounding atrophic GCs. LRCHL has a CD30+ immunophenotype, and is positive for EBV in 20%–40% of cases, unlike NLPHL.

20.4. Classical Hodgkin Lymphoma

20.4.1. Clinical Features

The differing histologic appearances of nodular sclerosis (NS)CHL and mixed cellularity (MC)HL are correlated with different clinical presentations and disease courses. NSCHL, representing 70% of HL in the United States, typically presents in younger patients with a mediastinal mass and/or peripheral adenopathy; bulky disease is present in 50%. NSCHL spreads primarily through the lymphatic system, so other sites of involvement usually radiate out from the presenting location and bone marrow, liver, lung and spleen involvement are uncommon at diagnosis [19]. Older patients with NSCHL often have atypical presentations, including at extranodal sites (e.g., bowel) and at a higher stage. Relapses in NSCHL can

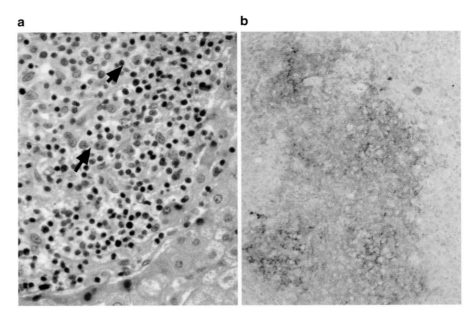

Fig. 20-9. T-cell rich large B-cell lymphoma in a patient with lymphocyte predominant Hodgkin lymphoma. (A) Liver biopsy shows a periportal infiltrate of small lymphocytes and scattered large tumor cells (*arrows*). (B) In contrast to background lymphocytes in NLPHL, the tumor-associated T cells in TCHRLBCL have an activated CD38+ immunophenotype

Table 20-2. Presenting features of Hodgkin lymphoma in the United States.

	NLPHL	**NSCHL**	**MCCHL**	**LRCHL**	**LDCHL**
Percentage of all cases (%)	3	73	18	4	2
Median age at diagnosis	40	32	38	48	30
Male: female	2.8:1	1:1	2.7:1	2.2:1	1.3:1
Stage I* (%)	53	10	21	46	4
Stage II (%)	28	47	32	24	52
Stage III (%)	14	29	35	24	17
Stage IV (%)	6	14	13	6	26
Mediastinal involvement (%)	7	80	40	15	35
B symptoms (%)	10	42	35	11	70
Epstein-Barr virus (%)	0	20	75	41	44

Stages refer to initial presentation, based on Ann Arbor classification (Table 21.1). Data is averaged from several large case series.

NLPHL nodular lymphocyte predominant Hodgkin lymphoma, *NS* nodular sclerosis classical Hodgkin lymphoma (CHL), *MC* mixed cellularity CHL, *LR* lymphocyte rich CHL, *LD* lymphocyte depleted CHL

occur rapidly following chemotherapy or radiation treatment, and may be either localized or at distant sites.

MCCHL presents at a slightly older age, usually affects peripheral lymph nodes rather than the mediastinum, and is more frequently high-stage with associated B-symptoms (Table 20-2) [6]. LRCHL comprises ~4% of HL and its demographic and presenting features are closer to those of NLPHL. Response to therapy is also similar to NLPHL, except for a higher relapse rate [20]. Lymphocyte-depleted (LD) CHL is a vanishingly rare entity (less than 1% of HL) but is commonly seen in HIV positive patients, where such cases are always associated with EBV. Bone marrow and retroperitoneal involvement are common in LDCHL, and the disease pursues an aggressive course, especially in immunodeficient patients.

20.4.2. Morphologic and Immunophenotypic Features

Well-developed NSCHL partially or completely replaces the lymph node with capsular thickening and tumor nodules rimmed by thick collagen bands. There are mixed infiltrates of inflammatory cells (eosinophils, neutrophils, histiocytes, plasma cells, and small lymphocytes) and variable numbers of binucleated or multinucleated Reed-Sternberg (R-S) cells with large eosinophilic central nucleoli, as well as mononuclear R-S variants (Fig. 20-10a, b). The lacunar cell, with its convoluted nuclei and clear retracted cytoplasm due to formalin-fixation artifact, is considered more specific for NSCHL (Fig. 20-10c). "Mummified" tumor cells with condensed chromatin are also commonly seen in NSCHL (Fig. 20-10d). The sclerosis surrounding nodules (Fig. 20-11) shows birefringence under polarized light [21].

The R-S cells and variants in NSHL and other CHL types are strongly, uniformly positive for CD30 (often with membrane and dot-like Golgi staining), and at least focally positive for CD15 using the LeuMI antibody (Fig. 20-12). CD45/LCA, CD43, and T-cell markers are negative but CD20 can be expressed in 20%–40% of the cases, usually focally. In the United States, NSHL is rarely positive for EBV. The background small lymphocytes are predominantly CD4 positive T cells.

Variant appearances of NSCHL can be related to the stage of the lesion, the histologic grade (see below), or to the effects of prior therapy. The nodules in the *syncytial variant* contain sheets of neoplastic cells with central necrosis; the early-stage parafollicular tumor aggregates in the *cellular phase* lack fibrotic bands (Fig. 20-13), and *fibrohistiocytic variants* have R-S cells embedded within the dense proliferations of reactive fibroblasts. Some cases of NSCHL may show such prominent neutrophilic or eosinophilic inflammation that R-S cells are easily overlooked.

Given the large variation in the density of tumor cells in NSCHL, there has been an ongoing debate over the prognostic utility of histologic grading. In 1989, Maclennan reported that the tumor cell-poor cases with lots of small lymphocytes had a better prognosis than lymphocyte-depleted cases or those with pleomorphic tumor cell morphology [22]. However, not all subsequent studies have confirmed these findings. Inclusion of additional histologic features in grading criteria, including the presence of eosinophilia (>5% of all cells or clusters in at least 5 high-power fields), lymphocyte depletion (<33% of cells in the entire section), and the presence of marked atypia in the R-S cells (>25% of R-S cells with bizarre or highly anaplastic features) has been reported to improve the predictive power [23]. However, due to the lack of consensus, the current guidance in the 4th Edition of the WHO Classification (2008) [2] is that grading is not required for routine clinical purposes.

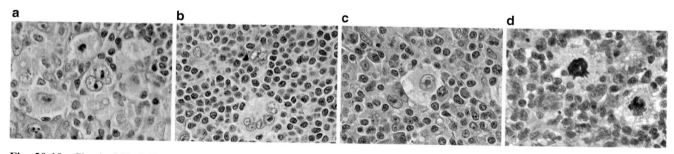

Fig. 20-10. Classical Hodgkin lymphoma, tumor cell morphology: (**a**) Classical Reed-Sternberg (R-S) cell with large eosinophilic nucleoli (center) with mononuclear variant at lower left; (**b**). Multinucleated R-S cell; (**c**) Lacunar cell; (**d**) Mummified tumor cells undergoing apoptosis

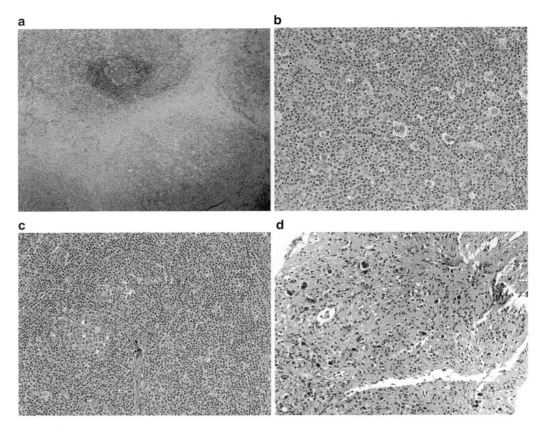

Fig. 20-11. Classical Hodgkin lymphoma, architectural features. (**a**) Nodular sclerosis type – thick fibrous bands encircling a mixed inflammatory nodule with scattered R-S cells. (**b**) Mixed Cellularity type – diffuse mixed inflammatory infiltrate with scattered H/R-S cells. (**c**) Lymphocyte Rich type – a nodular aggregate of small mature lymphocytes with eccentric small residual germinal center near the nodule border (*left*). Note rare Hodgkin cells in the lower left. (**d**) Lymphocyte Depleted type – fibrous background with scattered R-S cells and rare, small, mature lymphocytes

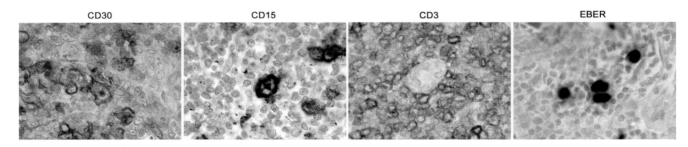

Fig. 20-12. Classical Hodgkin lymphoma, immunohistochemical staining. (**a**) CD30 showing cytoplasmic staining, highlighting the membrane and Golgi zone in an R-S cell. (**b**) CD15 immunostain shows cytoplasmic localization in R-S cells. (**c**) CD3 immunostain highlights the predominance of T cells surrounding the tumor cells. (**d**) EBER in situ hybridization shows multiple binucleated and mononuclear R-S forms that are positive for EBV

Several characteristic patterns of growth are noted with relapse or disease persistence in NSCHL. In one, R-S cells are sparse and embedded in dense reparative fibrosis resembling sclerosing lymphoma. In the other, there are sheet-like infiltrates of mononuclear tumor cells that can be indistinguishable from DLBCL. CD20 and other B-cell markers also tend to be upregulated in relapsed/recurrent CHL.

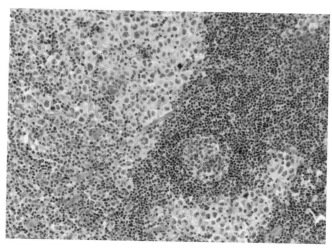

Fig. 20-13. Nodular sclerosis classical Hodgkin lymphoma, cellular phase. Early tumor nodules in NSCHL have a parafollicular location and lack surrounding collagen bands

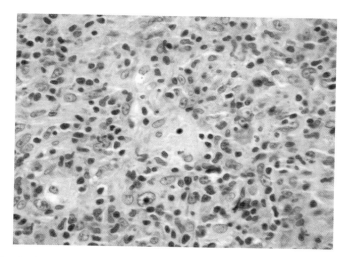

Fig. 20-14. Mixed cellularity classical Hodgkin lymphoma, histiocyte-rich

Lymph node involvement in MCCHL is interfollicular to diffuse and lacks the marked capsular thickening and sclerotic bands of NSCHL (Fig. 20-11). Admixed histiocytes and plasma cells are also more common in MCCHL and lacunar cells are absent. Variants include *histiocyte-rich* (Fig. 20-14) or granuloma-forming tumors resembling T-cell lymphoma [24]. MCCHL shows the typical CD15+ CD30+ R-S immunophenotype, but in contrast to typical NSCHL, is positive for EBV, using either LMP1 immunostaining or EBER in situ hybridization (Fig. 20-12), in 75% of cases in the United States.

LRCHL refers to cases that have an interfollicular or folliculocentric pattern of lymph node infiltration and in which the R-S cells are present in a background of small lymphocytes without many other inflammatory cells (Fig. 20-11c). In contrast to NLPHL, the folliculocentric infiltrate in LRCHL involves expanded mantle zones surrounding still-recognizable atrophic GCs (Fig. 20-15) [9]. The tumor cells have a typical R-S morphology and strongly express CD30, although CD20 may also be expressed and CD15 can be dim/negative (Table 20-3).

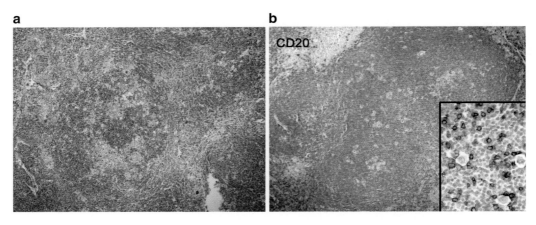

Fig. 20-15. Lymphocyte rich Hodgkin lymphoma, follicular variant. (**a**) Mantle zone of a disrupted germinal cells are markedly expanded by a mixed infiltrate of small lymphocytes and R-S tumor cells. (**b**) CD20 immunostain is positive in mantle zone lymphocytes but negative in tumor cells; CD57+ follicular T cells surround some of the tumor cells (*inset*)

Table 20-3. Comparison of immunophenotype in Hodgkin lymphoma and lymphoma subtypes.

Marker	NLPHL	NSCHL	MCCHL	LRCHL	LDCHL	TCRBCL	ALCL
CD15	0	75	75	74	90	0	52
CD30	0	100	100	98	100	20	100
CD20	98	13	26	27	0	100	0
CD79[a]	80	13	20	43	25	40	16
PAX5	100	100	100	100	100	73	0
MUM1/IRF4	0[a]	97	98	100	100	40	100
Oct-2 (GCB)	100	61	63	72	67	80	Rare
Bob-1 (GCB)	100	39	33	50	33	93	Rare
Pu.1	86	0	0	0	0	54	0 (ALK+) 23 (ALK−)
EBER	0	20	75	41	44	10	0
EBV-LMP1	0	18	33	10	60	9	0

Data is averaged from several large case series [12,14,18,44–50]
[a]30% of cases may have minimal positive staining (<10 cells)

LDCHL should be reserved for those cases with a CHL immunophenotype, but where the sheet-like nature of the infiltrate or the degree of tumor cell pleomorphism is so prominent that the tumor resembles a poorly differentiated sarcoma or carcinoma. The fibrotic variant of LDCHL has sparse pleomorphic tumor cells embedded in fibrosis, but without the nodular collagen seen in NSCHL. The reticular or sarcomatous variant has a diffuse proliferation of R-S cells which may appear "mummified" or sarcomatous (Fig. 20-11d). The immunophenotype must be typical of CHL and it is important to exclude (T-cell) anaplastic large cell lymphoma (ALCL) and anaplastic DLBCL by doing T-cell and B-cell gene rearrangement studies. Poorly differentiated carcinoma can be positive for CD15 and (focally) for CD30 so it should be excluded with appropriate immunostains.

20.4.3. Pathogenesis

Similar to L&H cells, R-S tumor cells carry rearranged and somatically-mutated Ig genes, but the Ig sequences often predict for non-functional or "crippled" B-cell receptor (BCR) which would not signal normally [2]. The mechanisms by which such crippled R-S cells avoid apoptosis without having a functional BCR are varied but include expression of EBV latency genes (particularly EBNA1 and LMP1) in some cases, and compensatory genetic alterations in the nuclear factor kappa (NF-k)B pathway in others. For example, REL, an NF-kB transcription factor, is amplified in ~50% of CHL, [25] and the NF-kB inhibitor kappa beta (IkB)-alpha and IkB-epsilon are inactivated by mutations in a substantial number of cases [26, 27]. Signaling through the tumor necrosis factor (TNF) family receptors CD30, CD40, and RANK further activates NF-kB. EBV LMP1 functions as a non-membrane mimic of activated CD40 [28].

Upregulation of nuclear NF-kB activity, by whatever mechanism, drives transcription of several anti-apoptotic genes such as c-FLIP/CFLAR, BCL2, BCLXL/BCL2L1 and XIAP. c-FLIP mediates signaling through CD95 and TRIAL which are the two major cell death pathways operative in GC B-cell selection [29]. Constitutive activation of the JAK-STAT pathways (through overexpression of STAT3, STAT5A/B and STAT6) may cooperate in overriding extrinsic and intrinsic apoptotic pathways allowing R-S cells to escape programmed cell death [30]. The absence of a functional BCR signal in CHL also apparently has significant effects in shifting the transcriptional program in R-S cells, with loss of many pan-B markers and transcription factors (e.g., POU2F2/Oct-2 and POU2AF1/Bob-1), acquisition of others (e.g., the post-GC marker IRF4/MUM-1), and activation of signaling though the NOTCH pathway. The cytokine IL-13 and its receptor are also highly expressed in Hodgkin cell lines and R-S cells likely functioning to promote autocrine growth.

Given the centrality of GCB signaling in CHL development, the presentation of most cases with NSCHL in the mediastinum (suggesting thymic origin) is paradoxical. It suggests that the proliferation of R-S cells is heavily dependent on particular microenvironmental factors which may be provided by trophic growth factors in lymph collecting at this site. Indeed, the shifts in gene expression in R-S produced by the genetic alterations detailed above also result in the abnormal production of large amounts of cytokines and chemotactic chemokines that have dramatic effects on the tissue microenvironment. Although each CHL case likely secretes different patterns of growth factors, recruitment and activation of CD4+ T cells is central. These T cells are recruited by several chemokines expressed by R-S cells, particularly TARC/CCL17 which is expressed in involved lymph nodes only by the tumor cells (Fig. 20-16). R-S cells also produce a number of cytokines including IL-5 and IL-10 which polarize the tumor-associated T cells to produce additional Th2 cytokines (IL-10 and IL-6) and chemokines (such as CCL11 and CCL27) that attract eosinophils and plasma cells [18].

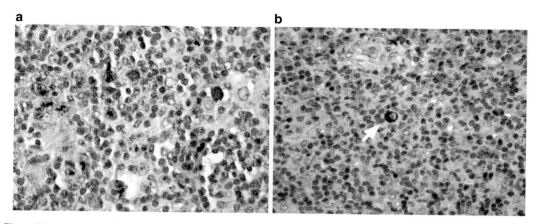

Fig. 20-16. Chemokine expression in classical Hodgkin lymphoma. (**a**) Selective expression of TARC/CCL17 in R-S tumor cells. (**b**) Reactive lymph node with only extremely rare CCL17+ immunoblasts (*arrow*); all other lymph node cells were negative for CCL17

20.4.4. Differential Diagnosis

Most cases of CHL are straightforward to diagnose, however cases with large numbers of tumor cells (particularly common at relapse) may be mistaken for large cell lymphomas. In small biopsies from patients with mediastinal masses, primary mediastinal large B-cell lymphoma (PMLBCL) is the most common differential because of its sclerotic background, and often weak/focal positivity for CD30. Helpful clues favoring PMLBCL are a clearing artifact around the tumor cells, the lack of significant pleomorphism, and the uniform positivity for CD20. The strong staining of PMLBCL for B-cell transcription factors (e.g., Bob-1, Oct-2 and PU.1), as opposed to the weak/focal positivity in CHL, can be helpful in difficult cases.

In the rare CHL cases with a sinusoidal growth pattern, [31] or those with sheet-like anaplastic tumor cell infiltrates (Fig. 20-17), CD30+ ALCL may be a consideration. There are even rare cases of ALCL that diffusely express CD15 [32]. However, despite the loss of expression of some T-cell markers, [33] almost all cases of ALCL will express one or more T-cell markers (particularly CD2 and CD43/MT-1), as well as ALK, CD45, and EMA in some cases, and are negative for PAX-5. Molecular studies for T-cell receptor gene rearrangements are helpful, as ALCL will demonstrate a monoclonal rearrangement in 90% of cases using newer PCR methods, [34] as is EBV staining which is almost always negative in ALCL [35].

Even with the use of multiple molecular and immunophenotypic markers, a handful of cases will be encountered where overlapping features preclude definitive distinction between CHL and ALCL ("Hodgkin-like ALCL") or between CHL and LBCL. These so-called grey zone lymphomas are best handled by correlation with clinical presentation (including degree of tumor bulk and site(s) of involvement) and with therapy selected based on an integrated approach.

Another problem in diagnosis of CHL is related to the propensity of tumor-associated inflammatory changes to obscure the underlying neoplasm. Staging bone marrows and extranodal sites (e.g., liver and spleen) will often show paraneoplastic granulomas implicating an infectious or autoimmune etiology. Marked blood eosinophilia (and occasionally eosinophilic tissue abscesses) may be mistaken for myeloproliferative neoplasms or infections. Lymph nodes draining sites of HL are usually mildly enlarged and show marked follicular hyperplasia with interfollicular plasmacytosis mimicking plasma cell Castleman disease, [36] due to the effects of tumor-associated cytokine production (Fig. 20-18). For this reason, rebiopsy is recommended for any such diagnosis of reactive plasmacytosis in younger patients presenting with a mediastinal mass.

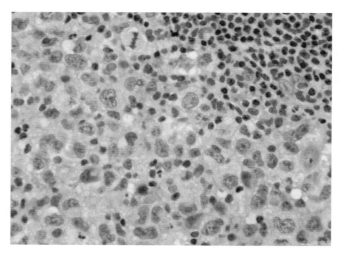

Fig. 20-17. Classical Hodgkin lymphoma, recurrent. Sheets of large tumor cells in a case of recurrent NSCHL resemble large cell lymphoma

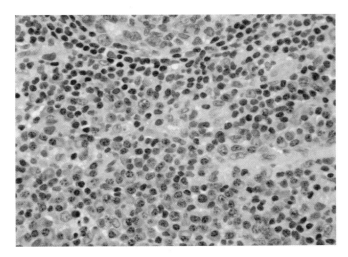

Fig. 20-18. Interfollicular plasmacytosis in a lymph node draining CHL. Hyperplastic follicles (one partially seen at top of figure) and marked interfollicular proliferations of reactive-appearing plasma cells resemble the plasma cell variant of Castleman disease. Followup lymph node biopsy from an adjacent area revealed NSCHL

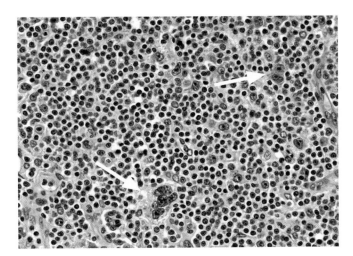

Fig. 20-19. Small lymphocytic lymphoma, with associated Reed-Sternberg cells. Flow cytometry revealed CD5+ B cells consistent with small lymphocytic lymphoma

20.5. HL-Like Proliferations in Other Lymphomas

Due to immunosuppressive effects of the tumor or its treatment, some types of B-cell and T-cell lymphomas can show proliferations of EBV+ large lymphocytes with a R-S morphology (Fig. 20-19) [37–40]. These proliferations are particularly common in patients with CLL treated with fludarabine and in angioimmunoblastic T-cell lymphomas, but can occur in any other lymphoma subtype. In most cases, these admixed EBV+ R-S cells are sparse and should simply be mentioned as an incidental finding since they are indicative of a clinically significant degree of tumor-associated immunosuppression. In other cases, the infiltrate become discrete and take on the inflammatory background of CHL and are best diagnosed as composite lymphoma. These EBV+ cases probably represent the majority of the 1%–2% of composite HL cases that have been reported. Rare composite lymphomas consisting of T-cell lymphoma and HL (with or without T-cell gene rearrangements) may occur. Concurrent DLBCL in NLPHL also always represents transformation and should not be diagnosed as composite lymphoma without molecular evidence of a distinct clonal origin.

20.6. Prognostic Factors and Treatment

The introduction in the 1960s of multi-drug chemotherapy containing alkylating agents dramatically improved survivals in CHL; further refinements, including the introduction of the ABVD, MOPP, and more recently the Stanford-5 and BEACOPP regimens (discussed in Chap. 21) have improved the overall survival in CHL to 70%–90% at 10 years [7,20]. A primary goal is now to stratify patients using clinical predictors (such as the International Prognostic Scoring System, IPSS), [41] tumor markers, and host genetic (pharmacogenetic) features to identify the 10%–20% of treatment-refractory cases and to determine which patients would benefit from adjuvant radiotherapy or targeted agents such as anti-CD20 antibodies or cellular immunotherapy in EBV+ cases.

Newer radiologic methods to assess tumor bulk and metabolic activity, such as 2-[18F] fluoro-2-deoxy-D-glucose positron emission tomography (FDG-PET), may identify poor-risk patients. A negative FDG-PET scan, defined as no pathologic uptake at any site, corresponded to 95% complete remission with treatment of ABVD, in one study [42]. Additionally, the two serum markers that have been consistently associated with poor outcomes in CHL are increased soluble CD30 (above 100–200 U/mL) and IL-10 (above 10 pg/mL) but are rarely monitored routinely at this time. Among tissue markers, an increase in tumor-infiltrating regulatory T cells expressing FOXP3 especially with respect to granzyme B+ T cells (ratio > 1) may correlate with a better prognosis [19]. However, currently, the only routinely-used tumor prognostic markers in HL include the clinical and hematologic parameters listed in Tables 21-5 and 21-8 (Chap. 21).

Suggested Readings

Kuppers R. The biology of Hodgkin's lymphoma. Nat Rev Cancer 2009; 9(1):15-27.
• A recent and through review of HL pathogenesis and the role of the microenvironment.

Pileri SA, Ascani S, Leoncini L, et al. Hodgkin's lymphoma: the pathologist's viewpoint. J Clin Pathol 2002; 55(3):162-76.
• Comprehensive review of the histopathologic classification of HL

Anagnostopoulos I, Hansmann ML, Franssila K, et al. European Task Force on Lymphoma project on lymphocyte predominance Hodgkin disease: histologic and immunohistologic analysis of submitted cases reveals 2 types of Hodgkin disease with a nodular growth pattern and abundant lymphocytes. Blood 2000; 96(5):1889-99.
• A paper summarizing a large series of NLPHL cases (n=563) highlighting the differential diagnosis with LRHL.

References

1. Khan G. Epstein-Barr virus, cytokines, and inflammation: a cocktail for the pathogenesis of Hodgkin's lymphoma? Exp Hematol 2006;34:399–406.
2. Swerdlow SH, Campo E, Harris NL, et al. WHO Classification of Tumour of Haematopoietic and Lymphoid Tissues. Lyon: IARC Press, 2008.
3. Hummel M. World Health Organization and beyond: new aspects in the pathology of an old disease. Hematol Oncol Clin North Am 2007;21:769–86.
4. Kuppers R, Rajewsky K, Zhao M, et al. Hodgkin disease: Hodgkin and Reed-Sternberg cells picked from histological sections show clonal immunoglobulin gene rearrangements and appear to be derived from B cells at various stages of development. Proc Natl Acad Sci U S A 1994;91:10962–6.

5. Kanzler H, Kuppers R, Hansmann ML, Rajewsky K. Hodgkin and Reed-Sternberg cells in Hodgkin's disease represent the outgrowth of a dominant tumor clone derived from (crippled) germinal center B cells. J Exp Med 1996;184:1495–505.

6. Stein H, Marafioti T, Foss HD, et al. Down-regulation of BOB.1/OBF.1 and Oct2 in classical Hodgkin disease but not in lymphocyte predominant Hodgkin disease correlates with immunoglobulin transcription. Blood 2001;97:496–501.

7. Marafioti T, Hummel M, Foss HD, et al. Hodgkin and reed-sternberg cells represent an expansion of a single clone originating from a germinal center B-cell with functional immunoglobulin gene rearrangements but defective immunoglobulin transcription. Blood 2000;95:1443–50.

8. Chang KC, Khen NT, Jones D, Su IJ. Epstein-Barr virus is associated with all histological subtypes of Hodgkin lymphoma in Vietnamese children with special emphasis on the entity of lymphocyte predominance subtype. Hum Pathol 2005;36:747–55.

9. Chang KC, Huang GC, Jones D, Tsao CJ, Lee JY, Su IJ. Distribution and prognosis of WHO lymphoma subtypes in Taiwan reveals a low incidence of germinal-center derived tumors. Leuk Lymphoma 2004;45:1375–84.

10. Nakatsuka S, Aozasa K. Epidemiology and pathologic features of Hodgkin lymphoma. Int J Hematol 2006;83:391–7.

11. Nogova L, Reineke T, Brillant C, et al. Lymphocyte-predominant and classical Hodgkin's lymphoma: a comprehensive analysis from the German Hodgkin Study Group. J Clin Oncol 2008;26:434–9.

12. Boudova L, Torlakovic E, Delabie J, et al. Nodular lymphocyte-predominant Hodgkin lymphoma with nodules resembling T-cell/histiocyte-rich B-cell lymphoma: differential diagnosis between nodular lymphocyte-predominant Hodgkin lymphoma and T-cell/histiocyte-rich B-cell lymphoma. Blood 2003;102:3753–8.

13. Lin P, Medeiros LJ, Wilder RB, Abruzzo LV, Manning JT, Jones D. The activation profile of tumour-associated reactive T-cells differs in the nodular and diffuse patterns of lymphocyte predominant Hodgkin's disease. Histopathology 2004;44:561–9.

14. Fan Z, Natkunam Y, Bair E, Tibshirani R, Warnke RA. Characterization of variant patterns of nodular lymphocyte predominant hodgkin lymphoma with immunohistologic and clinical correlation. Am J Surg Pathol 2003;27:1346–56.

15. Jones D. Dismantling the germinal center: comparing the processes of transformation, regression, and fragmentation of the lymphoid follicle. Adv Anat Pathol 2002;9:129–38.

16. Achten R, Verhoef G, Vanuytsel L, De Wolf-Peeters C. Histiocyte-rich, T-cell-rich B-cell lymphoma: a distinct diffuse large B-cell lymphoma subtype showing characteristic morphologic and immunophenotypic features. Histopathology 2002;40:31–45.

17. Khoury JD, Jones D, Yared MA, et al. Bone marrow involvement in patients with nodular lymphocyte predominant Hodgkin lymphoma. Am J Surg Pathol 2004;28:489–95.

18. Anagnostopoulos I, Hansmann ML, Franssila K, et al. European Task Force on Lymphoma project on lymphocyte predominance Hodgkin disease: histologic and immunohistologic analysis of submitted cases reveals 2 types of Hodgkin disease with a nodular growth pattern and abundant lymphocytes. Blood 2000;96:1889–99.

19. Hsi ED. Biologic features of Hodgkin lymphoma and the development of biologic prognostic factors in Hodgkin lymphoma: tumor and microenvironment. Leuk Lymphoma 2008;49:1668–80.

20. Diehl V, Behringer K. Could BEACOPP be the new standard for the treatment of advanced Hodgkin's lymphoma (HL)? Cancer Invest 2006;24:713–7.

21. Pileri SA, Ascani S, Leoncini L, et al. Hodgkin's lymphoma: the pathologist's viewpoint. J Clin Pathol 2002;55:162–76.

22. MacLennan KA, Bennett MH, Tu A, et al. Relationship of histopathologic features to survival and relapse in nodular sclerosing Hodgkin's disease. A study of 1659 patients. Cancer 1989;64:1686–93.

23. von Wasielewski S, Franklin J, Fischer R, et al. Nodular sclerosing Hodgkin disease: new grading predicts prognosis in intermediate and advanced stages. Blood 2003;101:4063–9.

24. Patsouris E, Noel H, Lennert K. Cytohistologic and immunohistochemical findings in Hodgkin's disease, mixed cellularity type, with a high content of epithelioid cells. Am J Surg Pathol 1989;13:1014–22.

25. Martin-Subero JI, Gesk S, Harder L, et al. Recurrent involvement of the REL and BCL11A loci in classical Hodgkin lymphoma. Blood 2002;99:1474–7.

26. Cabannes E, Khan G, Aillet F, Jarrett RF, Hay RT. Mutations in the IkBa gene in Hodgkin's disease suggest a tumour suppressor role for IkappaBalpha. Oncogene 1999;18:3063–70.

27. Emmerich F, Theurich S, Hummel M, et al. Inactivating I kappa B epsilon mutations in Hodgkin/Reed-Sternberg cells. J Pathol 2003;201:413–20.

28. Mosialos G, Birkenbach M, Yalamanchili R, VanArsdale T, Ware C, Kieff E. The Epstein-Barr virus transforming protein LMP1 engages signaling proteins for the tumor necrosis factor receptor family. Cell 1995;80:389–99.

29. Mathas S, Lietz A, Anagnostopoulos I, et al. c-FLIP mediates resistance of Hodgkin/Reed-Sternberg cells to death receptor-induced apoptosis. J Exp Med 2004;199:1041–52.

30. Kuppers R. The biology of Hodgkin's lymphoma. Nat Rev Cancer 2009;9:15–27.

31. Lee SS, Ryoo BY, Park YH, et al. Hodgkin lymphoma with unusual intrasinusoidal pattern of infiltration. Leuk Lymphoma 2004;45:2135–41.

32. Gorczyca W, Tsang P, Liu Z, et al. CD30-positive T-cell lymphomas co-expressing CD15: an immunohistochemical analysis. Int J Oncol 2003;22:319–24.

33. Bonzheim I, Geissinger E, Roth S, et al. Anaplastic large cell lymphomas lack the expression of T-cell receptor molecules or molecules of proximal T-cell receptor signaling. Blood 2004;104:3358–60.

34. Tan BT, Seo K, Warnke RA, Arber DA. The frequency of immunoglobulin heavy chain gene and T-cell receptor gamma-chain gene rearrangements and Epstein-Barr virus in ALK+ and ALK- anaplastic large cell lymphoma and other peripheral T-cell lymphomas. J Mol Diagn 2008;10:502–12.

35. Herling M, Rassidakis GZ, Jones D, Schmitt-Graeff A, Sarris AH, Medeiros LJ. Absence of Epstein-Barr virus in anaplastic large cell lymphoma: a study of 64 cases classified according to World Health Organization criteria. Hum Pathol 2004;35:455–9.

36. Maheswaran PR, Ramsay AD, Norton AJ, Roche WR. Hodgkin's disease presenting with the histological features of Castleman's disease. Histopathology 1991;18:249–53.

37. Petrella T, Yaziji N, Collin F, et al. Implication of the Epstein-Barr virus in the progression of chronic lymphocytic leukaemia/small lymphocytic lymphoma to Hodgkin-like lymphomas. Anticancer Res 1997;17:3907–13.

38. Momose H. Jaffe ES, Shin SS, Chen YY. Weiss LM. Chronic lymphocytic leukemia/small lymphocytic lymphoma with Reed-Sternberg-like cells and possible transformation to Hodgkin's disease. Mediation by Epstein-Barr virus. Am J Surg Pathol 1992;16:859–67.

39. Abruzzo LV, Rosales CM, Medeiros LJ, et al. Epstein-Barr virus-positive B-cell lymphoproliferative disorders arising in immunodeficient patients previously treated with fludarabine for low-grade B-cell neoplasms. Am J Surg Pathol 2002;26:630–6.

40. Higgins JP, van de Rijn M, Jones CD, Zehnder JL, Warnke RA. Peripheral T-cell lymphoma complicated by a proliferation of large B cells. Am J Clin Pathol 2000;114:236–47.

41. Hasenclever D, Diehl VA. prognostic score for advanced Hodgkin's disease. International Prognostic Factors Project on Advanced Hodgkin's Disease. N Engl J Med 1998;339:1506–14.

42. Gallamini A, Hutchings M, Rigacci L, et al. Early interim 2-[18F]fluoro-2-deoxy-D-glucose positron emission tomography is prognostically superior to international prognostic score in advanced-stage Hodgkin's lymphoma: a report from a joint Italian-Danish study. J Clin Oncol 2007;25:3746–52.

43. Parkin DM, Whelan SL, Ferlay J, Storm H. Cancer Incidence in Five Continents. Vol I to VIII IARC CancerBase. Lyon: IARC Press, 2005:45-173.

44. Benharroch D, Levy A, Gopas J, Sacks M. Lymphocyte-depleted classic Hodgkin lymphoma-a neglected entity? Virchows Arch 2008;453:611–6.

45. Garcia-Cosio M, Santon A, Martin P, et al. Analysis of transcription factor OCT.1, OCT.2 and BOB.1 expression using tissue arrays in classical Hodgkin's lymphoma. Mod Pathol 2004;17:1531–8.

46. Marafioti T, Mancini C, Ascani S, et al. Leukocyte-specific phosphoprotein-1 and PU.1: two useful markers for distinguishing T-cell-rich B-cell lymphoma from lymphocyte-predominant Hodgkin's disease. Haematologica 2004;89:957–64.

47. McCune RC, Syrbu SI, Vasef MA. Expression profiling of transcription factors Pax-5, Oct-1, Oct-2, BOB.1, and PU.1 in Hodgkin's and non-Hodgkin's lymphomas: a comparative study using high throughput tissue microarrays. Mod Pathol 2006;19:1010–8.

48. Niitsu N, Okamoto M, Tomita N, et al. Multicentre phase II study of the baseline BEACOPP regimen for patients with advanced-stage Hodgkin's lymphoma. Leuk Lymphoma 2006;47:1908–14.

49. Tamaru J, Tokuhira M, Nittsu N, et al. Hodgkin-like anaplastic large cell lymphoma (previously designated in the REAL classification) has same immunophenotypic features to classical Hodgkin lymphoma. Leuk Lymphoma 2007;48:1127–38.

50. Tzankov A, Zimpfer A, Pehrs AC, et al. Expression of B-cell markers in classical hodgkin lymphoma: a tissue microarray analysis of 330 cases. Mod Pathol 2003;16:1141–7.

Chapter 21

Treatment of Hodgkin Lymphoma

Samer A. Srour and Luis E. Fayad

Abstract/Scope of Chapter The presenting features and clinical workup of both classical and lymphocyte predominant Hodgkin lymphoma are discussed. The move away from the use of extended field radiotherapy and the advantages and disadvantages of ABVD (doxorubicin, bleomycin, vinblastine, dacarbazine) compared to other therapies are discussed. The response criteria used in the evaluation of treatment effects are summarized as are prognostic factors that may be broadly useful in patients with advanced stage disease. Finally, the therapy for relapsed disease is covered with a discussion on the role of high-dose chemotherapy and autologous hematopoietic stem cell transplantation.

Keywords Hodgkin lymphoma, treatment • Hodgkin lymphoma, ABVD • Hodgkin lymphoma, autologous stem cell transplant • Hodgkin lymphoma, antibody therapy • Hodgkin lymphoma, rituximab

21.1. Presenting Features

Hodgkin lymphoma (HL), formerly known as Hodgkin's disease (HD), accounts for approximately 1% of all cancers [1] and has two main subtypes, classical (C)HL, comprising 95% of cases, and the uncommon nodular lymphocyte predominant (NLP)HL [2]. CHL is further divided into four subtypes: nodular sclerosis, mixed cellularity, lymphocyte depleted, and lymphocyte rich variants. [3–5] Although each subtype has a different natural history and distinctive morphologic and immunophenotypic features, the diagnostic workup is similar for all cases.

The incidence of HL has been stable over the last few decades, with approximately 8,220 new cases and 1,350 deaths due to disease in the United States (US) in 2008. [6]. There has been recent progress in identifying risk factors for development of HL. These include a subset of cases with an identifiable hereditary genetic component, as evidenced by an increased incidence of HL in the first degree relatives (siblings, twins, and children) of HL patients and an increased incidence in certain ethnic populations (e.g., Jews of Eastern European ancestry) [7–10]. In the US, Epstein-Bar virus (EBV) infection is implicated in the etiology of the mixed cellularity variant of CHL, but rarely in other subtypes [184,185]. The presence of EBV in HL is especially common in cases arising in patients infected with human immunodeficiency virus (HIV) who often present with advanced stage disease due to extranodal involvement and usually have a poor response to initial therapy [11–15].

From: *Neoplastic Hematopathology*: Contemporary Hematology,
Edited by: D. Jones, DOI 10.1007/978-1-60761-384-8_21,
© Humana Press, a part of Springer Science+Business Media, LLC 2010

21.2. Diagnosis and Staging

Given that the sparse tumor cells in HL are often far outnumbered by reactive inflammatory cells, the initial diagnosis should always be established by tissue biopsy. A core needle biopsy may be adequate, but an excisional biopsy is preferred. Fine needle aspirate (FNA) alone is generally insufficient for the evaluation of architecture and for immunophenotyping. [16–18] Because the cytokines associated with HL can produce hyperplastic changes in adjacent lymph nodes, several biopsies may sometimes be required to obtain diagnostic material [19]. As discussed in Chap. 20, immunohistochemical stains are essential for the accurate diagnosis of any case of HL with atypical features, including many cases of NLPHL.

Staging of HL is based on the Ann Arbor staging system that was developed in 1971 [20] and further modified in 1989 through a consensus meeting in Cotswolds, England (Table 21-1) [21]. The staging workup in HL starts with a thorough history and physical examination. The history should focus on the presence or absence of systemic B symptoms (fever >38°C, drenching night sweats, and unexplained weight loss of >10% body weight within the preceding 6 months), performance status, pruritus, alcohol intolerance, and any history of prior cancers requiring chemotherapy or radiation treatment. About one third of patients with HL present with B symptoms, [19] and systemic symptoms, pruritus, and alcohol-induced pain are more common in CHL than NLPHL [22]. Physical examination should assess all sites of secondary lymphoid tissue as well as the size of the liver and spleen.

As per the most recent National Comprehensive Cancer Network (NCCN) guidelines, initial laboratory studies should include a complete blood count (CBC) with leukocyte differential, erythrocyte sedimentation rate (ESR), serum lactate dehydrogenase (LDH) levels, liver and kidney function tests, and a pregnancy test for women of childbearing age. Bone marrow (BM) biopsy should be done for all patients with stage IB-IV disease. To exclude a B-cell lymphoma, flow cytometric analysis of the BM or peripheral blood may be advisable. More invasive staging procedures such as liver biopsy, [23] diagnostic laparotomy, [24] or splenectomy are restricted to a very small subgroup of patients where the initial staging is inconclusive.

Radiographic studies should include chest X-ray and a computed tomography (CT) scan of the chest, abdomen, and pelvis. Recently, positron emission tomography (PET) scans have

Table 21-1. Modified Ann Arbor staging system for HL.

Stage definition/disease involvement	
I	Involvement of a single lymph node region (I) or a single extralymphatic site (IE).
II	Involvement of two or more lymph node regions on the same side of the diaphragm (II) or localized involvement of only one extranodal organ or site and of ≥1 lymph node regions on the same side of the diaphragm (IIE).
III	Involvement of lymph node regions on both sides of the diaphragm (III), which may also be accompanied by involvement of the spleen (III_S) or by localized involvement of an extranodal organ or site (IIIE) or both (III_{S+E}).
IV	Diffuse involvement of one or more extranodal organs or sites, with or without associated lymph node involvement.
Each stage may be subdivided into:	
A	No symptoms.
B	General symptoms include any of the following: fever (temperatures >38°C), drenching night sweats, unexplained loss of >10% body weight within the preceding 6 months.
X	Bulky disease which is defined by any nodal mass with a maximal dimension ≥10 cm or a mediastinal mass exceeding one third of the widest transverse transthoracic diameter measured on a standard PA chest radiography.
E	Involvement of a single extranodal site that is contiguous or proximal to the known nodal site.

also become integral to initial staging and follow-up assessment and are used at most centers. [27,28]. In a review done by Juweid et al., PET scans in HL resulted in a modification of the disease stage (usually upstaging) in about 15–20% of patients and influenced management in about 5–15% of patients [27]. However, it remains unclear whether these changes will have an impact on improved outcomes so the value of PET for initial staging of HL patients remains controversial [28]. On the other hand, as reviewed by Juweid et al., response assessment after completion of therapy is currently the most widely utilized application of restaging PET in HL and can be considered the standard of care for posttreatment assessment [27].

21.3. Treatment

21.3.1. Overview of Progress in Early Stage and Advanced HL

Treatment in HL is largely based on clinical stage, with early stage HL defined as stages I, II, and IIIA, and advanced HL as stage IIIB and stage IV, according to the Cotswolds modification of the Ann Arbor classification [183] (Table 21-1). HL is currently curable in 85–95% of patients, with the highest responses seen with localized disease [1]. In the H8-F trial, Ferme et al. reported a 10-year overall survival (OS) estimate of 97% for early stage disease [29]. Cure rates for HL are now so high for early stage disease that the overriding treatment considerations currently relate to minimizing long-term toxicity [2]. For patients presenting with disseminated disease, improvement in cure rates are still the focus of clinical trials, but the potential long-term effect of treatments are an important secondary consideration. New innovative treatment strategies are also clearly needed for the refractory and recurrent disease, as the cure rates for these patients are still low, [30] especially for those who relapse after autologous hematopoietic stem cell transplantation (AHSCT).

21.3.2. Definitions of Risk Groups in HL

In addition to stage, various prognostic factors that can predict the treatment outcome and affect the choice of treatment have been identified (Table 21-2). The most recently published NCCN guidelines define *early stage favorable (intermediate)* as stage I-II disease with no B symptoms or large mediastinal adenopathy; *early stage unfavorable* as stage I-II disease with large mediastinal mass, with or without B symptoms or stage I-II with B symptoms, numerous sites of disease, or significantly elevated ESR; and *advanced stage disease* as stage III-IV disease. However, some centers in the US define only two risk groups, namely limited stage (IA and IIA without bulky disease) and advanced stage HL [III and IV; B symptoms; bulky disease (≥10 cm)] [28]. Other risk stratification schemes used include the European Organization for Research and Treatment of Cancer (EORTC) criteria which are similar to those used by German HL Study Group (GHSG) [31–34]. The EORTC criteria differs by substituting age ≥50 years for the extra nodal disease criterion and specifying ≥4 involved regions rather than ≥3, as in GHSG [36]. Similarly, the National Cancer Institute of Canada (NCIC) and the Eastern Cooperative Oncology Group (ECOG) subdivided early stage HL into risk categories, with "low risk" comprising NLPHL and nodular sclerosis CHL, age <40 years, erythrocyte sedimentation rate (ESR) <50, and ≤3 disease regions. High-risk tumors were all other stage I-II cases, except those with bulky disease > 10 cm, which are classified as advanced-stage HL [36,37].

21.3.3. Treatment of Early Stage HL

Prior to the last 15–20 years, extended field radiotherapy (EF-RT) was the standard of care for treating early stage HL. However, EF-RT was complicated by high relapse rates [38] and serious long-term side effects, [39] including pulmonary dysfunction, [40] heart disease,

Table 21-2. Definitions of prognostic factors and treatment groups in the major HL study groups.

	GHSG	EORTC/GELA	NCIC/ECOG	NCCN
Risk factors	A Large mediastinal mass	A Large mediastinal mass	A Bulky disease >10 cm	A Large mediastinal mass or bulky disease
	B Extranodal disease	B Age ≥50 years	B Age ≥40	B ≥2 extranodal sites
	C ESR ≥50 or B[a] symptoms with ESR ≥30	C Same as for GHSG	C ESR ≥50 or any B[a] symptom	C ESR ≥50, if asymptomatic
	D ≥3 involved regions	D ≥4 involved regions	D >3 involved regions	D >3 involved regions
			E MCHL or LDHL	E B[a] symptoms
Treatment groups				
Lymphocyte predominant	NLPHL histology in CS I–II with no RF	NLPHL histology in supradiaphragmatic CS I–II	CS I–II with no RF	
Early stage favorable	CS I–II with no RF	CS I–II supradiaphragmatic with no RF	Low risk early stage	CS I–II with none of the RFs
Early stage unfavorable	CS I, CS IIA with any RF; CS IIB with C/D but without A/B	CS I–II supradiaphragmatic with any RF	High risk early stage	CS I–II with any of the RFs
Advanced stage	CS IIB with A/B; CS III–IV	CS III–IV	CS I–II with A; CS III–IV	CS III–IV

[a]B symptoms include fever with temperature >38°C, drenching night sweats, and unexplained weight loss of >10% body weight within 6 months

CS clinical stage, EORTC European Organization for Research and Treatment of Cancer, ESR erythrocyte sedimentation rate, GELA Groupe d'Etude des Lymphomes de l'Adulte, GHSG German Hodgkin Study Group, LDHL lymphocyte depleted Hodgkin's lymphoma, MCHL mixed cellnbority Holgkins lymphoma, NCIC/ECOG National Cancer Institute of Canada/Eastern Cooperative Oncology Group, NCCN National Comprehensive Cancer Network, NLPHL nodular lymphocyte predominant Hodgkin's lymphoma, RF risk factor

Table 21-3. Recommended treatments for early stage HL.

Histology	Prognostic group	Recommended treatment
Early stage CHL	Favorable[a]	Chemotherapy[b] + IFRT or Chemotherapy alone with ABVD × 6 cycles (category 2B)
	Unfavorable[a]	Chemotherapy[c] + IFRT
Early stage NLPHL	CS IA	Local LN excision or IFRT alone
	CS IIA	IFRT or regional RT alone[d]vs.
		Brief chemotherapy followed by IFRT as an alternative
	CS I–IIB	Chemotherapy[e] followed by IFRT

[a]See Table 21-2 for the definitions of favorable and unfavorable prognostic groups
[b]For favorable early stage CHL, the most commonly used regimens are the ABVD (two to four cycles) and the Stanford V regimen (two cycles) see Table 21-4 for dosage/schedule
[c]For unfavorable early stage CHL, either ABVD is given for four to six cycles or Stanford V for three cycles
[d]In the setting of nonbulky CS IIA NLPHL
[e]Given the rarity of NLPHL, no large randomized trials regarding the best chemotherapeutic regimen are done. ABVD is widely used based on data for CHL. Immunotherapy with rituximab has recently been shown to have excellent response rates in LPHL. Other suggested chemotherapy regimens with or without rituximab include CVP, CHOP, and EPOCH, *CS* clinical stage, *IFRT* involved field radiation therapy, *LN* lymph node, *RT* radiation therapy

[41] and secondary cancers [42–44]. Furthermore, treatment with combined modality therapy proved superior to treatment with radiation therapy alone, and has now become the standard therapy (Table 21-3 and Table 21-4) [45–52]. When using RT, the application of chemotherapy prior to irradiation not only led to better treatment results but also enabled the reduction of EF-RT to involved field (IF)-RT in this group of patients [46,50,53,54] permitting a significant reduction of up to 50% in the effective radiation dose [55].

There is still no consensus as to what chemotherapy should be used, how many cycles should be delivered, and how much RT should be administered, if at all. The most recent published NCCN guidelines for early stage HL recommend the use of either ABVD or the Stanford V (mechlorethamine, doxorubicin, vinblastine, prednisone, vincristine, bleomycin, VP-16) regimens as the first line treatment followed by consolidative irradiation. The choice of ABVD as a standard regimen was based on many studies that were conducted in Europe and the US that compared the combination of either EFRT or IFRT with different chemotherapy regimens like ABVD, MOPP (mechlorethamine, vincristine, procarbazine, prednisone), MOPP/ABV (doxorubicin, bleomycin, vinblastine), EBVP (epirubicin, bleomycin, vinblastine, prednisone), COPP (cyclophosphamide, vincristine, procarbazine, prednisone) and BEACOPP (bleomycin, etoposide, doxorubicin, cyclophosphamide, vincristine, procarbazine, prednisone) [29,46–48,51,56,57]. The Stanford V regimen, which incorporated the active agents from ABVD and MOPP into a brief dose-intense regimen, is one of the new regimens that also has been proven, combined with radiotherapy, to be highly effective in early stage favorable and unfavorable or locally extensive HL and has a low toxicity profile [58–62]. The number of chemotherapy cycles (2 to 6 ABVD vs. 2 to 3 Stanford V), and the intensity of radiation, depends on the favorable factors and the bulkiness of the disease.

In contrast to early stage CHL, patients with stage IA NLPHL can be treated with LN excision followed by a "watch and wait" approach or with IFRT only [63–67]. IFRT or regional RT has been also considered a valid choice in the setting of nonbulky stage II NLPHL, [2,66,67] although brief chemotherapy followed by IFRT is also an acceptable alternative management strategy [22].

The use of midtreatment PET scans has been proposed as one way in early stage HL to select those patients who can receive less therapy. In this model, patients with negative PET

Table 21-4. Common Chemotherapeutic regimens used for the treatment of HL in Europe and US.

Regimen	Dosage and schedule	Frequency/Duration[a]
ABVD[b]		
Doxorubicin	25 mg/m2 IV on days 1 and 15	
Bleomycin	10 units/m2 IV on days 1 and 15	Repeat cycle every 28 days
Vinblastine	6 mg/m2 IV on days 1 and 15	
Dacarbazine[b]	375 mg/m2 IV on days 1-5	
Standard BEACOPP[c]		
Bleomycin	10 units/m2 IV on day 8	
Etoposide	100 mg/m2 IV on days 1, 2, and 3	
Doxorubicin	25 mg/m2 IV on day 1	
Cyclophosphamide	650 mg/m2 IV on day 1	Repeat cycle every 21 days
Vincristine[d]	1.4 mg/m2 IV on day 8	
Procarbazine	100 mg/m2 PO on days 1-7	
Prednisone[e]	40 mg/m2 PO on days 1-14	
Esc-BEACOPP[c]		
Bleomycin	10 mg/m2 IV on day 8	
Etoposide	200 mg/m2 IV on days 1, 2, and 3	
Doxorubicin	35 mg/m2 IV on day 1	
Cyclophosphamide	1200 mg/m2 IV on day 1	Repeat cycle every 21 days
Vincristine[d]	1.4 mg/m2 IV on day 8	
Procarbazine	100 mg/m2 PO on days 1-7	
Prednisone	40 mg/m2 PO on days 1-14	
Filgrastim[e]	300 mcg/day starting on day 8	
STANFORD V[f]		
Doxorubicin	25 mg/m2 IV on days 1 and 15	
Vinblastine[g]	6 mg/m2 IV on days 1 and 15	Repeat cycle every 28 days for
Mechlorethamine	6 mg/m2 IV on day 1	a total of 2 to 3 cycles.
Vincristine[g]	1.4 mg/m2 IV on days 8 and 22	Radiotherapy to initial sites
Bleomycin	5 units/m2 IV on days 8 and 22	5 cm or larger starting
Etoposide	60 mg/m2 IV on days 15 and 16	2 weeks after completion of
Prednisone[h]	40 mg/m2 PO every other day	chemotherapy (dose: 36 Gy).

[a] The duration of chemotherapy/number of cycles is determined by the stage of the disease and the prognostic factors (see text for details)

[b] ABVD regimen was used first as described in the table by Bonadonna G et al. On subsequent studies, dacarbazine was administered on days 1 and 15 rather than on days 1-5 [85].

[c] Derived from Diehl V et al. 2003 [94]

[d] Maximum dose 2 mg.

[e] Filgrastrim is given subcutaneously starting on day 8 and continuing until WBC ≥13,000/mm3 on 3 consecutive days. The dose is 300 mcg/day for patients with body weight <75 kg and 400 mcg/day for those ≥75 kg

[f] Derived from Bartlett NL et al. 1995 [91]

[g] Vinblastine dose reduced to 4mg/m2 and vincristine dose to 1mg/m2 during cycle 3 for patients 50 years of age or older

[h] Prednisone is started on day 1 and continued every other day. It is tapered by 10 mg/dose every other day starting on day 14 of the third cycle

scans after two cycles of treatment could be considered for an abbreviated course of chemotherapy, whereas those with positive PET scan would be treated with standard combined modality therapy [19]. In this regard, it is important to note that PET shows an excellent negative predictive value between 91–95% in several studies, [68,69] but the positive predictive value is substantially lower and considerably more variable, averaging approximately 65% [27]. To decrease the false-positive results, the International Harmonization Project

(IHP) recommends that PET not be performed for at least 3 weeks following chemotherapy and preferably 8–12 weeks after completion of radiotherapy. [70].

There is an ongoing trial in the United Kingdom testing whether PET scanning can guide therapy in early HL after three cycles of chemotherapy; PET-negative patients are randomized to IFRT versus observation while PET-positive cases are treated with four-cycle ABVD followed by IFRT [36,71]. Also, the recently initiated EORTC/GELA H10 Intergroup trial is comparing "standard therapy" to PET-based response-adapted therapy (i.e., PET after two cycles of ABVD) for favorable and intermediate group patients with early stage HL [36].

21.3.4. Treatment of Advanced Stage HL

Since the development of the MOPP regimen, [72] intensive chemotherapy regimens have been the standard for treatment of advanced stage HL. However, the challenge is to select those patients that require more intensive regimens while minimizing the likelihood of long-term adverse effects by the use of standard therapies in the remainder of cases. The international prognostic score (IPS) reported by Hasencleaver et al. in 1998 [73] has been the most well-adopted prognostic scheme and has been incorporated into the current NCCN guidelines. Based on an analysis of 5,141 patients, the IPS incorporates seven variables which stratify the 5-year progression rate from 45 to 80% (Table 21-5) [73]. The IPS has been incorporated in many clinical trials and correlates with treatment efficacy in both the standard versus escalated BEACOPP versus COPP/ABVD arms in the HD9 trial [74,75].

PET scan has also emerged as an important tool for prognostication in advanced HL when performed after two [76–79] or three [80,81] courses of chemotherapy. In a large prospective study of 260 newly-diagnosed patients with advanced stage HL treated with ABVD, such early PET scans proved to be the most powerful of the known prognostic markers even compared to the IPS [82]. Indeed, IPS had no significant independent prognostic value when tested against early PET in a multivariate analysis [83]. In patients treated with standard therapy who had a negative early PET scan, 2-year progression-free survival rates were similar to patients treated with more aggressive (and more toxic) regimens such as esc-BEACOPP (escalated BEACOPP) [82]. However, the prognostic value of early PET after esc-BEACOPP is not yet determined. The HD-18 study of the German Hodgkin Study Group (GHSG) will specifically address this issue [83].

Table 21-5. The international prognostic score (IPS) for risk stratification in advanced HL.

Adverse prognostic factors	Relative risk
Serum albumin <4 g/dL	1.49
Hemoglobin <10.5 g/dL	1.35
Male sex	1.35
Stage IV disease	1.26
Age ≥45 years	1.39
White blood count ≥15,000/mm^3	1.41
Lymphocyte count <600/mm^3 or <8%	1.38

Outcome according to prognostic score

Number of factors	FFP at 5 years (%)	OS at 5 years (%)
0	84	89
1	77	90
2	67	81
3	60	78
4	51	61
≥5	42	56

Scoring criteria derived from Hasenclever and Diehl [73]. *FFP* freedom from progression, *OS* overall survival

Because of the high relapse rate and late toxicities experienced with MOPP, multiple other regimens have been developed in an attempt to improve the efficacy and decrease the toxicities from chemotherapy (Table 21-6 and Table 21-4). Several major randomized studies during the past 20 years have attempted to identify the regimen with the greatest activity and the most favorable side effect profile [19]. The most commonly used in Europe and the US are ABVD, Stanford V, and BEACOPP. ABVD has been the standard treatment for patients with advanced HL based on different studies comparing ABVD alternating with MOPP versus MOPP, [84] MOPP versus ABVD versus MOPP alternating with ABVD, [85] MOPP/ ABVD hybrid versus MOPP alternating with ABVD, [86,87] and MOPP/ABVD hybrid versus ABVD [88]. Overall, these studies revealed that ABVD by itself has better activities with less toxicities (acute pulmonary and hematologic toxicities, MDS, and leukemias) than MOPP or MOPP/ABVD and other multidrug regimens with 5-year OS around 82 - 90%, 5-year failure-free survival (FFS) around 63 - 78%, and 5-year freedom from progression (FFP) of 75 - 85% [88,89,90].

Stanford V and BEACOPP are the other two regimens developed to improve the outcome of patients with advanced disease [2]. The Stanford V regimen, which incorporated the active agents MOPP and ABVD into a brief and dose-intensive treatment, was first developed in 1989 [91]. In a phase II single-center trial, Stanford V was given weekly for 12 weeks combined with RT to sites of initial bulky disease (≥5 cm) [60,91]. Most recent updates from this study revealed 12-year FFP and OS rates of 83 and 95%, respectively, [62] with low toxicity profile (maintained fertility and no reported secondary leukemia or myelodysplasia). Similar results have been reported from the MSKCC study [59,92] and from a multi-institutional ECOG study [58,93]. However, a large European phase III randomized trial conducted by the Intergruppo Italiano Linfomi has shown that ABVD, and MOPPEBVCAD are superior to modified Stanford V in terms of response, FFS and FFP rates [89]. This study was criticized as a limited number of patients received consolidation radiotherapy and the timing for response evaluation was different among the three arms

Table 21-6. Recommended treatments for advanced HL.

Histology	Prognostic group	Recommended treatment
Advanced stage CHL		Six to 8 cycles of ABVD[a] ± IFRT[b] or 3 cycles of Stanford V ± RT[c] or Escalated BEACOPP[d] (especially if IPS ≥4) ± RT[e]
Advanced stage NLPHL	CS III-IVA	Observation (category 2B) or Local RT (palliation only) or Chemotherapy[f] ± RT
	CS III-IVB	Chemotherapy[f] ± RT

[a]ABVD is administered for four cycles followed by complete restaging. If complete remission (CR) is achieved two additional cycles are given. Another two cycles (total of eight) might be administered if the patient achieved a CR after six cycles not four cycles

[b]Consolidative RT might be considered for patients with bulky disease

[c]Consolidative RT is instituted to initial sites >5 cm and spleen (if focal nodules are present initially) or residual PET positive sites

[d]Escalated BEACOPP is given for 4 cycles followed by complete restaging. Another four cycles of esc-BEACOPP are given if partial remission (PR) is achieved, while four cycles of baseline BEACOPP are administered if CR is achieved see Table 21-4 for dosages/schedule

[e]RT to initial sites >5 cm or to residual PET positive sites

[f]Given the rarity of advanced stage NLPHL, the best chemotherapeutic regimen is yet to be determined. ABVD is widely used based on data for CHL treatment. Recent studies showed that rituximab has excellent activity either as a single agent or combined with other regimens. Other suggested chemotherapy regimens with or without rituximab include: CVP, CHOP, and EPOCH. *CS* clinical stage, *IFRT* involved field radiation therapy, *IPS* international prognostic score, *RT* radiation therapy

[2,28]. The ongoing E2496 Intergroup trial comparing the Stanford V regimen with ABVD combined with radiation therapy for bulky stage II and stages III-IV, might be able to decide which regimen is superior.

The BEACOPP regimen was introduced in 1992 by the GHSG based on a mathematical model that predicted a 10% improvement in tumor control with a moderate increase in dose of chemotherapy. The regimen contains the same drugs as COPP/ABVD, but replaces dacarbazine and vinblastine with etoposide [94,95]. The large phase III randomized study (HD9) compared COPP/ABVD versus standard-BECOPP versus esc-BEACOPP combined with radiotherapy for bulky disease at diagnosis and for residual disease after chemotherapy [94]. A recent update showed that the freedom from treatment failure (FFTF) and OS at 10 years were superior for esc-BEACOPP (82 and 86% respectively) compared to the other two regimens [96]. However, esc-BEACOPP was associated with the highest incidence of hematologic toxicities, including nine cases of AML/MDS versus four cases in the standard-BEACOPP arm and one case in the COPP/ABVD arm [94]. Therefore, the GHSG started to undertake two successive studies, HD12 and HD15, to de-escalate BEACOPP and reduce radiotherapy, hence reducing the toxic burden of this very effective principle [97]. An interim analysis from the HD12 trial, at a median follow-up of 30 months, showed no significant differences regarding the FFTF and OS rates between eight cycles of esc-BEACOPP versus four cycles of esc-BEACOPP followed by four additional cycles of baseline-BEACOPP (4+4) with or without IF-RT [98]. Another risk-adapted study using BEACOPP was published recently [99]. Patients with advanced stage HL and IPS ≥3 were treated with esc-BEACOPP versus standard-BEACOPP for low risk patients followed by restaging with PET after two cycles. Patients with positive PET scan were treated with four additional cycles of esc-BEACOPP, whereas four cycles of standard-BEACOPP were given to patients with negative PET scan. Five-year EFS and OS rates were similar in both risk groups [99]. As the GHSG compared BEACOPP to COPP/ABVD (not to ABVD), the EORTC is now conducting an ongoing intergroup trial (No. 20012) that addresses the question whether the BEACOPP (4+4 variant) is superior to eight cycles of ABVD [28,100]. However, two recent studies have been published and showed no significant difference in OS between ABVD and BEACOPP [186,187]. The first randomized trial, by Gianne et al, compared 6-8 cycles of ABVD to 4 cycles of esc-BEACOPP plus 4 cycles of standard BEACOPP. The 3-year outcome showed that BEACOPP has a superior FFP in 16% of patients, but showed a comparable FF2P and an identical OS rate, and was thus an overtreatment for the 71% already cured by ABVD-first [186].The second study, by Federico et al, reported results from the HD2000 Gruppo Italiano per lo Studio dei Linfomi Trial which showed also no significant 5-year OS difference between 6 cycles of ABVD versus 4 cycles of esc-BEACOPP plus 2 standard BEACOPP versus CEC (cyclophosphamide, lomustine, vindesine, melphalan, prednisone, epidoxirubicin, vincristine, procarbazine, vinblastine, bleomycin; COPP/EBV/CAD). BEACOPP did have higher rates of FFP, but was also associated with higher rates of acute toxicities [187].

Based on above studies, while awaiting results from the EORTC intergroup trial, esc-BEACOPP has been adopted by NCCN guidelines as one of the first line therapeutic options in advanced HL, especially for patients with IPS ≥4 [2]. This recommendation does not apply to elderly patients (over age 65) as they were excluded from the HD9 trial [94], and another HD9 elderly study showed unsatisfactory results in both arms (COPP/ABVD versus standard-BEACOPP) with patients 65 to 75 years old and unacceptable toxicity with standard-BEACOPP [75,101]. Consolidative HDCT (high dose chemotherapy)/ASCT therapy, after initial response for chemotherapy, has been also studied as an option for advanced stage and unfavorable HL. Final results from two European studies showed that conventional chemotherapy by itself might have equivalent or better outcomes than HDCT/ASCT [102,103].

Given the rarity of advanced stage LPHL, its optimal treatment is not yet well defined. In general, early unfavorable or advanced stage LPHL is treated similarly to CHL with ABVD being most widely used. Most recently, the anti-CD20 chimeric antibody rituximab has been shown to have excellent response rates as a single agent in patients with relapsed or previously untreated LPHL [104,105]. Thus, rituximab has been suggested to have a role in treatment of advanced stage LPHL, either as a single agent or combined with other regimens (Table 21-6). Other chemotherapy regimens seem to be effective, based on few small studies and on treatment regimens for B-cell NHL, include CHOP (cyclophosphamide, doxorubicin, vincristine, and prednisone), CVP (cyclophosphamide, vincristine and prednisone), and EPOCH (etoposide, prednisone, vincristine, cyclophosphamide, and doxorubicin). Regarding treatment outcome, the current published data show that patients with early unfavorable or advanced stage LPHL had similar outcomes as CHL [64,106].

21.4. Response Criteria

Uniform criteria for assessment of initial treatment response in HL are essential since they guide the use of additional therapy. To that end, the International Working Group (IWG) published guidelines in 1999, that have been adopted for HL, focusing on the size reduction of the enlarged LN/tumor mass (as measured with CT scan) and the extent of BM involvement [107,108]. However, repeat bone marrow aspirate and biopsy should only be performed to confirm a CR if they were initially positive or if it is clinically indicated by new abnormalities in the peripheral blood counts or blood smear [108].

Additionally, the International Harmonization Project proposed revised guidelines for treatment response in NHL and HL in 2007 incorporating PET, immunohistochemistry, and flow cytometry (Table 21-7) [107]. The categories were simplified to include complete response (CR), partial response (PR), stable disease (SD), relapsed disease, or progressive disease (PD), with the elimination of the Cru (complete response uncertain) category. This was based on the improved ability of PET to distinguish between viable tumor and necrosis or fibrosis in residual masses present after treatment [2,109–112]. The recent increase in the use of combined PET/CT scans may further help in this distinction [27,113–115].

21.5. Treatment of Relapsed or Progressive HL

21.5.1. Patterns of Relapse and Progression in HL

Relapsed HL is defined as a recurrence of the tumor after attaining a complete remission for at least 3 months. Relapse is further classified for the purpose of prognosis and treatment into early relapse (within 3–12 months) and late relapse (more than 12 months) [28]. Primary refractory or progressive disease is defined as progressive or nonresponse during induction treatment or within 90 days of completing treatment [19]. The risk of relapsed HL after achieving an initial complete remission is about 10–30%, while disease refractory to initial treatment with a progressive course is seen in approximately 5–10% of patients [116,117].

In patients with progressive disease or suspected relapse, rebiopsy and complete restaging studies should be done since 5–9% of patients with suspected relapse will actually have another neoplasm, typically NHL, [118,119] which could reflect composite lymphomas not recognized in the initial biopsy [120]. The accuracy of PET for restaging appears similar to pretreatment staging [121–123]. The role of PET scan for routine post therapy surveillance remains controversial [27,116,124] primarily because of the potential for a disproportionate fraction of false-positive findings, resulting in increasing cost without proven benefit from earlier PET detection of disease compared to standard surveillance methods [124].

Table 21-7. Revised response criteria/definitions for lymphoma.

Response	Definition	Nodal masses	Spleen, liver	Bone marrow
CR	Disappearance of all evidence of disease	(a) FDG-avid or PET positive prior to therapy; mass of any size permitted if PET negative(b) Variably FDG-avid or PET negative; regression to normal size on CT	Not palpable, nodules disappeared	Infiltrate cleared on repeat biopsy; if indeterminate by morphology, immunohisto-chemistry should be negative
PR	Regression of measurable disease and no new sites	≥50% decrease in SPD of up to six largest dominant masses; no increase in size of other nodes (a) FDG-avid or PET positive prior to therapy; one or more PET positive at previously involved site (b) Variably FDG-avid or PET negative; regression on CT	≥50% decrease in SPD of nodules (for single nodule in greatest transverse diameter); no increase in size of liver or spleen	Irrelevant if positive prior to therapy; cell type should be specified
SD	Failure to attain CR/PR or PD	(a) FDG-avid or PET positive prior to therapy; PET positive at prior sites of disease and no new sites on CT or PET (b) Variably FDG-avid or PET negative; no change in size of previous lesions on CT		
Relapsed disease or PD	Any new lesion or increase by ≥50% of previously involved sites from nadir	Appearance of a new lesion(s) >1.5 cm in any axis, ≥50% increase in SPD of more than one node, or ≥50% increase in longest diameter of a previously identified node >1 cm in short axis Lesions PET positive if FDG-avid lymphoma or PET positive prior to therapy	>50% increase from nadir in the SPD of any previous lesions	New or recurrent involvement

Data is derived from Table 2 in Cheson et al [107, 108]. *CR* complete remission, *FDG* [¹⁸F]fluorodeoxyglucose, *PET* positron emission tomography, *CT* computed tomography, *PR* partial remission, *SPD* sum of the product of the diameters, *SD* stable disease, *PD* progressive disease

21.5.2. Primary Refractory HL

In general, patients with primary progressive HL have the worst prognosis as virtually no patient survives more than 8 years with conventional chemotherapy [125]. The poor prognosis of HL with refractory disease has also been noted in a large Italian study [126]. For patients with primary progressive disease, a retrospective study analysis from GHSG identified the following adverse prognostic factors: Karnofsky performance score at progression (above or equal 90 versus less than 90), age (50 years or less versus more than 50 years), and attainment of a temporary remission to first-line chemotherapy [127]. Patients with no risk factors had a 3-year OS of 55%, compared with 0% for those with three-risk factors [127]. However, due to substantial improvements in first line therapy of HL, the number of patients with refractory HL has decreased over the last decade [28].

21.5.3. Outcome after Relapsed HL

It was first noticed in 1979 that a shorter length of remission on first-line chemotherapy had a marked effect on the ability of patients to respond to subsequent salvage treatment [97,128]. Other factors that have been shown to correlate with treatment resistance at relapse include advanced stage at presentation, B symptoms, and extranodal disease (Table 21-8). Moskowitz and colleagues prospectively identified three prognostic factors that correlated with higher rates of relapse and poor outcome including B symptoms, extranodal disease, and CR duration of less than 1 year. Event-free survival (EFS) rates in intention-to-treat analyses were 83% for patients with 0–1 factor, 27% for patients with two factors and 10% for patients with three factors [129]. The GHSG retrospectively identified three factors that correlated with poor outcome in relapsed HL, including duration of first remission, stage at relapse, and the presence or absence of anemia, with freedom from second failure (FF2F) rates estimated at 45, 32 and 18%, for patients with 0/1, 2 or 3 prognostic factors respectively [130]. On the other hand, patients with early stage disease who relapsed after primary radiotherapy had an excellent prognosis with salvage chemotherapy [131].

21.5.4. Treatment Options for Relapsed CHL

The treatment of recurrent disease must take into consideration the initial treatment, the duration of complete remission, the stage at recurrence, and the age of the patient [132]. In general, treatment options range from salvage RT to conventional chemotherapy to high-dose chemotherapy (HDCT), and hematopoietic stem cell transplantation (SCT) (Table 21-9). Salvage therapy with RT only is considered an option in treatment of recurrent/progressive disease in the instance of localized stages in previously nonirradiated areas [133,134]. The

Table 21-8. Prognostic factors for refractory/relapsed HL.

	Moskowitz et al. (n = 65)		Josting et al. (n = 422)		Brice et al. (n = 187)		Primary refractory HL[b]	
Risk factors[a]	A	CR duration <12 months	A	CR duration <12 months	A	CR duration <12 months	A	Temporary remission
	B	Extranodal disease	B	CS III-IV at relapse	B	Extranodal disease	B	Karnofsky performance
	C	B symptoms	C	Anemia[c]			C	Age

[a]The most relevant risk factors (RFs) in each study were combined into a prognostic score that predicts survival and recurrence rates. As per Moskowitz et al. study, the 5-year event-free and overall survival (OS) rates were 83 and 93% for patients with 0-1 RF versus 10 and 25% for patients with three RFs. As per Josting et al. study, the 4-year freedom from second failure and OS rates for patients with none of the RF were 48 and 83% versus to 17 and 27% for patients with 3 RFs. The same analysis was also done with Brice et al. and showed 4-year OS rates of 93, 59 and 43% for patients with 0, 1 and 2 RFs respectively [119,120,129]
[b]Primary refractory HL is considered a bad prognostic factor by itself compared to relapsed HL. The 3-year OS was estimated to reach 55% in patients with no RFs compared with 0% for patients with 3 RFs. Cutoffs for Karnofsky performance score is 90 or above or less than 90 and for age 50 years or less or more than 50 years [107].
[c]Anemia was considered a RF if Hb <12 g/dl in males or <10.5 g/dl in females
B symptoms include fever with temperature >38°C, drenching night sweats, and unexplained weight loss of >10% body weight within 6 months; *CR* complete remission *CS* clinical stage; *n* is the number of patients in each study

Table 21-9. Recommended treatments for primary refractory and relapsed HL[a].

Disease presentation	Suggested treatment
Primary refractory disease	Salvage chemotherapy + HDCT + ASCT±RT
Relapse/progression after first-line radiotherapy	Conventional chemotherapy as for primary advanced HL
Nodal relapse (CS IA-IIA) with no prior RT	Salvage RT alone or Non-cross resistant chemotherapy or Salvage chemotherapy + HDCT + ASCT±RT
All other relapses (early and late)	Salvage chemotherapy + HDCT + ASCT±RT
Multiple relapses after HDCT/ASCT	Reduced-intensity allogeneic transplantation or Experimental protocol/Novel agents[b] or Palliative regimen

[a]Refractory LPHL is much less common than CHL but the rate of relapse is the same (usually late onset relapses). Patients may be managed according to the same algorithm as mentioned above. However, some patients with LPHL might have an indolent course and observation alone is an option. Another advance in patients with relapsed/refractory LPHL is their response to rituximab, which also should be considered as an option in those patients.
[b]Many novel agents are under investigation and few of them have shown clinical benefits (see text for details). Patients are encouraged to be involved in more experimental trials especially those with multiple relapses.
ASCT autologous stem cell transplantation, *CS* clinical stage, *HDCT* high dose chemotherapy, *RT* radiation therapy

5-year freedom from second treatment failure and OS rates were 28 and 51% respectively [135]. Features reported to predict a favorable outcome have included age <40 years, initial response to treatment lasting at least one year, absence of B symptoms, limited stage disease, and Karnofsky performance status >90%.

Treatment with chemotherapy with or without RT is a treatment option for those initially treated with only RT or MOPP chemotherapy, those with localized recurrence who have been in complete remission for more than 12 months, or those older than 65 years of age [132]. In patients with late relapse, studies have shown that treatment with conventional chemotherapy by itself led to high second remission rates with a median survival of approximately 4 years [125]. However, despite the initial responses, patients often relapse and subsequently die of disease progression or complications of treatment. Hence, most eligible patients with relapsed disease, no matter what the duration of remission is, are now treated with HDCT/ASCT. PET scans can provide an accurate assessment of response to salvage therapy and also important prognostic information [136,137].

21.5.5. Hematopoietic Stem Cell Transplantation in Relapsed/Refractory Disease

A number of phase 2 studies and two small, randomized trials have shown that HDCT followed by ASCT can improve outcomes in relapsed/refractory HL compared to conventional chemotherapy, producing 30–70% long-term disease-free survival in selected patients [138–144]. The BNLI conducted the first randomized trial where the patients with relapsed or refractory disease were assigned to receive either conventional chemotherapy with the mini-BEAM (BCNU, etoposide, arabinoside, and melphalan) regimen only or HDCT with BEAM followed by ASCT (20 patients per group). The 3-year event-free survival rate was significantly better in patients who received high-dose chemotherapy and the study was terminated early (53 vs. 10%) [145]. The second trial, conducted by the GHSG and the European Group for Blood and Marrow Transplantation (EBMT), was similar but included many more patients. In this randomized multicenter study, patients with relapse after polychemotherapy were assigned to either four cycles of Dexa-BEAM (dexamethasone-BEAM) or two cycles of Dexa-BEAM followed by BEAM and ASCT. The results were published first in 2002 and showed that the failure-free survival at 3 years was significantly better for patients given BEAM-HDT (55 vs. 34%) but with no differences in the OS; [146] these results were further confirmed by an update with a 7-year follow up of that trial [147]. The lack of differences in the OS of these two trials is difficult to interpret and might reflect the small number of patients and events [148]. It might also be attributed to the fact that patients relapsing after conventional salvage therapy had subsequently undergone HDCT and ASCT [28,148].

Although chemosensitivity to the pretransplant regimen likely influences outcomes with HDCT-ASCT, [149] there have been no randomized studies to compare different salvage regimens. However, several nonrandomized studies have shown several effective cytoreduction second-line chemotherapy regimens before HDCT/ASCT [129,150]. These regimens were developed over years based on the assumption that the relapsed HL is resistant to the initially-used chemotherapeutic drugs [28]. Historically, aggressive regimens such as mini-BEAM, BEAM, ICE (ifosfamide, carboplatin, etoposide), ESHAP (etoposide/high-dose cytarabine/cis-platinum) and others have been favored [71,151–153]. More recently, platinum-based [143,154] and gemcitabine-containing regimens, such as gemcitabine, vinorelbine, and pegylated liposomal doxorubicin (GVD), have also been reported to have high response rates and a favorable side-effect profile [155–157]. Also, the vinorelbine/gemcitabine based regimen IGEV (ifosfamide, gemcitabine, vinorelbine) has been shown to have high response rates and has been adopted, as for the GVD regimen, by the recent NCCN guidlines [157,188]. Some studies have also suggested that patients with minimal residual disease at relapse may need no conventional-dose CT before HDCT [144,158].

Allogeneic (allo)-SCT has also been studied in relapsed/refractory HL with or without prior ASCT, but its role remains controversial. As allo-SCT is associated with high transplant-related mortality and poor outcomes in most series, [159,160] reduced-intensity conditioning (RIC) with allo-SCT has emerged as an alternative promising approach based on few studies [161–164]. More follow-up and further studies are needed to better define the role of allo-SCT in patients with relapsed/refractory HL.

21.5.6. Treatment Options for Recurrent LPHL

The rate of relapse of LPHL after initial treatment is similar to that for CHL, but primary refractory disease is extremely rare [106]. Relapses tend to occur late, often more than 10 years after completion of treatment [63]. Patients with relapsed LPHL may be managed according to the same algorithm as mentioned above, however, some patients with LPHL have an indolent course and observation only is an option [2]. Since L&H cells express CD20, the antibody rituximab has been studied in patients with relapsed LPHL and has shown very promising results [104,105]. Hence, single agent rituximab is considered an option in the treatment of relapsed LPHL.

21.5.7. Novel Treatments for HL

Several agents have been studied and others are still under investigation for the treatment of refractory/relapsed HL, especially for those patients who progress despite chemotherapy and relapse after ASCT.

Of the different chemotherapeutic agents that have been studied, Gemcitabine and vinorelbine have shown impressive results. Gemcitabine, a pyrimidine analogue, has been studied in heavily pretreated patients, either by itself or in combination with other drugs including rituximab, and the results from many phase II studies are promising, with an overall response rate of 53% [156,165–168]. Vinorelbine, a new vinca alkaloid derivative, has demonstrated also an impressive efficacy in heavily pretreated patients, either as a single agent or combined with other drugs [157,169,170].

Based on preclinical data from studies on genetic characteristics and the identification of the molecular basis of several transcriptional signaling pathways involved in the anti-apoptotic phenotype of lymphoma cells, many agents are being investigated now for these potential targets. Bortezomib, a proteasome inhibitor, was studied and showed a minimal single-agent activity in heavily pretreated refractory/relapsed HL patients [171]. However, bortezomib needs to be studied in less heavily-treated patients and as a combination therapy, as there is some evidence to suggest potential synergistic activity with other agents [172,173]. Histone deacetylase inhibitors are also being investigated, [174,175] as well as lenalidomide and other molecular targets [36,71].

Many monoclonal antibodies have been investigated in HL for several years but the results have not been as successful as for B-cell lymphomas [148]. The antigen CD30 is expressed in nearly all cases of classical HL, but has more limited expression in normal immune cells. Hence, different anti-CD30 antibodies are being studied. The results from two different studies investigating the chimeric anti-CD30 antibody SGN-30 and the humanized anti-CD30 monoclonal antibody MDX-060 were reported recently with disappointing outcomes [176,177]. On the other hand, the antibody-drug conjugate SGN-35, an anti-CD30 antibody that is conjugated to the anti-tubulin agent monomethylauristatin E, shows promise in preliminary clinical trials [178,179]. The anti-CD20 antibody rituximab has shown activity against refractory/relapsed LPHL and multiple relapsed CD20-positive classical HL, but unfortunately these responses have been of short duration [180,181]. Rituximab has also been studied in patients with relapsed classical HL independent of the CD20 expression of the H-RS cells and the results were not promising [182]. Other monoclonal antibodies being investigated are directed against CD25, CD40, and CD80 as well as bispecific monoclonal antibodies directed against both CD30 and CD64.

References

1. Diehl V. Hodgkin's disease – from pathology specimen to cure. N Engl J Med 2007;357: 1968–71.

2. Hoppe RT, Advani RH, Ambinder RF, et al. Hodgkin disease/lymphoma. J Natl Compr Canc Netw 2008;6:594–622.

3. Diehl V, Harris NL, Mauch PM. Hodgkin's disease. In: Devita VT, Hellman S, Rosenberg SA, eds. Cancer. Principles and practice in oncology. 7th ed. Philadelphia: Lippincott Williams & Wilkins, 2005

4. Harris NL, Jaffe ES, Diebold J, et al. World Health Organization classification of neoplastic diseases of the hematopoietic and lymphoid tissues: report of the Clinical Advisory Committee meeting-Airlie House, Virginia, November 1997. J Clin Oncol 1999;17:3835–49.

5. Jaffe ES, Harris N, Stein H. Tumors of hematopoietic and lymphoid tissues. Lyon: IARC, 2001

6. Jemal A, Siegel R, Ward E, et al. Cancer statistics, 2008. CA Cancer J Clin 2008;58:71–96.

7. Bernard SM, Cartwright RA, Darwin CM, et al. Hodgkin's disease: case control epidemiological study in Yorkshire. Br J Cancer 1987;55:85–90.

8. Glaser SL, Jarrett RF. The epidemiology of Hodgkin's disease. Baillieres Clin Haematol 1996;9:401–16.

9. Lynch HT, Marcus JN, Lynch JF. Genetics of Hodgkin's and non-Hodgkin's lymphoma: a review. Cancer Invest 1992;10:247–56.

10. Mack TM, Cozen W, Shibata DK, et al. Concordance for Hodgkin's disease in identical twins suggesting genetic susceptibility to the young-adult form of the disease. N Engl J Med 1995;332:413–8.

11. Andrieu JM, Roithmann S, Tourani JM, et al. Hodgkin's disease during HIV1 infection: the French registry experience. French Registry of HIV-associated Tumors. Ann Oncol 1993;4:635–41

12. Franceschi S, Dal Maso L, La Vecchia C. Advances in the epidemiology of HIV-associated non-Hodgkin's lymphoma and other lymphoid neoplasms. Int J Cancer 1999;83:481–5.

13. Lowenthal DA, Straus DJ, Campbell SW, Gold JW, Clarkson BD, Koziner B. AIDS-related lymphoid neoplasia. The Memorial Hospital experience. Cancer 1988;61:2325–37.

14. Tirelli U, Errante D, Dolcetti R, et al. Hodgkin's disease and human immunodeficiency virus infection: clinicopathologic and virologic features of 114 patients from the Italian Cooperative Group on AIDS and Tumors. J Clin Oncol 1995;13:1758–67.

15. Tirelli U, Vaccher E, Rezza G, et al. Hodgkin disease and infection with the human immunodeficiency virus (HIV) in Italy. Ann Intern Med 1988;108:309–10.

16. Caraway NP. Strategies to diagnose lymphoproliferative disorders by fine-needle aspiration by using ancillary studies. Cancer 2005;105:432–42.

17. Hehn ST, Grogan TM, Miller TP. Utility of fine-needle aspiration as a diagnostic technique in lymphoma. J Clin Oncol 2004;22:3046–52.

18. Meda BA, Buss DH, Woodruff RD, et al. Diagnosis and subclassification of primary and recurrent lymphoma. The usefulness and limitations of combined fine-needle aspiration cytomorphology and flow cytometry. Am J Clin Pathol 2000;113:688–99.

19. Ansell SM, Armitage JO. Management of Hodgkin lymphoma. Mayo Clin Proc 2006;81:419–26.

20. Carbone PP, Kaplan HS, Musshoff K, Smithers DW, Tubiana M. Report of the Committee on Hodgkin's Disease Staging Classification. Cancer Res 1971;31:1860–1.

21. Lister TA, Crowther D, Sutcliffe SB, et al. Report of a committee convened to discuss the evaluation and staging of patients with Hodgkin's disease: Cotswolds meeting. J Clin Oncol 1989;7:1630–6.

22. Fanale MA, Younes A. Nodular lymphocyte predominant Hodgkin's lymphoma. Cancer Treat Res 2008;142:367–81.

23. Lieberz D, Sextro M, Paulus U, Franklin J, Tesch H, Diehl V. How to restrict liver biopsy to high-risk patients in early-stage Hodgkin's disease. German Hodgkin's Lymphoma Study Group. Ann Hematol 2000;79:73–8.

24. Carde P, Hagenbeek A, Hayat M, et al. Clinical staging versus laparotomy and combined modality with MOPP versus ABVD in early-stage Hodgkin's disease: the H6 twin randomized trials from the European Organization for Research and Treatment of Cancer Lymphoma Cooperative Group. J Clin Oncol 1993;11:2258–72.

25. Isasi CR, Lu P, Blaufox MD. A metaanalysis of 18F–2-deoxy-2-fluoro-D-glucose positron emission tomography in the staging and restaging of patients with lymphoma. Cancer 2005;104:1066–74.

26. Seam P, Juweid ME, Cheson BD. The role of FDG-PET scans in patients with lymphoma. Blood 2007;110:3507–16.

27. Juweid ME. Utility of positron emission tomography (PET) scanning in managing patients with Hodgkin lymphoma. Hematology Am Soc Hematol Educ Program 2006;259–65:510–1.

28. Fuchs M, Diehl V, Re D. Current strategies and new approaches in the treatment of Hodgkin's lymphoma. Pathobiology 2006;73:126–40.

29. Ferme C, Eghbali H, Meerwaldt JH, et al. Chemotherapy plus involved-field radiation in early-stage Hodgkin's disease. N Engl J Med 2007;357:1916–27.

30. Oki Y, Pro B, Fayad LE, et al. Phase 2 study of gemcitabine in combination with rituximab in patients with recurrent or refractory Hodgkin lymphoma. Cancer 2008;112:831–6.

31. Carde P, Burgers JM, Henry-Amar M, et al. Clinical stages I and II Hodgkin's disease: a specifically tailored therapy according to prognostic factors. J Clin Oncol 1988;6:239–52.

32. Loeffler M, Pfreundschuh M, Ruhl U, et al. Risk factor adapted treatment of Hodgkin's lymphoma: strategies and perspectives. Recent Results Cancer Res 1989;117:142–62.

33. Mauch P, Tarbell N, Weinstein H, et al. Stage IA and IIA supradiaphragmatic Hodgkin's disease: prognostic factors in surgically staged patients treated with mantle and paraaortic irradiation. J Clin Oncol 1988;6:1576–83.

34. Tubiana M, Henry-Amar M, Carde P, et al. Toward comprehensive management tailored to prognostic factors of patients with clinical stages I and II in Hodgkin's disease. The EORTC Lymphoma Group controlled clinical trials: 1964–1987. Blood 1989;73:47–56.

35. Noordijk EM, Carde P, Dupouy N, et al. Combined-modality therapy for clinical stage I or II Hodgkin's lymphoma: long-term results of the European Organisation for Research and Treatment of Cancer H7 randomized controlled trials. J Clin Oncol 2006;24:3128–35.

36. Evens AM, Hutchings M, Diehl V. Treatment of Hodgkin lymphoma: the past, present, and future. Nat Clin Pract Oncol 2008;5:543–56.

37. Meyer RM, Gospodarowicz MK, Connors JM, et al. Randomized comparison of ABVD chemotherapy with a strategy that includes radiation therapy in patients with limited-stage Hodgkin's lymphoma: National Cancer Institute of Canada Clinical Trials Group and the Eastern Cooperative Oncology Group. J Clin Oncol 2005;23:4634–42.

38. Horwich A, Specht L, Ashley S. Survival analysis of patients with clinical stages I or II Hodgkin's disease who have relapsed after initial treatment with radiotherapy alone. Eur J Cancer 1997;33:848–53.

39. Ekstrand BC, Horning SJ. Hodgkin's disease. Blood Rev 2002;16:111–7.

40. Dubray B, Henry-Amar M, Meerwaldt JH, et al. Radiation-induced lung damage after thoracic irradiation for Hodgkin's disease: the role of fractionation. Radiother Oncol 1995;36:211–7.

41. Hancock SL, Tucker MA, Hoppe RT. Factors affecting late mortality from heart disease after treatment of Hodgkin's disease. JAMA 1993;270:1949–55.

42. Bhatia S, Yasui Y, Robison LL, et al. High risk of subsequent neoplasms continues with extended follow-up of childhood Hodgkin's disease: report from the Late Effects Study Group. J Clin Oncol 2003;21:4386–94.

43. Ng AK, Bernardo MV, Weller E, et al. Second malignancy after Hodgkin disease treated with radiation therapy with or without chemotherapy: long-term risks and risk factors. Blood 2002;100:1989–96.

44. van Leeuwen FE, Klokman WJ, Stovall M, et al. Roles of radiation dose, chemotherapy, and hormonal factors in breast cancer following Hodgkin's disease. J Natl Cancer Inst 2003;95:971–80.

45. Gospodarowicz MK, Meyer RM. The management of patients with limited-stage classical Hodgkin lymphoma. Hematology Am Soc Hematol Educ Program 2006:253–8.

46. Bonadonna G, Bonfante V, Viviani S, Di Russo A, Villani F, Valagussa P. ABVD plus subtotal nodal versus involved-field radiotherapy in early-stage Hodgkin's disease: long-term results. J Clin Oncol 2004;22:2835–41.

47. Engert A, Franklin J, Eich HT, et al. Two cycles of doxorubicin, bleomycin, vinblastine, and dacarbazine plus extended-field radiotherapy is superior to radiotherapy alone in early favorable Hodgkin's lymphoma: final results of the GHSG HD7 trial. J Clin Oncol 2007;25:3495–502.

48. Engert A, Schiller P, Josting A, et al. Involved-field radiotherapy is equally effective and less toxic compared with extended-field radiotherapy after four cycles of chemotherapy in patients with early-stage unfavorable Hodgkin's lymphoma: results of the HD8 trial of the German Hodgkin's Lymphoma Study Group. J Clin Oncol 2003;21:3601–8.

49. Ferme C, Eghbali H, Hagenbeek A, et al. MOPP/ABV hybrid and irradiation in unfavorable supradiaphragmatic clinical stages I-II Hodgkin's disease: comparison of three treatment modalities.

Preliminary results of the EORTC-GELA H8-U randomized trial in 995 patients (abstract). Blood 2000;96:A576

50. Hagenbeek A, Eghbali H, Fermé C, et al. Three cycles of MOPP/ABV hybrid and involved-field irradiation is more effective than subtotal nodal irradiation in favorable supra-diaphragmatic clinical stages I-II Hodgkin's disease: preliminary results of the EORTC-GELA H8-F randomized trial in 543 patients. Blood 2000;96:575a.

51. Press OW, LeBlanc M, Lichter AS, et al. Phase III randomized intergroup trial of subtotal lymphoid irradiation versus doxorubicin, vinblastine, and subtotal lymphoid irradiation for stage IA to IIA Hodgkin's disease. J Clin Oncol 2001;19:4238–44.

52. Specht L, Gray RG, Clarke MJ, Peto R. Influence of more extensive radiotherapy and adjuvant chemotherapy on long-term outcome of early-stage Hodgkin's disease: a meta-analysis of 23 randomized trials involving 3,888 patients. International Hodgkin's Disease Collaborative Group. J Clin Oncol 1998;16:830–43.

53. Diehl V, Engert A, Mueller RP, et al. HD10: investigating reduction of combined modality treatment intensity in early stage Hodgkin's lymphoma. Interim analysis of a randomized trial of the German Hodgkin Study Group. J Clin Oncol 2005;23:561S.

54. Noordijk EM, Thomas J, Fermé C, et al. First results of the EORTC-GELA H9 randomized trials: the H9-F trial (comparing 3 radiation dose levels) and H9-U trial (comparing 3 chemotherapy schemes) in patients with favorable or unfavorable early stage Hodgkin's lymphoma. J Clin Oncol 2005;23:561S.

55. Yahalom J. Favorable early-stage Hodgkin lymphoma. J Natl Compr Canc Netw 2006;4:233–40.

56. Horning SJ, Hoppe R, Advani RH, et al. A prospective trial of involved field radiation (IFRT) + chemotherapy compared to extended field (EFRT) radiation for favorable Hodgkin disease: survival differences and implications of mature follow-up for current combined modality therapy. J Clin Oncol 2007;25:Abstract no. 8014.

57. Santoro A, Bonadonna G, Valagussa P, et al. Long-term results of combined chemotherapy-radiotherapy approach in Hodgkin's disease: superiority of ABVD plus radiotherapy versus MOPP plus radiotherapy. J Clin Oncol 1987;5:27–37.

58. Aversa SM, Salvagno L, Soraru M, et al. Stanford V regimen plus consolidative radiotherapy is an effective therapeutic program for bulky or advanced-stage Hodgkin's disease. Acta Haematol 2004;112:141–7.

59. Edwards-Bennett SM, Moskowitz C, Jacobs J, et al. A non-Stanford mature experience with Stanford V +- RT regimen for locally extensive and advanced Hodgkin's lymphoma (HL). Int J Radiat Oncol Biol Phys 2007:S18–9.

60. Horning SJ, Hoppe RT, Breslin S, Bartlett NL, Brown BW, Rosenberg SA. Stanford V and radiotherapy for locally extensive and advanced Hodgkin's disease: mature results of a prospective clinical trial. J Clin Oncol 2002;20:630–7.

61. Horning SJ, Rosenberg SA, Hoppe RT. Brief chemotherapy (Stanford V) and adjuvant radiotherapy for bulky or advanced Hodgkin's disease: an update. Ann Oncol 1996;7(Suppl 4):105–8.

62. Horning SJ, Hoppe R, Advani RH, et al. Efficacy and late effects of Stanford V chemotherapy and radiotherapy in untreated Hodgkin's disease: mature data in early and advanced stage patients [abstract]. Blood 2004:Abstract no. 308.

63. Diehl V, Sextro M, Franklin J, et al. Clinical presentation, course, and prognostic factors in lymphocyte-predominant Hodgkin's disease and lymphocyte-rich classical Hodgkin's disease: report from the European Task Force on Lymphoma Project on Lymphocyte-Predominant Hodgkin's Disease. J Clin Oncol 1999;17:776–83.

64. Nogova L, Reineke T, Eich HT, et al. Extended field radiotherapy, combined modality treatment or involved field radiotherapy for patients with stage IA lymphocyte-predominant Hodgkin's lymphoma: a retrospective analysis from the German Hodgkin Study Group (GHSG). Ann Oncol 2005;16:1683–7.

65. Schlembach PJ, Wilder RB, Jones D, et al. Radiotherapy alone for lymphocyte-predominant Hodgkin's disease. Cancer J 2002;8:377–83.

66. Wilder RB, Schlembach PJ, Jones D, et al. European Organization for Research and Treatment of Cancer and Groupe d'Etude des Lymphomes de l'Adulte very favorable and favorable, lymphocyte-predominant Hodgkin disease. Cancer 2002;94:1731–8.

67. Wirth A, Yuen K, Barton M, et al. Long-term outcome after radiotherapy alone for lymphocyte-predominant Hodgkin lymphoma: a retrospective multicenter study of the Australasian Radiation Oncology Lymphoma Group. Cancer 2005;104:1221–9.

68. de Wit M, Bohuslavizki KH, Buchert R, Bumann D, Clausen M, Hossfeld DK. 18FDG-PET following treatment as valid predictor for disease-free survival in Hodgkin's lymphoma. Ann Oncol 2001;12:29–37.

69. Weihrauch MR, Re D, Scheidhauer K, et al. Thoracic positron emission tomography using 18F-fluorodeoxyglucose for the evaluation of residual mediastinal Hodgkin disease. Blood 2001;98:2930–4.

70. Juweid ME, Stroobants S, Mottaghy FM. Recommendations of the imaging committee of the International Harmonization Project (IHP) for FDG-PET (PET) use in patients with lymphoma. J Nucl Med 2006;47(Suppl 1):452.

71. Bartlett NL. Modern treatment of Hodgkin lymphoma. Curr Opin Hematol 2008;15:408–14.

72. Longo DL, Young RC, Wesley M, et al. Twenty years of MOPP therapy for Hodgkin's disease. J Clin Oncol 1986;4:1295–306.

73. Hasenclever D, Diehl V. A prognostic score for advanced Hodgkin's disease. International Prognostic Factors Project on Advanced Hodgkin's Disease. N Engl J Med 1998;339:1506–14.

74. Diehl V, Franklin J, Tesch H, et al. Dose escalation of BEACOPP chemotherapy for advanced Hodgkin's disease in the HD9 trial of the German Hodgkin's Lymphoma Study Group (GHSG). ASCO 19:2000;Abstract no. 7.

75. Horning SJ. Risk, cure and complications in advanced hodgkin disease. Hematology Am Soc Hematol Educ Program 2007;2007:197–203.

76. Gallamini A, Rigacci L, Merli F, et al. The predictive value of positron emission tomography scanning performed after two courses of standard therapy on treatment outcome in advanced stage Hodgkin's disease. Haematologica 2006;91:475–81.

77. Haioun C, Itti E, Rahmouni A, et al. [18F]fluoro-2-deoxy-D-glucose positron emission tomography (FDG-PET) in aggressive lymphoma: an early prognostic tool for predicting patient outcome. Blood 2005;106:1376–81.

78. Hutchings M, Loft A, Hansen M, et al. FDG-PET after two cycles of chemotherapy predicts treatment failure and progression-free survival in Hodgkin lymphoma. Blood 2006;107:52–9.

79. Torizuka T, Nakamura F, Kanno T, et al. Early therapy monitoring with FDG-PET in aggressive non-Hodgkin's lymphoma and Hodgkin's lymphoma. Eur J Nucl Med Mol Imaging 2004;31:22–8.

80. Hutchings M, Mikhaeel NG, Fields PA, Nunan T, Timothy AR. Prognostic value of interim FDG-PET after two or three cycles of chemotherapy in Hodgkin lymphoma. Ann Oncol 2005;16:1160–8.

81. Mikhaeel NG, Hutchings M, Fields PA, O'Doherty MJ, Timothy AR. FDG-PET after two to three cycles of chemotherapy predicts progression-free and overall survival in high-grade non-Hodgkin lymphoma. Ann Oncol 2005;16:1514–23.

82. Gallamini A, Hutchings M, Rigacci L, et al. Early interim 2-[18F]fluoro-2-deoxy-D-glucose positron emission tomography is prognostically superior to international prognostic score in advanced-stage Hodgkin's lymphoma: a report from a joint Italian-Danish study. J Clin Oncol 2007;25:3746–52.

83. Gallamini A, Hutchings M, Avigdor A, Polliack A. Early interim PET scan in Hodgkin lymphoma: where do we stand? Leuk Lymphoma 2008;49:659–62.

84. Bonadonna G, Valagussa P, Santoro A. Alternating non-cross-resistant combination chemotherapy or MOPP in stage IV Hodgkin's disease. A report of 8-year results. Ann Intern Med 1986;104:739–46.

85. Canellos GP, Anderson JR, Propert KJ, et al. Chemotherapy of advanced Hodgkin's disease with MOPP, ABVD, or MOPP alternating with ABVD. N Engl J Med 1992;327:1478–84.

86. Connors JM, Klimo P, Adams G, et al. Treatment of advanced Hodgkin's disease with chemotherapy – comparison of MOPP/ABV hybrid regimen with alternating courses of MOPP and ABVD: a report from the National Cancer Institute of Canada clinical trials group. J Clin Oncol 1997;15:1638–45.

87. Viviani S, Bonadonna G, Santoro A, et al. Alternating versus hybrid MOPP and ABVD combinations in advanced Hodgkin's disease: ten-year results. J Clin Oncol 1996;14:1421–30.

88. Duggan DB, Petroni GR, Johnson JL, et al. Randomized comparison of ABVD and MOPP/ABV hybrid for the treatment of advanced Hodgkin's disease: report of an intergroup trial. J Clin Oncol 2003;21:607–14.

89. Gobbi PG, Levis A, Chisesi T, et al. ABVD versus modified stanford V versus MOPPEBVCAD with optional and limited radiotherapy in intermediate- and advanced-stage Hodgkin's lymphoma: final results of a multicenter randomized trial by the Intergruppo Italiano Linfomi. J Clin Oncol 2005;23:9198–207.

90. Johnson PW, Radford JA, Cullen MH, et al. Comparison of ABVD and alternating or hybrid multidrug regimens for the treatment of advanced Hodgkin's lymphoma: results of the United Kingdom Lymphoma Group LY09 Trial (ISRCTN97144519). J Clin Oncol 2005;23:9208–18.

91. Bartlett NL, Rosenberg SA, Hoppe RT, Hancock SL, Horning SJ. Brief chemotherapy, Stanford V, and adjuvant radiotherapy for bulky or advanced-stage Hodgkin's disease: a preliminary report. J Clin Oncol 1995;13:1080–8.

92. Moskowitz CH, Yahalom J, Straus D, et al. The use of Stanford V overcomes poor prognostic features in patients with advanced-stage Hodgkin's disease. Blood 1998:2579a

93. Horning SJ, Williams J, Bartlett NL, et al. Assessment of the stanford V regimen and consolidative radiotherapy for bulky and advanced Hodgkin's disease: Eastern Cooperative Oncology Group pilot study E1492. J Clin Oncol 2000;18:972–80.

94. Diehl V, Franklin J, Pfreundschuh M, et al. Standard and increased-dose BEACOPP chemotherapy compared with COPP-ABVD for advanced Hodgkin's disease. N Engl J Med 2003;348: 2386–95.

95. Diehl V, Sieber M, Ruffer U, et al. BEACOPP: an intensified chemotherapy regimen in advanced Hodgkin's disease. The German Hodgkin's Lymphoma Study Group. Ann Oncol 1997;8:143–8.

96. Diehl V, Franklin J, Pfistner B. German Hodgkin Study Group. Ten-year results of a German Hodgkin Study Group randomized trial of standard and increased dose BEACOPP chemotherapy for advanced Hodgkin lymphoma (HD9). J Clin Oncol 2007;25: Abstract no. LBA8015

97. Kuppers R, Yahalom J, Josting A. Advances in biology, diagnostics, and treatment of Hodgkin's disease. Biol Blood Marrow Transplant 2006;12:66–76.

98. Diehl V, Brillant C, Franklin J, et al. BEACOPP chemotherapy for advanced Hodgkin's disease: results of further analyses of the HD9- and HD12-trials of the German Hodgkin Study Group (GHSG). Blood 2004;104(11):307a

99. Dann EJ, Bar-Shalom R, Tamir A, et al. Risk-adapted BEACOPP regimen can reduce the cumulative dose of chemotherapy for standard and high-risk Hodgkin lymphoma with no impairment of outcome. Blood 2007;109:905–9.

100. Raemaekers J, Kluin-Nelemans H, Teodorovic I, et al. The achievements of the EORTC Lymphoma Group. European Organisation for Research and Treatment of Cancer. Eur J Cancer 2002;38(Suppl 4):S107–13

101. Ballova V, Ruffer JU, Haverkamp H, et al. A prospectively randomized trial carried out by the German Hodgkin Study Group (GHSG) for elderly patients with advanced Hodgkin's disease comparing BEACOPP baseline and COPP-ABVD (study HD9elderly). Ann Oncol 2005;16:124–31.

102. Federico M, Bellei M, Brice P, et al. High-dose therapy and autologous stem-cell transplantation versus conventional therapy for patients with advanced Hodgkin's lymphoma responding to front-line therapy. J Clin Oncol 2003;21:2320–5.

103. Proctor SJ, Mackie M, Dawson A, et al. A population-based study of intensive multi-agent chemotherapy with or without autotransplant for the highest risk Hodgkin's disease patients identified by the Scotland and Newcastle Lymphoma Group (SNLG) prognostic index. A Scotland and Newcastle Lymphoma Group study (SNLG HD III). Eur J Cancer 2002;38:795–806

104. Schulz H, Rehwald U, Morschhauser F, et al. Rituximab in relapsed lymphocyte-predominant Hodgkin lymphoma: long-term results of a phase 2 trial by the German Hodgkin Lymphoma Study Group (GHSG). Blood 2008;111:109–11.

105. Horning SJ, Bartlett N, Breslin S, et al. Results of a prospective phase II trial of limited and extended rituximab treatment in nodular lymphocyte predominant Hodgkin's disease (NLPHD). Blood (ASH Annual Meeting Abstracts), 2007;110: 644.

106. Nogova L, Rudiger T, Engert A. Biology, clinical course and management of nodular lymphocyte-predominant hodgkin lymphoma. Hematology Am Soc Hematol Educ Program 2006:266–72

107. Cheson BD, Pfistner B, Juweid ME, et al. Revised response criteria for malignant lymphoma. J Clin Oncol 2007;25:579–86.

108. Cheson BD, Horning SJ, Coiffier B, et al. Report of an international workshop to standardize response criteria for non-Hodgkin's lymphomas. NCI Sponsored International Working Group. J Clin Oncol 1999;17:1244

109. Buchmann I, Reinhardt M, Elsner K, et al. 2-(fluorine-18)fluoro-2-deoxy-D-glucose positron emission tomography in the detection and staging of malignant lymphoma. A bicenter trial. Cancer 2001;91:889–99.

110. Jerusalem G, Beguin Y, Fassotte MF, et al. Whole-body positron emission tomography using 18F-fluorodeoxyglucose for posttreatment evaluation in Hodgkin's disease and non-Hodgkin's

lymphoma has higher diagnostic and prognostic value than classical computed tomography scan imaging. Blood 1999;94:429–33.

111. Jerusalem G, Warland V, Najjar F, et al. Whole-body 18F-FDG PET for the evaluation of patients with Hodgkin's disease and non-Hodgkin's lymphoma. Nucl Med Commun 1999;20:13–20.

112. Wirth A, Seymour JF, Hicks RJ, et al. Fluorine-18 fluorodeoxyglucose positron emission tomography, gallium-67 scintigraphy, and conventional staging for Hodgkin's disease and non-Hodgkin's lymphoma. Am J Med 2002;112:262–8.

113. Allen-Auerbach M, Quon A, Weber WA, et al. Comparison between 2-deoxy-2-[18F]fluoro-D-glucose positron emission tomography and positron emission tomography/computed tomography hardware fusion for staging of patients with lymphoma. Mol Imaging Biol 2004;6:411–6.

114. Hutchings M, Loft A, Hansen M, et al. Position emission tomography with or without computed tomography in the primary staging of Hodgkin's lymphoma. Haematologica 2006;91:482–9.

115. Schaefer NG, Hany TF, Taverna C, et al. Non-Hodgkin lymphoma and Hodgkin disease: coregistered FDG PET and CT at staging and restaging–do we need contrast-enhanced CT? Radiology 2004;232:823–9.

116. Diehl V, Mauch PM, Harris NL. Hodgkin's disease In: Devita VT, Hellman S, Rosenberg SA, eds. Cancer. Principles and practice of oncology. Sixth ed. Philadelphia: Lippincott Williams & Wilkins, 2001

117. Horning SJ. Hodgkin's disease. 2nd ed. London: Martin Dunitz, 2000.

118. Borchmann P, Behringer K, Josting A, et al. Secondary malignancies after successful primary treatment of malignant Hodgkin's lymphoma. Pathologe 2006;27:47–52.

119. Rueffer U, Josting A, Franklin J, et al. Non-Hodgkin's lymphoma after primary Hodgkin's disease in the German Hodgkin's Lymphoma Study Group: incidence, treatment, and prognosis. J Clin Oncol 2001;19:2026–32.

120. Hansmann ML, Fellbaum C, Hui PK, Lennert K. Morphological and immunohistochemical investigation of non-Hodgkin's lymphoma combined with Hodgkin's disease. Histopathology 1989;15:35–48.

121. Freudenberg LS, Antoch G, Schutt P, et al. FDG-PET/CT in re-staging of patients with lymphoma. Eur J Nucl Med Mol Imaging 2004;31:325–9.

122. Jerusalem G, Beguin Y, Fassotte MF, et al. Whole-body positron emission tomography using 18F-fluorodeoxyglucose compared to standard procedures for staging patients with Hodgkin's disease. Haematologica 2001;86:266–73.

123. Naumann R, Beuthien-Baumann B, Reiss A, et al. Substantial impact of FDG PET imaging on the therapy decision in patients with early-stage Hodgkin's lymphoma. Br J Cancer 2004;90:620–5.

124. Jerusalem G, Beguin Y, Fassotte MF, et al. Early detection of relapse by whole-body positron emission tomography in the follow-up of patients with Hodgkin's disease. Ann Oncol 2003;14:123–30.

125. Longo DL, Duffey PL, Young RC, et al. Conventional-dose salvage combination chemotherapy in patients relapsing with Hodgkin's disease after combination chemotherapy: the low probability for cure. J Clin Oncol 1992;10:210–8.

126. Tarella C, Cuttica A, Vitolo U, et al. High-dose sequential chemotherapy and peripheral blood progenitor cell autografting in patients with refractory and/or recurrent Hodgkin lymphoma: a multicenter study of the intergruppo Italiano Linfomi showing prolonged disease free survival in patients treated at first recurrence. Cancer 2003;97:2748–59.

127. Josting A, Rueffer U, Franklin J, Sieber M, Diehl V, Engert A. Prognostic factors and treatment outcome in primary progressive Hodgkin lymphoma: a report from the German Hodgkin Lymphoma Study Group. Blood 2000;96:1280–6.

128. Fisher RI, DeVita VT, Hubbard SP, Simon R, Young RC. Prolonged disease-free survival in Hodgkin's disease with MOPP reinduction after first relapse. Ann Intern Med 1979;90:761–3.

129. Moskowitz CH, Nimer SD, Zelenetz AD, et al. A 2-step comprehensive high-dose chemoradiotherapy second-line program for relapsed and refractory Hodgkin disease: analysis by intent to treat and development of a prognostic model. Blood 2001;97:616–23.

130. Josting A, Franklin J, May M, et al. New prognostic score based on treatment outcome of patients with relapsed Hodgkin's lymphoma registered in the database of the German Hodgkin's lymphoma study group. J Clin Oncol 2002;20:221–30.

131. Roach M 3rd, Brophy N, Cox R, Varghese A, Hoppe RT. Prognostic factors for patients relapsing after radiotherapy for early-stage Hodgkin's disease. J Clin Oncol 1990;8:623–9.

132. Ferme C, Cosset JM, Fervers B, et al. Hodgkins disease. Br J Cancer 2001;84(Suppl 2):55–60.

133. Brada M, Eeles R, Ashley S, Nichols J, Horwich A. Salvage radiotherapy in recurrent Hodgkin's disease. Ann Oncol 1992;3:131–5.

134. Pezner RD, Nademanee A, Forman SJ. High-dose therapy and autologous bone marrow transplantation for Hodgkin's disease patients with relapses potentially treatable by radical radiation therapy. Int J Radiat Oncol Biol Phys 1995;33:189–94.

135. Josting A, Nogova L, Franklin J, et al. Salvage radiotherapy in patients with relapsed and refractory Hodgkin's lymphoma: a retrospective analysis from the German Hodgkin Lymphoma Study Group. J Clin Oncol 2005;23:1522–9.

136. Jabbour E, Hosing C, Ayers G, et al. Pretransplant positive positron emission tomography/gallium scans predict poor outcome in patients with recurrent/refractory Hodgkin lymphoma. Cancer 2007;109:2481–9.

137. Schot BW, Zijlstra JM, Sluiter WJ, et al. Early FDG-PET assessment in combination with clinical risk scores determines prognosis in recurring lymphoma. Blood 2007;109:486–91.

138. Bierman PJ, Bagin RG, Jagannath S, et al. High dose chemotherapy followed by autologous hematopoietic rescue in Hodgkin's disease: long-term follow-up in 128 patients. Ann Oncol 1993;4:767–73.

139. Brice P, Bouabdallah R, Moreau P, et al. Prognostic factors for survival after high-dose therapy and autologous stem cell transplantation for patients with relapsing Hodgkin's disease: analysis of 280 patients from the French registry. Societe Francaise de Greffe de Moelle. Bone Marrow Transplant 1997;20:21–6.

140. Jones RJ, Piantadosi S, Mann RB, et al. High-dose cytotoxic therapy and bone marrow transplantation for relapsed Hodgkin's disease. J Clin Oncol 1990;8:527–37.

141. Josting A, Katay I, Rueffer U, et al. Favorable outcome of patients with relapsed or refractory Hodgkin's disease treated with high-dose chemotherapy and stem cell rescue at the time of maximal response to conventional salvage therapy (Dex-BEAM). Ann Oncol 1998;9:289–95.

142. Josting A, Reiser M, Rueffer U, Salzberger B, Diehl V, Engert A. Treatment of primary progressive Hodgkin's and aggressive non-Hodgkin's lymphoma: is there a chance for cure? J Clin Oncol 2000;18:332–9.

143. Josting A, Rudolph C, Reiser M, et al. Time-intensified dexamethasone/cisplatin/cytarabine: an effective salvage therapy with low toxicity in patients with relapsed and refractory Hodgkin's disease. Ann Oncol 2002;13:1628–35.

144. Sweetenham JW, Taghipour G, Milligan D, et al. High-dose therapy and autologous stem cell rescue for patients with Hodgkin's disease in first relapse after chemotherapy: results from the EBMT. Lymphoma Working Party of the European Group for Blood and Marrow Transplantation. Bone Marrow Transplant 1997;20:745–52

145. Linch DC, Winfield D, Goldstone AH, et al. Dose intensification with autologous bone-marrow transplantation in relapsed and resistant Hodgkin's disease: results of a BNLI randomised trial. Lancet 1993;341:1051–4.

146. Schmitz N, Pfistner B, Sextro M, et al. Aggressive conventional chemotherapy compared with high-dose chemotherapy with autologous haemopoietic stem-cell transplantation for relapsed chemosensitive Hodgkin's disease: a randomised trial. Lancet 2002;359:2065–71.

147. Schmitz N, Haverkamp H, Josting A, et al. Long term follow up in relapsed Hodgkin's disease (HD): updated results of the HD-R1 study comparing conventional chemotherapy (cCT) to high-dose chemotherapy (HDCT) with autologous haemopoietic stem cell transplantation (ASCT) of the German Hodgkin Study Group (GHSG) and the Working Party Lymphoma of the European Group for Blood and Marrow Transplantation (EBMT). J Clin Oncol 2005;23:567s.

148. Brice P. Managing relapsed and refractory Hodgkin lymphoma. Br J Haematol 2008;141:3–13.

149. Reece DE, Connors JM, Spinelli JJ, et al. Intensive therapy with cyclophosphamide, carmustine, etoposide +/- cisplatin, and autologous bone marrow transplantation for Hodgkin's disease in first relapse after combination chemotherapy. Blood 1994;83:1193–9.

150. Phillips JK, Spearing RL, Davies JM, et al. VIM-D salvage chemotherapy in Hodgkin's disease. Cancer Chemother Pharmacol 1990;27:161–3.

151. Hagemeister FB, Tannir N, McLaughlin P, et al. MIME chemotherapy (methyl-GAG, ifosfamide, methotrexate, etoposide) as treatment for recurrent Hodgkin's disease. J Clin Oncol 1987;5:556–61.

152. Pfreundschuh MG, Rueffer U, Lathan B, et al. Dexa-BEAM in patients with Hodgkin's disease refractory to multidrug chemotherapy regimens: a trial of the German Hodgkin's Disease Study Group. J Clin Oncol 1994;12:580–6.

153. Pfreundschuh MG, Schoppe WD, Fuchs R, Pfluger KH, Loeffler M, Diehl V. Lomustine, etoposide, vindesine, and dexamethasone (CEVD) in Hodgkin's lymphoma refractory to cyclophosphamide, vincristine, procarbazine, and prednisone (COPP) and doxorubicin, bleomycin, vinblastine, and dacarbazine (ABVD): a multicenter trial of the German Hodgkin Study Group. Cancer Treat Rep 1987;71:1203–7.

154. Rodriguez J, Rodriguez MA, Fayad L, et al. ASHAP: a regimen for cytoreduction of refractory or recurrent Hodgkin's disease. Blood 1999;93:3632–6.

155. Bartlett NL, Niedzwiecki D, Johnson JL, et al. Gemcitabine, vinorelbine, and pegylated liposomal doxorubicin (GVD), a salvage regimen in relapsed Hodgkin's lymphoma: CALGB 59804. Ann Oncol 2007;18:1071–9.

156. Kuruvilla J, Nagy T, Pintilie M, Tsang R, Keating A, Crump M. Similar response rates and superior early progression-free survival with gemcitabine, dexamethasone, and cisplatin salvage therapy compared with carmustine, etoposide, cytarabine, and melphalan salvage therapy prior to autologous stem cell transplantation for recurrent or refractory Hodgkin lymphoma. Cancer 2006;106:353–60.

157. Santoro A, Magagnoli M, Spina M, et al. Ifosfamide, gemcitabine, and vinorelbine: a new induction regimen for refractory and relapsed Hodgkin's lymphoma. Haematologica 2007;92:35–41.

158. Bierman PJ, Anderson JR, Freeman MB, et al. High-dose chemotherapy followed by autologous hematopoietic rescue for Hodgkin's disease patients following first relapse after chemotherapy. Ann Oncol 1996;7:151–6.

159. Freytes CO, Loberiza FR, Rizzo JD, et al. Myeloablative allogeneic hematopoietic stem cell transplantation in patients who experience relapse after autologous stem cell transplantation for lymphoma: a report of the International Bone Marrow Transplant Registry. Blood 2004;104:3797–803.

160. Peniket AJ, Ruiz de Elvira MC, Taghipour G, et al. An EBMT registry matched study of allogeneic stem cell transplants for lymphoma: allogeneic transplantation is associated with a lower relapse rate but a higher procedure-related mortality rate than autologous transplantation. Bone Marrow Transplant 2003;31:667–78

161. Alvarez I, Sureda A, Caballero MD, et al. Nonmyeloablative stem cell transplantation is an effective therapy for refractory or relapsed hodgkin lymphoma: results of a spanish prospective cooperative protocol. Biol Blood Marrow Transplant 2006;12:172–83.

162. Khouri IF, Keating M, Korbling M, et al. Transplant-lite: induction of graft-versus-malignancy using fludarabine-based nonablative chemotherapy and allogeneic blood progenitor-cell transplantation as treatment for lymphoid malignancies. J Clin Oncol 1998;16:2817–24.

163. Peggs KS, Hunter A, Chopra R, et al. Clinical evidence of a graft-versus-Hodgkin's-lymphoma effect after reduced-intensity allogeneic transplantation. Lancet 2005;365:1934–41.

164. Sureda A, Robinson S, Canals C, et al. Reduced-intensity conditioning compared with conventional allogeneic stem-cell transplantation in relapsed or refractory Hodgkin's lymphoma: an analysis from the Lymphoma Working Party of the European Group for Blood and Marrow Transplantation. J Clin Oncol 2008;26:455–62.

165. Baetz T, Belch A, Couban S, et al. Gemcitabine, dexamethasone and cisplatin is an active and non-toxic chemotherapy regimen in relapsed or refractory Hodgkin's disease: a phase II study by the National Cancer Institute of Canada Clinical Trials Group. Ann Oncol 2003;14:1762–7.

166. Santoro A, Bredenfeld H, Devizzi L, et al. Gemcitabine in the treatment of refractory Hodgkin's disease: results of a multicenter phase II study. J Clin Oncol 2000;18:2615–9.

167. Venkatesh H, Di Bella N, Flynn TP, Vellek MJ, Boehm KA, Asmar L. Results of a phase II multicenter trial of single-agent gemcitabine in patients with relapsed or chemotherapy-refractory Hodgkin's lymphoma. Clin Lymphoma 2004;5:110–5.

168. Younes A, Fayad L, Pro B, et al. Gemcitabine plus rituximab therapy of patients with relapsed and refractory classical Hodgkin lymphoma. Blood 2005;1498a.

169. Devizzi L, Santoro A, Bonfante V, et al. Vinorelbine: an active drug for the management of patients with heavily pretreated Hodgkin's disease. Ann Oncol 1994;5:817–20.

170. Ferme C, Bastion Y, Lepage E, et al. The MINE regimen as intensive salvage chemotherapy for relapsed and refractory Hodgkin's disease. Ann Oncol 1995;6:543–9.

171. Younes A, Pro B, Fayad L. Experience with bortezomib for the treatment of patients with relapsed classical Hodgkin lymphoma. Blood 2006;107:1731–2.

172. Boll B, Hansen H, Heuck F, et al. The fully human anti-CD30 antibody 5F11 activates NF-{kappa}B and sensitizes lymphoma cells to bortezomib-induced apoptosis. Blood 2005;106:1839–42.

173. Georgakis GV, Li Y, Humphreys R, et al. Activity of selective fully human agonistic antibodies to the TRAIL death receptors TRAIL-R1 and TRAIL-R2 in primary and cultured lymphoma cells: induction of apoptosis and enhancement of doxorubicin- and bortezomib-induced cell death. Br J Haematol 2005;130:501–10.

174. O'Connor OA, Heaney ML, Schwartz L, et al. Clinical experience with intravenous and oral formulations of the novel histone deacetylase inhibitor suberoylanilide hydroxamic acid in patients with advanced hematologic malignancies. J Clin Oncol 2006;24:166–73.

175. Younes A Fayad M, Pro B, et al. A phase II study of a novel oral isotype-selective histone deacetylase (HDAC) inhibitor in patients with relapsed or refractory Hodgkin lymphoma. J Clin Oncol 2007;25:441s

176. Ansell SM, Horwitz SM, Engert A, et al. Phase I/II study of an anti-CD30 monoclonal antibody (MDX-060) in Hodgkin's lymphoma and anaplastic large-cell lymphoma. J Clin Oncol 2007;25:2764–9.

177. Bartlett NL, Younes A, Carabasi MH, et al. A phase 1 multidose study of SGN-30 immunotherapy in patients with refractory or recurrent CD30+ hematologic malignancies. Blood 2008;111:1848–54.

178. Francisco JA, Cerveny CG, Meyer DL, et al. cAC10-vcMMAE, an anti-CD30-monomethyl auristatin E conjugate with potent and selective antitumor activity. Blood 2003;102:1458–65.

179. Younes A, Forero-Torres A, Bartlett NL, et al. A novel antibody-drug conjugate, SNG-35 (Anti-CD30-Auristatin), induces objective responses in patients with relapsed or refractory Hodgkin lymphoma: preliminary results of a phase I tolerability study. Haematologica 2007:64

180. Ekstrand BC, Lucas JB, Horwitz SM, et al. Rituximab in lymphocyte-predominant Hodgkin disease: results of a phase 2 trial. Blood 2003;101:4285–9.

181. Rehwald U, Schulz H, Reiser M, et al. Treatment of relapsed CD20+ Hodgkin lymphoma with the monoclonal antibody rituximab is effective and well tolerated: results of a phase 2 trial of the German Hodgkin Lymphoma Study Group. Blood 2003;101:420–4.

182. Younes A, Romaguera J, Hagemeister F, et al. A pilot study of rituximab in patients with recurrent, classic Hodgkin disease. Cancer 2003;98:310–4.

183. Josting A, Wolf J, Diehl V. Hodgkin disease: prognostic factors and treatment strategies. Curr Opin Oncol 2000;12:403–11.

184. Pallesen G, Hamilton-Dutoit SJ, Rowe M, et al. Expression of Epstein-Barr virus latent gene products in tumour cells of Hodgkin's disease. Lancet 1991;337:320–2.

185. Murray PG, Young LS, Rowe M, et al. Immunohistochemical demonstration of the Epstein-Barr virus-encoded latent membrane protein in paraffin sections of Hodgkin's disease. J Pathol 1992;166:1–5.

186. Gianni AM, Rambaldi A, Zinzani P, et al. Comparable 3-year outcome following ABVD or BEACOPP first-line chemotherapy, plus pre-planned high-dose salvage, in advanced Hodgkin lymphoma (HL): A randomized trial of the Michelangelo, GITIL and IIL cooperative groups. J Clin Oncol 26: 2008 (suppl; abstr 8506).

187. Federico M, Luminari S, Iannitto E, et al. ABVD compared with BEACOPP compared with CEC for the initial treatment of patients with advanced Hodgkin's lymphoma: results from the HD2000 Gruppo Italiano per lo Studio dei Linfomi Trial. J Clin Oncol. 2009;27:805–11.

188. Magagnoli M, Spina M, Balzarotti M, et al. IGEV regimen and a fixed dose of lenograstim: an effective mobilization regimen in pretreated Hodgkin's lymphoma patients. Bone Marrow Transplant. 2007 ;40:1019–25.

Chapter 22

Classification of T-cell and NK-cell Malignancies

Dan Jones

Abstract/Scope of Chapter This chapter provides an overview of mature T-cell malignancies, including those presenting in lymph nodes (e.g., angioimmunoblastic T-cell lymphoma), extranodal sites (e.g., hepatosplenic T-cell lymphoma), and leukemias (e.g., Sézary syndrome). The role of the two prototypic mature T-cell oncogenes, ALK kinase in anaplastic large cell lymphoma and TCL1 in T-cell prolymphocytic leukemia, is discussed. A general model for T-cell tumor initiation involving canonical and aberrant signaling through the T-cell receptor is presented. The clinical presentation and morphologic range of NK-cell malignancies are also discussed.

Keywords Lymphoblastic lymphoma, precursor T • NOTCH1 • HOX genes • Angioimmunoblastic T-cell lymphoma • CXCL13 • PD-1, CD10, T-cell lymphoma • BCL-6, T-cell lymphoma • PTCL, NOS • Peripheral T-cell lymphoma, not otherwise specified • Lennert lymphoma • T-cell lymphoma, interfollicular • T-cell lymphoma, central memory type • T-cell lymphoma, paracortical • T-cell lymphoma, follicular variant • Anaplastic large cell lymphoma ALK-positive • ALCL • Anaplastic large cell lymphoma, null type • Anaplastic large cell lymphoma, hallmark cell • Anaplastic large cell lymphoma, ALK-negative • Anaplastic large cell lymphoma, small cell type • Anaplastic large cell lymphoma, neutrophil-rich • Anaplastic large cell lymphoma, lymphohistiocytic type • Enteropathy-associated T-cell lymphoma • Enteropathy-associated T-cell lymphoma, low-grade component • Hepatosplenic T-cell lymphoma • Hepatosplenic T-cell lymphoma, alpha-beta type • T-cell lymphoma, bone marrow involvement • T-cell prolymphocytic leukemia • T-cell prolymphocytic leukemia, TCL1 expression • TCL1 • Large granular lymphocyte leukemia • Sezary syndrome • Adult T-cell leukemia/lymphoma • Human T-cell lymphotropic virus • T-cell receptor, Vbeta typing • T-cell receptor, signaling in lymphoma • NK receptors, role in diagnosis • T-cell lymphoma, alternate classification • EBV, role in T-cell lymphomas • Large B-cell lymphoma, secondary in T-cell lymphomas • Extranodal NK/T-cell lymphoma, nasal type • Extranodal NK/T-cell lymphoma, non-nasal type • EBV, role in NK-cell tumors • NK-cell leukemia • Aggressive NK-cell leukemia

22.1. General Features of T-cell Neoplasms

The 2008 WHO classification divides tumors of T-cell lineage into precursor/thymic and post-thymic/mature subgroups. The pathogenesis and clinical behavior of precursor-T lymphoblastic lymphoma/acute lymphoblastic leukemia (T-LBL/ALL) is easy to understand compared with mature T-cell neoplasms and is briefly summarized here and in Chap. 13. Thymocytes, or occasionally more primitive bone marrow (BM) T-cell progenitors, transform to LBL/ALL after acquiring reciprocal chromosomal translocations that activate one of many different transcription factors (such as the HOX genes) which block T-cell maturation at a particular stage [1]. In at least 50% of cases, T-LBL/ALL also acquires activating mutations of the growth regulator NOTCH1, which promotes proliferation [2]. These tumors, which mostly arise in children and young adults during the period of maximal thymocyte production, then expand the thymus producing a mediastinal mass and spill over into the peripheral blood (PB) and BM (see Chaps. 13 and 27).

In contrast, the pathogenesis and clinical behavior of mature (post-thymic) T-cell malignancies are much more complex. Such peripheral T-cell lymphomas and leukemias (PTCL/L) can present at nearly any tissue site, have a variety of phenotypes, and display complex patterns of tumor progression. Furthermore, most PTCL/L, unlike mature B-cell tumors and LBL/ALL, lack reciprocal chromosomal translocations [3] complicating diagnosis and posttreatment monitoring. As a result, most of the PTCL/L entities in the 2008 WHO classification represent syndromes such as the cutaneous T-cell lymphoma (CTCL, covered in Chap. 24) or enteropathy-associated intestinal T-cell lymphoma (EATL), which show molecular and immunophenotypic heterogeneity. Fortunately, PTCL/L are rare, comprising approximately 5% of all hematolymphoid malignancies in the United States [4].

One of the likely reasons that PTCL/L are so complex is that the biology of non-neoplastic T cells lacks the linear schema of differentiation evident in B cells. Instead, there are many fully or partially differentiated functional subsets of T cells with considerable plasticity. Nonetheless, shared features of the most common types of PTCL/L can help in understanding which factors drive outgrowth of these tumors.

- Most PTCL/L are positive for CD4 with cytokine/growth factor receptor expression patterns consistent with a persistently activated helper T-cell phenotype.
- Molecular evidence of precedent polyclonal and oligoclonal T-cell proliferations supports a stepwise process of transformation in T-cell tumors such as angioimmunoblastic T-cell lymphoma (AITL), CTCL, T-cell large granular lymphocyte leukemia (T-LGLL), and adult T-cell leukemia/lymphoma (ATLL).
- The pathogenesis of many of these slowly evolving cases shows a strong role for (exogenous or autoimmune) antigen stimulation, in that long-standing inflammatory lesions precede neoplastic transformation. Examples include chronic dermatitis in CTCL, enteropathy in EATL, and autoimmune cytotoxic T-cell expansions in T-LGLL.

22.2. Clinical Features

Mature T-cell malignancies are rare in the United States, with higher incidences in most Asian countries [4–6]. With the exceptions of ALK-translocated anaplastic large cell lymphoma (ALCL) and hepatosplenic T-cell lymphoma (HSTCL), PTCL/L are tumors of the middle-aged and elderly. The demographic features, sites of involvement, and presentation features of the PTCL/L subtypes listed in the 2008 WHO classification are summarized in Chaps. 23 (Tables 23-1/2) and 24 (Tables 24-5/6/7).

One of the most important clinical features of many subtypes of PTCL/L is that the tumor cells are functional and produce cytokines that drive tumor-associated proliferation of other immune cell types such as B cells and dendritic cells. These properties interfere with hematopoiesis (producing cytopenias), damage immune function (leading to immunosuppression), cause end-organ damage, and are a major cause of mortality in PTCL/L (Table 22-1). A consequence of these immune effects is that many PTCL/L have a clinical impact that is disproportionate to their tumor burden and are thus diagnosed earlier in the (oligoclonal) phase of development. The impact of these features on the appropriate methods for staging PTCL/L and for follow-up monitoring are discussed in Chap. 23.

Table 22-1. Paraneoplastic and symptomatic presentations of mature T-cell neoplasms.

Type	Sign(s)	Symptom(s)	Laboratory finding	Complications during course	Pathogenetic cause
Predominantly nodal					
AITL	Skin rash after drug, small adenopathy, ascites	B-symptoms neuropathy, arthritis	Hypergammaglobulinemia, hemolytic anemia (cold agglutins), autoantibodies	Secondary EBV+ DLBCL	Follicular or Th2-like T cells secrete cytokines that drives B-cell expansion
PTCL, NOS	Adenopathy	B-symptoms	Eosinophilia (subset)	Secondary plasma cell neoplasm Secondary EBV+ DLBCL	Various
ALCL, ALK-translocated	Tumor masses	B-symptoms	Rare leukemic variants	Extranodal spread or recurrence	ALK transformation of activated cytotoxic T cells
ALCL, non-ALK	Adenopathy	B-symptoms	Cytopenias (subset)	As above	Unknown
Predominantly extranodal					
ATLL	Skin rash, adenopathy	B-symptoms, pruritis	Hypercalcemia, eosinophilia, lytic bone lesions	Opportunistic infections, exfoliative skin rash	HTLV-1 tax gene transformation with secondary genetic changes
Enteropathy-associated TCL	Intestinal perforation	Malabsorption	Anti-gliadin antibodies	Recurrent bowel ulcers, perforation at anastomosis	Autoimmune expansions of gut-homing T cells
NK/TCL, nasal type	Ulcerating mass	B-symptoms	Lymphopenia	Erosion into facial bones, other organs	EBV transformation with secondary genetic changes
HSTCL	Organomegaly	Splenomegaly	Pancytopenia	Severe cytopenias	Expansions of Vδ1 γ/δ-T cells
Predominantly leukemic					
SS	Erythroderma	Pruritis	Eosinophilia	Large cell transformation, spread to organs	MF transformation or primary expansions of Th2 T cells
T-PLL	Edema	Fatigue	High WBC	Pancytopenia	Naïve T-cells that acquire TCL1 activation
T-LGLL	Bruising	Fatigue, infection	Cytopenia(s), rheumatic diseases	Secondary MDS, infections	Autoimmune expansions of cytotoxic T cells

Other rarer types of cutaneous types of TCL/L are discussed in Chap. 24

22.3. Diagnostic Features of T-cell Lymphomas

In lymph node (LN), most PTCL have a nodular paracortical or interfollicular pattern of involvement in the early stage, but diffusely replace the LN as the disease progresses (Table 22-2) [7].

AITL in LN: This is a morphologically distinctive type of CD4+ PTCL that is associated with polymorphous proliferations of non-neoplastic lymphocytes and immune accessory cells due to tumor cell expression of growth-promoting cytokines [8]. As a result, AITL evolves through a number of different histologic appearances with the initial stage usually showing focal tumor cell infiltration into hyperplastic germinal centers (GCs) (Fig. 22-1a). These tumor aggregates are visible as clusters of clear cells highlighted by T-cell immunostains within the B-cell follicles (Fig. 22-1b and c). The phenotype of the neoplastic T

Table 22-2. Morphogenetic features of the T-cell lymphomas/leukemias.

Type	Pattern of growth in lymph node	Tumor cell morphology	Histologic variants	Most common immunophenotype of tumor T cells (all are usually CD2+CD3+ except ALCL)
Predominantly nodal				
AITL	Germinotropic and interfollicular	Large with clear cytoplasm	Histiocyte-rich	Positive: PD-1, CXCL13, CD10 (w), BCL6(w) Negative: cytotoxic granule proteins CD4+ ≫ CD8+
PTCL, NOS	Interfollicular, paracortical, diffuse	Variable, often clear cytoplasm	Lymphoepithelioid, nodular, follicular	Positive: CD5, CD7, TCR-β, CD30 (subset) Negative: CD8 (most), CD10, CXCL13 CD4+ ≫ CD8+
ALCL	Intrasinusoidal to diffuse	"Hallmark" cells with abundant cytoplasm	Small cell, Hodgkin-like, inflammatory, lymphohistiocytic, sarcomatoid	Positive: CD30, CD43, CD45, clusterin, ALK (70%), cytotoxic granule proteins Negative: PAX5, CD15 (most), EBER Variable: EMA, CD56, pan-T markers CD4 ≫ CD8
Predominantly extranodal				
ATLL	Nodular to diffuse	Varying size, polylobate nuclei	Smoldering, acute, lymphoma	Positive: CD4, CD5, CD25, CCR4, FOXP3 Negative: CD7, CD8
Enteropathy-associated TCL	Interfollicular to diffuse	Variable size, pale cytoplasm	Monomorphic (CD8+, Type II)	Positive: CD7, CD103, TCR-β, CD30 (LCT) Negative: CD5 CD4−CD8−> CD8+
NK/TCL, nasal type	Paracortical to diffuse	Variable size, necrosis	Extranasal, EBV-cases, leukemic forms	Positive: CD2, cCD3, CD30 (LCT), CD56, EBER Negative: CD4, CD5, CD8, CD16, CD57 T-cell type will be sCD3+CD5+CD8+v
HSTCL	Paracortical	Medium-sized with blastic chromatin	BM interstitial. BM sinusoidal/blastic	Positive: CD56, TCR-γ/δ, TIA−1 Negative: CD4, CD5, granzyme B, perforin Variable: CD8, CD94
Predominantly leukemic				
SS	Paracortical to diffuse	Variable including large cell forms	Secondary from MF, de novo (primary SS)	Positive: CD4, TCR-β Negative: CD8, CD26 50% of de novo cases are CD7+
T-PLL	Interfollicular to diffuse	Distinct nucleoli, variable nuclear irregularities	Small cell	Positive: TCL1, CD5, CD7, CD45RA (40%) Negative: CD25 (most) CD4+CD8−> CD4+CD8+ > CD4−CD8+
T-LGLL	Intrasinusoidal	Abundant granular cytoplasm	Rare CD4+ and NK phenotypes	Positive: CD8, CD16, CD57,TCR-β, cytotoxic granule proteins Negative: CD5 (or dim), CD7 (dim), CD56 Variable: CD99

Abbreviations: as in text and (*w*): weak/dim expression; *v*: variable expression; *LCT*: large cell transformation

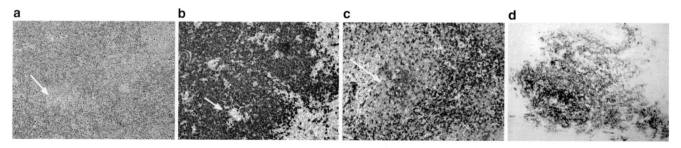

Fig. 22-1. Angioimmunoblastic T-cell lymphoma, folliculocentric growth. (**a**) The lymph node is effaced by a polymorphous infiltrate of inflammatory cells and clusters of large tumor cells with clear cytoplasm (*arrow*). (**b**) CD20 immunostain highlights expansions of B cells within the altered follicle as well as in the surrounding marginal zone areas. (**c**) CD3 immunostain highlights a cluster of tumor cells within the follicle (*arrow*). (**d**) CD21 immunostain highlights the expanded follicular dendritic cell network outside of the B-cell follicle surrounding a blood vessel

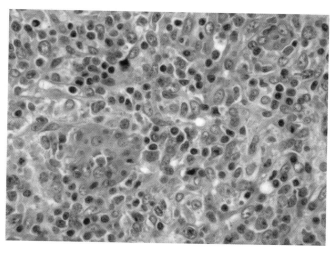

Fig. 22-2. Angioimmunoblastic T-cell lymphoma. Polymorphous infiltrate of lymphocytes of various sizes, with eosinophils and plasma cells. A prominent high endothelium venule (HEV) with sclerotic adluminal membrane is present at *bottom left*

cells in AITL resembles that of normal follicular homing T cells, with expression of BCL6, CD10, the chemokine CXCL13 [9], and the immunoregulatory molecule PD-1 [10]. Fully developed AITL is always associated with extrafollicular proliferations of follicular dendritic cells (Fig. 22-1d) and plump high-endothelial blood vessels (Fig. 22-2). However, depending on the disease course, AITL can also show prominent plasma cells, eosinophils, or histiocytes [11]. Given the tumor-associated immune dysfunction, Epstein–Barr virus (EBV)-infected B cells are almost always increased and their detection by EBER in situ hybridization is a helpful diagnostic feature. These virally-infected B cells can transform into diffuse large B-cell lymphoma, which is diagnosed whenever sheet-like EBV+ B cells are present, a complication seen in approximately 20% of patients with AITL [12]. EBV-negative clonal plasma cell proliferations can be seen in 5–10% of cases [13]. Rare T-cell tumors with a CD8+ immunophenotype resemble AITL.

PTCL, NOS in LN: This category contains a number of distinctive histogenetic subgroups with differing histological appearances, genetic findings, chemotactic properties and cytokine secretion patterns. The histiocyte-rich lymphoepithelioid variant of PTCL, NOS (also known as Lennert lymphoma) shows rows of epithelioid histiocytes surrounded by numerous small B cells and usually only a small number of enlarged tumor T cells which may have a CD8+ immunophenotype (Fig. 22-3). The nodular paracortical type of PTCL, NOS shows pale-staining CD4+ T-cell proliferations that expand in the LN paracortex adjacent to the mantle zones of B-cell follicles (Fig. 22-4) [14]. PTCL, NOS with a T-zone pattern shows interfollicular growth with minimal disruption of the B-cell compartment (Fig. 22-5). This tumor type may arise from nonactivated recirculating memory T cells accounting for the subtle nondestructive manner of nodal infiltration [15]. Finally, rare PTCL, NOS cases may preferentially colonize reactive germinal centers, without the FDC disruption and inflammatory cell proliferations characteristic of AITL, and have been referred to as follicular T-cell lymphoma [16].

Anaplastic large cell lymphoma: ALCL is a neoplasm of large cells with either T cell or null immunophenotype (but with evidence of TCR gene rearrangement) and uniform expression of CD30 [17]. The most common ALCL subtype shows activation of the ALK kinase by chromosome translocation [usually t(2;5)/ALK-NPM1] and is the only mature T-cell tumor that commonly occurs in pediatric patients [18]. ALCL involves the LN with an intrasinusoidal, focal, or diffuse growth pattern; ALCL also involves many different extranodal sites.

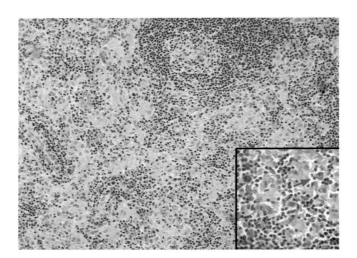

Fig. 22-3. Nodal peripheral T-cell lymphoma, lymphoepithelioid variant. Interfollicular infiltrate comprised of a polymorphous infiltrate including small lymphocytes (B cells), and epithelioid histiocytes arranged in rows. A reactive germinal center is in *upper right*. *Inset* shows scattered large nucleolated tumor cells (*arrows*) that were positive for CD8 (not shown)

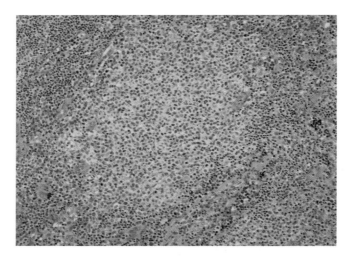

Fig. 2-4. Nodal peripheral T-cell lymphoma, nodular (paracortical) variant. A nodular aggregate of pale-staining tumor cells, in the paracortex of an involved lymph node

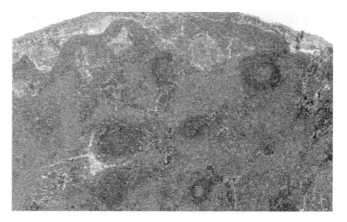

Fig. 22-5. Nodal peripheral T-cell lymphoma, interfollicular. Marked lymph node expansion by an infiltrate of large tumor lymphocytes that do not disrupt the overall architecture

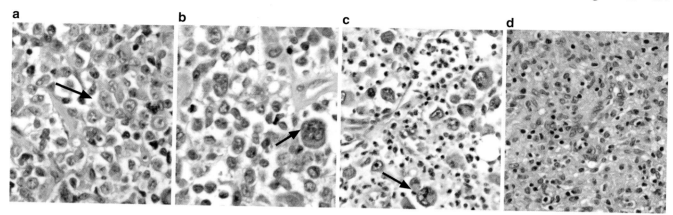

Fig. 22-6. Anaplastic large cell lymphoma, ALK-positive. A variety of histological appearances are evident including: (**a**) Classical type. (**b**) Small cell variant. (**c**) Neutrophil-rich case (with edematous stroma). (**d**) Lymphohistocytic type. Hallmark cells are indicated with *arrows*

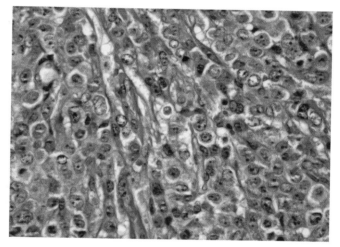

Fig. 22-7. Anaplastic large cell lymphoma, ALK-negative. Tumor morphology is similar to the case in 22.6A, but lacks expression of the ALK protein

There are several distinct clinical presentations and cytologic variants of ALK-translocated ALCL [19]. The classical morphology is that of uniformly large tumor cells with abundant eosinophilic cytoplasm and vesicular (cleared-out) nuclei with prominent nucleoli. Such cells that also show perinuclear cytoplasmic inclusions are referred to as "Hallmark" cells. Morphologic variants of ALCL include the small cell type with only rare classical ALCL cells [20] neutrophil- and/or eosinophil-rich cases, and a lymphohistiocytic type in which the epithelioid histiocytes nearly obscure the tumor cells (Fig. 22-6). The 30% of ALCL cases lacking detectable ALK-translocation are morphologically indistinguishable from ALK-translocated ALCL cases, are largely restricted to adults, and have more aggressive clinical behavior (Fig. 22-7) [21].

Enteropathy-associated T-cell lymphoma: EATL is a rare intestinal lymphoma arising from precursor epitheliotropic T cells; most cases present with intestinal perforation or blockage due to a transmural, diffuse large cell tumor infiltrate. Multifocal involvement of the jejunum or ileum with accompanying ulceration is most common (see Chap. 27).

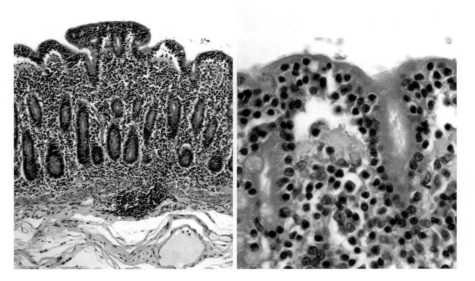

Fig. 22-8. Enteropathy-associated lymphoma, low-grade component. (**a**) Small epitheliotropic neoplastic lymphocytes in small bowel are associated with enteropathic changes including villous blunting and an increase in lymphocytes in the lamina propria. The lifting off of the epithelium due to the destructive lymphocyte infiltration is a typical feature of EATL distinguishing it from enteritis. (**b**) Intraepithelial tumor lymphocytes are predominantly small, and had a TCR-β+ CD8+ T-cell immunophenotype in this case (not shown)

Areas away from the site of the transformed tumor will often show a low-grade T-cell lymphomatous component infiltrating into the mucosa and/or enteropathy-associated epithelial changes such as villous blunting and crypt hyperplasia (Fig. 22-8). Most commonly EATL shows a CD4−CD8− T-cell phenotype with expression of the intestine homing adhesion molecules CD103 (αE integrin) and α4β7 integrin, but a minority of cases express CD8. Most cases show genomic amplification at chromosome 9q33–q34 [22]. Some intestinal TCL with a similar appearance and immunophenotype occur in patients without evidence of enteropathy. Rare EATL cases present in the stomach, liver or as extensive mesenteric infiltrates.

Hepatosplenic T-cell lymphoma (liver and spleen): HSTCL is an extremely aggressive neoplasm arising, in most cases, from T cells expressing TCR-gamma/delta. It shows red pulp infiltration in the spleen, intrasinusoidal infiltrates in the liver, and intrasinusoidal or interstitial BM involvement, with typically medium-sized tumor lymphocytes with irregular nuclear contours and blastoid chromatin (Fig. 22-9). HSTCL almost always shows low-level PB and BM involvement at diagnosis as well as focal infiltration in the perisplenic LNs. In the BM, it may be mistaken for high-grade MDS given its blastoid appearance. Extramedullary dissemination of HSTCL occurs late in the disease course, including to skin and other mucosal sites.

PTCL in the bone marrow and peripheral blood: The BM is commonly involved in all T-cell lymphoma types (60–80%), except for ALCL, EATL, and most CTCL variants. Commonly, loose, vaguely-defined fibrotic lymphoid aggregates are randomly distributed throughout the BM (see Chap. 5) [23]. Exceptions to this pattern include ALCL which shows single-cell or rarely diffuse infiltration particularly in pediatric cases, [24] and HSTCL which usually shows an intrasinusoidal pattern [25]. Significant PB involvement in PTCL is usually only seen in the terminal stage of dissemination or in the rare leukemic forms of ALCL [26]. AITL often shows an increase in circulating plasmacytoid B cells.

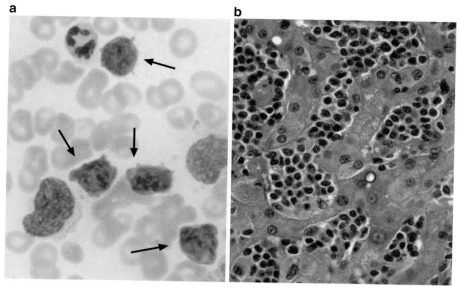

Fig. 22-9. Hepatosplenic T-cell lymphoma. (**a**) Tumor cells in BM are medium-sized with irregular nuclear contours and blastoid chromatin (*arrows*). (**b**) Intrasinusoidal liver infiltrate is composed of medium-sized blastoid lymphocytes

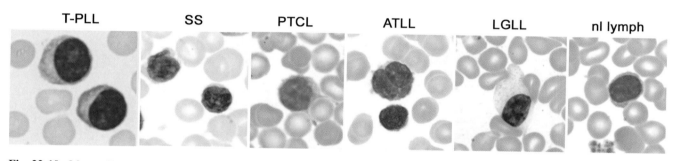

Fig. 22-10. Mature T-cell leukemias, morphologic comparisons. (**a**) T-PLL shows round to irregular nuclei with prominent nucleoli and abundant agranular cytoplasm. (**b**) Sézary syndrome can show larger lymphocytes with minimal atypia or more classical small cells with cerebriform nuclei. (**c**) Peripheralized nodal T-cell lymphoma can resemble Sézary cells. (**d**) Adult T-cell leukemia/lymphoma with large cells with multilobate nuclei (normal lymphocyte is shown below). (**e**) LGL leukemia with abundant cytoplasmic granules. (**f**) Normal (nonactivated) lymphocyte

22.4. Morphological Features of T-cell Leukemias

The mature T-cell neoplasms with a predominant leukemic pattern are T-cell prolymphocytic leukemia (T-PLL), Sézary syndrome (SS), T-LGLL, and ATLL. Morphologic features are extremely helpful in narrowing the differential (Fig. 22-10).

T-cell large granular lymphocyte leukemia: T-LGLL is an extremely indolent disorder of CD8+ cytotoxic T-cells that presents with often marked BM LGL infiltration, low-to-moderate levels of LGLs in the PB, and red pulp infiltration in the spleen (Fig. 22-11). In BM, LGLL shows interstitial and intrasinusoidal infiltration, but there are typically also multiple reactive B-cell aggregates [27]. LGLL tumor cells are typically positive for CD8 and TCR-α/β and show expression of cytotoxic granule proteins. Suppression of hematopoiesis (due to cytolytic or immune-mediated attack on marrow elements) can manifest as neutropenia, anemia, or multilineage hypoplasia. Marrow dysplastic changes mimicking or progressing to MDS are often noted in long-standing LGLL [28]. Most cases show only modest tumor cell atypia, so distinguishing polyclonal LGL lymphocytosis from oligoclonal and monoclonal

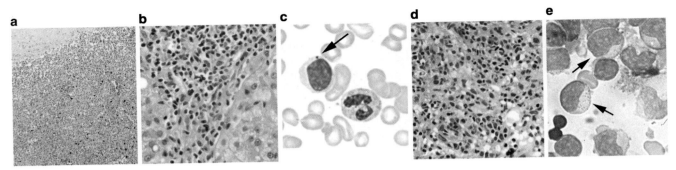

Fig. 22-11. Large granular lymphocyte (LGL) leukemia. (**a**) Involvement of the splenic red pulp. (**b**) Higher magnification showing LGLL within sinusoids and cords. (**c**) Appearance of LGLL in blood resembling a normal LGL except for coarse granules (*arrow*). (**d**) Extensive LGL leukemia BM infiltration with fibrosis, myeloid hypoplasia, and erythroid dysplasia. (**e**) Bone marrow aspirate shows increased enlarged LGL tumor cells with a morphologic appearance that can overlap with maturing myeloid elements (*arrows*)

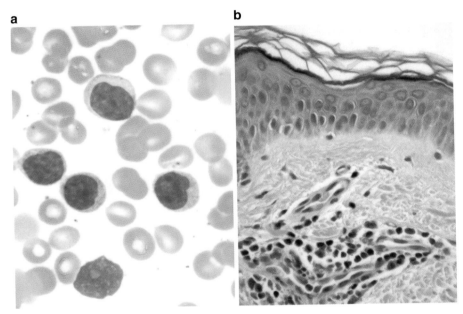

Fig. 22-12. T-cell prolymphocytic leukemia. (**a**) Many cases of T-PLL show a spectrum of morphology in blood and BM with few classical prolymphocytes. (**b**) Skin involvement manifested as sparse perivascular infiltrates. Immunostain for TCL1 was positive (not shown)

LGLL can be difficult, [29] and relies on the use of TCR molecular clonality studies. TCR-Vbeta profiling by FC, [30] or expression profiling of the natural killer receptors (NKRs), such as CD94 and CD158, has also been used for clonality assessment. In contrast to the variable expression of NKRs in reactive LGL populations, most LGLL tumor cells will show a consistent pattern of antigen expression or loss [31]. Atypical immunophenotypic variants of LGLL (such as CD4+, CD4−CD8−, and TCR-g/d+) are more commonly encountered in association with other neoplasms, or in post-therapy and post-transplant settings [32].

  T-cell prolymphocytic leukemia: T-PLL almost always presents with very high WBC counts (>100×10⁹/L), diffuse replacement of the BM and splenomegaly; only rare cases have low levels of lymphocytosis [33]. Although some T-PLL cases show a predominance of classical prolymphocytes (Fig. 22-10, left), a mixture of small and large irregular forms is more typical (Fig. 22-12a). Cutaneous infiltration, often in a subtle perivascular pattern, is seen in at least 50% of patients at some point during the disease course (Fig. 22-12b),

a b

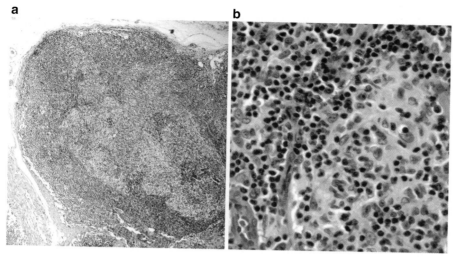

Fig. 22-13. Mycosis fungoides involving lymph node. (**a**) Nodular paracortical infiltrate with dermatopathic appearance. (**b**) At high magnification, atypical cerebriform lymphocytes are admixed with the dendritic cells

but lymphadenopathy is typically modest. In 70–80% of cases, T-PLL will demonstrate chromosomal rearrangements activating TCL1 by TCRA, which can be detected by karyotype [inversion or translocation (14;14)(q11;q32)], FISH, or IHC for TCL1 that is not expressed in mature T cells or other mature T-cell tumors [33].

Sézary syndrome: SS, defined as a T-cell leukemia with skin and LN involvement associated with erythroderma, may arise as a distinctive de novo leukemia [33–36] or as extracutaneous spread of long-standing mycosis fungoides [33]. The marrow infiltration is often subtle requiring flow cytometry for adequate detection, with a CD4+CD7+ T-cell phenotype showing one or more aberrancies in the level of expression of pan-T-cell markers found in nearly all cases. Lymph node involvement by SS (or MF) shows interfollicular to diffuse involvement usually with dermatopathic change due to pruritis-associated skin breakdown (Fig. 22-13).

Adult T-cell leukemia/lymphoma: ATLL is a heterogeneous entity comprising the mature T-cell tumors arising following T-cell transformation by the retrovirus human T-cell lymphotropic virus (HTLV)-1. The lymphoid malignancies comprising ATLL normally have an unusual T-cell regulatory phenotype characterized by high-level expression of CD25 and FOXP3 [37] due to the effects of the HTLV-1-encoded multifunctional transcriptional regulator TAX. Other HTLV-1-associated diseases include tropical spastic paraparesis/myelopathy and diffuse dermatitis, and all are largely restricted to endemic areas such as Japan and the Caribbean basin but rarely seen in the United States and Europe. ATLL usually presents in late adulthood (median age 55 years) with lymphadenopathy (75%), skin lesions (50%), hepatosplenomegaly (25–50%), and hypercalcemia (30%). This variability in ATLL presentation has been grouped into four subtypes: acute, lymphoma, chronic, and smoldering [38]. The acute and lymphoma subtypes have the worst prognosis, with median survival of approximately 6 months [39]. Histological clues to the diagnosis of ATLL include an extensively epidermotropic cutaneous infiltrate with frequent tumor cell apoptosis, and tumor cells with highly irregular and polylobated nuclear contours and/or multinucleation. Immunophenotyping will reveal bright CD25 positivity with a CD4+ immunophenotype in most cases. Southern blot analysis to look for clonal HTLV-1 proviral integration is the gold standard for ATLL diagnosis, but in nonendemic areas, viral etiology is usually inferred from HTLV-1 seropositivity.

22.5. Ancillary Studies in Diagnosis

Given the subtlety of the histologic findings in many mature T-cell tumors, immunophenotyping is essential and the mainstay of diagnosis (Table 22-2). Whenever possible, flow cytometry (FC) is the preferred method, since it will detect discrete populations of tumor cells that have complete loss or dimmer or brighter expression of one or more pan-T-cell markers. An appropriate FC marker panel would include CD2, CD3, CD4, CD5, CD7, CD8, and TCR-α/β as well as the B-cell marker CD19 and the NK-cell marker combination CD16+CD56. If no TCR-α/β expression is seen, TCR-γ/δ should be tested as well as TdT to exclude T-LBL/ALL. If the tumor is positive for CD2, but negative for surface CD3 and CD5, NK-cell tumors should be considered with the addition of markers such as CD94 and cytotoxic granule proteins (by IHC). CD30 should be tested in all T-cell tumors with large size or anaplastic morphology, and CD25 (or FOXP3) added if there is clinical suspicion of ATLL, due to hypercalcemia or serologic evidence of HTLV-1 infection. Finally, T-PLL should be considered in those tumors presenting with very high white blood counts or those with coexpression of CD4 and CD8, and can be evaluated using TCL1 antibodies by FC or IHC.

When performing immunostaining on paraffin sections, antibodies against all of the above markers can be utilized except for TCR-δ, which does not stain reliably in fixed material. ALK immunostaining should be done in any CD30+ tumor, and TdT performed in any tumor with blastoid features and a high mitotic rate. Additional immunostaining for cytotoxic granule proteins (TIA-1, granzyme B, and perforin) can be useful in the diagnosis of ALCL, and in separating HSTCL (typically TIA-1+, granzyme B-, perforin-) from T-LGLL (positive for all three markers).

Polymerase chain reaction (PCR) studies for TCR-beta and TCR-gamma gene rearrangements are extremely useful in supporting a diagnosis of PTCL/L, if used judiciously. Molecular studies can definitively assign T-cell lineage in those PTCL and ALCL that show extensive loss of pan-T-cell antigens [40]. The major limitations of the T-cell PCR clonality assays are the frequent findings of false-positive oligoclonal TCR rearrangements in the PB or BM that are unrelated to the neoplastic clone (see Chap. 4). The routine use of TCR PCR for staging at these sites needs further evaluation [41].

Cytogenetic studies can be used to demonstrate clonality but are typically complex in PTCL/L without diagnostically helpful changes. Three exceptions are the t(2;5)(p23;q35) / ALK-NPM1 (or other translocations involving chr 2p23) seen in ALK+ ALCL, isochromosome 7q seen in HSTCL (often along with +8), and t(14;14)(q11;q32) or inv(14)(q11q32)/TCRA-TCL1 seen in T-PLL. All three changes can also be detected by commercially available fluorescence in situ hybridization (FISH) probes. Other recurrent chromosomal changes occur more rarely in PTCL/L [42].

22.6. Differential Diagnosis

In diagnosing any T-cell tumor, it is important to correlate the histologic features with the clinical presentation, pre-existing conditions, and the predominant site(s) of involvement. For example, EATL, T-PLL, MF, or SS may present in LN morphologically resembling PTCL-NOS (Fig. 22-13). Similarly, AITL may present in the skin with sparse perivascular infiltrates resembling SS or CTCL variants. Also, since many PTCL/L categories are defined based on their sites of involvement and functional properties, immunophenotypic variants will be encountered and are usually grouped with the cases that have the more characteristic markers. Examples include HSTCL expressing TCR-α/β (instead of TCR-γ/δ), [43] LGLL expressing CD4 or TCR-γ/δ (instead of CD8 and TCR-α/β), [44] or T-PLL lacking TCL1 activation.

The functional properties of many T-cell tumors also result in dysplastic changes in the surrounding hematopoiesis in BM infiltration that can mimic myelodysplastic syndromes. This is particularly evident in HSTCL, [45] T-LGLL, [28] and AITL [46].

22.7. Pathogenesis of Mature T-cell Malignancies

22.7.1. The Role of TCR Signaling in PTCL/L

Mature T cells are difficult to transform as evidenced by the dearth of experimental models, [47] the rarity of mature T-cell tumor cell lines, [48] and the low incidence of T-cell malignancies as compared to B-cell tumors [5]. However, the two well-established classical transforming oncogenes in mature T-cell tumors (ALK and TCL1) reveal an important element of transformation, namely dysregulated TCR pathway signaling.

ALK, a transmembrane receptor tyrosine kinase which is normally expressed only in the central nervous system, is abnormally expressed in ALCL by fusion to a range of different proteins that alter its subcellular localization. In synergy with CD30, this leads to altered signaling through JAK-STAT, PI3K/AKT/FOXO3a, and RAS/MAPK pathways substituting for the stimulatory effects of TCR engagement (see Chap. 35) [49,50]. Not surprisingly, many ALCLs downregulate many of the components of the TCR/antigen receptor signal complex, including CD3 and TCR itself. In contrast, the TCL1 protein activated in T-PLL functions to boost TCR growth signals by binding to and upregulating the kinase activity of the TCR-associated kinase AKT [51].

The oncogenic function of both the TCL1 and ALK oncogenes highlights the importance of TCR pathway signaling in modulating the transformation process. Further evidence comes from the frequent activation of LCK and other TCR-associated kinases such as ZAP70 in most T-cell tumors [52,53]. Recent evidence suggests that partial interruption of the TCR pathway by kinase inhibitors that target the TCR-proximal tyrosine kinases (e.g., LYN) can block T-cell growth in vitro and have functional activity in vivo.

22.7.2. Alternate Classification Strategies

The influence of new directions in treatment (i.e., immunotherapy and growth kinase targeting) has highlighted the need for different approaches to classification of T-cell tumors that may be more therapeutically useful. As detailed above, the functional immune properties of T-cell tumors result in many harmful paraneoplastic immune phenomena [54]. One approach is to classify tumors by their functional roles in the immune system. This is particularly apparent for the follicle-associated phenotype of AITL, but such functional differentiation is also evident for subsets of PTCL, NOS, CTCL, HSTCL, and EATL. Indeed, even for PTCL/L subtypes that do not have clear functional roles in immune dysregulation, tumor modulation by infiltrating non-neoplastic immune cells may have major important effects on outcome that can be exploited for therapy. An example is the effects of intratumoral FOXP3-positive regulatory T-cells on outcome in ALCL.

In this regard, our initial efforts to classify PTCL/L based on their cytokine or chemokine receptor expression [55,56] likely will be replaced by more sophisticated efforts that capitalize on advances in understanding of functional T-cell subsets (Fig. 22-14 and Chap. 38).

22.8. Prognosis and Patterns of Progression/Transformation

As discussed in Chap. 23, clinical staging systems (e.g., Ann Arbor) and prognostic models (e.g., IPI) developed for B-cell lymphomas perform poorly for PTCL/L because many of these tumors are high-stage at diagnosis or have a nearly uniform aggressive disease course. The time to progression, pattern of spread, and morphologic changes seen are different for most PTCL/L subtypes. Common findings include a shift to a large tumor cell size, and propensity for leukemic dissemination.

A large number of genomic and gene expression profiling studies have now been published for a variety of different PTCL/L types [57–66]. A commonality of these studies is the

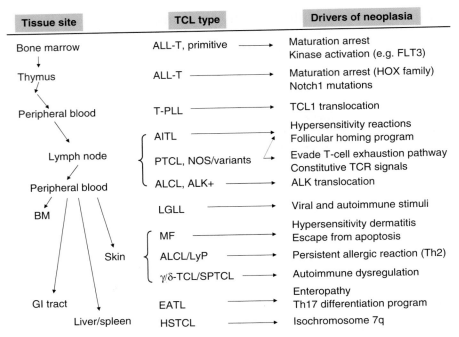

Fig. 22-14. Models of transformation in TCL/L. Mature stages and functional (organ-specific) subsets of T cells are mapped onto the T-cell lymphoma subtypes they most resemble. For additional details, see Chap. 37

large number of different chromosomal gains and losses that occur. Although there is some selectivity for particular tumor types, these studies implicate G1-S cell cycle progression factors (such as loss of cyclin-dependent kinase inhibitors), apoptosis defects, [67,68] and NF-kappa B pathway upregulation [69] in tumor progression.

Another common feature of tumor progression in T-cell neoplasms that deserves special mention is the frequent development of secondary B-cell neoplasms, especially among the "functional" subsets of tumors including AITL, PTCL, NOS, and ALK-negative ALCL. These tumors arise as a result of tumor-associated immune dysregulation and are usually, but not always, driven by EBV infection [12,70].

22.9. NK-Cell Leukemias and Lymphomas

22.9.1. Clinical Features

The NK-cell entities recognized as distinct in the WHO classification are:

- Extranodal NK/T-cell lymphoma, nasal type (ENKTL)
- Aggressive NK-cell leukemia
- Chronic lymphoproliferative disorders of NK cells (provisional)

However, natural killer (NK) cell malignancies are rare (especially in the United States) so experience with, and classification of, these malignancies has received less attention [71]. Most NK-cell lymphomas occur at extranodal sites, with presentations in the nasal mucosa, salivary glands, and oropharynx, most commonly. Skin and lung presentations are also seen. Epstein–Barr virus (EBV) is present in the majority of NK-cell tumors but EBV-negative tumors are being increasingly recognized. Presentation of NK-cell lymphoma in LN is rare [72]. A phenotypically related group of cytotoxic lymphomas show rearrangements of the TCR receptor and have been dubbed "NK-like" leading to the designation of ENKTL [73].

Most ENKTL are less aggressive (stage-for-stage) than PTCL/L, with a median survival 30–60 months, and a 5-year survival rate approaching 40% [4,74].

22.9.2. Morphological Features

Extranodal: ENKTL, at every tissue site, has a sheet-like or infiltrative pattern of growth with zonal necrosis, preferential perivascular growth (angiocentricity), and ulceration of overlying mucosa common. Some cases of ENKTL exhibit bland lymphoid appearance (Fig. 22-15), whereas others present with cellular pleomorphism and high mitotic rate. However, progression to uniformly large blastoid cell morphology occurs over time (Fig. 22-16). In mucosal tumors, invasion of underlying tissues, such as bone, should be noted, as it is associated with adverse prognosis.

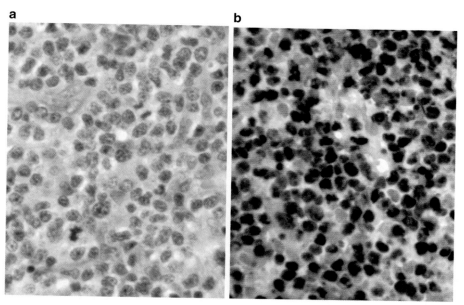

Fig. 22-15. Extranodal NK/T-cell lymphoma, nasal type. (**a**) Tumor cells are small with some pleomorphic forms and increased mitoses. (**b**) In situ hybridization demonstrates uniform staining for EBER

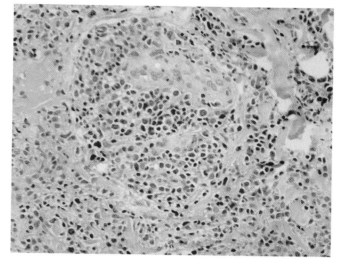

Fig. 22-16. Extranodal NK/T-cell lymphoma, nasal type. Tumor cells have a uniformly blastoid appearance

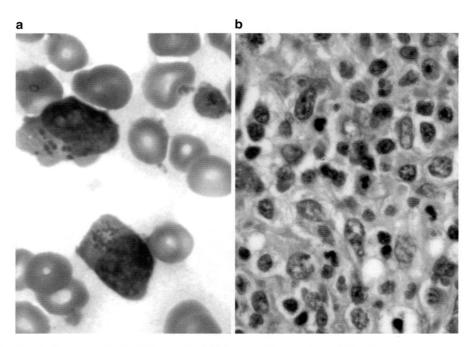

Fig. 22-17. Aggressive NK-cell leukemia. (**a**) Tumor cells in peripheral blood are large with coarse, eosinophilic cytoplasmic granules, and blastoid chromatin. (**b**) Leukemia infiltrating spleen shows a red pulp distribution with effacement of the white pulp

NK-cell lymphoma (BM)   cCD3   EBER

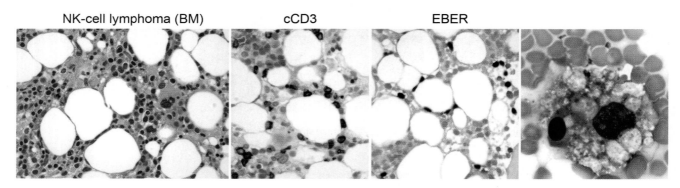

Fig. 22-18. EBV+ NK-cell lymphoma, bone marrow. (**a**) Rare enlarged atypical interstitial lymphocytes in BM biopsy; cytoplasmic (c)CD3 is positive by immunostain, and EBV is detected in tumor cells by in situ hybridization for EBER transcripts. Tumor-associated hemophagocytosis is illustrated in a large histiocyte showing erythrocyte debris in the cytoplasm (BM aspirate, *right panel*) (Images provided by Roberto Miranda)

Lymph node: Infiltration is typically diffuse, with the same range of cytologic features and areas of necrosis as seen in extranodal cases.

Peripheral blood and bone marrow: Two morphologic patterns of NK-cell leukemia have been recognized. In the indolent form, the tumor cells resemble LGL leukemias of the T-cell type. In the more common aggressive form, tumor cells have blastoid nuclear features (Fig. 22-17), can form focal aggregates in the BM, and are often associated with hemophagocytosis (Fig. 22-18).

22.9.3. Laboratory Testing for Diagnosis

The characteristic phenotype for NK cells includes immunopositivity for CD2, cytoplasmic CD3 (epsilon chain), CD16, CD56, and cytotoxic granule proteins (e.g., TIA-1, granzyme B, perforin). NK cells are negative for surface CD3 (as detected by FC antibodies) and for CD5, in most cases [37,75]. Most ENKTL and most NK-cell leukemias are positive for EBV, which can be demonstrated with EBER ISH, or with immunostaining for the EBV-LMP1 protein. CD30 is often expressed in large cells in both leukemia and lymphoma cases. The expression patterns of the polymorphic NKRs can be used in diagnosis of NK-cell malignancies by FC [76] as they have been for T-cell LGLL [31]. However, interpretation of these studies is not always straight forward.

22.9.4. Differential Diagnosis

Given their frequent blastoid appearance, the differential diagnosis of NK-cell malignances includes other high-grade lymphomas, small cell carcinomas, and myeloid sarcomas. However, some cases presenting in the nasal area can be extremely low-grade in appearance, mimicking chronic inflammation, so careful attention to the degree of nuclear atypia and the use of EBV in situ hybridization is recommended for all diffuse mucosal CD2+ CD5- lymphoid proliferations in the head and neck. CD56 (neural cell adhesion molecule, NCAM) expression is not specific for NK cells, as it is seen in a subset of acute leukemias, in the plasmacytoid dendritic cell tumor, plasma cell neoplasms, and a large number of nonhematopoietic tumors particularly those with neuroendocrine differentiation. Therefore, a complete panel of antibodies, as described above, should be used to distinguish NK-cell tumors from PTCL/L and primitive hematopoietic tumors.

22.9.5. Etiology and Pathogenesis

Natural killer (NK) cells function in the innate immune system to recognize altered-self or foreign antigens on the surface of other cells as well as participating in regulatory networks by secretion of cytokines which act on T cells. Antigen recognition by NK cells lacks the fine specificity of the TCR/BCR system and operates through the germline-encoded pattern-recognition toll-like receptors that recognize general classes of foreign antigens, such as bacterial polysaccharides, and double-stranded RNA [77]. The cytotoxic effector functions of NK cells sometimes require priming by dendritic cells [78] and are mediated by NKRs that include the inhibitory and activating killer immunoglobulin-like receptors (KIRs) [79]. The trigger for cytolysis by an NK cell depends on detection of a shift in the pattern of HLA class and other polymorphic ligands for the KIRs versus the growth stimulatory NKRs on an abnormally activated host cell or one presenting foreign antigen.

Given their requirement for DC priming, NK cell proliferation is normally tightly regulated. EBV infection of NK cells at mucosal sites may promote proliferation through EBV-EBNA1, facilitating escape from regulation, and lead to outgrowth of low-grade ENKTL [80]. The necrosis associated with NK-cell tumors may result from abnormal activation of the KIR system. The later stages in the pathogenesis of NK-cell tumors show molecular similarity to transformation in other lymphomas. Differential localization patterns (e.g., nasal versus extranasal) may be related to expression of different adhesion molecules [75]. The drivers for emergence of EBV-negative NK cell tumors are not currently known.

22.9.6. Prognostic Factors and Treatment

Cases of ENKTL presenting outside of the head and neck typically do worse [81]. The clinical predictors used for B-cell lymphomas have shown promise in outcome stratification in ENKTL, including LDH level, B symptoms, performance status, and stage [82–84]. Nuclear medicine scans show promise in highlighting more aggressive cases of ENKTL as gallium positivity has been associated with local tumor invasion [85].

Radiation therapy remains a mainstay of treatment for ENKTL, [74] with chemotherapy [86] and autologous SCT [87] having roles in managing tumor recurrence. Recently, adoptive (T cell) immunotherapy has been successfully used for ENKTCL [88]. In EBV+ cases, serial measurements of EBV viral load by quantitative PCR in the serum or plasma is helpful in detecting relapse [89]. The prognosis in aggressive NK-cell leukemias is typically dire.

22.9.7. Patterns of Progression/Transformation

There is not yet a well-established tumor grading scheme for NK-cell malignancies, although clinical progression is invariably associated with increases in the mitotic rate [31] and average tumor cell size. Several large comparative genomic hybridization studies analyzing NKTCL have shown complex genomic gains and losses suggesting a pattern of acquired genetic instability as seen with other aggressive lymphomas [90]. Cell cycle alterations in advanced stage tumors are also similar to other lymphomas [91].

Suggested Readings

Amin HM, Lai R. Pathobiology of ALK+ anaplastic large-cell lymphoma. Blood 2007;110:2259–67.
- A comprehensive overview of ALK signaling.

de Leval L, Bisig B, Thielen C, Boniver J, Gaulard P. Molecular classification of T-cell lymphomas. Crit Rev Oncol Hematol Feb 2009.
- An overview of the advances in molecular dissection of T-cell malignancies in the last 5 years.

References

1. Baleydier F, Decouvelaere AV, Bergeron J, et al. T cell receptor genotyping and HOXA/TLX1 expression define three T lymphoblastic lymphoma subsets which might affect clinical outcome. Clin Cancer Res 2008;14:692–700.
2. Weng AP, Ferrando AA, Lee W, et al. Activating mutations of NOTCH1 in human T cell acute lymphoblastic leukemia. Science 2004;306:269–71.
3. Leich E, Haralambieva E, Zettl A, et al. Tissue microarray-based screening for chromosomal breakpoints affecting the T-cell receptor gene loci in mature T-cell lymphomas. J Pathol 2007; 213:99–105.
4. Armitage J, Vose J, Weisenburger D. International peripheral T-cell and natural killer/T-cell lymphoma study: pathology findings and clinical outcomes. J Clin Oncol 2008;26:4124–30.
5. Abouyabis AN, Shenoy PJ, Lechowicz MJ, Flowers CR. Incidence and outcomes of the peripheral T-cell lymphoma subtypes in the United States. Leuk Lymphoma 2008;49:2099–107.
6. Stewart BW, Kleihues P Global burden of cancer. World Cancer Report. Lyon, France: IARC Press, 2003:12–9.
7. Jones D, Weissmann DJ, Kraus MD, Hasserjian RP, Shahsafaei A, Dorfman DM. Recurrences in nodal T-cell lymphoma. Changes in histologic appearance and immunophenotype over the course of disease. Am J Clin Pathol 2000;114:438–47.
8. Jones D, Jorgensen JL, Shahsafaei A, Dorfman DM. Characteristic proliferations of reticular and dendritic cells in angioimmunoblastic lymphoma. Am J Surg Pathol 1998;22:956–64.
9. Grogg KL, Attygalle AD, Macon WR, Remstein ED, Kurtin PJ, Dogan A. Expression of CXCL13, a chemokine highly upregulated in germinal center T-helper cells, distinguishes angioimmunoblastic T-cell lymphoma from peripheral T-cell lymphoma, unspecified. Mod Pathol 2006;19:1101–7.
10. Dorfman DM, Brown JA, Shahsafaei A, Freeman GJ. Programmed death-1 (PD-1) is a marker of germinal center-associated T cells and angioimmunoblastic T-cell lymphoma. Am J Surg Pathol 2006;30:802–10.
11. Ottaviani G, Bueso-Ramos CE, Seilstad K, Medeiros LJ, Manning JT, Jones D. The role of the perifollicular sinus in determining the complex immunoarchitecture of angioimmunoblastic T-cell lymphoma. Am J Surg Pathol 2004;28:1632–40.
12. Attygalle AD, Kyriakou C, Dupuis J, et al. Histologic evolution of angioimmunoblastic T-cell lymphoma in consecutive biopsies: clinical correlation and insights into natural history and disease progression. Am J Surg Pathol 2007;31:1077–88.
13. Balague O, Martinez A, Colomo L, et al. Epstein-Barr virus negative clonal plasma cell proliferations and lymphomas in peripheral T-cell lymphomas: a phenomenon with distinctive clinicopathologic features. Am J Surg Pathol 2007;31:1310–22.

14. Rudiger T, Ichinohasama R, Ott MM, et al. Peripheral T-cell lymphoma with distinct perifollicular growth pattern: a distinct subtype of T-cell lymphoma? Am J Surg Pathol 2000;24:117–22.

15. Rudiger T, Geissinger E, Muller-Hermelink HK. 'Normal counterparts' of nodal peripheral T-cell lymphoma. Hematol Oncol 2006;24:175–80.

16. Jiang L, Jones D, Medeiros LJ, Orduz YR, Bueso-Ramos CE. Peripheral T-cell lymphoma with a "follicular" pattern and the perifollicular sinus phenotype. Am J Clin Pathol 2005;123:448–55.

17. Medeiros LJ, Elenitoba-Johnson KS. Anaplastic large cell lymphoma. Am J Clin Pathol 2007;127:707–22.

18. D'Amore E, Menin A, Bonoldi E, et al. Anaplastic large cell lymphomas: a study of 75 pediatric patients. Pediatr Dev Pathol 2007;10(3):181–91.

19. Falini B, Pileri S, Zinzani PL, et al. ALK+ lymphoma: clinico-pathological findings and outcome. Blood 1999;93:2697–706.

20. Kinney MC, Collins RD, Greer JP, Whitlock JA, Sioutos N, Kadin ME. A small-cell-predominant variant of primary Ki-1 (CD30)+ T-cell lymphoma. Am J Surg Pathol 1993;17:859–68.

21. ten Berge RL, Oudejans JJ, Ossenkoppele GJ, Meijer CJ. ALK-negative systemic anaplastic large cell lymphoma: differential diagnostic and prognostic aspects – a review. J Pathol 2003;200:4–15.

22. Zettl A, Ott G, Makulik A, et al. Chromosomal gains at 9q characterize enteropathy-type T-cell lymphoma. Am J Pathol 2002;161:1635–45.

23. Dogan A, Morice WG. Bone marrow histopathology in peripheral T-cell lymphomas. Br J Haematol 2004;127:140–54.

24. Massimino M, Gasparini M, Giardini R. Ki-1 (CD30) anaplastic large-cell lymphoma in children. Ann Oncol 1995;6:915–20.

25. Vega F, Medeiros LJ, Bueso-Ramos C, et al. Hepatosplenic gamma/delta T-cell lymphoma in bone marrow. A sinusoidal neoplasm with blastic cytologic features. Am J Clin Pathol 2001;116:410–9.

26. Grewal JS, Smith LB, Winegarden JD 3rd, Krauss JC, Tworek JA, Schnitzer B. Highly aggressive ALK-positive anaplastic large cell lymphoma with a leukemic phase and multi-organ involvement: a report of three cases and a review of the literature. Ann Hematol 2007;86:499–508.

27. Osuji N, Beiske K, Randen U, et al. Characteristic appearances of the bone marrow in T-cell large granular lymphocyte leukaemia. Histopathology 2007;50:547–54.

28. Huh YO, Medeiros LJ, Ravandi F, Konoplev S, Jorgensen JL, Miranda RN. T-cell large granular lymphocyte leukemia associated with myelodysplastic syndrome: a clinicopathologic study of nine cases. Am J Clin Pathol 2009;131:347–56.

29. Wlodarski MW, Nearman Z, Jankowska A, et al. Phenotypic differences between healthy effector CTL and leukemic LGL cells support the notion of antigen-triggered clonal transformation in T-LGL leukemia. J Leukoc Biol 2008;83:589–601.

30. Lima M, Almeida J, Santos AH, et al. Immunophenotypic analysis of the TCR-Vbeta repertoire in 98 persistent expansions of CD3(+)/TCR-alphabeta(+) large granular lymphocytes: utility in assessing clonality and insights into the pathogenesis of the disease. Am J Pathol 2001;159:1861–8.

31. Morice WG, Kurtin PJ, Leibson PJ, Tefferi A, Hanson CA. Demonstration of aberrant T-cell and natural killer-cell antigen expression in all cases of granular lymphocytic leukaemia. Br J Haematol 2003;120:1026–36.

32. Airo P, Rossi G, Facchetti F, et al. Monoclonal expansion of large granular lymphocytes with a CD4+ CD8dim+/- phenotype associated with hairy cell leukemia. Haematologica 1995;80:146–9.

33. Herling M, Khoury JD, Washington LT, Duvic M, Keating MJ, Jones D. A systematic approach to diagnosis of mature T-cell leukemias reveals heterogeneity among WHO categories. Blood 2004;104:328–35.

34. Klemke CD, Fritzsching B, Franz B, et al. Paucity of FOXP3+ cells in skin and peripheral blood distinguishes Sezary syndrome from other cutaneous T-cell lymphomas. Leukemia 2006;20:1123–9.

35. Matutes E, Keeling DM, Newland AC, et al. Sezary cell-like leukemia: a distinct type of mature T cell malignancy. Leukemia 1990;4:262–6.

36. Mao X, McElwaine S. Functional copy number changes in Sezary syndrome: toward an integrated molecular cytogenetic map III. Cancer Genet Cytogenet 2008;185:86–94.

37. Karube K, Aoki R, Nomura Y, et al. Usefulness of flow cytometry for differential diagnosis of precursor and peripheral T-cell and NK-cell lymphomas: analysis of 490 cases. Pathol Int 2008;58:89–97.

38. Shimoyama M. Diagnostic criteria and classification of clinical subtypes of adult T-cell leukaemia-lymphoma. A report from the Lymphoma Study Group (1984-87). Br J Haematol 1991;79:428–37.

39. Matutes E. Adult T-cell leukaemia/lymphoma. J Clin Pathol 2007;60:1373–7.

40. Tan BT, Seo K, Warnke RA, Arber DA. The frequency of immunoglobulin heavy chain gene and T-cell receptor gamma-chain gene rearrangements and Epstein-Barr virus in ALK+ and ALK- anaplastic large cell lymphoma and other peripheral T-cell lymphomas. J Mol Diagn 2008;10:502–12.

41. Schutzinger C, Esterbauer H, Hron G, et al. Prognostic value of T-cell receptor gamma rearrangement in peripheral blood or bone marrow of patients with peripheral T-cell lymphomas. Leuk Lymphoma 2008;49:237–46.

42. Feldman AL, Law M, Remstein ED, et al. Recurrent translocations involving the IRF4 oncogene locus in peripheral T-cell lymphomas. Leukemia 2009;23(3):574–80.

43. Macon WR, Levy NB, Kurtin PJ, et al. Hepatosplenic alphabeta T-cell lymphomas: a report of 14 cases and comparison with hepatosplenic gammadelta T-cell lymphomas. Am J Surg Pathol 2001;25:285–96.

44. Bourgault-Rouxel AS, Loughran TP Jr, Zambello R, et al. Clinical spectrum of gammadelta+ T cell LGL leukemia: analysis of 20 cases. Leuk Res 2008;32:45–8.

45. Takaku T, Miyazawa K, Sashida G, et al. Hepatosplenic alphabeta T-cell lymphoma with myelodysplastic syndrome. Int J Hematol 2005;82:143–7.

46. Gaulier A, Jary-Bourguignat L, Serna R, Pulik M, Davi F, Raphael M. Occurrence of angioimmunoblastic T cell lymphoma in a patient with chronic myelomonocytic leukemia features. Leuk Lymphoma 2000;40:197–204.

47. Newrzela S, Cornils K, Li Z, et al. Resistance of mature T cells to oncogene transformation. Blood 2008;112:2278–86.

48. MacLeod RA, Nagel S, Scherr M, et al. Human leukemia and lymphoma cell lines as models and resources. Curr Med Chem 2008;15:339–59.

49. Amin HM, Lai R. Pathobiology of ALK+ anaplastic large-cell lymphoma. Blood 2007;110:2259–67.

50. Turner SD, Yeung D, Hadfield K, Cook SJ, Alexander DR. The NPM-ALK tyrosine kinase mimics TCR signalling pathways, inducing NFAT and AP-1 by RAS-dependent mechanisms. Cell Signal 2007;19:740–7.

51. Herling M, Patel KA, Teitell MA, et al. High TCL1 expression and intact T-cell receptor signaling define a hyperproliferative subset of T-cell prolymphocytic leukemia. Blood 2008;111:328–37.

52. Feldman AL, Sun DX, Law ME, et al. Overexpression of Syk tyrosine kinase in peripheral T-cell lymphomas. Leukemia 2008;22:1139–43.

53. Admirand J, Rassidakis G, Medeiros LJ, Jones D. CD3-independent activation of downstream effectors ZAP-70 and Syk in T-cell lymphomas. Lab Invest 2004;84:237A.

54. Zhang T, Barber A, Sentman CL. Chimeric NKG2D modified T cells inhibit systemic T-cell lymphoma growth in a manner involving multiple cytokines and cytotoxic pathways. Cancer Res 2007;67:11029–36.

55. Jones D, Fletcher CD, Pulford K, Shahsafaei A, Dorfman DM. The T-cell activation markers CD30 and OX40/CD134 are expressed in nonoverlapping subsets of peripheral T-cell lymphoma. Blood 1999;93:3487–93.

56. Jones D, Dorfman DM. Phenotypic characterization of subsets of T cell lymphoma: towards a functional classification of T cell lymphoma. Leuk Lymphoma 2001;40:449–59.

57. Ballester B, Ramuz O, Gisselbrecht C, et al. Gene expression profiling identifies molecular subgroups among nodal peripheral T-cell lymphomas. Oncogene 2006;25:1560–70.

58. Martinez-Delgado B. Peripheral T-cell lymphoma gene expression profiles. Hematol Oncol 2006;24:113–9.

59. de Leval L, Rickman DS, Thielen C, et al. The gene expression profile of nodal peripheral T-cell lymphoma demonstrates a molecular link between angioimmunoblastic T-cell lymphoma (AITL) and follicular helper T (TFH) cells. Blood 2007;109:4952–63.

60. Pitini V, Arrigo C, Altavilla G. Gene expression profiling does not identify molecular subgroup among nodal peripheral T-cell lymphomas. J Clin Oncol 2007;25:4851. author reply 4851–2.

61. Piccaluga PP, Agostinelli C, Califano A, et al. Gene expression analysis of angioimmunoblastic lymphoma indicates derivation from T follicular helper cells and vascular endothelial growth factor deregulation. Cancer Res 2007;67:10703–10.

62. Booken N, Gratchev A, Utikal J, et al. Sezary syndrome is a unique cutaneous T-cell lymphoma as identified by an expanded gene signature including diagnostic marker molecules CDO1 and DNM3. Leukemia 2008;22:393–9.

63. Shah MV, Zhang R, Irby R, et al. Molecular profiling of LGL leukemia reveals role of sphingolipid signaling in survival of cytotoxic lymphocytes. Blood 2008;112:770–81.

64. Cuadros M, Dave SS, Jaffe ES, et al. Identification of a proliferation signature related to survival in nodal peripheral T-cell lymphomas. J Clin Oncol 2007;25:3321–9.

65. Agostinelli C, Piccaluga PP, Went P, et al. Peripheral T cell lymphoma, not otherwise specified: the stuff of genes, dreams and therapies. J Clin Pathol 2008;61:1160–7.

66. Miyazaki K, Yamaguchi M, Imai H, et al. Gene expression profiling of peripheral T-cell lymphoma including gammadelta T-cell lymphoma. Blood 2009;113:1071–4.

67. Martinez-Delgado B, Melendez B, Cuadros M, et al. Expression profiling of T-cell lymphomas differentiates peripheral and lymphoblastic lymphomas and defines survival related genes. Clin Cancer Res 2004;10:4971–82.

68. Rassidakis GZ, Jones D, Thomaides A, et al. Apoptotic rate in peripheral T-cell lymphomas. A study using a tissue microarray with validation on full tissue sections. Am J Clin Pathol 2002;118:328–34.

69. Martinez-Delgado B, Cuadros M, Honrado E, et al. Differential expression of NF-kappaB pathway genes among peripheral T-cell lymphomas. Leukemia 2005;19:2254–63.

70. Higgins JP, van de Rijn M, Jones CD, Zehnder JL, Warnke RA. Peripheral T-cell lymphoma complicated by a proliferation of large B cells. Am J Clin Pathol 2000;114:236–47.

71. Huang Q, Chang KL, Gaal KK, Weiss LM. An aggressive extranodal NK-cell lymphoma arising from indolent NK-cell lymphoproliferative disorder. Am J Surg Pathol 2005;29:1540–3.

72. Ng WK, Lee CY, Li AS, Cheung LK. Nodal presentation of nasal-type NK/T-cell lymphoma. Report of two cases with fine needle aspiration cytology findings. Acta Cytol 2003;47:1063–8.

73. Tao J, Shelat SG, Jaffe ES, Bagg A. Aggressive Epstein-Barr virus-associated, CD8+, CD30+, CD56+, surface CD3-, natural killer (NK)-like cytotoxic T-cell lymphoma. Am J Surg Pathol 2002;26:111–8.

74. Wu X, Li P, Zhao J, et al. A clinical study of 115 patients with extranodal natural killer/T-cell lymphoma, nasal type. Clin Oncol (R Coll Radiol) 2008;20:619–25.

75. Schwartz EJ, Molina-Kirsch H, Zhao S, Marinelli RJ, Warnke RA, Natkunam Y. Immunohistochemical characterization of nasal-type extranodal NK/T-cell lymphoma using a tissue microarray: an analysis of 84 cases. Am J Clin Pathol 2008;130:343–51.

76. Sawada A, Sato E, Koyama M, et al. NK-cell repertoire is feasible for diagnosing Epstein-Barr virus-infected NK-cell lymphoproliferative disease and evaluating the treatment effect. Am J Hematol 2006;81:576–81.

77. Lehner T. Special regulatory T cell review: the resurgence of the concept of contrasuppression in immunoregulation. Immunology 2008;123:40–4.

78. Granucci F, Zanoni I, Ricciardi-Castagnoli P. Central role of dendritic cells in the regulation and deregulation of immune responses. Cell Mol Life Sci 2008;65:1683–97.

79. Boyton RJ, Altmann DM. Natural killer cells, killer immunoglobulin-like receptors and human leucocyte antigen class I in disease. Clin Exp Immunol 2007;149:1–8.

80. Ian MX, Lan SZ, Cheng ZF, Dan H, Qiong LH. Suppression of EBNA1 expression inhibits growth of EBV-positive NK/T cell lymphoma cells. Cancer Biol Ther 2008;7:1602–6.

81. Kim TM, Lee SY, Jeon YK, et al. Clinical heterogeneity of extranodal NK/T-cell lymphoma, nasal type: a national survey of the Korean Cancer Study Group. Ann Oncol 2008;19:1477–84.

82. Li YX, Fang H, Liu QF, et al. Clinical features and treatment outcome of nasal-type NK/T-cell lymphoma of Waldeyer ring. Blood 2008;112:3057–64.

83. Au WY, Weisenburger DD, Intragumtornchai T, et al. Clinical differences between nasal and extranasal NK/T-cell lymphoma: a study of 136 cases from the International Peripheral T-cell Lymphoma Project. Blood 2009;113(17):3931–7.

84. Na II, Kang HJ, Park YH, et al. Prognostic factors for classifying extranodal NK/T cell lymphoma, nasal type, as lymphoid neoplasia. Eur J Haematol 2007;79:1–7.

85. Suh C, Kang YK, Roh JL, et al. Prognostic value of tumor 18F-FDG uptake in patients with untreated extranodal natural killer/T-cell lymphomas of the head and neck. J Nucl Med 2008;49:1783–9.

86. Yong W, Zheng W, Zhu J, et al. L-Asparaginase in the treatment of refractory and relapsed extranodal NK/T-cell lymphoma, nasal type. Ann Hematol 2009;88(7):647–52.

87. Lee J, Au WY, Park MJ, et al. Autologous hematopoietic stem cell transplantation in extranodal natural killer/T cell lymphoma: a multinational, multicenter, matched controlled study. Biol Blood Marrow Transplant 2008;14:1356–64.

88. Merlo A, Turrini R, Dolcetti R, Zanovello P, Amadori A, Rosato A. Adoptive cell therapy against EBV-related malignancies: a survey of clinical results. Expert Opin Biol Ther 2008;8:1265–94.

89. Suwiwat S, Pradutkanchana J, Ishida T, Mitarnun W. Quantitative analysis of cell-free Epstein-Barr virus DNA in the plasma of patients with peripheral T-cell and NK-cell lymphomas and peripheral T-cell proliferative diseases. J Clin Virol 2007;40:277–83.

90. Nakashima Y, Tagawa H, Suzuki R, et al. Genome-wide array-based comparative genomic hybridization of natural killer cell lymphoma/leukemia: different genomic alteration patterns of aggressive NK-cell leukemia and extranodal Nk/T-cell lymphoma, nasal type. Genes Chromosomes Cancer 2005;44:247–55.

91. Kawamata N, Inagaki N, Mizumura S, et al. Methylation status analysis of cell cycle regulatory genes (p16INK4A, p15INK4B, p21Waf1/Cip1, p27Kip1 and p73) in natural killer cell disorders. Eur J Haematol 2005;74:424–9.

Chapter 23

Clinical Management of Non-cutaneous T-cell and NK-cell Malignancies

Marco Herling

Abstract/Scope of Chapter The uncommon but heterogeneous group of peripheral T-cell lymphomas and leukemias are now recognized to be derived from various functional subsets of post-thymic (mature) T cells. Conventional multi-agent chemotherapeutic regimens, developed primarily for B-cell tumors, generally work poorly for T-cell tumors. In this chapter, we outline the current clinical approaches to staging, outcome prediction, and therapy in T-cell and NK-cell malignancies presenting in the lymph node, peripheral blood, bone marrow and at extranodal sites with the exception of cutaneous T-cell lymphomas and Sézary syndrome which are covered in Chap. 25. We describe frontline and salvage therapies, introduce prognostic models, and evaluate the role of autologous and allogeneic stem cell transplantation. Finally, an overview of novel T-cell selective therapeutic agents is presented.

Keywords T-cell lymphoma, treatment • T-cell malignancies, staging • T-cell malignancies, prognosis • Peripheral T-cell lymphoma, treatment • T-cell leukemia, treatment • Anaplastic large cell lymphoma, treatment • Angioimmunoblastic T-cell lymphoma, treatment • Nasal NK-/T-cell lymphoma, treatment • Enteropathy-type T-cell lymphoma, treatment • Hepatosplenic T-cell lymphoma, treatment • T-cell prolymphocytic leukemia, treatment • Adult T-cell leukemia/lymphoma, treatment • T-cell large granular lymphocytic leukemia, treatment • Lymphoblastic leukemia/lymphoma, treatment

23.1. Introduction

As outlined in Chaps. 1 and 22, classification strategies for T-cell and natural killer (NK)-cell malignancies are in the process of evolution with a trend away from clinically-defined disease entities (e.g. intestinal T-cell lymphoma) toward more target-based and genetic approaches. However, this new approach is still incomplete and thus the terminology and diagnostic criteria used here will be those of the 2008 WHO classification. To emphasize their shared features, we will utilize the abbreviation TCL/L to refer generically to mature (post-thymic/peripheral) T-cell malignancies presenting as either lymphoma or leukemia and distinguish subtypes as relevant. Strategies for the treatment of cutaneous T-cell lymphomas (CTCL) are presented separately in Chap. 25.

Most therapies currently used for TCL/L were adapted from those applied for B-cell lymphomas, but many of these agents are not particularly well-suited to the unique biology of T cells. This may be one reason why the outcome of TCL/L is, with few exceptions, worse than even that of the most aggressive B-cell lymphomas at a similar clinical stage. In addition

From: *Neoplastic Hematopathology*: Contemporary Hematology,
Edited by: D. Jones, DOI 10.1007/978-1-60761-384-8_23,
© Humana Press, a part of Springer Science+Business Media, LLC 2010

to an apparent intrinsic resistance of TCL/L to conventional cytotoxic chemotherapy, at least the ones traditionally used, they are more likely than B-cell tumors to present with high-risk clinical features, such as advanced stage, extranodal involvement, and in patients with poor performance status (PS). Finally, TCL/L are rare, representing only 5–10% of lymphoid malignancies in the United States and Europe, making clinical trials in a controlled/randomized fashion difficult to conduct. Consequently, most prospective trials still enroll various TCL/L entities despite their demonstrable heterogeneity. For these reasons, most efforts in TCL/L focus on evaluating responses to newer, more T-cell specific drugs and toward implementing innovative trial designs.

Here, we summarize the challenging clinical management of TCL/L. We describe the most common current approaches to TCL/L risk assessment and therapy, with the recognition that there is no consensus on the optimal treatment for most subtypes, in contrast to the situation in B-cell malignancies. The role and timing of high-dose therapy (HDT) followed by stem cell transplantation (SCT) as frontline treatment and salvage therapy are discussed as well. We also introduce a new generation of T-cell active compounds and discuss when such targeted agents may be appropriate.

23.2. Clinical Presentations of TCL/L and NK-cell Tumors

Most TCL/L and NK-cell tumors involve multiple organ sites at the time of diagnosis due to the preserved migratory properties of the particular subset of transformed lymphocytes. The most common presenting sign is systemic lymph node enlargement. Skin rash, hepatosplenomegaly, gastrointestinal (GI) tract infiltration, involvement of the nasal sinuses, or a leukemic presentation are less frequent, but represent the principal clinical manifestation of certain tumor subsets. Cytopenias due to bone marrow (BM) infiltration are less common than in B-cell tumors and, if present, are very often a result of hemophagocytic syndrome (HPS) or other aggressive auto-immune mechanisms. Signs of central nervous system (CNS) or lung involvement are rare.

23.2.1. Lymph Node Presentations

The most common TCL/L subtypes presenting primarily in lymph node are angioimmunoblastic T-cell lymphoma (AITL), anaplastic large cell lymphoma (ALCL), and the remainder category of peripheral T-cell lymphoma-not otherwise specified (PTCL-NOS), with incidences of ~22%, ~10% and ~34%, respectively, in the Western countries (Table 23-1) [1]. AITL, slightly more often encountered in Europe than in the United States, is the most homogeneous category with a characteristic clinical presentation in elderly patients, with findings such as hypergammaglobulinemia, Coombs-positive hemolytic anemia, cytokine syndromes, and severe immunodeficiency [2]. AITL frequently shows involvement of the skin (rash), GI tract (diarrhea), and BM, with widespread but typically small lymphadenopathy. Its course is typically aggressive with deaths due to infections, end-organ dysfunction, or secondary development of EBV+ B-cell lymphomas [2].

Anaplastic large cell lymphoma (ALCL) has two variants including one with aberrant expression of the anaplastic lymphoma kinase (ALK) by chromosomal translocation and a poorly-characterized variant seen mostly in older adults that does not express ALK [3]. The overall survival (OS) rates of ALK-negative ALCL are superior to those in PTCL-NOS (Fig. 23-1). ALK+ ALCL typically presents in children and young adults, also involves extranodal sites (commonly bone, bowel and skin), is chemosensitive, and has a good prognosis. Leukemic presentations of ALK+ ALCL are more aggressive and have a poor outcome.

PTCL-NOS is the most common TCL/L and is an aggressive systemic disease typically presenting at advanced stage with frequent extranodal manifestations in middle-aged to eld-

Table 23-1. Primarily nodal and extranodal (non-CTCL) T-cell tumors and their key features (also see Chap. 22).

Category	Characteristics
Peripheral T-cell lymphoma-not otherwise specified [1,4,6–8]	*Epidemiology*: 25.9% of all TCL/L (34% in Western countries); median age 60 years, slight male predilection (66%)
	Presentation: systemic nodal (75% AA stage III/IV), 63% extranodal (27% BM, 14% skin, 19% liver), B-symptoms in 47%
	Treatment: CHOP-resistance, advanced stage, and PS ≥2 in 32% with limited frontline treatment success; currently no good stratification criteria to select those for HDT-SCT
	Outcome: 5-year OS rate ≈32%; better stratification by new prognostic IPI-based models but may need to include tumor features to achieve a successful risk-adapted treatment approach
Angioimmunoblastic T-cell lymphoma [1,2]	*Epidemiology*: North America/Asia 17% vs. Europe 29% of TCL/L; median age 65 years, equal male/female ratio
	Presentation: generalized adenopathy (89% AA stage III/IV), hepatosplenomegaly, skin rash, BM (29%), dysproteinemia
	Treatment: anthracyclines ineffective; new strategies include cyclosporine, thalidomide, interferon, anti-VEGF, anti-CD20, and anti-CD52 immunotherapy
	Outcome: 5-year OS rate ≈32%; opportunistic infections are the leading cause of death which limit use of immunosuppressive therapies
Anaplastic large cell lymphoma, ALK+ [1,3]	*Epidemiology*: 6.6% of TCL/L worldwide (16% in North America), uncommon in Asia; median age 34 years, male/female 1.7
	Presentation: 65% advanced stage, 60% B-symptoms, 10–14% BM, bone, subcutaneous involvement, 21% bulky disease
	Treatment: good sensitivity (88%) to CHOP regimens, age and extranodal sites >1 are the best predictors; good responses to salvage chemotherapy
	Outcome: 5-year OS rate ≈70%, 29% IPI score 3–5, IPI provides the best stratification, significant drop in 5-year OS (37%) in stage IV (36% of pts)
Anaplastic large cell lymphoma, ALK-negative [1,3]	*Epidemiology*: 5.5% of TCL/L worldwide (9.4% in Europe), uncommon in Asia; median age 58 years, male/female 1.5
	Presentation: 58% advanced stage, 57% B-symptoms, 39% IPI score 3–5 (high than in ALK+ cases mostly due to higher LDH and older age)
	Treatment: 76% respond to CHOP regimens; salvage still effective; role for HDT-SCT in frontline or salvage not established
	Outcome: 5-year OS rate ≈49%; IPI provides best stratification with the OS difference between ALK+ vs. ALK-negative cases being primarily age-related
Enteropathy-associated T-cell lymphoma [9]	*Epidemiology*: North America 5.8% vs. Europe 9.1% of TCL/L; median age 61 years, 2.1–6.6 rR after past/recent sprue
	Presentation: positive history (>90%) of abdominal pain, vomiting, diarrhea, malabsorption with anemia; other sites of involvement except regional LNs are rare
	Treatment: surgical resection; poor chemo-sensitivity; SCT sporadically successful; earlier detection through PET
	Outcome: 5-year OS rate ≈20%; aggressive treatment limited by poor PS and acute intestinal obstruction (23%) or perforation (37%)
Hepatosplenic T-cell lymphoma [10]	*Epidemiology*: 1.4% of all TCL/L; median age 34 years, 68% males, overrepresented in immunocompromised hosts including following SCT
	Presentation: splenomegaly (100%), hepatomegaly (80%), cytopenia (85%), BM almost always involved with low-level PB involvement, HPS, B-symptoms
	Treatment: not yet established; poor sensitivity to CHOP-type regimens, initial splenectomy/irradiation may slow disease progression
	Outcome: 5-year OS rate ≈7%; transient responses to purine analogues and alemtuzumab; role of HDT-SCT in first remission?

erly patients [1]. Molecular studies clearly distinguish PTCL-NOS from ALCL and AITL [3–5]. Although heterogeneous at the molecular level, PTCL-NOS is currently not subclassified, but markers like the proliferative index, EBV-status, and/or NF-kB pathway profiling are likely to improve on the clinically-based prognostic models [6–8].

23.2.2. Extranodal Presentations

The varieties of different CTCL are discussed in Chaps. 24 and 25. These also include the relatively indolent subcutaneous panniculitis-like T-cell lymphoma expressing the αβ T-cell

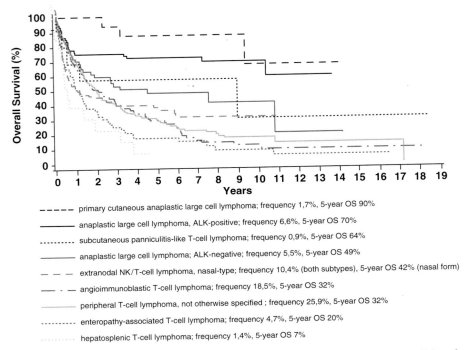

Fig. 23-1. *Overall survival (OS) in primarily nodal and extra-nodal peripheral T-cell lymphoma.* Outcomes for 1,300 peripheral T-cell lymphomas collected by the multi-center International T-cell Lymphoma Project (22 institutions across the world) is significantly different across specific subtypes. The frequencies of each subtype represent the average distribution across all continents. However, incidence varies with geographical region, with angioimmunoblastic T-cell lymphoma and enteropathy-associated T-cell lymphoma more frequently seen in the European centers, extranodal NK/T-cell lymphoma, nasal-type (NK/TCL) being more common in Asia, and ALK+ anaplastic large cell lymphoma diagnosed more often in North America. The 5-year OS of NK/TCL is different between the "nasal" and "extra-nasal"(not charted here) variants (42% vs. 9%). Modified and reprinted from Savage KJ. Hematology 2008;280–8, original data from J Clin Oncol. 2008;26:4124–4130; with permission, © the American Society of Hematology

receptor and the distinctive and highly aggressive cutaneous γδ T-cell lymphoma. Other primarily extranodal TCL/L include enteropathy-associated (intestinal) T-cell lymphoma (EATL), which often manifests as intestinal obstruction or perforation of the jejunum due to transmural tumor infiltration requiring surgical intervention. The majority of cases have a preceding or coincident history of malabsorption and related disorders, including classical (refractory) celiac disease with or without dermatitis herpetiformis [9]. Intestinal T-cell lymphomas without enteropathy also occur. Given the dismal results of conventional chemotherapy, ongoing efforts try to more aggressively intervene at the stage of celiac disease. HSTCL, often associated with iatrogenic immunosuppression, presents in spleen, liver, BM, and peripheral blood (PB) of young males without adenopathy and is usually rapidly fatal [10].

23.2.3. Leukemic Presentations

The most common leukemic T-cell malignancies are summarized in Table 23-2. The immature precursor T-lymphoblastic leukemia/lymphoma (T-ALL/LBL) is discussed in Chaps. 13 and 27. T-cell prolymphocytic leukemia (T-PLL), predominantly associated with chromosomal translocations involving the T-cell leukemia 1 (TCL1) oncogene, has the most aggressive course with high presenting white blood cell counts (WBC), rapid lymphocyte doubling times, and frequent effusions and skin involvement (rashes and purpura) [11,12]. Adult T-cell leukemia/lymphoma, (ATLL) is highly geographically-restricted and is driven by the human

Table 23-2. Leukemic T-cell malignancies and their key features (for diagnostic approach see Chap. 22).

Category	Characteristics
Precursor T-cell lymphoblastic leukemia/lymphoma [40]	*Epidemiology*: 20% of ALL, 80% of LBL; ALL vs. LBL determined by arbitrary cutoff of >25% BM involvement; median age 28 years *Presentation*: typically high WBC, bulky adenopathy, mediastinal mass, effusions, CNS involvement; male predominance *Treatment*: highly intensive chemotherapy, CNS-prophylaxis (irradiation, liquor instillation), outcome following allo-SCT may be determined by HOX expression profiles *Outcome*: 5-year OS rate ≈65%; poor survival after first relapse; better prognosis for cases with certain cortical thymocyte phenotypes
T-cell prolymphocytic leukemia [11,12,26]	*Epidemiology*: most common mature T-cell leukemia, 2% of all "CLL" cases; median age 63 years; increased in children with ataxia-telangiectasia *Presentation*: often discovered as an incidental finding, rapidly rising WBC, splenomegaly, generalized adenopathy, effusions, skin lesions *Treatment*: purine analogues ineffective, alemtuzumab most effective agent (RR ≈80%), particularly in front-line regimens *Outcome*: median OS 27 months; 5-year OS 21%, cures observed after allo-SCT (consider as option in first complete response)
Adult T-cell leukemia/lymphoma [13,26]	*Epidemiology*: 100% HTLV-1+, arises in 2-4% of carriers after a viral latency of ≈10–30 years, endemic distribution; median age 58 years *Presentation*: acute leukemic (60%) and lymphoma (18%) subtypes show organomegaly and hypercalcemia that are not seen in chronic form (18%) or smoldering form (4%) *Treatment*: low efficacy of conventional agents; best if combined with zidovudine and/or IFNα; allo-SCT for young patients *Outcome*: chronic/smoldering variants progress into acute form, overall 5-year OS in the ITLP series was 14%, median OS 12 months
T-cell/NK-cell large granular lymphocytic leukemia [11,26]	*Epidemiology*: wide age range, median 55–60 years, association with autoimmune disorders, i.e. RA, AIHA, AA *Presentation*: ≈30% asymptomatic, majority with bacterial infections, neutropenia (85%), anemia (50%), splenomegaly (50%) *Treatment*: objective is improving cytopenias, using low-dose methotrexate, cyclosporine A, cyclophosphamide, alemtuzumab *Outcome*: median OS ≈10 years; more aggressive chemoresistant NK-cell variant without associated autoimmune conditions
Aggressive NK-cell leukemia [16]	*Epidemiology*: 71% of cases in Asians, 25% of cases in Caucasians; median age ≈40 years; no sex predilection *Presentation*: fever with septic complications (100%), anemia (100%), liver dysfunction (80%); skin lesions are uncommon *Treatment*: severely reduced performance status impedes therapy, among the few responders (incl. after SCT) essentially all relapse *Outcome*: near-uniform mortality, OS of days-weeks (median <2 months), less aggressive course for the rare EBV-negative cases

Common abbreviations used in Tables 23-1 and 23-2:
TCL/L mature T-cell lymphoma/leukemia (non-cutaneous as per this Chapter), *AA* Ann Arbor, *BM* bone marrow, *CHOP* cyclophosphamide, doxorubicin, vincristine, prednisone, *PS* performance status, *HDT-SCT* high-dose therapy with stem cell transplantation, *OS* overall survival, *IPI* International Prognostic Index, *EBV* Epstein-Barr virus, *VEGF* vascular endothelial growth factor, *ALK* anaplastic lymphoma kinase, *LDH* lactate dehydrogenase, *rR* relative risk, *HLA* human leukocyte antigen, *PET* positron emission tomography, *TCR* T-cell receptor, *PB* peripheral blood, *HPS* hemophagocytic syndrome, *ALL* acute lymphoblastic leukemia, *LBL* lymphoblastic lymphoma, *WBC* white blood count, *CNS* central nervous system, *allo-SCT* allogeneic stem cell transplantation, *SLL* small lymphocytic leukemia/lymphoma, *AT* ataxia telangiectasia, *T-CLL* T-cell chronic lymphocytic leukemia, *HTLV-1* human T-cell leukemia virus type 1, *IFNα* interferon-alpha, *ITLP* International T-cell Lymphoma Project, *RA* rheumatoid arthritis, *AIHA* autoimmune hemolytic anemia, *AA* aplastic anemia, *KIR* killing inhibitory receptor

T-cell lymphotropic virus 1 (HTLV-1) [13]. ATLL shows indolent and aggressive presentations but almost always terminates in fulminant leukemias with spread to lymph nodes and skin. Sézary leukemia occurs both de novo and as a transformation of mycosis fungoides (see Chap. 24), and is characterized by diffuse erythema, concomitant BM and nodal involvement and frequent pruritis due to tumor-associated eosinophilia [11]. The indolent T-cell large granular lymphocyte leukemia (T-LGL) usually presents with often profound neutropenia or bi-/tri-lineage cytopenias and their consequences as well as with mild to moderate splenomegaly. An association with autoimmune diseases is very common. T-LGL rarely transforms into an aggressive tumor, but a more aggressive NK-cell variant exists.

23.2.4. T-cell Neoplasms Arising in Immunocompromised Patients

Comprising only 3% of lymphomas associated with human immunodeficiency virus (HIV) infection, TCL/L are formally not an AIDS-defining diagnosis, but are increased in HIV-infected individuals with a relative risk ratio of 15.0 after AIDS onset [14]. A wide variety of histologic subtypes have been identified including T-ALL/LBL, CTCL, PTCL-NOS, AITL, ALK-negative AITL, and ATLL. Highest risk is seen in patients with low CD4 T-cell counts or who have other risk factors such as injection drug use or exposure to HTLV-1. As with B-cell lymphomas, the use of highly active anti-retroviral therapy (HAART) reduces the risk of developing TCL/L and is synergistic with chemotherapy once lymphoma develops. The role of SCT (including eligibility criteria) is even less well-defined than in immunocompetent TCL/L patients. Rarely, T-cell tumors may occur after solid organ transplantation or SCT. These include HSTCL and T-LGL. They show a very aggressive course and unlike the more common B-cell lymphomas in that setting, they usually lack EBV and HHV8 (see Chap. 30) [15].

23.2.5. NK-cell Tumors

Mature NK-cell tumors are more common in Asia than in the Western countries. They include both primarily extranodal and leukemic presentations [16]. Most of them are associated with EBV infection, have an aggressive course, and can present with complications of tumor-associated HPS. The most common category is extranodal NK/T-cell lymphoma, nasal-type (NK/TCL). It is most prevalent in Asia, Mexico, and Central and South America, and typically afflicts males in their fifth decade. Although histologic features are similar, nasal and extra-nasal NK/TCL cases have different clinical presentations and outcomes. Nasal NK/TCL is largely confined to the nose and the midline structures of the upper aerodigestive tract, causing symptoms of obstruction and erosion, whereas extranasal cases typically involves skin, GI tract, salivary glands, testes, and lung and has a inferior prognosis [17]. Aggressive NK-cell leukemia is an invariably fatal systemic disease of PB and BM without significant tissue involvement (Table 23-2).

23.3. Clinical Workup of T-cell and NK-cell Malignancies

A guideline for a comprehensive clinical staging strategy for TCL/L is presented in Table 23-3. Given the difficulties in subclassification of TCL/L, an open tissue biopsy is far superior to core needle biopsy or fine needle aspiration for diagnosis. Cytologic sampling almost never provides enough material for the extensive immunophenotypic and molecular studies required. Low-level PB involvement is typical in HSTCL and PTCL-NOS, so flow cytometric analysis of PB, is the method of choice for leukemic TCL/L, but is also helpful in the phenotypic characterization of other TCL/L. Computed tomography (CT), the standard imaging procedure for patients with nodal / bulky disease, may not accurately detect extent of disease in some TCL/L due to their frequent extranodal presentation. Positron emission tomography (PET) shows superior sensitivity when compared with CT in TCL/L at extranodal non-cutaneous sites, but despite the detection of additional sites in ≈30% of cases, upstaging occurs in only 10% of patients [18–20]. PET is currently not part of standard TCL/L staging because of its expense and the small percentage of cases in which it alters management or outcome.

23.4. Initial Therapies for Newly-Diagnosed TCL/L and NK-cell Tumors

There is little consensus on the optimal frontline therapy for most TCL/L. CHOP (cyclophosphamide, doxorubicin, vincristine, prednisone)-like chemotherapy is widely used for T-cell lymphomas but is not particularly effective, except for ALK+ ALCL [1]. Dose- or time-intensified protocols (like Mega-CHOP and CHOP-14, respectively) have provided

Table 23-3. The diagnostic and staging work up of patients with T-cell and NK-cell lymphoma/leukemia.

Assessment approach	Specific tests/details
History	Including B-symptoms, intestinal, neurologic, skin, or musculoskeletal symptoms; chemical or infectious exposures; family history of autoimmune disorders, cancer; siblings for SCT donor; comorbid conditions
Physical examination	Including documentation of sizes and features of all nodal or other lesions; spleen; liver; signs of anemia, thrombocytopenia, effusions, edema; neurologic signs
Blood tests	Whole and differential blood counts with smear (flow cytometry only if suspicious); routine chemistries including uric acid, LDH (tumor burden); β2-micro-globulin (prognosis), α-fetoprotein, and β-human chorionic gonadotropin in patients with a mediastinal mass (differential with germ cell tumor); coagulation; viral serology (CMV, EBV, HBV, HCV, HIV, HTLV-1); cellular and humoral immune status
Biopsy (lymph node, other tissues)	Morphology, immunohistochemistry (including ALK), classical karyotyping, FISH, T-cell receptor rearrangement (clonality)
Bone marrow biopsy	Unilateral is sufficient, with aspirate smear, further studies (above) if suspicious
Imaging studies	Chest X-ray, CT (chest, abdomen, pelvis), ultrasonography (followup of suspicious lesions)
Special procedures	MRI and lumbar puncture (morphologic and flow cytometric assessment) in patients with neurologic symptoms, MRI in bone disease that is equivocal by radiographs, endoscopy (with biopsy) in certain conditions (intestinal, nasal), PET is not standard of practice yet but useful for extranodal non-cutaneous lesions
Pre-treatment comorbidity/ organ function	As above, with electrocardiogram, trans-thoracic echocardiography, pulmonary function testing, glomerular filtration rate, liver enzymes, as indicated; dental status

LDH lactate dehydrogenase, *CMV* cytomegalovirus, *EBV* Epstein-Barr virus, *HBV* hepatitis B virus, *HCV* hepatitis C virus, *HIV* human immunodeficiency virus, *HTLV-1* human T-cell leukemia virus type 1, *ALK* anaplastic lymphoma kinase, *FISH* fluorescence in-situ hybridization, *CT* computed tomography, *MRI* magnetic resonance imaging, *PET* positron emission tomography

limited additive benefits and the inclusion of more drugs (such as etoposide in CHOEP) may benefit only younger, good-risk patients [21]. Dose-escalated cyclophosphamide plus methotrexate, etoposide and dexamethasone (CMED) has shown higher complete remission (CR) rates and prolonged OS when compared with conventional CHOP in a phase III study of PTCL-NOS [22]. More aggressive anthracycline-containing regimens such as hyper-CVAD (fractionated and alternating cyclophosphamide, vincristine, doxorubicin, dexamethasone, methotrexate, and cytarabine) do not appear superior to CHOP but have significantly more toxicities [23]. The International T-cell Lymphoma Project (ITLP), which collected retrospective data on approximately 1,300 TCL/L cases, concluded that such anthracycline-based regimens are not associated with improved outcomes, at least in the PTCL-NOS and AITL subtypes [1]. All of these studies highlight the need for novel approaches to primary therapy of T-cell lymphomas.

In contrast, investigational use of new agents is much more common in frontline treatment of T-cell leukemias and variants of CTCL and has provided encouraging results for more T-cell-selective agents such as the anti-CD52 monoclonal antibody alemtuzumab, and nucleoside analogues such as pentostatin, or the antifolate pralatrexate that are especially active in T cells [24,25]. A successful incorporation of HDT-SCT procedures into primary therapy requires such more efficient induction protocols so that more patients with TCL/L actually reach transplant (below). Treatment modalities for NK-cell malignancies include chemotherapy with local radiation, especially in nasal-type NK/TCL.

23.5. Prognostic Models for TCL/L

The particular TCT/L subtypes based on the WHO criteria encode important prognostic information for both T-cell lymphomas (Fig. 23-1) and T-cell leukemias (Fig. 23-2). Among non-cutaneous TCL/L, ALK+ ALCL has the most favorable outcome, with a 70% 5-year OS rate that is slightly superior to that of diffuse large B-cell lymphoma. PTCL-NOS, AITL, and ALK-negative systemic ALCL comprise an intermediate to poor prognostic group with

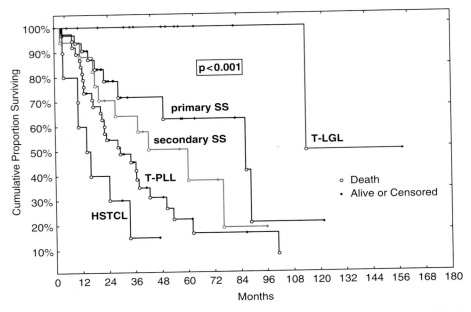

Fig. 23-2. *Survival in mature leukemic T-cell tumors.* Disease-specific overall survival (OS) of leukemic T-cell tumors diagnosed at the M. D. Anderson Cancer Center during 1996–2003 shows significant (*p* = 0.0002) differences between T-cell prolymphocytic leukemia (T-PLL), primary (no preceding patch/plaque skin disease) Sézary syndrome (SS), secondary (pre-existing mycosis fungoides) SS, T-cell large granular lymphocytic leukemia (T-LGL) and hepatosplenic T-cell lymphoma (HSTCL) with leukemic presentation. Reprinted with permission from Herling M et al. Blood 2004;104(2):328–35

OS rates of 32%, 32%, and 49% at 5 years, respectively. Very poor outcomes are seen in extranasal NK/TCL, EATL, and HSTCL, with 5-year OS rates of 9%, 20%, and 7%, respectively. Although treatments are much more variable in mature T-cell leukemias, we noted in a series from M. D. Anderson Cancer Center that T-LGL has, despite severe symptoms, a good outcome, while Sézary leukemia is of intermediate prognosis, and T-PLL has a poor outcome [11]. Anti-viral therapy is of central prognostic importance in ATLL [13,26].

No single prognostic model using clinical criteria is useful for all TCL/L cases since the characteristics of each subtype differ so widely [7,17,27·28]. The Ann Arbor staging system widely used for B-cell lymphoma (see Chap. 18) appears less useful than the IPI and a newly-developed Prognostic Index for T-cell lymphoma (PIT) for the nodal categories (Table 23-4). Both, however, provide limited stratification, partly because so many TCL/L cases have high-risk features at presentation when compared with B-cell lymphomas [1,29]. Importantly, the IPI and PIT seem to be of no use in the highest risk TCL/L types, namely EATL, HSTCL, and NK/TCL.

Other prognostic studies have explored the significance of immunophenotypic or biologic markers [6–8,30]. In general, unfavorable tumor markers include the presence of EBV or cytotoxic granule proteins, an increased BCL-2/BCL-xL ratio, and expression of CCR4, CD26, or glutathione-S-transferase. Markers of increased proliferation, such as more large transformed cells (>70% of cellularity), increased Ki-67 expression (>80% of cells), high topoisomerase 2α and CCND2 levels, or loss of the cell cycle regulators p53 and p21 correlate with aggressive clinical features. A more favorable prognosis seems to be associated with a particular "T-helper"-like phenotype defined by expression of the chemokine receptors CCR3, CCR5, and CXCR3. However, all of these studies are provisional and additional knowledge from gene expression data will likely be incorporated into more comprehensive phenotypic prognostic models [4,5].

Table 23-4. Prognostic factor scoring systems used in peripheral T-cell lymphomas.

Parameter	International prognostic index (IPI)[a][1]	Prognostic index for T-cell lymphoma (PIT) [29]	M. D. Anderson tumor score[b] [23]
Age	>60 years	>60 years	–
Performance status	ECOG>2	ECOG≥2	–
Lactate dehydrogenase	>Normal upper limit	>Normal upper limit	>250 IU/L
Extranodal sites	>1 site	–	Bulk>7 cm
Ann Arbor stage	III or IV	–	III or IV
β2-microglobulin	–	–	>3.0 mg/L
B-symptoms	–	–	Present
Bone marrow involvement	–	Present	–
Risk score groups in PTCL	0/1; 2; 3; 4/5	0; 1; 2; 3/4	0–2; ≥3

[a]The age adjusted (aa) IPI for patients <60 years includes Eastern Cooperative Oncology Group Performance Status (ECOG PS) > 2, LDH (lactate dehydrogenase) > normal, and Ann Arbor stage >2; in combination with β2-microglobulin the adjusted IPI predicts the outcome after autologous stem cell transplantation (Ref. 35)
[b]Developed at the M. D. Anderson Cancer Center, Houston, TX

23.6. Response Evaluation and Post-therapy Monitoring

Standardized minimal residual disease monitoring is not yet established for TCL/L. The timing and extent of response evaluation and follow up depends on the specific risk of failure/relapse and the consequences of a positive finding in the context of availability of effective (curative) rescue or salvage options. Based on the treatment responses and OS following mostly CHOP-like chemotherapy with or without loco-regional modalities, TCL/L with higher and lower risk for relapse can be identified [1]. The tests of primary response evaluation should be of appropriate sensitivity and generate comparable data. As for B-cell tumors, a role of PET in initial response assessment has yet to be determined in prospective studies [31]. PB blood flow cytometry using standardized 4- or 6- color TCL/L panels is important for tumor types that initially showed blood involvement or whenever lymphocytosis is detected. BM biopsy with immunophenotyping should be done when marrow infiltration initially existed or whenever cytopenias seemingly unrelated to therapy are noted.

How patients are followed in clinical practice is often different than in trials, but the minimal post-treatment monitoring comprises careful history, physical examination, complete blood count and serum chemistries including serial lactate dehydrogenase (LDH) measurements. This general approach better detects relapses with altered disease manifestation than assessing only the site of initial presentation. Although specific studies directed at TCL/L have not been done, routine CT or PET post-therapy surveillance has not proven beneficial in detecting the pre-clinical relapses in the majority of patients with lymphoma. To ensure comparability, clinical trials in TCL/L should optimally use well-defined endpoints including uniform criteria for progression free survival (PFS), equally sensitive tests, and standardized follow up intervals.

23.7. Therapeutic Options for Relapsed Disease and Developing Experimental Therapies for TCL/L and NK-cell Tumors

Traditional therapies for relapsed/refractory TCL/L have also been borrowed from those for aggressive B-cell lymphoma, including salvage/rescue regimens with at least one or two non cross-resistant agents when compared with the primary protocol (e.g. ifosfamide, etoposide, platinum-derivatives, cytarabine, and gemcitabine). There is, however, a growing number of new substances with marked activity in T-cell neoplasms (Table 23-5) [20,25,32,33]. Many of them are being tested in international multicenter registration trials. They will hopefully soon find their way into salvage or even primary protocols, ideally applied before HDT regimens in order to evaluate the most active of them. In PTCL-NOS, new exploitable targets such as PDGFR have been identified [3,4]. In AITL, a prominent vascular network, B-cell proliferations, and a high VEGF expression provide a rationale for approaches using immunomodulators (i.e. cyclophosphamide, thalidomide derivates), bevacizumab (anti-VEGF antibody), or rituximab. Based on the current treatment options, a risk-adapted therapy algorithm for TCL/L is presented in Fig. 23-3.

Table 23-5. Novel agents for T-cell malignancies and their characteristics.

Category/mechanism	Substance	Comments, see references [20, 24, 25, 32, 33]
Immunotherapy		
IL2 fusion toxin	Denileukin diftitox	Approved in CTCL, very active in other TCL/L, favorable toxicity profile supports use in combinations (i.e. trials ongoing with CHOP), some activity seen in CD25-negative cases
Anti-CD52 moAB	Alemtuzumab	55–75% RR in pretreated CTCL and T-cell leukemias, powerful single-agent activity in T-PLL, fewer concerns of opportunistic infections in frontline setting (i.e. combination with CHOP), CD52 expression varies across entities
Anti-CD2 moAB	Siplizumab	Ongoing phase I studies (≈10% CR rates)
Anti-CD4 moAB	Zanolimumab	Significant activity in CTCL, limited data in other TCL/L
Anti-CD25 (Tac) moAB	Daclizumab	Only partial responses in CD25+ATLL, combinations being tested
Anti-CD30 moAB	SGN-30, MDX-060	Use in ALCL with , encouraging phase I/II results
Anti-CCR4 moAB	KW-0761	Ongoing early testing in ATLL and other TCL/L
Anti-metabolites		
Pyrimidine analogue	Gemcitabine	Low toxicity, high RR in pretreated CTCL and TCL/L, commonly included in frontline regimens for TCL/L
Purine analogue	Pentostatin	High RR but short duration as a single agent in TCL/L; role of CD26 as a response predictor not fully established
Purine analogue	Nelarabine	Highest activity in pediatric and adult T-ALL/LBL
PNP inhibitor	Forodesine	Ongoing phase I/II trials in TCL/L; i.v. and oral formulation
Folate antagonist	Pralatrexate	Impressive >60% RR in pretreated TCL/L, exploration as a single agent or in combination with gemcitabine
Asparagine deprivation	Asparaginase	Highly active in T-ALL/LBL, recent studies in NK/TCL
HDAC inhibitors		
Pan-HDAC inhibitors	Vorinostat, Romidepsin, Belinostat	High RR and durable remissions in refractory CTCL (≈30%) and TCL/L (≈25%), cardiac toxicity (QT-prolongation)
Immunomodulators		
Cyclophilin binder	Cyclosporin	≈75% RR in AITL
Multi-effector	Lenalidomide	Promising activity in refractory CTCL
Proteasome inhibitors		
	Bortezomib	NF-kB-inhibition, ≈75% RR in CTCL, ongoing trials in TCL/L as single agent or in combination
Kinase inhibitors		
ALK, PKC, SYK, mTOR	Various compounds	Activity established for some compounds in small numbers of target-expressing TCL/L

IL2 interleukin 2, *CTCL* cutaneous T-cell lymphoma, *TCL/L* mature T-cell lymphoma/leukemia (non-cutaneous), *CHOP* cyclophosphamide, doxorubicin, vincristine, prednisone, *moAB* monoclonal antibody, *T-PLL* T-cell prolymphocytic leukemia, *ATLL* adult T-cell leukemia/lymphoma, *ALCL* anaplastic large cell lymphoma, *RR* response rate, *CR* complete remission, *T-ALL/LBL* precursor T-cell lymphoblastic leukemia/lymphoma, *PNP* purine nucleoside phosphorylase, *i.v.* intravenous, *NK/TCL* extranodal NK/T-cell lymphoma, nasal type, *HDAC* histone deacetylase, *AITL* angioimmunoblastic T-cell lymphoma

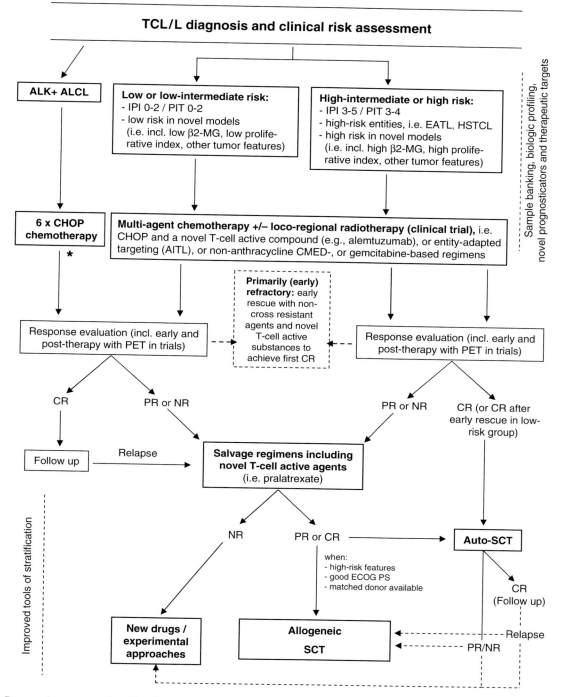

Fig. 23-3. *Proposed treatment algorithm for peripheral T-cell lymphomas.* T-cell lymphoma/leukemia (TCL/L) of primarily nodal and extranodal non-cutaneous subtypes should be risk-stratified and treated within clinical trials. *(asterisk) indicates that ALK+ anaplastic large cell lymphoma (ALCL) of high-intermediate or high risk; they are normally seen at a low-risk constellation at presentation; should be evaluated for consolidating autologous (auto) stem cell transplantation (SCT) in the first complete remission (CR), as these tend to progress early. The particular aspects of treatment of primarily leukemic forms are mentioned in Table 23-2. The goal should be an introduction of novel T-cell specific agents early into therapy. *IPI* International Prognostic Index, *PIT* Prognostic Index for Peripheral T-cell Lymphoma, *β2-MG* β2-microglobulin, *AITL* angioimmunoblastic T-cell lymphoma, *PET* positron emission tomography *PR* partial remission, *NR* no response, *EATL* enteropathy-associated T-cell lymphoma, *HSTCL* hepatosplenic T-cell lymphoma, *ECOG* Easten Cooperative Oncology Group, *PS* performance status

23.8. The Role of Stem Cell Transplantation in TCL/L

HDT followed by autologous (auto) SCT has been investigated as primary therapy of TCL/L in several retrospective analyses [34–36]. However, interpretation of most studies is limited by a positive selection bias due to preferential inclusion of patients with more favorable chemo-sensitive tumors such as ALK+ ALCL, and the exclusion of patients with refractory disease. Conclusions drawn primarily from the few prospective studies with intent-to-transplant designs include: (1) auto-SCT related mortality is consistently as low as 5–10%; (2) primary chemo-response to induction therapy (i.e. achievement of CR) is the strongest predictor of positive outcomes after consolidating auto-SCT; (3) only 40-70% of patients are transplantable, primarily due to refractory disease; (4) comparing equally chemo-sensitive TCL/L subtypes, consolidating auto-SCT appears to offer an additional 2–3 fold reduction in relapse risk. Overall, although frontline auto-SCT is currently the most effective approach for prolonging OS in good-response TCL/L but the data does not yet support its use as a standard therapy for all high-risk TCL/L. One limiting factor is that there is insufficient stratification of patients who would get benefits from this procedure by current predictive models [37,38]. Another problem is the need for more effective TCL/L-specific frontline protocols which limit the extent of residual disease pre-transplant in order to facilitate a larger proportion of patients being considered for SCT. Thus, routine incorporation of auto-SCT into primary therapy for certain TCL/L categories will await the development of these improved predictive and therapeutic tools.

Outcomes of auto-SCT as part of a salvage regimen are variable, with patients with chemosensitive tumors generally having a similar outcome as those transplanted in first partial remission. Auto-SCT after salvage therapy is most successful in patients with relapsed ALK+ ALCL but in only a minority of patients with other TCL/L types [35,37,39]. More sensitive tools of stratification will have to identify which TCL/L subtypes will benefit. Currently, the most powerful risk predictor is the sensitivity of the tumor to the salvage regimen.

Data on the success of allogeneic (allo) SCT in TCL/L are based primarily on retrospective studies of highly-selected relapsed or refractory patients, including those who had failed a prior auto-SCT [35]. Despite these inherent positive and negative selection biases and the non-uniform SCT procedures used, the reported 43–64% 5-year OS rates are very encouraging. Observations on the efficacy of allo-SCT include: (1) there is evidence of a graft-versus-lymphoma effect; (2) there is a plateau in the OS curves after approximately 2 years; (3) cures are accomplished in 70% of patients who are transplanted in CR; (4) ~30% of patients with residual chemo-resistant disease prior to transplant experience long-standing responses; (5) treatment-related mortality rates are variable (10–36%) without an obvious difference between the reduced conditioning and fully myeloablative regimens. There are ongoing prospective randomized trials that compare auto-SCT to allo-SCT after myeloablative conditioning as consolidating frontline therapy in TCL/L.

23.9. Currents Problems and Future Directions in the Treatment of T-cell and NK-cell Malignancies

Thanks to the recent advances in the recognition and classification of TCL/L, our concepts of specific disease management are evolving quickly. Unfortunately, for most patients with TCL/L, the prognosis considering all available treatments is still very poor. There are now a large number of novel compounds with encouraging preliminary data in TCL/L, however, one common denominator for nearly all categories is the lack of treatment guidelines. Developing better therapies for TCL/L will thus require closer interaction of biologists, pathologists, clinicians, and patients than has occurred to date.

Key priorities include:

1. Design of multi-center clinical trials to compensate for the rarity of TCL/L;
2. Development of frontline protocols that are superior to CHOP in inducing higher response rates and better long-term tumor control for the more common poor-risk subtypes;

3. Introduction of refined prognostic/predictive models that merge clinical features and tumor-associated factors to select patients for dose intensification and SCT;
4. Use of biomarker studies to direct targeted therapies.

Suggested Readings

Savage KJ. Prognosis and primary therapy in peripheral T-cell lymphomas. Hematology 2008;280–8.
- Reviews the most current aspects of clinical and tumor associated prognostic factors in TCL/L subsets and how to optimize therapy.

Rodríguez J, Gutiérrez A, Martínez-Delgado B, Perez-Manga G. Current and future aggressive peripheral T-cell lymphoma treatment paradigms, biological features and therapeutic molecular targets. Crit Rev Oncol Hematol 2009;71:181–98.
- Comprehensively addresses problematic issues in therapy including variation in frontline regimens, novel agents, and the role of SCT.

Molina AM, Horwitz SM. Rare T-cell lymphomas. Cancer Treat Res 2008;142:331–47.
- Overview of EATL, HSTCL, and SCPTCL. The article highlights the problem of limited treatment experience in three of the rarest T-cell lymphomas.

References

1. Armitage J, Vose J, Weisenburger D. International peripheral T-cell and natural killer/T-cell lymphoma study: pathology findings and clinical outcomes. J Clin Oncol 2008;26(25):4124–30.
2. Dunleavy K, Wilson WH, Jaffe ES. Angioimmunoblastic T cell lymphoma: pathobiological insights and clinical implications. Curr Opin Hematol 2007;14(4):348–53.
3. Savage KJ, Harris NL, Vose JM, et al. ALK- anaplastic large-cell lymphoma is clinically and immunophenotypically different from both ALK+ ALCL and peripheral T-cell lymphoma, not otherwise specified: report from the International Peripheral T-Cell Lymphoma Project. Blood 2008;111(12):5496–504.
4. Piccaluga PP, Agostinelli C, Califano A, et al. Gene expression analysis of peripheral T cell lymphoma, unspecified, reveals distinct profiles and new potential therapeutic targets. J Clin Invest 2007;117(3):823–34.
5. de Leval L, Rickman DS, Thielen C, et al. The gene expression profile of nodal peripheral T-cell lymphoma demonstrates a molecular link between angioimmunoblastic T-cell lymphoma (AITL) and follicular helper T (TFH) cells. Blood 2007;109(11):4952–63.
6. Rodriguez-Abreu D, Filho VB, Zucca E. Peripheral T-cell lymphomas, unspecified (or not otherwise specified): a review. Hematol Oncol 2008;26(1):8–20.
7. Lee Y, Uhm JE, Lee HY, et al. Clinical features and prognostic factors of patients with "peripheral T cell lymphoma, unspecified". Ann Hematol 2009;88(2):111–9.
8. Agostinelli C, Piccaluga PP, Went P, et al. Peripheral T cell lymphoma, not otherwise specified: the stuff of genes, dreams and therapies. J Clin Pathol 2008;61(11):1160–7.
9. Zettl A, deLeeuw R, Haralambieva E, Mueller-Hermelink HK. Enteropathy-type T-cell lymphoma. Am J Clin Pathol 2007;127(5):701–6.
10. Weidmann E. Hepatosplenic T cell lymphoma. A review on 45 cases since the first report describing the disease as a distinct lymphoma entity in 1990. Leukemia 2000;14(6):991–7.
11. Herling M, Khoury JD, Washington LT, Duvic M, Keating MJ, Jones D. A systematic approach to diagnosis of mature T-cell leukemias reveals heterogeneity among WHO categories. Blood 2004;104(2):328–35.
12. Herling M, Patel KA, Teitell MA, et al. High TCL1 expression and intact T-cell receptor signaling define a hyperproliferative subset of T-cell prolymphocytic leukemia. Blood 2008;111(1):328–37.
13. Matutes E. Adult T-cell leukaemia/lymphoma. J Clin Pathol 2007;60(12):1373–7.
14. Biggar RJ, Engels EA, Frisch M, Goedert JJ. Risk of T-cell lymphomas in persons with AIDS. J Acquir Immune Defic Syndr 1999, 2001;26(4):371–6.
15. Jamali FR, Otrock ZK, Soweid AM, et al. An overview of the pathogenesis and natural history of post-transplant T-cell lymphoma (corrected and republished article originally printed in Leukemia & Lymphoma, June 2007; 48(6): 1237–1241). Leuk Lymphoma 2007;48(9):1780–4.

16. Liang X, Graham DK. Natural killer cell neoplasms. Cancer 2008;112(7):1425–36.

17. Kim TM, Lee SY, Jeon YK, et al. Clinical heterogeneity of extranodal NK/T-cell lymphoma, nasal type: a national survey of the Korean Cancer Study Group. Ann Oncol 2008;19(8):1477–84.

18. Suh C, Kang YK, Roh JL, et al. Prognostic value of tumor 18F-FDG uptake in patients with untreated extranodal natural killer/T-cell lymphomas of the head and neck. J Nucl Med 2008;49(11):1783–9.

19. Bishu S, Quigley JM, Schmitz J, et al. F-18-fluoro-deoxy-glucose positron emission tomography in the assessment of peripheral T-cell lymphomas. Leuk Lymphoma 2007;48(8):1531–8.

20. Horwitz SM. Management of peripheral T-cell non-Hodgkin's lymphoma. Curr Opin Oncol 2007;19(5):438–43.

21. Pfreundschuh M, Trumper L, Kloess M, et al. Two-weekly or 3-weekly CHOP chemotherapy with or without etoposide for the treatment of young patients with good-prognosis (normal LDH) aggressive lymphomas: results of the NHL-B1 trial of the DSHNHL. Blood 2004;104(3):626–33.

22. Aviles A, Castaneda C, Neri N, et al. Results of a phase III clinical trial: CHOP versus CMED in peripheral T-cell lymphoma unspecified. Med Oncol 2008;25(3):360–4.

23. Escalon MP, Liu NS, Yang Y, et al. Prognostic factors and treatment of patients with T-cell non-Hodgkin lymphoma: the M. D. Anderson Cancer Center experience. Cancer 2005;103(10):2091–8.

24. Dearden C. The role of alemtuzumab in the management of T-cell malignancies. Semin Oncol 2006;33(2 Suppl 5):S44–52.

25. O'Leary HM, Savage KJ. Novel therapies in peripheral T-cell lymphomas. Curr Oncol Rep 2008;10(5):404–11.

26. Ravandi F, Kantarjian H, Jones D, Dearden C, Keating M, O'Brien S. Mature T-cell leukemias. Cancer 2005;104(9):1808–18.

27. Mourad N, Mounier N, Briere J, et al. Clinical, biologic, and pathologic features in 157 patients with angioimmunoblastic T-cell lymphoma treated within the Groupe d'Etude des Lymphomes de l'Adulte (GELA) trials. Blood 2008;111(9):4463–70.

28. Lee J, Suh C, Park YH, et al. Extranodal natural killer T-cell lymphoma, nasal-type: a prognostic model from a retrospective multicenter study. J Clin Oncol 2006;24(4):612–8.

29. Gallamini A, Stelitano C, Calvi R, et al. Peripheral T-cell lymphoma unspecified (PTCL-U): a new prognostic model from a retrospective multicentric clinical study. Blood 2004;103(7):2474–9.

30. Went P, Agostinelli C, Gallamini A, et al. Marker expression in peripheral T-cell lymphoma: a proposed clinical-pathologic prognostic score. J Clin Oncol 2006;24(16):2472–9.

31. Cheson BD. New staging and response criteria for non-Hodgkin lymphoma and Hodgkin lymphoma. Radiol Clin North Am 2008;46(2):213–23. vii.

32. Morris JC, Waldmann TA, Janik JE. Receptor-directed therapy of T-cell leukemias and lymphomas. J Immunotoxicol 2008;5(2):235–48.

33. Chen AI, Advani RH. Beyond the guidelines in the treatment of peripheral T-cell lymphoma: new drug development. J Natl Compr Canc Netw 2008;6(4):428–35.

34. Shustov AR, Savage KJ. Does high-dose therapy and autologous hematopoietic stem cell transplantation have a role in the primary treatment of peripheral T-cell lymphomas? Hematology Am Soc Hematol Educ Program 2008;2008:39–41.

35. Gutierrez A, Caballero MD, Perez-Manga G, Rodriguez J. Hematopoietic SCT for peripheral T-cell lymphoma. Bone Marrow Transplant 2008;42(12):773–81.

36. Paolo C, Lucia F, Anna D. Hematopoietic stem cell transplantation in peripheral T-cell lymphomas. Leuk Lymphoma 2007;48(8):1496–501.

37. Kim MK, Kim S, Lee SS, et al. High-dose chemotherapy and autologous stem cell transplantation for peripheral T-cell lymphoma: complete response at transplant predicts survival. Ann Hematol 2007;86(6):435–42.

38. Reimer P, Rudiger T, Geissinger E, et al. Autologous stem-cell transplantation as first-line therapy in peripheral T-cell lymphomas: results of a prospective multicenter study. J Clin Oncol 2009;27(1):106–13.

39. Yang DH, Kim WS, Kim SJ, et al. Prognostic factors and clinical outcomes of high-dose chemotherapy followed by autologous stem cell transplantation in patients with peripheral T cell lymphoma, unspecified: complete remission at transplantation and the prognostic index of peripheral T cell lymphoma are the major factors predictive of outcome. Biol Blood Marrow Transplant 2009;15(1):118–25.

40. Aljurf M, Zaidi SZ. Chemotherapy and hematopoietic stem cell transplantation for adult T-cell lymphoblastic lymphoma: current status and controversies. Biol Blood Marrow Transplant 2005;11(10):739–54.

Chapter 24

Cutaneous T-cell Lymphomas

Pranil Chandra, Mauricio P. Oyarzo, and Dan Jones

Abstract/Scope of Chapter T-cell malignancies presenting in the skin include mycosis fungoides, primary cutaneous anaplastic large cell lymphoma, and the related regressing lesion lymphomatoid papulosis as well as viral-associated adult T-cell leukemia/lymphoma. Rarer and more aggressive primary cutaneous lymphomas include extranodal natural killer cell/T-cell lymphoma, nasal type, subcutaneous panniculitits-like T-cell lymphoma, cutaneous gamma-delta T-cell lymphoma, and cutaneous aggressive epidermotropic CD8+ cytotoxic T-cell lymphoma. Systemic T-cell lymphomas that frequently involve the skin secondarily, such as angioimmunoblastic T-cell lymphoma, systemic anaplastic large cell lymphoma, and peripheral T-cell lymphoma, unspecified, are covered in Chap. 22.

Keywords Cutaneous T-cell lymphoma, classification • Mycosis fungoides • Mycosis fungoides, staging • Mycosis fungoides, CD8+ • Granulomatous slack skin disease • Sézary syndrome, primary • Sézary syndrome, staging • Sézary syndrome, transformation of MF • Pagetoid reticulosis • Mycosis fungoides, folliculotropic • Nasal type NK/T-cell lymphoma • Anaplastic large cell lymphoma, cutaneous • Lymphomatoid papulosis • Types A, B and C • Lymphomatoid papulosis • Model of regression • Gamma-delta T-cell lymphoma • T-cell lymphoma, subcutaneous panniculitits-like • Cutaneous T-cell lymphoma, CD4+ small/medium-sized pleomorphic T-cell lymphoma • Cutaneous T-cell lymphoma, NK/T-cell lymphoma, nasal type • Cutaneous T-cell lymphoma, gamma-delta • Cutaneous T-cell lymphoma, CD8+ aggressive epidermotropic cytotoxic T-cell lymphoma

24.1. Background

Cutaneous T-cell lymphoma (CTCL) is the umbrella term for the range of tumors presenting in the skin that remain predominantly at that site for at least 6 months. CTCL was first recognized over 200 years ago by Jean Louis Alibert [1] and is now known to comprise a range of both indolent and highly aggressive subtypes (Table 24-1)[2]. For that reason, correct classification of CTCL is extremely important for patient management, but can be difficult since it requires clinical correlation and knowledge of the histologic spectrum of each entity [3]. The World Health Organization (WHO) and the related European Organization for Research and Treatment of Cancer (EORTC) have provided a standardized diagnostic approach which will be used as the basis for this chapter [2,4,5].

From: *Neoplastic Hematopathology*: Contemporary Hematology,
Edited by: D. Jones, DOI 10.1007/978-1-60761-384-8_24,
© Humana Press, a part of Springer Science+Business Media, LLC 2010

Table 24-1. Indolent and aggressive types of primary cutaneous T-cell lymphomas.

Indolent clinical behavior
   Mycosis fungoides
   Folliculotropic mycosis fungoides
   Pagetoid reticulosis
   Granulomatous slack skin
   Primary cutaneous anaplastic large cell lymphoma
   Lymphomatoid papulosis
   Subcutaneous pannculitits-like T-cell lymphoma
   Primary cutaneous CD4+ small/medium-sized pleomorphic T-cell lymphoma (provisional entity)
Aggressive clinical behavior
   Sézary syndrome
   Primary cutaneous NK/T-cell lymphoma, nasal type
   Primary cutaneous CD8+ aggressive epidermotropic cytotoxic T-cell lymphoma
   Primary cutaneous γ/δ T-cell lymphoma
   Primary cutaneous peripheral T-cell lymphoma, unspecified

24.2. Mycosis Fungoides (MF)

24.2.1. Clinical Features

MF and its variants represent the majority of CTCL and arise from pre-existing dermatosis in the vast majority of patients [3]. There is a male-to-female ratio of 2:1, with a median age of 55–60 years at definitive diagnosis, but a preceding long history of rash and atopic dermatitis or allergy is often elicited. Well-developed MF rarely presents in children and adolescents [6, 7]. Given its subtlety, diagnosis of early-stage MF depends on many factors including perhaps the degree of access to medical care, as rising rates of diagnosis of MF in the United States are correlated with physician density, higher family income, education, and even home values [8].

In its classical presentation, MF begins as localized patches that can be hypopigmented, scaly, or erythrodermic. These patches then become more generalized and progress to raised plaques, and eventually to tumors before extracutaneous dissemination, as reflected in the staging system (Table 24-2). Initial skin lesions in MF have a predilection for the buttocks and other sun-protected areas. *Sézary syndrome*, defined as erythroderma with blood and lymph node MF involvement, is one characteristic pattern of progression. However, the vast majority of patients with MF do not progress and those with limited patch/plaque-stage MF generally have a similar life expectancy to age-, sex-, and race-matched control populations [6, 7].

24.2.2. Histological Features

Classically, MF is characterized by an epidermotropic and superficial dermal infiltration of small to medium-sized T cells with cerebriform nuclei and minimal spongiosis. Intraepidermal collections of tumor lymphocytes (*Pautrier microabscesses*) are a highly specific finding in MF but *basal layer seeding* of the epidermis by tumor cells is much more common (Fig. 24-1) [9]. However, there is a wide range of lymphocytic infiltration and epidermal reaction patterns seen in MF, including psoriasiform, acantholytic, and hyperkeratotic changes. Because MF arises frequently in dermatitis, the earliest patch stage of disease frequently shows reactive epidermal patterns including spongiosis, with only the degree of lymphocyte atypia distinguishing it from inflammatory changes. As MF proceeds, epidermal breakdown with concomitant bacterial infection frequently occurs and the associated acute inflammation can obscure the diagnosis. Such skin breakdown also produces increased lymph node drainage and *dermatopathic lymphadenitis* which is one cause for benign lymph node enlargement associated with Stage II MF.

Table 24-2. Clinical staging system for mycosis fungoides and Sézary syndrome (ISCL/EORTC, 2007) [52].

Stage I A	Disease confined to skin with patches/papules/plaques affecting < 10% of skin surface (T1)
B	Disease confined to skin with patches/papules/plaques affecting ≥ 10% of skin surface (T2)
Stage II A	Extensive skin involvement with patch/plaque and enlarged but not diffusely involved lymph nodes (N1, N2)
B	Extensive skin involvement with one or more tumors (>1 cm in size) (T3)
Stage III	Erythroderma (T4) with enlarged but minimally involved lymph node (N0-2) and low blood tumor burden (<1,000/μL circulating Sézary cells)
Stage IV	High blood tumor burden (>1,000/μL circulating Sézary cells) and/or extensive lymph node (N3) or visceral involvement (M1)

T (tumor), *N* (lymph node), *M* (organ spread) classification as per ISCL/EORTC criteria

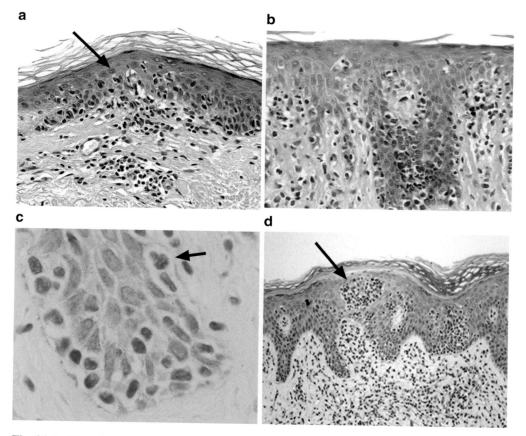

Fig. 24-1. Mycosis fungoides, early stage. (**a**) Early-stage MF often shows discrete foci of infiltration into the epidermis resembling spongiotic dermatitis (*arrow*). (**b**) Basal layer seeding of neoplastic lymphocytes is common with extensive patch stage disease. (**c**) High magnification shows atypical small and large (*arrow*) cerebriform lymphocytes seeding the basal layer of epidermis with minimal spongiosis. (**d**) Plaque stage disease is usually associated with atypical lymphoid infiltrates extending into the reticular dermis below the rete ridges. A psoriasiform epidermal reaction pattern is noted, with a Pautrier microabscess indicated by *arrow*

As MF progresses clinically, the infiltrate often shifts to the dermis with loss of epidermotropism, and the average tumor cell size increases (Fig. 24-2). *Large cell transformation* is diagnosed when greater than 25% of the infiltrate is composed of large cells. However, the association of morphological transformation with clinical progression is not absolute. A morphologic shift to blastoid-appearing hyperchromatic but still small lymphocytes is also occasionally observed with clinical progression (Fig. 24-3).

24.2.3. Laboratory Testing for Diagnosis and Staging

The neoplastic cells in MF are nearly always CD3+ CD45RO+ memory T cells that have a skin homing phenotype [i.e. cutaneous lymphocyte antigen (CLA)+, CD7-negative [10], with the vast majority expressing CD4, and only rare cases expressing CD8. Therefore, CD4 and CD8 immunostaining are critical to the differentiation of MF from reactive lesions, where mixed CD4+ and CD8+ infiltrates predominate, and from unusual CTCL subtypes, which are usually positive for CD8 or negative for both CD4 and CD8. Although changes in the level of other T-cell markers occur commonly in MF, complete loss of pan–T-cell antigens such as CD2, CD3, or CD5 is usually only detected by immunohistochemistry in late-stage MF or those with large cell transformation [11]. T-cell activation markers such as CD25 are variably expressed in both MF and reactive dermatoses and so are usually not helpful in diagnosis, however they may identify cases where targeted therapy is useful (See Chap. 25) [12].

CD8+ lesions that otherwise resemble classic MF (e.g. small cell morphology, lymphocyte atypia and basal layer seeding) have the same clinical behavior and prognosis as CD4+ cases [13], but CD8+ CTCL with ulceration, large cell morphology, deep infiltration, or necrosis likely represent one of the variants described below.

Although it has a limited role in skin biopsies, flow cytometric monitoring (FCM) is extremely useful to detect MF in lymph nodes and peripheral blood, with changes in the surface expression of CD3, CD4, and complete loss of CD26 expression representing the most common aberrations permitting quantitation of MF/SS levels in nearly all cases [14,15].

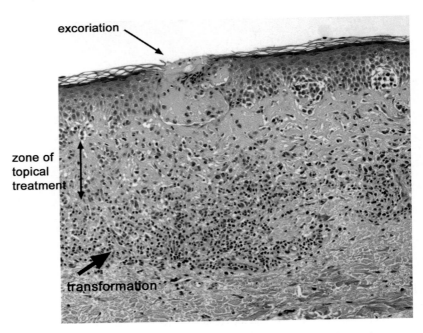

Fig. 24-2. Effects of treatment and progression in mycosis fungoides. Blisters due to excoriation/ pruritis can lead to skin breakdown, with associated spongiosis. Superficial dermal fibrosis is due to chronic use of topical agents. Large cell transformation usually occurs in deeper dermis

Fig. 24-3. Transformed MF with blastoid nuclear features

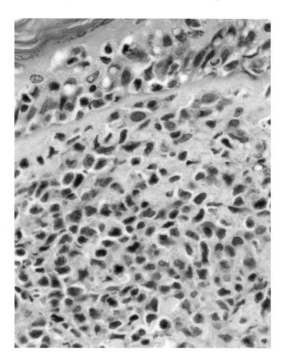

FCM on needle aspirate material from enlarged lymph nodes is thus largely replacing the prior histological staging systems (Table 24-3). Similarly, the ability of FCM to quantitate neoplastic cells in blood has led to a classification based on absolute tumor cell numbers. Identification of the particular T-cell receptor (TCR) beta variable chain expressed by the tumor cells at diagnosis using a panel of TCR-beta antibodies can also be used to search for low levels of MF/SS by FCM in follow-up samples.

Greater than 95% of MF cases show clonal rearrangement of the TCR-gamma and/or TCR-beta loci by PCR analysis but "clonal" TCR rearrangement can also be seen in the reactive dermatoses (See Chap. 4 for discussion of the difficulties around interpreting these clonality assays). The most helpful use of molecular studies in workup of MF is to compare the PCR patterns observed from two different sites or in sequential biopsies, with the finding of an identical TCR gene rearrangement at both sites indicative of systemic disease with a higher risk of progression [16]. Such an approach is also helpful in staging peripheral blood, where false-positive TCR PCR results are frequently seen due to T-cell pseudoclones unrelated to the MF population.

24.2.4. Prognostic and Predictive Factors

The prognosis of patients with MF is most dependent on clinical stage, with large cell transformation (particularly extracutaneous transformation), visceral involvement, and high blood tumor burden representing the most adverse prognostic factors [6,7,17]. Upregulation of a number of immunophenotypic markers are weakly correlated with progression and poor outcome including CD30, cytotoxic proteins such as T-cell intracellular antigen-1 (TIA-1) and granzyme B[18], and some cytokines and chemokine receptors [19]. More promising as a predictive model in later-stage MF is genomic profiling by comparative genomic hybridization (CGH). Chromosomal abnormalities seen with progression include gain of chromosome 7q26 region (involving the FASTK gene) [20], chromosomal deletions involving 5q13, 9p21, 10q [21], and 13q14, and amplification at chromosome 19p13.2 spanning the JUNB transcription factor [22,23]. Loss of expression of the tumor suppressors

Table 24-3. Comparison of methods for histopathological staging of clinically abnormal lymph nodes (>1.5 cm) in mycosis fungoides and Sézary syndrome.

Dutch system (1980)[53]	NCI/navy system (1985) [54]	ISCL/EORTC (2005) [52]
Grade 1: DL, no atypical CMC	LN0: no atypical lymphocytes	N1
	LN1: occasional, isolated atypical lymphocytes	(a) No clonal TCR
		(b) Clonal TCR
	LN2: clusters (3–6 cells) of atypical lymphocytes	
Grade 2: DL with early involvement with scattered atypical CMC	LN3: aggregates of atypical lymphocytes, but architecture preserved	N2
		(a) No clonal TCR
		(b) Clonal TCR
Grade 3: partial effacement of nodal architecture with many CMC	LN4: partial or complete efface-ment of nodal architecture by frankly atypical lymphocytes	N3
Grade 4: complete effacement of nodal architecture		

DL dermatopathic lymphadenopathy, *CMC* cerebriform mononuclear cells with nuclei > 7.5 μm, *TCR* T-cell receptor gene rearrangement

Table 24-4. Most common molecular alterations associated with progression or transformation in MF.

Gene	Chromosome	% Affected	Molecular mechanism
p16/INK4a (CDKN2A)	9p21	18–73%	Hypermethylation and/or LOH
p14/ARF (CDKN2A)	9p21	Up to 18%	Hypermethylation and/or LOH
p15/INK4b (CDKN2B)	9p21	5–27%	Hypermethylation and/or LOH
PTEN	10q23–24	10–45%	LOH or homozygous deletion
TP53 (p53)	17p13	Up to 66%	Point mutation
JUNB	19p13	50–91%	Genomic amplification Transcriptional regulation
HLA-G	6p	Up to 28%	Transcriptional upregulation
FAS	10q24.1	14–59%	Point mutation
FASLG (Fas ligand)	1q23	50–83%	Transcriptional upregulation
NAV3	12q14	10–85%	Genomic deletion

LOH loss of heterozygosity. For details, see references [23,25,55–61]

CDKN2A, RB1, and TP53 by deletion or methylation silencing represent some of the most common molecular changes found in advanced stage MF/SS (Table 24-4) [24–26]

24.2.5. Differential Diagnosis and Variants of MF

Given that some of the rarer CTCL types have aggressive clinical behavior, it is important to be alert to features that suggest lymphomas other than MF. Apoptosis, necrosis, and angioinvasion are rare in classical low-grade MF and should trigger consideration of other CTCL types. If only tumor lesions are present without preceding or concurrent patches or plaques, a diagnosis of MF is unlikely and the CD30+ T-cell disorders or a systemic lymphoma should be considered.

For more indolent lesions, a wide variety of localized and/or non-epidermotropic CTCLs have been described that are generally grouped as variants of MF (Table 24-5) [3]. The most common of these is *folliculotropic MF*, which partially spares the epidermis, with often dense and destructive adnexal infiltration with or without mucinosis (Fig. 24-4). This variant has preferential involvement of the head and neck area, and its adnexal involvement imparts a micropapular nature to the infiltrate clinically resembling folliculitis. In several studies, folliculotropic MF has been reported to have a worse prognosis than plaque stage MF [27], but this may be due to reporting bias. Many cases, in our experience, have an indolent course.

Table 24-5. MF and its variants.

Variant	Synonyms	Clinical features	Morphological and immunophenotypic features
Classical MF	Alibert-Bazin	– Patches, plaques, and tumors – Usually precedent chronic dermatitis	– Colonization of the basal layer of the epidermis – Pautrier microabscesses seen in a minority (10–40%) – Shift to superficial dermis in plaque and tumor stage – Minimal lymphocyte apoptosis – Degree of spongiosis and epidermal reaction less than in reactive dermatitis
Folliculotropic MF	Pilotropic Follicular MF Syringotropic	– Grouped follicular papules, acneiform lesions, indurated plaques, on head and neck area – Associated with alopecia and mucinorrhea – Pruritis may be a sign of disease progression. – Secondary bacterial infections common – Less amenable to topical agents but antibiotics used – Both aggressive and indolent variants occur	– Periadnexal and/or peri-eccrine localization – Infiltration of follicle and sparing of the epidermis – Mucinous degeneration of follicle (follicular mucinosis), best seen with Alcian blue staining. – Admixed eosinophils and plasma cells.
Pagetoid reticulosis	Woringer–Kolopp disease	– Solitary psoriasiform or hyper-keratotic patch or plaque, stable for years or slowly progressive – Most common on extremities	– Localized raised intraepidermal infiltration by nests of atypical lymphocytes with vacuolated cytoplasm – Associated hyperplastic epidermis – Most are CD8+; uniform CD25 or CD30 expression can be seen
Granulomatous slack skin disease		– Very rare, with indolent but relentless course – Slow development of circum-scribed areas of pendulous lax skin of the axillae and groin – May be seen in patients with Hodgkin lymphoma	– Dense granulomatous dermal infiltrates containing mildly atypical T cells, many multinucleated giant cells containing elastic tissue (elastolysis) – Minimal epidermotropism – Overwhelmingly CD4+ T cells
Primary Sézary syndrome (SS)		– Presentation with erythroderma and lymphadenopathy due to neoplastic T cells in blood, skin and lymph node – Must be distinguished from sec-ondary SS in MF – Erythrodermic flare of derma-titis, particularly psoriasis, can mimic primary SS	– Perivascular skin infiltrates, usually minimal epidermotropism – Lymph node involvement interfollicular to diffuse – Blood Sézary counts $> 1 \times 10^9$/L; if lower, it is best diagnosed as "pre-SS" or "low-level involvement" – CD4+ but often CD7+ in contrast to MF – Bone marrow involvement is subtle but can be documented by flow cytometry in most cases

Pagetoid reticulosis is one of the best characterized patterns of unilesional MF [28]. This entity is composed of extremely slow-growing localized plaques on the extremities with a CD8+ tumor immunophenotype in most cases (Fig. 24-5). *Granulomatous slack skin disease* is an unusual dermal-based CTCL of the axillae and groin that shows large numbers of multinucleated giant cells and mildly atypical T cells, manifesting as slow development of lax skin in the major skin folds (Fig. 24-6). It is distinct from *granulomatous MF*, which is a histiocyte-rich dermal-based CTCL variant that can occur at any site [29]. *Primary Sézary syndrome* is a variant of CTCL that presents with erythroderma, lymph node, and blood involvement that lacks significant epidermo-tropism, but instead has a largely perivascular pattern of skin involvement (Fig. 24-7) [30]. Recent evidence suggests that it may be genetically distinct from classical MF [20].

24.2.6. Pathogenesis and Patterns of Progression

Although it is clear that the majority of cases of MF arise from pre-existing dermatitis, little is known about the molecular pathogenesis of early-stage lesions. Reaction to bacterial superantigens

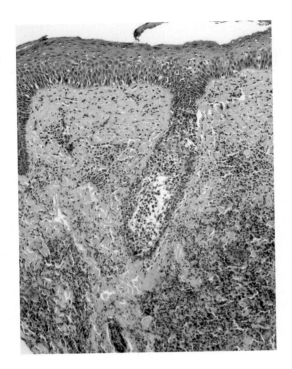

Fig. 24-4. Folliculotropic mycosis fungoides. Atypical lymphoid infiltrate in dermis and infiltrating adnexa with mucinous degeneration of the hair follicle. Minimal epidermotropism is present

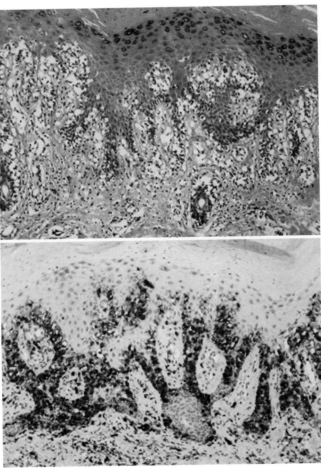

Fig. 24-5. Pagetoid reticulosis. (**Top**) Localized plaque with highly epidermotropic infiltrate of large lymphocytes with clear cytoplasm, associated with spongiosis and hyperkeratosis. (**Bottom**) CD8 immunostain is positive in neoplastic T cells

has been suggested,[31,32] as has alterations in the epidermal microenvironment from activated keratinocytes which can promote neoplastic transformation of infiltrating lymphocytes. [33,34]. What we do know is that the early-stage MF cells show (a) resistance to apoptosis [35] and (b) distinct patterns of chemokine and cytokine receptor expression [10,36].

Progression in MF is associated with shifts in the functional phenotype of the tumor cells reflected in expression of markers such as CD25, CD30, and cytotoxic granule markers [37].

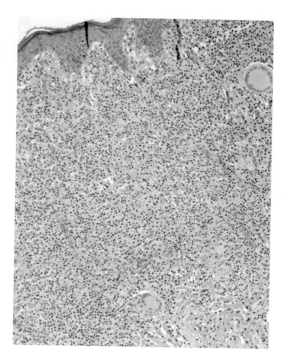

Fig. 24-6. Granulomatous slack skin disease. Dense dermal infiltrate of predominantly small, irregular lymphocytes with admixed multinucleated histiocyte giant cells

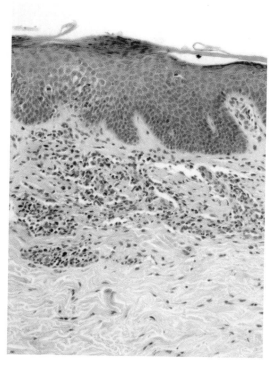

Fig. 24-7. Primary Sézary syndrome. Infiltrate is composed of atypical enlarged lymphocytes and eosinophils in a tight perivascular pattern with minimal epidermotropism

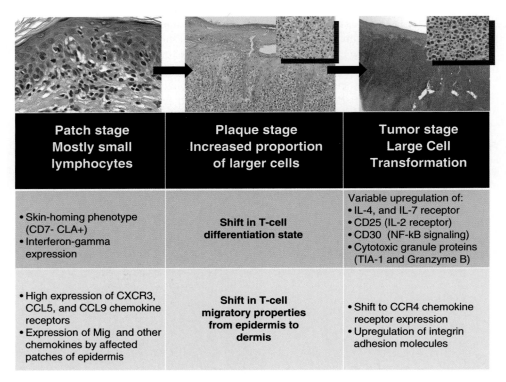

Patch stage Mostly small lymphocytes	Plaque stage Increased proportion of larger cells	Tumor stage Large Cell Transformation
• Skin-homing phenotype (CD7- CLA+) • Interferon-gamma expression	**Shift in T-cell differentiation state**	Variable upregulation of: • IL-4, and IL-7 receptor • CD25 (IL-2 receptor) • CD30 (NF-kB signaling) • Cytotoxic granule proteins (TIA-1 and Granzyme B)
• High expression of CXCR3, CCL5, and CCL9 chemokine receptors • Expression of Mig and other chemokines by affected patches of epidermis	**Shift in T-cell migratory properties from epidermis to dermis**	• Shift to CCR4 chemokine receptor expression • Upregulation of integrin adhesion molecules

Fig. 24-8. Model of molecular transformation in MF. Shift in phenotype and functional properties of tumor cells during tumor progression

These changes generally reflect a switch in gene expression during progression from a mixed patterns or one more similar to type 1 helper T cells (Th1) to one more uniformly resembling type 2 helper T cells (Th2) (Fig. 24-8) [38–40]. The genetic events described above (e.g. loss of tumor suppressor genes) are mostly seen in later-stage MF.

24.3. Primary Cutaneous CD30 Positive T-cell Lymphoproliferative Disorders

24.3.1. Clinical Features

Primary cutaneous CD30+ T-cell lymphoproliferative disorders include *primary cutaneous anaplastic large cell lymphoma* (cALCL), *lymphomatoid papulosis* (LyP), and borderline cases. Together, they account for approximately 30% of CTCL. Lymphomatoid papulosis is a chronic recurrent skin disease characterized by multifocal, spontaneously regressing papules, which appear and disappear over 1–3 months. This clonal T-cell disease almost always has a benign but unremitting course and usually presents when patients are older children or young adults. LyP can be grouped into three histologic subtypes (Table 24-6), but different lesions in the same patient can have multiple appearances. cALCL presents as a solitary ulcerated tumor, or as several grouped, localized nodules without evidence of regression. In our experience, patients with long-standing LyP will usually have one or more non-regressing lesions, and patients with cALCL sometimes give a history of prior regressing lesions suggesting that the two entities are closely related. Borderline cases are those where a definite distinction between cALCL and LyP cannot be made despite careful clinicopathological evaluation.

Table 24-6. Diagnosis of CD30+ lymphoproliferative disorders in skin.

Entity	Clinical Features	Morphological and immunophenotypic features
Lymphomatoid papulosis (LyP)	– Wide age range (median 45 years) – Male to female ratio, 1.5:1 – Waxing and waning papulonodular eruptions – 20% transform to overt lymphoma – Very indolent, 98% 5-year survival	– *Type A*: Wedge-shaped, polymorphous infiltrate (large lymphocytes, neutrophils and eosinophils) inflammatory infiltrate with few CD30+ cells – *Type B*: similar to MF with epidermotropic T-lymphocytes and cerebriform nuclei – *Type C/Borderline*: Dense CD30+ infiltrates similar to cALCL
Primary cutaneous ALCL	– Wide age range (median 60 years) – Male to female ratio, 2–3:1 – Solitary or localized crops of nodules – May be a variant of LyP since many patients also have regressing lesions – Very indolent, >90% 5-year survival	– Cohesive sheets of large, non-epidermotropic and anaplastic CD30+ tumor cells, diffusely distributed – Anaplastic morphology with round, oval, or irregularly-shaped nuclei, and Hallmark cells with prominent eosinophilic nucleoli and abundant cytoplasm – May have pleomorphic or immunoblastic morphology – Admixed inflammatory cells uncommon, ALK–
Transformed MF	– Clinical history of/evolution from patches/plaques disease	– Frequent loss of epidermotropism so may be histologically indistinguishable from cALCL
Systemic ALCL	– Usually associated lymphadenopathy or other sites	– Can be morphologically identical to cALCL – CD30+, higher rate of EMA positivity than cALCL – Expression of ALK in most cases infiltrating skin

24.3.2. Histological and Immunophenotypic Features

Both cALCL and LyP are characterized by the presence in the dermis of large, nucleolated T cells expressing the cytokine receptor CD30 (also known as Ki-1). Histological appearances in LyP include the wedge-shaped type A lesion with perivascular accentuation (Fig. 24-9), the MF-like type B (Fig. 24-10), and the ALCL-like type C (Fig. 24-11), whereas cALCL tends to have a more sheet-like infiltrate (Fig. 24-12). Most LyP and cALCL are CD4+ with less than 10% expressing CD8; rare cases coexpress CD4 and CD8 or are negative for both. LyP cases usually have more admixed small CD4+ and CD8+ lymphocytes, eosinophils, and plasma cells, whereas cALCL has a higher density of CD30+ T cells that can extend into the subcutis. Loss of T cell antigens (commonly CD3 and TCR/βF1) and expression of fascin and clusterin are more common in cALCL but can be seen in LyP; clonal and oligoclonal TCR gene rearrangements are present in both lesions and are similarly not helpful in differentiation.

24.3.3. Differential Diagnosis

If there is any clinical evidence of systemic, extracutaneous disease, the diagnoses of cALCL and LyP are totally excluded and the diagnosis of transformed MF, systemic ALCL, or Hodgkin lymphoma (HL) should be considered. Immunohistochemistry for the ALK kinase should always be done in younger patients to exclude systemic ALCL (Fig. 24-13), although ALK-negative ALCL, CD30+ peripheral T-cell lymphoma, and transformed MF are more difficult to exclude by morphology or immunohistochemistry alone. Classical HL will only involve the skin in advanced stage cases, usually by extension, and show tumor cells that express both CD30 and CD15. There is a rare overlap syndrome of LyP-ALCL-HL where the recurrences in skin and lymph node can have a variety of appearances.

The differential diagnosis of early lesions of LyP with few CD30+ cells includes MF-like localized inflammatory lesions such as pityriasis lichenoides et varioliformis acuta (PLEVA), and particularly insect bite reactions and drug reactions.

24.3.4. Pathogenesis

A small subset of cALCL have a known molecular pathogenesis, including translocations involving the IRF4 locus [41]. But for most cases, it remains unclear why LyP lesions rapidly

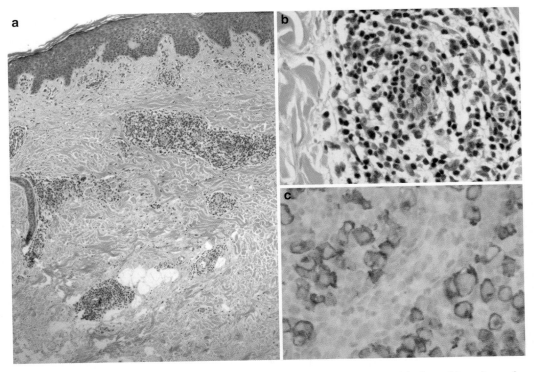

Fig. 24-9. Lymphomatoid papulosis, type A lesion. (**a**) Wedge-shaped dermal lesion with perivascular accentuation. (**b**) Small lymphocytes are admixed with large nucleolated lymphocytes. (C) CD30 immunostain highlights the large cell component

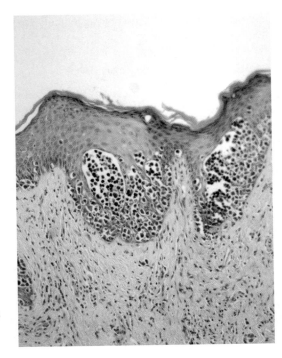

Fig. 24-10. Lymphomatoid papulosis, type B lesion. Extensive epidermotropism in a case of LyP resembling MF

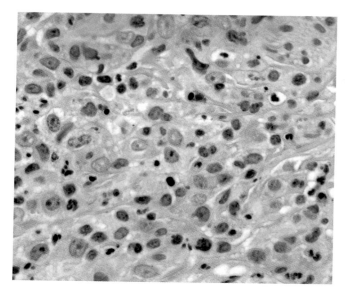

Fig. 24-11. Lymphomatoid papulosis, type C lesion. Tumor cells are uniformly large, resembling ALCL, and were uniformly positive for CD30. However, all of this patient's lesions showed typical regression over several months. The presence of numerous apoptotic cells may be indicative of impending regression in a late-stage LyP lesion

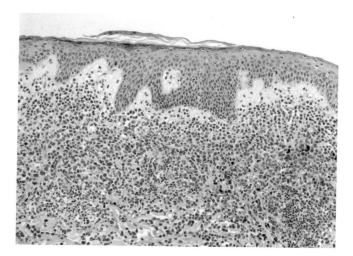

Fig. 24-12. Primary cutaneous anaplastic large cell lymphoma. Dense dermal infiltrate of uniformly large tumor cells, that were positive for CD30 and the T-cells markers CD2 and CD45RO (not shown)

appear and regress and cALCLs do not. Persistence in cALCL is likely due to balances between growth, apoptosis, and immune control of each lesion. Interactions of tumor cell CD30 with stromal expressed CD30 ligand may play a role (Fig. 24-14) [42]. Further work needs to be done on discovering the specific trophic dermal growth signals, apoptotic mechanisms [43], and immunoregulatory mechanisms that divide LyP and ALCL [44].

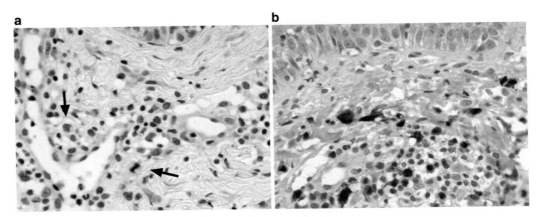

Fig. 24-13. Systemic cutaneous anaplastic large cell lymphoma presenting in skin. (**a**) Perivascular dermal infiltrate of sparse large lymphocytes with prominent nucleoli (arrows). (**b**) ALK immunostain is positive

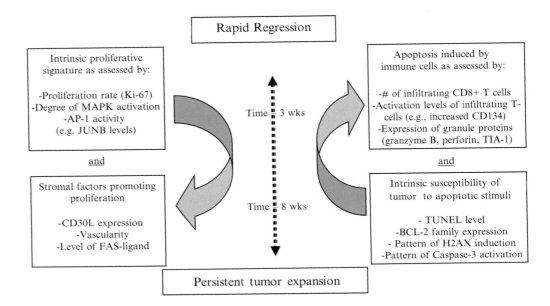

Fig. 24-14. Model of regression and growth persistence in CD30+ cutaneous lymphoproliferative disorders. A multi-factorial model of regression integrating apoptotic and growth parameters in predicting behavior may be helpful

24.4. Uncommon T-cell Lymphomas Involving Skin

The remaining 20% of primary CTCL represent a range of rare tumor types that often have extremely aggressive clinical features (Table 24-7) [3]. Clues to the diagnosis of these rare tumors include marked pleomorphic or blastoid nuclear features, presence of angioinvasion, involvement of subcutaneous tissue, zonal necrosis, the absence of CD4 and CD8 expression in a T-cell infiltrate, or a CD8+ cytotoxic immunophenotype. A secondary marker panel including TCR subunits (BetaF1 and gamma), CD56, EBV-encoded RNA in situ hybridization (EBER), and cytotoxic granule antigens (e.g., TIA-1, granzyme B or perforin) is useful for distinguishing these tumors.

Adult T-cell leukemia/lymphoma (ATLL) is a systemic T-cell neoplasm etiologically associated with infection by human T-cell leukemia virus 1 (HTLV-1). ATLL is almost always CD4+ with strong CD25 expression, and can have dermal or extensively epidermotropic patterns

Table 24-7. Uncommon cutaneous T-cell lymphomas.

CTCL Type	Clinical Presentation	Histological Features	Immunophenotype (all cytoplasmic CD3+)	Behavior
Predominantly epidermotropic and dermal				
Adult T-cell leukemia/lymphoma	– HTLV-1 seropositivity – Endemic to Caribbean, Japan, South America, and Central Africa – Skin lesions in 50% (nodules, papules, or plaques)	– Highly pleomorphic or polylobated cells – Tumor apoptosis often prominent unlike in MF	CD4+, CD8–, CD25+	– Highly variable but usually terminates in fatal leukemia – Hypercalcemia is a poor prognostic sign
Primary cutaneous CD8+ epidermotropic cytotoxic T-cell lymphoma	– Localized or disseminated papules, plaques or tumors – Central ulceration	– Pronounced epidermotropism with pagetoid spread – Angioinvasion and necrosis in dermis	CD8+, TCR-beta+, Cytotoxic proteins+ EBV–, often CD2–, CD5–	– Few cases reported but generally poor outcome (2–3 years median survival) – Needs to be distinguished from indolent localized CD8+ pagetoid reticulosis and CD8+ MF
Predominantly dermal				
Extranodal NK/T-cell lymphoma, nasal type	– Seen in Asia, Central/South America, rare in US – Multiple plaques/tumors or mid-facial destructive lesion (midline granuloma)	– Dense pleomorphic infiltrate in dermis – Angioinvasive, with necrosis.	CD56+, EBER+, CD2+, cytotoxic proteins+, surface CD3–, CD5– in NK cell cases (80%)	– Variable course with rapid demise in 50%, radiosensitive – Systemic spread common including leukemia and HPS can be seen
Cutaneous gamma-delta T-cell lymphoma	– Disseminated plaques and/or ulcerating tumors, on extremities – HPS	– Mid-dermal/adnexal extending into subcutis and epidermis – Admixed reactive T cells	CD56+/–, CD2+, CD5v, TCR-beta-, most CD4– and CD8–	– Poor response to chemotherapy, median survival 1–3 years despite lack of extracutaneous spread
Hydroa vacciniforme-like lymphoma	– Children and adolescents with chronic EBV infection – Asia, Central/South America – Papulovesicular eruption which proceeds to ulceration and scarring – Fever, wasting, HSM	– Small to medium-sized lymphocytes in dermis extending to ulcerated epithelium and subcutis – Necrosis, angioinvasion	CD8+, EBER+CD56v Some may be CD4+	– Progression from reactive infiltrates to frank lymphoma – Systemic symptoms late in the course of disease.
Restricted to subcutaneous tissue				
Subcutaneous panniculitits-like T-cell lymphoma	– Multiple nodules and plaques, legs and trunk – Systemic HPS rare	– Limited to subcutis – Polymorphous lymphocytes with apoptosis and rimming of adipocytes – Macrophages with ingested debris (Bean-bag appearance)	CD8+, CD4–, cytotoxic proteins+, EBER–, usually CD56–	– Variable course (median survival 5–7 years), with frequent relapses

HSM hepatosplenomegaly, *HPS* hemophagocytic syndrome, *EBER* Epstein Barr virus (EBV)-encoded RNA transcripts detected by in situ hybridization, *v* variable expression

including large Pautrier microabscesses (Fig. 24-15). A clue to ATLL is the frequent presence of apoptosis which is unusual in MF. Skin lesions are generally a manifestation of widely disseminated disease, but a slowly progressive form with only skin lesions can occur [45].

Extranodal NK/T-cell lymphoma, nasal type is a dermal-based EBV+ lymphoma with pleomorphic cytology (including frequent small, irregular cells), zonal necrosis, and angiocentric growth (Fig. 24-16). Tumors are usually of NK-cell lineage (CD2+, CD5–) but

Fig. 24-15. Adult T-cell leukemia/lymphoma, in skin. Pautrier microabscess with a uniform blastoid appearance to tumor cells. Image courtesy of Roberto Miranda

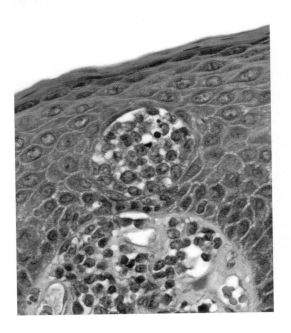

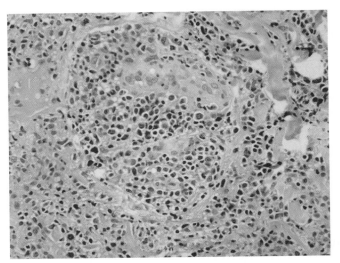

Fig. 24-16. Extranodal NK/T-cell lymphoma, nasal type, in skin

can also be CD8+ T cells; both types express cytotoxic markers (TIA-1, granzyme B, and perforin) and EBV LMP1 and EBER. Skin involvement may be primary or secondary and skin is the second most common site of involvement after the nasal cavity/nasopharynx [46]. Differentiation of nasal type lymphoma from the rare *hydroa vacciniforme-like lymphoma* is based on the presence of a characteristic recurrent papulovesicular rash and the absence of extensive epidermal involvement and edema in the latter [47]. Another tumor type with propensity to cause ulceration and necrosis is primary cutaneous aggressive epidermotropic CD8+ cytotoxic T-cell lymphoma (Fig. 24-17).

Subcutaneous panniculitis-like T-cell lymphoma is a lymphoma derived from cytotoxic T cells that is primarily localized to the subcutis, frequently affects the legs and abdomen, and mimics the board-like skin seen with panniculitits. There is pleomorphic cytomorphology, rimming of the subcutaneous fat, high numbers of apoptotic cells, and many macrophages filled with cell debris (Fig. 24-18). The phenotype is CD8+ EBV− with the expression of cytotoxic markers and high expression of the pro-apoptotic BAX protein [48]. Numerous admixed reactive T and B cells can make definitive phenotyping of the tumor cells difficult in some cases. CD4+ tumors with a similar pattern usually represent spread from a systemic lymphoma. The clinical course is indolent except when systemic hemophagocytic syndrome occurs, usually in patients with high tumor burden.

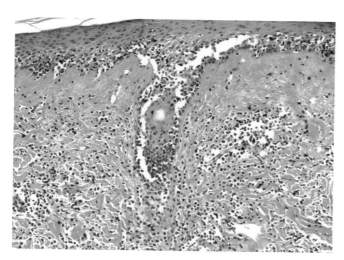

Fig. 24-17. Primary cutaneous CD8+ aggressive epidermotropic cytotoxic T-cell lymphoma. Highly epitheliotropic infiltrate of tumor cells with clear cytoplasm produces breakdown of the skin. Immunostains were positive for CD8 and granzyme B in the tumor cells

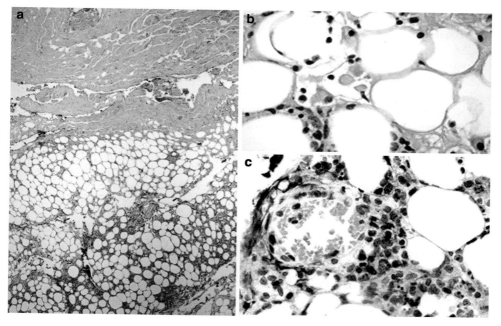

Fig. 24-18. Subcutaneous panniculitits-like T-cell lymphoma. (**a**) Sparse lymphoid infiltrate is confined to the subcutaneous tissue. (**b**) Hyperchromatic lymphocytes are admixed with histiocytes with apoptotic debris. (**c**) CD8 immunostain is positive in the atypical hyperchromatic lymphocytes

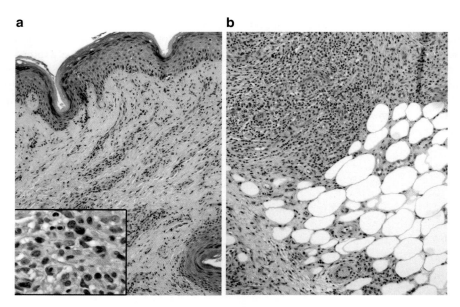

Fig. 24-19. Cutaneous gamma-delta T-cell lymphoma. (**a**) Early lesion shows dermal-based monomorphic perivascular lymphoid infiltrate. (**b**) A case with more extensive involvement shows extension of blastoid lymphocytes into subcutis

Cutaneous gamma-delta T-cell lymphoma is a very rare, extremely aggressive, multifocal, tumor-forming dermal-based neoplasm [49,50]. It is unrelated to hepatosplenic T-cell lymphoma. Most cases have a small cell appearance with blastoid nuclei, and typically start as a mid-dermal perivascular/periadnexal infiltrate that becomes diffuse and spreads into the subcutis and into the ulcerated epidermis (Fig. 24-19). Tumor cells express gamma/delta TCR (detectable by FCM or IHC using TCR-delta antibodies in fresh/frozen and TCR-gamma in fixed sections), are usually negative for both CD4 and CD8 (although admixed reactive T cells are common), and are negative for EBV. This tumor almost never disseminates outside the skin, but median survival is only 1–3 years due to the extensive ulcerated/necrotic lesions and cytokine effects, including frequent hemophagocytic syndrome.

The diagnosis of CD4+ dermal-based lymphomas that don't resemble MF or one of its recognized variants is still a matter of study. The WHO classification lists two provisional entities: primary cutaneous CD4+ small/medium T-cell lymphoma and the default primary cutaneous peripheral T-cell lymphoma, unspecified for such cases. Systemic T-cell lymphomas also frequently involve the skin with *angioimmunoblastic T-cell lymphoma* being the most common and subtle, usually forming sparse perivascular polymorphous infiltrates, but occasionally showing epidermal infiltration. *T-cell prolymphocytic leukemia* involves the skin in up to 50% of cases, often resembling the appearance of the tight perivascular aggregates of primary Sézary syndrome but with much higher blood tumor counts [51].

24.5. Other Tumors Mimicking Cutaneous T-cell Lymphoma

B-cell lymphomas involving the skin are summarized in Chap. 27; most are easily distinguished from T-cell tumors. T-cell-rich B-cell lymphomas, particularly *lymphomatoid granulomatosis*, can involve the skin and should be considered whenever interspersed large B cells are present in a dense dermal T-cell rich infiltrate. The blastoid plasmacytoid dendritic cell neoplasm, which often resembles lymphoid cells, and leukemia cutis are the most critical differential diagnoses (Chap. 26). Finally, small cell melanoma and Merkel cell carcinoma can resemble lymphoma and should be considered in any cutaneous tumor that is negative for CD3, CD20, CD30, and CD45.

Selected Reviews

Hwang ST, Janik JE, Jaffe ES, Wilson WH. Mycosis fungoides and Sezary syndrome. Lancet 2008;371:945–57.
- Recent clinicopathologic summary of MF.

Kinney MC, Jones D. Cutaneous T-cell and NK-cell lymphomas: the WHO-EORTC classification and the increasing recognition of specialized tumor types. Am J Clin Pathol 2007;127:670–86.
- A summary of findings at a workshop on T-cell and NK-cell malignancies held in 2005.

Willemze R, Jaffe ES, Burg G, et al. WHO-EORTC classification for cutaneous lymphomas. Blood 2005;105:3768–85.
- Brief summaries of the current cutaneous lymphoma subtypes.

References

1. Willemze R, Meijer CJ. Classification of cutaneous T-cell lymphoma: from Alibert to WHO-EORTC. J Cutan Pathol 2006;33(Suppl. 1):18–26.
2. Willemze R, Jaffe ES, Burg G, et al. WHO-EORTC classification for cutaneous lymphomas. Blood 2005;105:3768–85.
3. Kinney MC, Jones D. Cutaneous T-cell and NK-cell lymphomas: the WHO-EORTC classification and the increasing recognition of specialized tumor types. Am J Clin Pathol 2007;127:670–86.
4. Swerdlow SH, Campo E, Harris NL, et al. WHO classification of tumour of haematopoietic and lymphoid tissues. Lyon: IARC Press, 2008.
5. LeBoit PE. Pathology and genetics of skin tumors. Lyon, France: IARC Press, 2006.
6. Kim YH, Liu HL, Mraz-Gernhard S, Varghese A, Hoppe RT. Long-term outcome of 525 patients with mycosis Fungoides and Sezary syndrome: clinical prognostic factors and risk for disease progression. Arch Dermatol 2003;139:857–66.
7. Zackheim H, Amin S, Kashani-Sabet M, McMillan A. Prognosis in cutaneous T-cell lymphoma by skin stage: long-term survival in 489 patients. J Am Acad Dermatol 1999;40:418–25.
8. Criscione VD, Weinstock MA. Incidence of cutaneous T-cell lymphoma in the United States, 1973–2002. Arch Dermatol 2007;143:854–9.
9. Shapiro PE, Pinto FJ. The histologic spectrum of mycosis fungoides/Sezary syndrome (cutaneous T-cell lymphoma). A review of 222 biopsies, including newly described patterns and the earliest pathologic changes. Am J Surg Pathol 1994;18:645–67.
10. Lu D, Duvic M, Medeiros LJ, Luthra R, Dorfman DM, Jones D. The T-cell chemokine receptor CXCR3 is expressed highly in low-grade mycosis fungoides. Am J Clin Pathol 2001;115:413–21.
11. Ralfkiaer E. Controversies and discussion on early diagnosis of cutaneous T-cell lymphoma. Phenotyping. Dermatol Clin 1994;12:329–34.
12. Jones D, Ibrahim S, Patel K, Luthra R, Duvic M, Medeiros LJ. Degree of CD25 expression in T-cell lymphoma is dependent on tissue site: implications for targeted therapy. Clin Cancer Res 2004;10:5587–94.
13. Lu D, Patel KA, Duvic M, Jones D. Clinical and pathological spectrum of CD8-positive cutaneous T-cell lymphomas. J Cutan Pathol 2002;29:465–72.
14. Jones D, Dang NH, Duvic M, Washington LT, Huh YO. Absence of CD26 expression is a useful marker for diagnosis of T-cell lymphoma in peripheral blood. Am J Clin Pathol 2001;115:885–92.
15. Washington LT, Huh YO, Powers LC, Duvic M, Jones D. A stable aberrant immunophenotype characterizes nearly all cases of cutaneous T-cell lymphoma in blood and can be used to monitor response to therapy. BMC Clin Pathol 2002;2:5.
16. Vega F, Luthra R, Medeiros LJ, et al. Clonal heterogeneity in mycosis fungoides and its relationship to clinical course. Blood 2002;100:3369–73.
17. van Doorn R, Van Haselen CW, van Voorst Vader PC, et al. Mycosis fungoides: disease evolution and prognosis of 309 Dutch patients. Arch Dermatol 2000;136:504–10.

18. Vermeer MH, Geelen FA, Kummer JA, Meijer CJ, Willemze R. Expression of cytotoxic proteins by neoplastic T cells in mycosis fungoides increases with progression from plaque stage to tumor stage disease. Am J Pathol 1999;154:1203–10.

19. Jones D, O'Hara C, Kraus MD, et al. Expression pattern of T-cell-associated chemokine receptors and their chemokines correlates with specific subtypes of T-cell non-Hodgkin lymphoma. Blood 2000;96:685–90.

20. van Doorn R, van Kester MS, Dijkman R, et al. Oncogenomic analysis of mycosis fungoides reveals major differences with Sezary syndrome. Blood 2009;113:127–36.

21. Smoller BR, Santucci M, Wood GS, Whittaker SJ. Histopathology and genetics of cutaneous T-cell lymphoma. Hematol Oncol Clin North Am 2003;17:1277–311.

22. Kari L, Loboda A, Nebozhyn M, et al. Classification and prediction of survival in patients with the leukemic phase of cutaneous T cell lymphoma. J Exp Med 2003;197:1477–88.

23. Mao X, Orchard G, Lillington DM, Russell-Jones R, Young BD, Whittaker SJ. Amplification and overexpression of JUNB is associated with primary cutaneous T-cell lymphomas. Blood 2003;101:1513–9.

24. Mao X, Orchard G, Vonderheid EC, et al. Heterogeneous abnormalities of CCND1 and RB1 in primary cutaneous T-Cell lymphomas suggesting impaired cell cycle control in disease pathogenesis. J Invest Dermatol 2006;126:1388–95.

25. Navas IC, Algara P, Mateo M, et al. p16(INK4a) is selectively silenced in the tumoral progression of mycosis fungoides. Lab Invest 2002;82:123–32.

26. Zhang C, Toulev A, Kamarashev J, Qin JZ, Dummer R, Dobbeling U. Consequences of p16 tumor suppressor gene inactivation in mycosis fungoides and Sezary syndrome and role of the bmi-1 and ras oncogenes in disease progression. Hum Pathol 2007;38:995–1002.

27. Klemke CD, Dippel E, Assaf C, et al. Follicular mycosis fungoides. Br J Dermatol 1999;141:137–40.

28. Cerroni L, Fink-Puches R, El-Shabrawi-Caelen L, Soyer HP, LeBoit PE, Kerl H. Solitary skin lesions with histopathologic features of early mycosis fungoides. Am J Dermatopathol 1999;21:518–24.

29. Kempf W, Ostheeren-Michaelis S, Paulli M, et al. Granulomatous mycosis fungoides and granulomatous slack skin: a multicenter study of the Cutaneous Lymphoma Histopathology Task Force Group of the European Organization For Research and Treatment of Cancer (EORTC). Arch Dermatol 2008;144:1609–17.

30. Diwan AH, Prieto VG, Herling M, Duvic M, Jones D. Primary Sezary syndrome commonly shows low-grade cytologic atypia and an absence of epidermotropism. Am J Clin Pathol 2005;123:510–5.

31. Jackow CM, Cather JC, Hearne V, Asano AT, Musser JM, Duvic M. Association of erythrodermic cutaneous T-cell lymphoma, superantigen-positive Staphylococcus aureus, and oligoclonal T-cell receptor V beta gene expansion. Blood 1997;89:32–40.

32. Talpur R, Bassett R, Duvic M. Prevalence and treatment of Staphylococcus aureus colonization in patients with mycosis fungoides and Sezary syndrome. Br J Dermatol 2008;159:105–12.

33. Sarris AH, Esgleyes-Ribot T, Crow M, et al. Cytokine loops involving interferon-gamma and IP-10, a cytokine chemotactic for CD4+ lymphocytes: an explanation for the epidermotropism of cutaneous T-cell lymphoma? Blood 1995;86:651–8.

34. Tensen CP, Vermeer MH, van der Stoop PM, et al. Epidermal interferon-gamma inducible protein-10 (IP-10) and monokine induced by gamma-interferon (Mig) but not IL-8 mRNA expression is associated with epidermotropism in cutaneous T cell lymphomas. J Invest Dermatol 1998;111:222–6.

35. Wu J, Nihal M, Siddiqui J, Vonderheid EC, Wood GS. Low FAS/CD95 Expression by CTCL correlates with reduced sensitivity to apoptosis that can be restored by FAS upregulation. J Invest Dermatol 1009;129:1165–73.

36. Yagi H, Seo N, Ohshima A, et al. Chemokine receptor expression in cutaneous T cell and NK/T-cell lymphomas: immunohistochemical staining and in vitro chemotactic assay. Am J Surg Pathol 2006;30:1111–9.

37. Talpur R, Jones DM, Alencar AJ, et al. CD25 expression is correlated with histological grade and response to denileukin diftitox in cutaneous T-cell lymphoma. J Invest Dermatol 2006;126:575–83.

38. Hahtola S, Tuomela S, Elo L, et al. Th1 response and cytotoxicity genes are down-regulated in cutaneous T-cell lymphoma. Clin Cancer Res 2006;12:4812–21.

39. Lee BN, Duvic M, Tang CK, Bueso-Ramos C, Estrov Z, Reuben JM. Dysregulated synthesis of intracellular type 1 and type 2 cytokines by T cells of patients with cutaneous T-cell lymphoma. Clin Diagn Lab Immunol 1999;6:79–84.

40. Papadavid E, Economidou J, Psarra A, et al. The relevance of peripheral blood T-helper 1 and 2 cytokine pattern in the evaluation of patients with mycosis fungoides and Sezary syndrome. Br J Dermatol 2003;148:709–18.

41. Feldman AL, Law M, Remstein ED, et al. Recurrent translocations involving the IRF4 oncogene locus in peripheral T-cell lymphomas. Leukemia 2009;23:574–80.

42. Mori M, Manuelli C, Pimpinelli N, et al. CD30–CD30 ligand interaction in primary cutaneous CD30(+) T-cell lymphomas: a clue to the pathophysiology of clinical regression. Blood 1999;94:3077–83.

43. Goteri G, Simonetti O, Rupoli S, et al. Differences in survivin location and Bcl-2 expression in CD30+ lymphoproliferative disorders of the skin compared with systemic anaplastic large cell lymphomas: an immunohistochemical study. Br J Dermatol 2007;157:41–8.

44. Gjerdrum LM, Woetmann A, Odum N, et al. FOXP3 positive regulatory T-cells in cutaneous and systemic CD30 positive T-cell lymphoproliferations. Eur J Haematol 2008;80:483–9.

45. Shimoyama M. Diagnostic criteria and classification of clinical subtypes of adult T-cell leukaemia–lymphoma. A report from the Lymphoma Study Group (1984–87). Br J Haematol 1991;79:428–37.

46. Chan JK, Sin VC, Wong KF, et al. Nonnasal lymphoma expressing the natural killer cell marker CD56: a clinicopathologic study of 49 cases of an uncommon aggressive neoplasm. Blood 1997;89:4501–13.

47. Iwatsuki K, Ohtsuka M, Harada H, Han G, Kaneko F. Clinicopathologic manifestations of Epstein–Barr virus-associated cutaneous lymphoproliferative disorders. Arch Dermatol 1997;133:1081–6.

48. Sen F, Rassidakis GZ, Jones D, Medeiros LJ. Apoptosis and proliferation in subcutaneous panniculitis-like T-cell lymphoma. Mod Pathol 2002;15:625–31.

49. Toro JR, Liewehr DJ, Pabby N, et al. Gamma-delta T-cell phenotype is associated with significantly decreased survival in cutaneous T-cell lymphoma. Blood 2003;101:3407–12.

50. Jones D, Vega F, Sarris AH, Medeiros LJ. CD4-CD8-"Double-negative" cutaneous T-cell lymphomas share common histologic features and an aggressive clinical course. Am J Surg Pathol 2002;26:225–31.

51. Valbuena JR, Herling M, Admirand JH, Padula A, Jones D, Medeiros LJ. T-cell prolymphocytic leukemia involving extramedullary sites. Am J Clin Pathol 2005;123:456–64.

52. Olsen E, Vonderheid E, Pimpinelli N, et al. Revisions to the staging and classification of mycosis fungoides and Sezary syndrome: a proposal of the International Society for Cutaneous Lymphomas (ISCL) and the cutaneous lymphoma task force of the European Organization of Research and Treatment of Cancer (EORTC). Blood 2007;110:1713–22.

53. Scheffer E, Meijer CJ, Van Vloten WA. Dermatopathic lymphadenopathy and lymph node involvement in mycosis fungoides. Cancer 1980;45:137–48.

54. Sausville EA, Worsham GF, Matthews MJ, et al. Histologic assessment of lymph nodes in mycosis fungoides/Sezary syndrome (cutaneous T-cell lymphoma): clinical correlations and prognostic import of a new classification system. Hum Pathol 1985;16:1098–109.

55. Dereure O, Levi E, Vonderheid EC, Kadin ME. Infrequent Fas mutations but no Bax or p53 mutations in early mycosis fungoides: a possible mechanism for the accumulation of malignant T lymphocytes in the skin. J Invest Dermatol 2002;118:949–56.

56. Karenko L, Hahtola S, Paivinen S, et al. Primary cutaneous T-cell lymphomas show a deletion or translocation affecting NAV3, the human UNC-53 homologue. Cancer Res 2005;65:8101–10.

57. Nagasawa T, Takakuwa T, Takayama H, et al. Fas gene mutations in mycosis fungoides: analysis of laser capture-microdissected specimens from cutaneous lesions. Oncology 2004;67:130–4.

58. Scarisbrick JJ, Woolford AJ, Calonje E, et al. Frequent abnormalities of the p15 and p16 genes in mycosis fungoides and Sezary syndrome. J Invest Dermatol 2002;118:493–9.

59. Scarisbrick JJ, Woolford AJ, Russell-Jones R, Whittaker SJ. Loss of heterozygosity on 10q and microsatellite instability in advanced stages of primary cutaneous T-cell lymphoma and possible association with homozygous deletion of PTEN. Blood 2000;95:2937–42.

60. Urosevic M, Willers J, Mueller B, Kempf W, Burg G, Dummer R. HLA-G protein up-regulation in primary cutaneous lymphomas is associated with interleukin-10 expression in large cell T-cell lymphomas and indolent B-cell lymphomas. Blood 2002;99:609–17.

61. van Doorn R, Dijkman R, Vermeer MH, Starink TM, Willemze R, Tensen CP. A novel splice variant of the Fas gene in patients with cutaneous T-cell lymphoma. Cancer Res 2002;62:5389–92.

Chapter 25

Treatment of Cutaneous T-cell Lymphomas

Katherine M. Cox and Madeleine Duvic

Abstract/Scope of the Chapter Cutaneous T-cell lymphomas (CTCLs) are a diverse group of non-Hodgkin's lymphomas presenting as skin lesions containing malignant, skin-homing T cells. Mycosis fungoides (MF) and the leukemic variant, Sézary Syndrome (SS), are the most common CTCLs and the main focus of this chapter. Skin-directed therapy is sufficient for early patch/plaque MF which may remain indolent for many years. Biological response modifiers and phototherapy are added for SS, and for refractory or progressive MF. Experimental agents that block key pathways and targeted therapies are under development and will provide more options.

Keywords Cutaneous T-cell Lymphoma, treatment • Mycosis fungoides, staging • Mycosis fungoides, treatment • Sézary syndrome, treatment • CD25, immunotherapy

25.1. Pathogenesis of Cutaneous T-Cell Lymphoma (CTCL)

Mycosis fungoides (MF) and its leukemic variant, Sézary syndrome (SS), are clonal expansions of skin-homing helper/memory T cells, hypothesized to emerge in genetically susceptible individuals following persistent exposure to self or extrinsic antigens (e.g. infections or chemicals) [1]. The CD4+CD45RO+ helper-like T cells characterizing MF lack FAS ligand-induced programmed cell death, and often express Th2 cytokines which can depress cellular immunity and deplete the T-cell repertoire of normal Th1 effector cells and CD8 cytotoxic cells [2]. As a result, restoration of normal T-lymphocyte subset homeostasis may be a reasonable goal for targeted therapies. More effective treatments for CTCLs may arise as we better understand its etiology and pathogenesis.

25.2. Clinical Workup for CTCL at the Time of Diagnosis

MF skin lesions most often appear in sun-shielded areas and are highly pleomorphic with various shapes, colors, and degrees of exfoliation. Although a pink and scaly appearance is most common, MF can be hypopigmented or hyperpigmented, have telangectasias (i.e. poikiloderma), or present as confluent pink patches (i.e. erythroderma). Itching may or may not be present. Skin biopsy must be taken from persistent, *untreated* lesions and must show epidermotropic, atypical T cells for the unequivocal diagnosis of MF. Immunohistochemical stains showing CD4+>> CD8+ T cells with loss one or more pan-T-cell antigens as well as clonal T-cell receptor gene rearrangement are other characteristic features (see Chap. 24).

From: *Neoplastic Hematopathology*: Contemporary Hematology,
Edited by: D. Jones, DOI 10.1007/978-1-60761-384-8_25,
© Humana Press, a part of Springer Science+Business Media, LLC 2010

Once a histological diagnosis of MF is obtained, the patient is staged according to the tumor, node, metastasis, and blood (TNMB) system. T stage is determined by extent of patch/plaque/tumor lesions for each body area using the severity weighted assessment (SWAT) score. The T scoring is T1 [patch/plaque of <10% body surface area (BSA)], T2 (patches/plaques of >10% BSA), T3 (tumors present), and T4 (erythroderma), with 1% BSA equal to an area equivalent to the size of a patient's palm. The dimensions of significant tumors should be measured and photography is useful to follow the response of skin lesions to therapy. Early MF is difficult to distinguish from chronic dermatitis, but using the International Society of Cutaneous Lymphomas (ISCL) point-based algorithm is helpful as it combines clinical and histological criteria [3].

Lymph nodes greater than 1.5 cm in the longest transverse diameter or with abnormal palpable qualities (firm, irregular, fixed, clustered) are regarded as clinically significant, and should be sampled by needle aspiration or excisional biopsy (See classification criteria in Chap. 24). Imaging by computed tomography (CT) scan or by tandem positron emission tomography (PET)-CT should be performed at baseline in patients who have lymphadenopathy.

Routine recommended laboratory testing include complete blood count (CBC) with differential, and serum chemistries including magnesium and lactic dehydrogenase, rapid plasmin reagin (RPR) test, human T-cell lymphotropic virus (HTLV)-1 serology, and quantitative immunoglobulin levels for patients with advanced disease. If SS is suspected from a high white blood cell count, flow cytometry of peripheral blood should be ordered to determine the absolute CD4+ and CD8+ T cell numbers and the percentage of presumed neoplastic T-cells (for MF, often represented by a CD4+CD26- phenotype). The criteria for blood involvement were revised in the 2007 guidelines as: B0 (≤5% Sezary cells), B1 (>5% Sezary cells), or B2 (positive T-cell receptor gene clonal rearrangement **and** either ≥1000/μL Sezary cells **or** one of the following: (a) CD4/CD8 ratio ≥10 **or** (b) increased CD4 cells with a CD7- or CD26- immunophenotype. The current staging uses the ISCL/ European Organization for Research and Treatment of Cancer (EORTC) 2007 guidelines [3].

Bone marrow biopsy should be done whenever there is confirmed blood involvement (especially B2) or with unexplained hematologic abnormalities [3]. No specific staging system for bone marrow involvement yet exists, but patients with major bone marrow involvement may be classified as stage IVB; whereas patients with minimal bone marrow involvement may be classified as stage IVA. Visceral involvement can be assumed when there is splenomegaly on exam or by imaging that shows focal splenic defects not considered to be cystic or vascular, even without biopsy confirmation. Suspected disease in the liver, lungs, or other organs should be confirmed by biopsy or needle aspirate to rule out other malignancies or infectious causes.

25.3. Standard Therapy Options for Newly Diagnosed CTCL

Appropriate treatment is selected based on overall clinical stage, TNMB classification, and other prognostic variables, such as folliculocentric involvement, or large cell transformation [4]. The EORTC published consensus treatment recommendations in 2006, [5] but these are becoming outdated as more agents become available [6–16].

Approximately, two thirds of newly diagnosed patients present with stage I [patch/ plaque] disease and have an excellent prognosis not different from age-matched controls [4]. Stage I MF patients require only skin-directed therapy initially, and many may never require systemic treatment unless their disease progresses or is refractory. The most common skin-directed therapies (Table 25-1), outlined in the National Comprehensive Cancer Network (NCCN) guidelines (available at www.nccn.org), include corticosteroids, retinoids, phototherapy, mustargen ointment, or electron beam radiation, and should be used in that order unless there are mitigating circumstances. Narrow-band UVB (nbUVB) is effective

Table 25-1. Skin-directed therapies for CTCL.

Treatment	Mechanism of action	Recommended stage	Dosing	Response	Side effects
Corticosteroids (Class I–III) [6]	Immune suppression to epidermis with minimal effects in dermis	Common initial tx for early MF Adjunct palliative agent in all stages	Triamcinolone 0.1% cream with warm wet wraps	ORR 67–100% CR 25–67%	Skin atrophy, striae
Retinoids [7]	Ligands for RAR + RXR retinoid receptors that form nuclear transcription complexes	Refractory early MF	Tazarotene 1% gel/cream	ORR 58% CR 35%	Erythema/desquamation Burning/pruritus Dryness/irritation Teratogenic potential
Rexinoids [7]	Ligands for RXR retinoid receptors only to form nuclear transcription complexes	Refractory early MF	Bexarotene 1% gel	ORR 44–63% CR 8–21%	Pruritus/irritation Pain Teratogenic potential
Ultraviolet B (UVB) [8]	290–320 nm; Induces apoptosis of T cells	Early MF: patch disease (not effective for plaques) Combination with topicals	Depends on skin type Increase duration gradually	CR: 74% Better response in lighter skin types	Burning Non-melanoma skin cancer Actinic damage
Narrow-band UVB (nbUVB) [8]	311 nm; induces apoptosis of T cells	Early MF Combination with topicals	Depends on skin type Increase duration gradually	CR 75% All skin types respond	Burning Non-melanoma skin cancer Actinic damage
Psoralen + Ultraviolet A (PUVA) [8]	320–400 nm; suppresses DNA synthesis by DNA-crosslinking; selective immunosuppression	Early MF Adjuvant tx for later stages	Depends on skin type- Combine with IFN or bexarotene	ORR 95% CR 74%	Nausea/headaches Lightheadedness Non-melanoma skin cancer
Nitrogen Mustard (NM) (Mustargen) [6]	Donates alkyl groups to DNA, disrupts DNA synthesis	Early MF Maintenance tx after CR cALCL/LyP	NM 10% in aquaphor daily NM 20%a NM 40%a	ORR 63–93% CR 26–80%	Contact/allergic dermatitis Squamous cell carcinoma
Carmustine (BCNU)[6]	Forms electrophiles that cross-link DNA, disrupts DNA synthesis	Second/third-line tx for refractory early MF	BCNU topically daily or BID x 1–4 mo (aqueous) or 6–12 mo (ointment)	ORR 85–100% CR 48–86%	Erythema/Tenderness Telangiectasias Contact/allergic dermatitis Myelosuppression
Imiquimoid	Immune response modifier via toll receptor interaction (TLR7)	Refractory early MF	Imiquimoid 5% 3x/wk x 12 weeks	Anecdotal evidence	Erythema/irritation
Photodynamic therapy (PDT)	Photosensitizer activation leads to reactive oxygen species → apoptosis and tumor reduction	Early MF	Wavelength specific to photosensitizer	Anecdotal CR for hypericin + D-Aminolevulinic acid (ALA)	Erythema Burning sensation Crusting Vesicles
Total body skin electron beam (TSEB)[8]	High energy electrons directed towards entire body; mechanism of action is unknown	Preparation for transplant Extensive patch/plaque disease Spot radiation to single lesion MF or cALCL/LyP Palliation for stage IV	Combine with ECP Prior to transplant to ↑ disease free survival	CR 70% (T1: CR 95%)	Radiation dermatitis Dry/moist exfoliation Erythema/tenderness Blistering/anhidrosis Loss of nails

aDenotes experimental use; early stage MF is stage IA, IB, and IIA

ORR overall response rate. CR complete response, tx treatment, cALCL primary cutaneous anaplastic large cell lymphoma, LyP lymphomatoid papulosis, BCNU bischlorethylnitrosurea

against patch disease with thin plaques. Thicker plaques respond better to psoralen plus UVA (PUVA) although this treatment has a greater risk for non-melanoma skin carcinomas than nbUVB and the known side-effects of psoralen. Total skin electron beam (TSEB) is reserved for patients with extensive generalized disease and severe skin symptoms [4].

Systemic therapies are usually reserved for advanced disease [stage IIB – IV] or in less extensive disease [stage IB – IIA] that is refractory to skin-directed therapies (Table 25-2). Biological response modifying modifiers (BRMs), such as interferon (IFN) and retinoids, enhance the anti-tumor response and lack cumulative toxicity, but may take longer to act; most show partial response rates of around 50% [4]. Unfortunately, comparative trials are not yet available to guide the initial therapy choice.

Patients with additional poor prognostic factors can receive an intensified treatment regimen with a combination of skin-directed therapies or a combination of skin-directed plus systemic BRM agents. For example, patients with infiltrated plaques could be treated with PUVA to which either IFN-alpha or an oral retinoid can be added to shorten the course or achieve a complete response (Figure 25-1).

Radiation is used for single tumors, including transformed MF and ALCL. Patients with multiple cutaneous tumors [stage IIB] who fail combined PUVA and BRM may be treated with TSEB followed by maintenance therapy; however, denileukin diftitox (anti-CD25 immunotoxin, Ontak) or mono-chemotherapy agents (e.g. gemcitabine or doxil) may be very effective in debulking tumors. Young patients who have large cell transformation within 2 years of the initial MF diagnosis have a worse prognosis and could be considered for a non-ablative allogeneic stem cell transplant.

All patients with blood involvement should be considered for systemic therapy (Figure 25-2). Patients with Sézary syndrome (T4B2, stage IVA) have a worse prognosis and therefore require intensive systemic therapy, such as BRMs or antibody immunotherapy. In erythrodermic MF and SS, a combination of topical steroids, extracorporeal photopheresis (ECP), IFN-alpha +/- an oral retinoid gives a high response rate ranging from 57 to 100% overall response rate (ORR) and 13–80% complete response (CR) [7]. Second line therapy with the histone deacetylase (HDAC) inhibitor vorinostat (suberoylanilide hydroxamic acid, SAHA) has a response rate of 30%.

Patients with bulky lymph nodes or visceral disease may benefit from chemotherapy both as a primary therapy or salvage therapy. Gemcitabine and liposomal doxorubicin are two very active single agents with minimal toxicity and response rates of 70% and 80%, respectively. They are particularly effective for patients with tumors. Combination chemotherapy regimens are reserved for patients at stage IV and may be associated with worsening skin disease and infection. After tumor reduction occurs, maintenance therapy with BRMs (e.g., the retinoid bexarotene or IFN) should be considered to optimize response duration. As a general guideline, patients who later experience disease relapse after achieving a complete response generally respond well to the same regimen that had been previously successful [4].

Patients with MF often have severe, intractable pruritus and are frequently colonized with *Staphylococcus aureus*. Diligent skin care (i.e. acidification with vinegar rinses) is helpful, as are supportive anti-histamines, including gabapentin, or mirtazapine. Infections or even sepsis from loss of skin integrity or central lines are common. Cultures should be used to guide the choice of antibiotics and to treat methicillin-resistant *Staphylococcus aureus*. As patients become immunocompromised, as judged by their blood CD4 T cell count, they should be protected against opportunistic infections.

Nitrogen mustard, TSEB, and localized radiation therapy are treatment options for primary cutaneous anaplastic large cell lymphoma (cALCL) and lymphomatoid papulosis (LyP). For rare cases of cALCL and LyP that are refractory to topical treatments, anti-CD30 immunotherapy (e.g. SGN-30) or T-cell selective chemotherapy (e.g. pralatrexate) may be options.

Table 25-2. General systemic therapies for CTCL.

Treatment	Mechanism of action	Recommended stage	Dosing	Response	Side effects
Interferons (IFNs) IFN-alpha (α) [8] IFN-beta IFN-gamma	Antiproliferative Cytotoxic ↑TH1 immune response	Second line tx for relapsed or refractory skin disease Sézary syndrome	IFN-alpha: 1-5 million units SQ 3x/week Optimal combination with PUVA (T1, T2) or ECP (T4)	IFN-α alone: ORR: 54%, CR: 17% IFN-α ± PUVA: ORR:90–96%, CR:62–80% Better response in earlier stages	Flu-like symptoms Leukopenia Thrombocytopenia Hepatitis, diarrhea Fatigue, hypothyroidism Mental status changes
Oral Retinoids (Isotretin, Acitetin, Etretinate) [7,8]	Ligands for RAR + RXR retinoid receptors that form nuclear transcription complexes	Second line tx for relapsed or refractory skin disease Sézary syndrome	Combine with PUVA = Combine with ECP / IFN	Alone: ORR: 50% With PUVA: same as PUVA alone With IFN-alpha: ORR: 60%, CR: 11%	Dryness Alopecia Arthritis Hepatitis Bone spurs Central hypothyroidism Hyperlipidemia Pancreatitis
Oral Rexinoids (Bexarotene) [7]	Ligands for RXR retinoid receptors only to form nuclear transcription complexes Alters T-cell trafficking to shift them from the skin to the periphery (154)	Any stage Large cell transformation	Bexarotene 300 mg/m²/day Can combine with PUVA, ECP, IFN, and denileukin difitox Keep free T4 normal with synthroid dose Use lipid lowering agents, but NOT gemfibrozil	Dose-dependentEarly stage ORR: >300 mg/m²/day: 67% <300 mg/m²/day: 54% Late stage ORR: >300 mg/m²/day: 55% <300 mg/m²/day: 45%	Headache Asthenia Pruritus Leukopenia
Extracorporeal Photopheresis (ECP) [8]	Phototherapy with leukopheresis (photoactivated 8-MOP crosslinks DNA after ex vivo UVA irradiation; then reinfused into pt) Exact MOA unknown	Erythrodermic MF Sézary Syndrome Stage III and IV MF Maintenance tx after TSEB Do before chemotherapy as requires intact immune system	Two consecutive days of tx weekly to monthly Combine with IFN +/- bexarotene	Alone:ORR: 20–88%, CR: 14–25%	Increased erythema x 24 h Injection site ecchymosis
HDAC inhibitors (Class I – IV) [9,10]	Block deacetylation of histones that contain tumor suppressors and cell cycle regulatory genes, leading to apoptosis	Late stage Relapsed/refractory MF Clinical radiation sensitizers/protectors	Vorinostat: 400 mg PO daily (FDA approved) Belinostat[a] Panobinostat[a] Romidepsin [depsipeptide][a]	Vorinostat: ORR: 24–30 Romidepsin: ORR: 34%	Thrombocytopenia GI symptoms Dehydration Fatigue Altered taste Pulmonary embolism Heart block
Pralatrexate [10][a]	Competitive antagonist for dihydrofolate reductase → stops DNA/RNA synthesis; greater affinity or internalization than methotrexate	cALCL/LyP Late stages MF	Give with folic acid daily and B12 shots q6-8 weeks 10–30 mg/m² weekly	ORR: 50%	Thrombocytopenia Ulcerative stomatitis Diarrhea/vomiting Acute pneumonitis

[a]Denotes experimental use

tx treatment; CR complete response; PUVA psoralen and ultraviolet A; TSEB total skin electron beam; HDAC histone deacetylase; LyP lymphomatoid papulosis; cALCL primary cutaneous anaplastic large cell lymphoma; ECP extracorporeal photopheresis; AMS altered mental status; CMI cell-mediated immunity; ORR overall response rate; 8-MOP 8-methoxypsoralen; pt patient; tx treatment

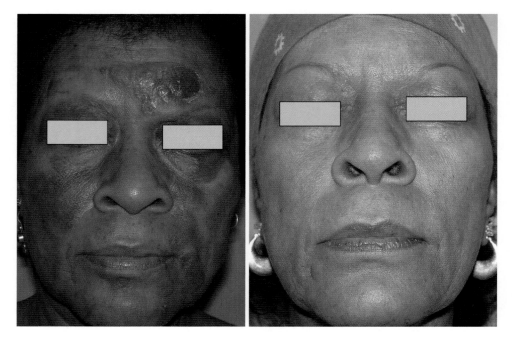

Fig. 25-1. Patient with extensive MF plaques who showed complete resolution of skin disease on PUVA and bexarotene treatment over 2 years

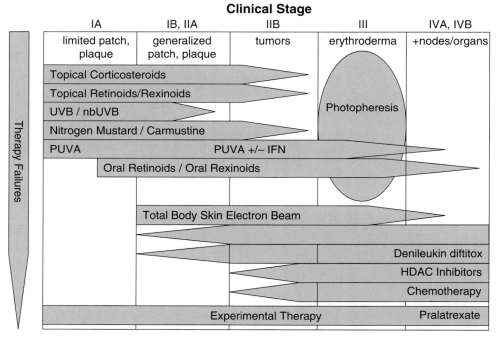

Fig. 25-2. Treatment map for newly-diagnosed and therapy-resistant MF. Abbreviations as in Table25-1

25.4. Assessing Response to Treatment

Treatment response should be measured in all compartments: skin (by SWAT), blood (by flow cytometry), lymphadenopathy (by CT or PET), and pruritus [by visual analog scale (VAS) scale]. To achieve a partial response (PR) (i.e. 50% improvement from baseline), the skin SWAT must improve to PR, and with no worsening of disease at other sites. Complete remissions (CR) with no clinical evidence of disease, or biopsy-confirmed CRs are rare and difficult to achieve in patients at advanced stage. Metrics for measurement of progressive disease (PD) remain controversial but PD should be considered whenever there is >25% worsening from original baseline (if no PR has been reached), or for patients who have had a prior PR but subsequently progressed.

Blood involvement can be assessed by serial flow cytometry. A 50% decrease in the absolute CD4 T-cell count or in the percentage of CD4+/CD26- T cells is considered a PR. Rising absolute numbers of CD8+ T cells or decrease in the CD4 to CD8 ratios are usually favorable prognostic indicators. Lymph node responses are difficult to determine by clinical exam alone but can be measured by serial CT scans or full body PET/CT scans more accurately. Symptomatic relief or exacerbation can be measured through quality of life instruments or by the patient's subjective grading (on a scale of 1–10) of pain, pruritus, and general well being.

25.5. Experimental Therapeutics for CTCL

New treatments that have received FDA approval in the past 10 years include denileukin diftitox, bexarotene, romidepsin, and vorinostat. However, all patients with disease refractory to multiple treatments should be considered candidates for clinical trials. For skin-directed therapy, two formulations of topical nitrogen mustard are currently under investigation. The

Table 25-3. Targeted systemic therapies for CTCL.

Treatment	Mechanism of action	Recommended stage	Dosing	Response	Side effects
Denileukin diftitox (Ontak®) [10]–[12]	Recombinant IL-2-diptheria toxin fusion protein targeted to IL-2 receptor on T lymphocytes → endocytosed → inhibits protein synthesis	Failed IFN/bexarotene- Have tumors and nodes CD25 positivity >20%	Pre-medicate w/ steroids to ↓ hypersensitivity Saline bolus after dose Dose: 9 or 18 mcg/kg	ORR 30–60%, CR 10% No clear difference between doses	Capillary leak syndrome Constitutional symptoms Hypersensitivity rash Thrombosis-related events Infusion reactions
Alemtuzumab [8] (Campath-H1 ®)[a]	Anti-CD52 monoclonal antibody that targets T and B lymphocytes.	Sézary syndrome Erythrodermic MF NOT useful for tumors or lymphadenopathy	3, 5, 10, 30 mg/kg IV/SQ	ORR 50–70% [13] CR 25%	Immunosuppression → CMV reactivation + opportunistic infections Arrhythmias Flu-like symptoms Tumor lysis syndrome
Zanolimumab [14] (HuMax-CD4 ®)	Anti-CD4 monoclonal antibody that blocks receptor-mediated T-cell signaling + cell-mediated toxicity of CD4+ T lymphocytes	Erythrodermic MF Sézary syndrome	Doses in trials: 280 mg/m^2 560 mg/m^2 980 mg/m^2	ORR: 280 mg/m^2 = 25% 980 mg/m^2 = 75%	Immunosuppression → reactivation of CMV + opportunistic infections
SGN-30 [15][a]	Anti-CD30 monoclonal antibody	CD30+ MF with large cell transformation cALCL/LyP	Short infusions q2–3 weeks	ORR 87%	Immunosuppression → reactivation of CMV + opportunistic infections
Forodesine [16] (BCX-1777 ®)[a]	Inhibits purine nucleoside phosphorylase (PNP) Requires cyclin-dependent kinase (CDK)	Refractory MF Failed 3 other systemic tx	Optimal dose: 80 mg/m^2 IV	ORR: 37%	Diarrhea Fluid retention

[a]Denotes experimental use

cALCL primary cutaneous anaplastic large cell lymphoma; *LyP* lymphomatoid papulosis; *tx* treatments

most exciting class of agents under investigation are the HDAC inhibitors which seem to be generally active in CTCL. In addition to the newly-approved oral agents romidepsin and vorinostat, two other inhibitors, panibinostat, and belinostat, are also being tested. Targeted therapies (e.g. antibodies, fusion toxins, or specific enzyme inhibition by small molecules) offer the hope of greater response rates without toxicity. In particular, the PNP inhibitor forodesine, the AKT inhibitor enzastaurin, and the tumor necrosis factor pathway inhibitor revlimid have also been studied in oral formulations. Targeted antibodies against CD52 (Campath H1) and CD4 (Humax-CD4) are active, but may be too immunosuppressive for use in MF (Table 25-3).

25.6. The Role of Stem Cell Transplantation in CTCL

Non-ablative, allogeneic hematopoietic stem cell transplant (HSCT) has been used in a limited number of CTCL patients but is promising since there may be a demonstrable graft-versus-T-cell lymphoma effect [17]. Therefore, HSCT should be considered in young healthy patients with advanced disease (i.e. stage IIB – IV) that is refractory to all primary and salvage therapy options, and who have matched donors. Limited data suggest the potential for long-term remissions and curative outcomes,[17] however the timing of transplant remains controversial. Exposing patients to the required immunosuppression is not advisable for patients with early stage MF given their good prognosis. However, delaying HSCT until after the patient's disease has advanced and is rapidly progressive, raises the risk of infection, rapid relapse, and death. We have found that the use of non-immunosuppressive monochemotherapy (if needed) followed by TSEB to debulk the skin disease is helpful to obtain preparing the patient undergoing transplant to obtain the best response.

Suggested Readings

Olsen E., Vonderheid E., Pimpinelli N., Willemze R., Kim Y., Knobler R., Zackheim H., Duvic M., Estrach T., Lamberg S., Wood G., Dummer R., Ranki A., Burg G., Heald P., Pittelkow M., Bernengo M. G., Sterry W., Laroche L., Trautinger F., and Whittaker S. (2007) Revisions to the staging and classification of mycosis fungoides and Sézary syndrome: a proposal of the International Society for Cutaneous Lymphomas (ISCL) and the cutaneous lymphoma task force of the European Organization of Research and Treatment of Cancer (EORTC) *Blood* **110(6)**, 1713-22.

Horwitz S. M., Olsen E. A., Duvic M., Porcu P., Kim Y. H. (2008) Review of the treatment of mycosis fungoides and Sezary syndrome: A stage-based approach *J Natl Compr Canc Netw* **6(4)**, 436-42.

References

1. Tan RS, Butterworth CM, McLaughlin H, Malka S, Samman PD. Mycosis fungoides: a disease of antigen persistence Br J Dermatol 1974;91:607–16.
2. Olsen EA, Bunn PA Jr. Interferon in the treatment of cutaneous T-cell lymphoma. Hematol Oncol Clin NorthAm 1995;9:1089–107.
3. Olsen E, Vonderheid E, Pimpinelli N, et al. Revisions to the staging and classification of mycosis fungoides and Sézary syndrome: a proposal of the International Society for Cutaneous Lymphomas (ISCL) and the cutaneous lymphoma task force of the European Organization of Research and Treatment of Cancer (EORTC). Blood 2007;110(6):1713–22.
4. Horwitz SM, Olsen EA, Duvic M, Porcu P, Kim YH. Review of the treatment of mycosis fungoides and Sezary syndrome: A stage-based approach J Natl Compr Canc Netw 2008;6(4):436–42.
5. Trautinger F, Knobler R, Willemze R, et al. EORTC consensus recommendations for the treatment of mycosis fungoides/Sézary syndrome Eur J Cancer 2006;42:1014–30.
6. Berthelot C, Rivera A, Duvic M. Skin directed therapy for mycosis fungoides: a review. J Drug Dermatol 2008;7(7):655–66.
7. Zhang C, Duvic M. Treatment of cutaneous T-cell lymphoma with retinoids dermatol therapy 2006;19:264–71.
8. Apisarnthanarax N, Talpur R, Duvic M. Treatment of cutaneous T cell lymphoma: current status and future directions. Am J Clin Dermatol 2002;3(3):193–215.

9. Duvic M, Talpur R, Ni X, et al. Phase II trial of oral vorinostat (suberoylanilide hydroxamic acid, SAHA) for refractory cutaneous T-cell lymphoma (CTCL). Blood 2007;109(1):31–9.

10. Horwitz SM. Novel therapies for cutaneous T-cell lymphomas. Clin Lymphoma Myeloma 2008;8(Suppl 5):S187–92.

11. Olsen EA, Duvic M, Frankel A, et al. Pivotal phase III trial of two dose levels of denileukin diftitox for the treatment of cutaneous T-cell lymphoma. J Clin Oncol 2001;19:376–88.

12. Chin KM, Foss FM. Biologic correlates of response and survival in patients with cutaneous T-cell lymphoma treated with denileukin diftitox. Clin Lymphoma Myeloma 2006;7(3):199–204.

13. Lundin J, Hagberg H, Repp R, et al. Phase 2 study of alemtuzumab (anti-CD52 monoclonal antibody) in patients with advanced mycosis fungoides/Sézary syndrome. Blood 2003;101:4267–72.

14. Kim YH, Duvic M, Obitz E, et al. Clinical efficacy of zanolimumab (HuMax-CD4): Two phase II studies in refractory cutaneous T-cell lymphoma. Blood 2007;109(11):4655–62.

15. Forero-Torres A, Bernstein SH, Gopal A. SGN-30 (Anti-CD30 mAb) has a single-agent response rate of 21% in patients with refractory or recurrent systemic anaplastic large cell lymphoma (ALCL). Blood 2006;108:768a. abstr 2718.

16. Kicska GA, Long L, Hörig H, et al. Immucillin H, a powerful transition state analog inhibitor of purine nucleoside phosphorylase selectively inhibits human T lymphocytes. Proc Nat Acad Sci USA 2001;98:4593–8.

17. Molina A, Zain J, Arber DA, et al. Durable clinical, cytogenetic, and molecular remissions after allogeneic hematopoietic cell transplantation for refractory Sezary syndrome and mycosis fungoides. J Clin Oncol 2005;23:6163–71.

Chapter 26

Histiocytic and Dendritic Cell Neoplasms

Kedar V. Inamdar and Dan Jones

Abstract/Scope of Chapter This chapter covers tumors of the monocytic and dendritic cell lineage and those that arise from the reticular network of lymph node and extranodal lymphoid tissues (i.e. Waldeyer's ring and gut lymphoid tissue), including follicular dendritic cell sarcoma and fibroblastic reticular cell sarcoma. Mature/fully-differentiated histiocytic/dendritic cell neoplasms include Langerhans cell histiocytosis, its malignant counterpart Langerhans cell sarcoma, and the related S100-negative histiocytoses. Immature malignancies in this group include myeloid and monocytic leukemia presenting first in extramedullary tissues, and the newly recognized blastic plasmacytoid dendritic cell neoplasm.

Keywords Histiocyte • Monocyte • Langerhans cell • Langerhans cell histiocytosis (LCH) • Eosinophilic granuloma • Langerhans cell sarcoma • Juvenile xanthogranuloma • Non-LC histiocytosis • Erdheim–Chester disease • Kikuchi–Fujimoto disease • Subacute necrotizing lymphadenitis • Sinus histiocytosis with massive lymphadenopathy (SHML) • Rosai–Dorfman disease • Hemophagocytic syndrome • Plasmacytoid dendritic cell • Blastic plasmacytoid dendritic cell neoplasm • Hematodermic tumor • Myeloid sarcoma • Histiocytic sarcoma • Extramedullary myeloid tumor • Chloroma • Follicular dendritic cell • Castleman disease, hyaline vascular type • Castleman disease, myoid tumor • Follicular dendritic cell sarcoma • Reticular cell • Reticular cell sarcoma • Interdigitating dendritic cell • Interdigitating dendritic cell sarcoma • Sarcoma, lymph node • Inflammatory myofibroblastic tumor

26.1. Introduction

No group of tumors better demonstrates the dangers of basing a classification on histogenesis before the relationships between normal cell lineages are clearly established than the histiocyte, dendritic cell (DC) and reticular cell neoplasms described here. There have been great advances in the understanding of DC biology in the last decade with the recognition of several new subsets, a reevaluation of the lineage differentiation schemes (Fig. 26-1), and increasing understanding that mature monocytic and DC subsets have great plasticity capable of functional redifferentiation under the influence of a variety of tissue microenvironments [1,2]. This naturally has led to a reevaluation of the boundaries and proper nomenclature for tumors derived from these cells. Since there is still minimal understanding of the resident stromal cell populations in secondary lymphoid tissues, nodal stromal tumor classification will likely continue to undergo refinement in the coming years.

From: *Neoplastic Hematopathology*: Contemporary Hematology,
Edited by: D. Jones, DOI 10.1007/978-1-60761-384-8_26,
© Humana Press, a part of Springer Science+Business Media, LLC 2010

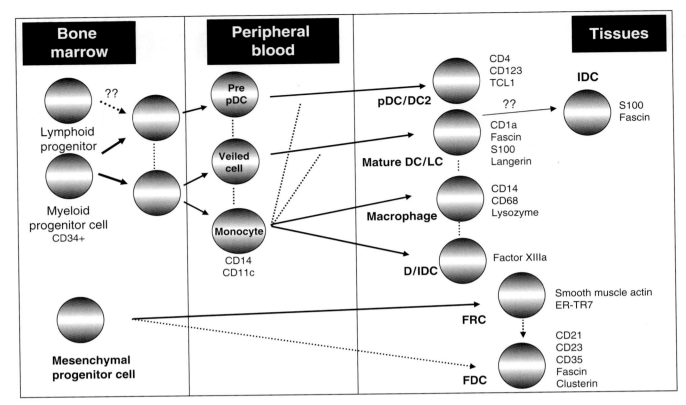

Fig. 26-1. Schematic of histiocytic, dendritic cell, and LN stromal cell types. The postulated cell of origin and interrelationship of various ancillary immune cell types is based in vitro differentiation data. Abbreviations are *pDC* plasmacytoid dendritic cell, *LC* Langerhans cell, *IDC* interdigitating dendritic cells, *I/DDC* interstitial/dermal dendritic cells, *FDC* follicular dendritic cell, and *FRC* fibroblastic reticular cell

26.2. Stromal and Dendritic Cell Biology and Their Relationship to Tumor Types

Monocytes represent the bone marrow-derived precursors of the antigen-processing, antigen-presenting and biosynthetic populations of tissue-associated macrophages and histiocytes. Most blood-derived and mucosal dendritic cell populations are also closely related to monocytes since these populations can be derived from each other following in vitro culture with different growth factors such as FLT3 ligand and granulocyte-macrophage colony stimulating factor (GM-CSF). Langerhans cells (LCs) are one particularly well-studied population of antigen-presenting dendritic cells that normally reside along the basal layer of the skin. When activated by antigen, they migrate within hours to regional lymph nodes via lymphatics in association with lymphocytes.

The plasmacytoid dendritic cell precursor in blood (pDC, previously known as the lymphoid DC) and its mature "DC2" form found in lymph node and mucosal sites (previously known as the plasmacytoid monocyte) comprise interferon-producing cell populations that show a different marker profile from other DC types [3,4] The pDC/DC2 lineage cells function predominantly in viral immunity and recent evidence suggests that they may be related developmentally to bone marrow monocytic precursors as well.

The normal biology and histogenesis of the non-motile lymph node stromal elements have, by comparison, attracted relatively little attention. The origin of follicular dendritic cells (FDC), the cell type that traps and presents antigen to B cells and helper T cells in the germinal center, is still under study, but local differentiation from the pre-existing fibroblastic reticular cell (FRC) network is favored. As discussed in Chapter 12, FRCs extend from the subcapsular sinus to the high endothelial venules in the lymph node hilum providing two closely opposed corridors for solute and cell trafficking. The histogenesis of the S100+ interdigitating dendritic cells (IDCs) and the possibly related factor XIII+ interstitial/dermal dendritic cells (I/DDC) is not clear but they could evolve either from localized nodal stromal populations or more likely from variably differentiated migrating DC populations [5]. The most useful paraffin-section antibody markers for each histiocytic, DC, and stromal cell population are summarized in Table 26-1. The term "histiocyte" is occasionally used to refer to all types of the dendritic cell/monocytic lineage.

Tumors arising from the supporting stroma of lymph node and the antigen-presenting DC and histiocytic cells are rare when compared with lymphomas. The reasons for this are likely related to the low proliferative capacity of many of these cell types when compared with the marked and rapid expansions of lymphocytes thus providing expanded pools of cells that might undergo neoplastic transformation. Also, DC, LC and histiocytes are terminally differentiated cell types and thus transformation and tumor formation in these lineages much more commonly occur in immature precursors and present as monocytic or mixed lineage leukemias (Table 26-2).

Table 26-1. Immunohistochemical profile of dendritic cell, histiocyte and stromal cell types.

Cell type	Immunohistochemical marker															
	CD45	CD21	CD23	CD35	S100	CD1a	Langerin	Fascin	Clusterin	CD68	CD123	CD163	CD4	FXIIIa	TCL1	Lysozyme
LC	+	−	−	−	+	+	+	LCH only[a]	−	+	−	−	+	−	−	+/−
IDC	+	−	−	−	+	−	−	+	−/+	+/−	−	−	+	−	−	−
Macrophage or histiocyte	+	−	−	+/−	+/−	−	−	+/−	−	+	−	+	+	−	−	+
I/DDC	+	−	−	−	−/+	−	−	+	−	+	−	−	+/−	+	−	−
pDC	+	−	−	−	−	−	−	−	−	+	+	−	+	−	+	−
FDC[a]	−	+	+	+	+/−	−	−	+	+	−/+	−	−	+	v	−	−
FRC	+	−	−	−	−	−	−	−	−	+	−	−	−	−	−	−

LC Langerhans, *IDC* interdigitating dendritic cells, *I/DDC* interstitial/dermal dendritic cells, *pDC* plasmacytoid dendritic cell, *FDC* follicular dendritic cell, and *FRC* fibroblastic reticular cell

Immunostaining graded as +: strongly positive; +/−: subset positive; −/+: focally positive; −: negative; v: variable staining and as in text.
[a]*FDC* may accumulate antigens on their surface released by other cells including CD20, CD45, and immunoglobulins from B cells

Table 26-2. Classification of histiocytic, dendritic cell and lymph node stromal cell tumors.

Monocyte and/or dendritic cell origin	Stromal tumors involving secondary lymphoid tissues
Terminally differentiated tumors	Follicular dendritic cell sarcoma
Langerhans cell histiocytosis	Inflammatory pseudo-tumor-like variant (liver/spleen)
Langerhans cell sarcoma	
Non-Langerhans cell histiocytosis	Tumors arising out of HVCD
Juvenile xanthogranuloma group	Stromal-rich variant of HVCD
Non-JXG group	Myoid tumor
Histiocytic sarcoma	Fibroblastic reticular cell tumor/sarcoma
	Inflammatory myofibroblastic tumor
Mixed/immature/primitive tumors	*Indeterminate cell types*
Extramedullary myeloid tumors	Interdigitating dendritic cell sarcoma
AML, CML, CMML	
Blastic plasmacytoid dendritic cell neoplasm	

JXG juvenile xanthogranuloma, *AML* acute myeloid leukemia, *CML* chronic myelogenous leukemia, *CMML* chronic myelomonocytic leukemia, *HVCD* hyaline vascular Castleman disease

26.3. Mature Histiocytic and Dendritic Cell Tumors

26.3.1. Langerhans Cell Histiocytosis

26.3.1.1. Incidence, Demographics and Clinical Features

LCH, previously known as *histiocytosis X*, comprises several clinicopathologic entities having clonal proliferation of tumor cells with morphologic, immunophenotypic and ultrastructural features of Langerhans cells. Recognized variants of LCH include localized lesions (solitary eosinophilic granuloma), unisystem multifocal disease (Hand-Schüller-Christian Disease), multifocal multisystem disease (Letterer-Siwe disease), and the Hashimoto–Pritzker syndrome (spontaneously resolving cutaneous LCH seen in infants). Other synonyms for LCH variants include self-healing histiocytosis, pure cutaneous histiocytosis, Langerhans cell granulomatosis, and Type II histiocytosis [6].

Depending on the subtype, LCH has a broad age range, but is most common in male children between 1–4 years, with an overall incidence of 2–5 new cases per million per year. Children are more likely to present with involvement of multiple organ systems, including bone, skin, liver, spleen, lung, and lymph node, whereas in adults LCH is often localized to a single organ. In contrast, the multifocal/multisystem presentation of LCH is mostly seen in adults and in very young children. Primary pulmonary LCH which occurs predominantly in adult female smokers, [7] may be a reactive lesion since some cases regress with smoking cessation, and only one third are reported to be clonal [8].

Regardless of its mode of presentation, LCH most frequently involves the skeletal system in particular bones of skull, mandible, femur, pelvis and vertebrae. Besides constitutional symptoms, such as fever, weight loss, malaise and night sweats, signs and symptoms depend on the organ system involved and thus may include, but are not limited to rash or cutaneous tumor nodules, pancytopenia, hepatosplenomegaly, and diabetes insipidus [7].

26.3.1.2. Pathologic Features

LCH, at any site, is characterized by a proliferation of LC with their characteristic pale eosinophilic cytoplasm and reniform, indented, grooved or folded nucleus in a polymorphous background composed of neutrophils, eosinophils, small histiocytes, lymphocytes, and multinucleated giant cells. Sometimes eosinophils can be so numerous that the lesions resemble eosinophilic abscesses. Cytologic atypia is minimal and generally the appearance is that of a bland-appearing benign histiocytic proliferation. Within the lymph node, LC primarily involves the sinuses (Fig. 26-2), with extracapsular extension usually only seen

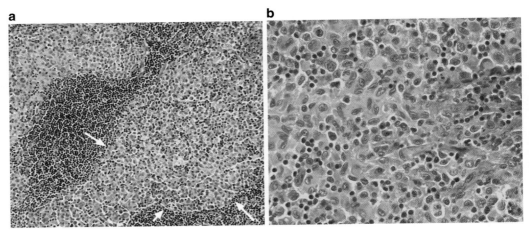

Fig. 26-2. Langerhans cell histiocytosis, lymph node. (**a**) Intrasinusoidal infiltrate of Langerhans cells, eosinophils and small lymphocytes. (**b**) Nuclear grooves in tumor cells are apparent on high magnification

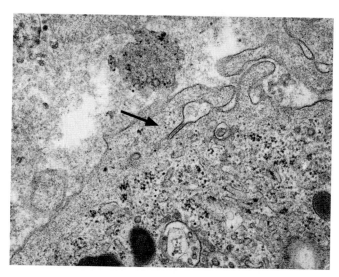

Fig. 26-3. Birbeck granules in LCH. Electron microscopy reveals an intracellular striated Birbeck granule with bulbous shape at one end (tennis racquet-shaped inclusion, *arrow*) Photograph courtesy of Bruce Jones, MD

in widely disseminated cases. Splenic lesions preferentially involve red pulp whereas in the liver the Langerhans cells plug intrahepatic biliary ducts leading to sclerosing cholangitis.

26.3.1.3. Laboratory Testing for Diagnosis

LCH must be strongly positive for at least one specific LC marker such as langerin (CD207) or CD1a and also positive for CD68, S-100, and vimentin, and negative (or dim) for the histiocyte marker lysozyme. LCH is negative for B-cell, T-cell, and FDC markers [9,10] but is positive for fascin unlike nonneoplastic LC [11]. Ultrastructural demonstration of *Birbeck granules*, which are elongated membranous bodies with a striated appearance and a bulbous tip shaped like a tennis racquet, can also confirm the diagnosis (Fig. 26-3).

LCH in all forms except possibly localized pulmonary presentations (Fig. 26-4) are clonal proliferations, as determined by the human androgen receptor (HUMARA) X-chromosome inactivation assay [12]. Genomic analysis of LCH have not yet shown a characteristic chromosomal abnormality, with CGH often showing losses on chromosomes 1p, 5, 6, 7, 9, 16, 17, and 22q, and gains on chromosomes 2q, 4q, and 12 [13]. A recent whole genome gene expression by the SAGE technique has identified several genes known to be highly expressed in Langerhans cells such as CD1A, LYZ, and CD207 (langerin), in addition to other genes not previously known to be expressed, such as GSN, MMP12, CCL17, and CCL2 [14].

26.3.1.4. Differential Diagnosis

Nodal LCH must be differentiated from other tumors with sinusoidal infiltration and from reactive histiocytic-DC disorders, including Rosai-Dorfman disease (sinus histiocytosis with massive lymphadenopathy, SHML), Kikuchi's disease (subacute necrotizing lymphadenitis) and dermatopathic lymphadenitis. Some immune regulatory disorders such as macrophage activation or hemophagocytic syndromes may have large numbers of sinus histiocytes (with variable hemophagocytosis), but they have an acute presentation and/or association with Epstein-Barr virus infection. SHML, discussed in more detail below, is characterized by sheets of large histiocytes with occasionally vacuolated cytoplasm and rounded nuclei that lack nuclear grooves and Birbeck granules, and show lymphocyte emperipolesis. Kikuchi's disease, which shows zonal collections of crescentic histiocytes (with C-shaped nuclei) with associated karyorrhexis without neutrophils, is a self-limited lymphadenitis occurring mostly in younger women that may be related to autoimmune diseases such as lupus. Dermatopathic-type lymphadenitis is LN

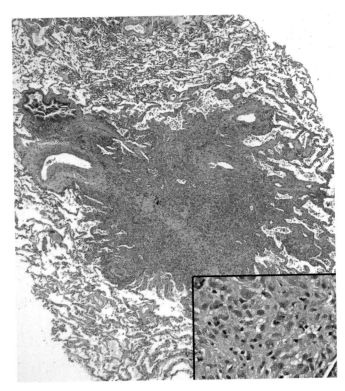

Fig. 26-4. Langerhans cell histiocytosis, lung. (**a**) Stellate lesions invading into lung parenchyma shows a mixed infiltrate of LCs and numerous eosinophils (*inset*). Photograph courtesy of Roberto Miranda, MD

engorgement due to increased DC drainage where LCs can be quite prominent, but there are usually admixed melanin-laden and/or hemosiderin-laden histiocytes and minimal distortion of the LN architecture. Among tumors, metastatic well-differentiated carcinoma and CD30+ anaplastic large cell lymphoma (ALCL) should be considered because of their preferential sinusoidal pattern of lymph node infiltration.

The pulmonary form of LCH needs to be distinguished from histiocyte-rich reactive lesions such as sarcoidosis as well as tuberculosis and fungal infections. The differential diagnosis of bone LCH includes myeloma, metastatic carcinoma, infections, and chronic osteomyelitis.

26.3.1.5. Prognosis and Treatment

Prognosis of LCH is dictated by clinical stage at presentation. Single organ disease has an excellent prognosis with long-term survival rates over 95%. With the involvement of multiple organ systems, the mortality rate rises sharply and multisystem multifocal disease carries the worst prognosis. Factors predictive of disease progression and poor prognosis include involvement of multiple systems at presentation, more than 3 bone lesions, hepatosplenomegaly, and failure to respond to chemotherapy. Age at presentation does not significantly influence prognosis except in cases of multiorgan presentations, as children younger that 3 years have high mortality [7,15].

The choice of treatment is based on the pattern of disease presentation. Skin disease may be treated with topical steroids while solitary bone lesions may be subjected to curetting with or without steroids, or localized radiation. Single or multi-agent chemotherapy is reserved for multisystem multifocal disease [16].

26.3.2. Langerhans Cell Sarcoma

Langerhans cell sarcoma (LCS), also known as malignant histiocytosis X, is a rare entity with approximately 20 cases reported to date. LCS, which may be defined as a tumor with LC immunophenotype and appearance but having high mitotic rate, and anaplastic cytologic features, is usually seen in lymph nodes and skin but may also affect liver, spleen and lung [17,18]. The immunophenotype should be similar to LCH (CD1a+, S100+, langerin+) and at least some cells should have the characteristic LC features with grooved nuclei and/or Birbeck granules. LCS is reported to be an aggressive malignancy with a high mortality rate, despite aggressive treatments.

26.3.3. Interdigitating Dendritic Cell (IDC) Sarcoma

IDC sarcoma is an exceedingly rare primary nodal neoplasm that appears to be histogenetically related to the S100+ IDC populations of lymph node which may be derived from LC. IDC sarcoma has been reported most commonly in older males with median age of 71 years; however, pediatric cases have also been reported in a single series [19,20]. Localized lymphadenopathy is most common, however extranodal presentation involving liver, spleen, skin, soft tissue, nasopharynx, testis and gastrointestinal tract has been reported. Constitutional symptoms such as fatigue, weight loss, and night sweats can occur in rare cases.

IDC sarcoma shows complete to partial paracortical replacement of the LN by fascicles or whorls of spindled cells, with a background of small lymphocytes (Figure 26-5). Some cases will show areas of tumor more closely resembling LC or histiocytes. By definition, tumor cells are uniformly positive for S-100 and are negative for CD1a, CD163, and FDC markers (CD21, CD23 and CD35), but can show variable expression of CD11c, CD14, CD45, CD68, HLA-DR, and vimentin. IDC sarcomas lack clonal IgH or TCR gene rearrangements. Distinction from FDC sarcoma is based on lack of expression of FDC markers and the absence of well-formed desmosomes by electron microscopy. Metastatic desmoplastic melanoma and sarcomatoid carcinoma represent important diagnoses of exclusion.

IDC sarcoma behaves more aggressively than FDC sarcoma, with 35–40% mortality within 1–2 years from the initial diagnosis. Bulky disease at presentation, extranodal spread and involvement of CNS are reported as poor prognostic indicators. Treatment is quite variable as in FDC sarcoma and has included a combination of surgery, chemotherapy and radiation.

26.3.4. Non-LC Mature Histiocytic Tumors

The classification of systemic non-LC histiocytoses is confusing and needs improvement. This category includes tumors that resemble LCH clinically, with bone, LN, and cutaneous

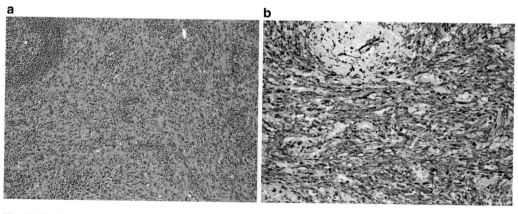

Fig. 26-5. Interdigitating dendritic cell sarcoma. (**a**) Interfollicular malignant spindle cell infiltrate with admixed small lymphocytes. (**b**) S100 immunostain is diffusely positive

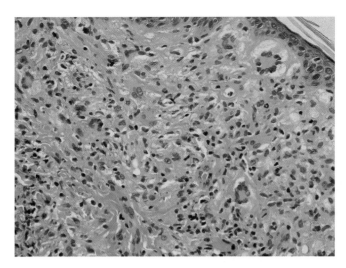

Fig. 26-6. Juvenile xanthogranuloma. Dermal infiltrate of Touton-type giant cells and foamy histiocytes

involvement, but are negative for CD1a and S100. These can occur both in children and adults and likely are a mixture of genetically-determined and acquired neoplastic lesions. Like LCH, there are three modes of presentation, including cutaneous lesions only, skin involvement with systemic disease, or predominantly extracutaneous presentation.

Juvenile xanthogranuloma (JXG) is a dermal-based nodular proliferation of round to spindle-shaped histiocytes that have a background of inflammatory cells and admixed Touton-type (wreath-like nuclei) giant cells (Fig. 26-6) [21–23]. Foamy histiocytes are common at the periphery of JXG nodules. JXG histiocytes are positive for CD14, CD68 (PGM1 clone), CD163, factor XIIIa, and fascin but lack CD1a, S100, and langerin. The classical presentation of JXG occurs in childhood at a median age of 24 months. Neurofibromatosis type I and juvenile myelomonocytic leukemia can sometimes occur in association with JXG suggesting a genetic origin. However, the clonal origin of these lesions has not been well studied.

Other non-LC histiocytoses include benign cephalic histiocytosis (cutaneous lesions in the head and neck region of young children), generalized eruptive histiocytosis (multiple cutaneous lesions in non-hyperlipidemic patients), progressive nodular histiocytosis (multiple cutaneous nodules with spindled histiocytes), xanthoma disseminatum (visceral, mucosal involvement in addition to skin in young adults) and the systemic Erdheim-Chester disease (bilateral multifocal osseous lesions and often lung involvement). There have not been enough studies to fully understand the clinical behavior and pathogenetic features of any of these disorders, but an indolent and relapsing course is common. Cases with multiple lesions and/or CNS involvement can occasionally be fatal. Besides LCH and ALCL, the differential diagnoses for many of these lesions include immunodeficiency states producing poorly formed granulomas, and B-cell disorders such as lymphomatoid granulomatosis.

26.3.5. Histiocytic Sarcoma (HS)

HS refers to a cytologically malignant neoplasm with the morphologic and immunophenotypic features of mature histiocytes. If extramedullary presentation of acute monocytic leukemia is excluded, these tumors are extremely rare and limited data in the modern era exists on their clinical course and optimal treatments [24]. The true incidence of this tumor is unclear since it has now been reported that some cases of HS may actually represent poorly differentiated B-cell malignancies that have lost multiple B-cell antigens or differentiated from common stem/precursor cells. In some of these cases, usually occurring in patients with follicular lymphoma, both tumors have been shown to be clonally related [25,26].

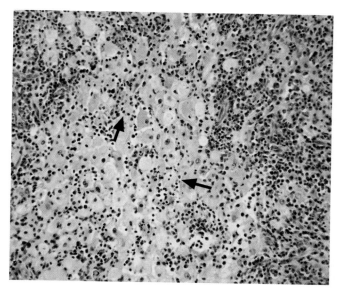

Fig. 26-7. Rosai–Dorfman disease. Lymph node expanded by a proliferation of large histiocytes with pale cytoplasm containing intact lymphocytes (*arrows*)

26.3.6. Sinus Histiocytosis with Massive Lymphadenopathy (Rosai–Dorfman Disease)

SHML, originally described by Juan Rosai and Ronald Dorfman, [27] is a tumor-forming lesion of reactive, activated histocytes characterized by often massive sheet-like collections of large distended clear to pink histiocytes with some cytoplasmic vacuoles and intact lymphocytes within their cytoplasm (emperipolesis) (Fig. 26-7). Lesions at extranodal sites, usually involving soft tissue, often show more fibrosis and less frequent emperipolesis. The histiocytes of SHML are positive for CD68, CD163, and S100 but lack expression of CD1a [9,28].

The most common presenting symptom in SHML is painless lymphadenopathy, frequently in the cervical region followed by axillary, mediastinal, and para-aortic sites. Extranodal sites of involvement include skin, upper respiratory tract, genitourinary tract, soft tissue, bone, and oral cavity. Clinically, constitutional symptoms are common as are coexisting immune regulatory disorders such as rheumatoid arthritis, polymyalgia rheumatica, asthma, and diabetes mellitus. Many patients also have chronic disease-type anemia, elevated white blood cell count and ESR, and polyclonal hypergammaglobulinemia suggesting a transient hyperimmune response possibly related to recurrent viral infections.

SHML is a non-clonal disorder [29] with spontaneous resolution occurring in the majority of patients. Various treatment strategies including steroids, antibiotics, single-agent chemotherapy or radiation have been tried and are usually reserved for cases that show organ dysfunction or that pose a high risk of mortality due to massive immune activation [30].

26.4. Extramedullary Immature Myeloid, Monocytic and Dendritic Cell Tumors

The terminology for immature myeloid, monocyte, and DC tumors presenting in extramedullary tissues is confusing with both old and new terms continuing to be in wide use. However, whatever name is used, this group of tumors is extremely important to recognize because of their aggressive course which nearly always terminates in leukemic dissemination if left untreated.

26.4.1. Extramedullary Myeloid Tumors (EMT)

EMT, also known as granulocytic sarcoma, myeloid sarcoma, or chloroma, is a discrete proliferation of blasts with or without maturing myeloid and/or monocytic precursors presenting at extramedullary sites, including skin, bone, lymph node, and gastrointestinal tract, in decreasing order of frequency [31,32]. Given the frequent absence of bone marrow or peripheral blood data, EMT is one of the most frequently misdiagnosed lesions, and should be considered whenever an immature mononuclear infiltrate of unclear origin is encountered (Fig. 26-8).

All types of myeloid and monocytic leukemias can present as an EMT including acute myeloid leukemia (AML) particularly of monocytic type, chronic myeloproliferative neoplasms (MPN) particularly chronic myeloid leukemia (CML), and myeloproliferative/myelodysplastic diseases particularly chronic myelomonocytic leukemia (CMML). However, there are particular patterns of EMT associated with each disease. CMML and acute monocytic leukemia have a high rate of skin and mucosal involvement often manifested clinically as gum hypertrophy, skin nodules, or palpable purpura [33]. Such lesions may precede bone marrow involvement by many months. EMT in CML frequently involves soft tissues of the extremities, is usually seen at time of relapse, and often heralds blast phase transformation.

The morphologic features of EMT are related to the underlying disorder but single cell infiltration in skin and mucosal biopsies is common, along with predilection for perivascular locations, and sparing of the epithelium. In LN, EMT infiltrates are initially interfollicular but may diffusely efface the node. Immunostaining with myeloid markers such as CD15, CD34, CD117, or myeloperoxidase (MPO), monocytic markers such as CD68 (KP1 and PGM1) and lysozyme, and megakaryocytic markers (CD61 and factor VIII-related antigen) are useful in paraffin sections to distinguish various EMT subtypes. It is important to consider that EMT cases like conventional AML can show expression of B-cell (CD19, CD20, CD22, and CD79a), T-cell (CD2, CD3, CD7) or natural killer (NK) cell markers (CD56). CD4 and CD43/Leu22 are expressed in both T cells and monocytes and should not be used as lineage-specific markers. EMT is usually treated identically to typical presentations of AML, CMML or MPNs, although radiotherapy may be used for refractory tumor lesions.

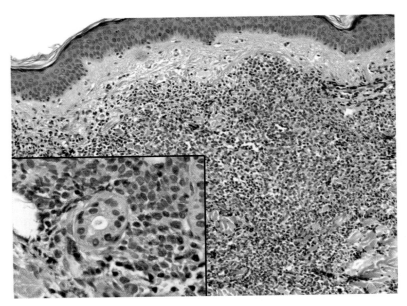

Fig. 26-8. Myeloid sarcoma. (**a**) Soft tissue infiltrate of blasts with a nested growth pattern. MPO and CD68 were both positive by IHC consistent with a myelomonocytic blast phenotype (not shown)

26.4.2. Blastic Plasmacytoid Dendritic Cell (BPDC) Neoplasm

BPDC neoplasm is a recently renamed tumor which arises from plasmacytoid dendritic cells or their precursors. The confusion surrounding the histogenesis and immunophenotype of this entity led to its reporting previously under various names including blastic NK-cell lymphoma, NK-cell leukemia/lymphoma, agranular CD4+ NK cell leukemia and CD4+, CD56+ hematodermic neoplasm.

26.4.2.1. Incidence, Demographics and Clinical Features

BPDC neoplasm can present in both children and adults, but has a median age of 67 years and is roughly 3 times more common in males [34,35]. Skin is the most common site of involvement (95–100%), followed by the bone marrow and peripheral blood (60–90%). Lymphadenopathy occurs in 50% while splenomegaly is seen in about 20% of cases. Skin lesions include solitary or multifocal patches, plaques, or bruises with or without ulceration. BM involvement originally manifests as cytopenias with only minimal tumor infiltration requiring immunophenotyping to detect, but usually rapidly progresses to leukemia if therapy is not promptly initiated. BPDC tumors may precede or occur concurrently with *isolated monocytosis* or myelodysplastic syndrome and may transform to acute myelomonocytic leukemia supporting the close relationship of the pDC lineage to myeloid precursors [36].

26.4.2.2. Pathologic Features

Skin lesions in BPDC neoplasm show sparing of epidermis with dermal involvement often in a perivascular or periadnexal pattern (Fig. 26-9); lymph node involvement is interfollicular to diffuse. Tumor cells are typically monomorphous but can range from medium-sized to large with immature blast-like chromatin and variably prominent nucleoli. Mitoses are often seen but necrosis and angioinvasion is uncommon. Involvement of bone marrow at presentation is often subtle and difficult to detect without the aid of immunostains, such as CD123 or TCL1. On smears and touch imprints, tumor cells often show small cytoplasmic vacuoles and bulbous cytoplasmic extensions (i.e. pseudopods).

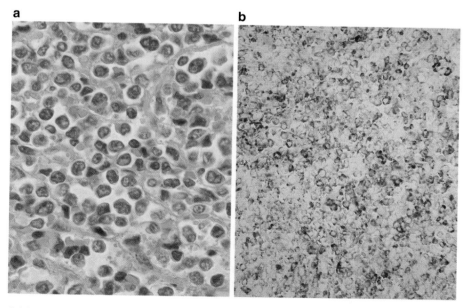

Fig. 26-9. Blastic plasmacytoid dendritic cell neoplasm. Dense dermal based tumor with periadnexal and perivascular accentuation. (**a**) Tumor cells are typically large with variably prominent nucleoli and blastoid chromatin (**b**) Uniform CD123 positivity is the most specific immunophenotypic finding

26.4.2.3. Laboratory Testing for Diagnosis

BPDC neoplasms express CD4 and CD56 along with more specific pDC markers such as CD123 (interleukin-3 receptor alpha chain) and BDCA-2 (blood dendritic cell antigen 2). Expression of TCL1 can help confirm the diagnosis in cases with weak expression of CD4, CD56, or CD123. CD43, CD45RA (4KB5 clone), and CD68 are positive in nearly all cases, and CD33 and CD7 are positive in a subset. TdT shows variable nuclear expression, which is often the strongest in lymph node. BPDC tumor cells are negative for B-cell (CD19, CD20), T-cell (CD3, CD5), and myelomonocytic antigens (CD34, CD117, myeloperoxidase and lysozyme).

Multiple chromosomal aberrations are quite common in BPDC and resemble those seen in high-risk AML, including deletion 5q, seen in 50–70%, followed by abnormalities of chromosome regions 12p13, 13q, 6q, 15q, and 9p, in decreasing order of frequency. Clonal immunoglobulin heavy chain gene rearrangements are absent, but occasional cases show clonal rearrangement of the T-cell receptor gamma chain by PCR.

26.4.2.4. Differential Diagnosis

The blastoid appearance and expression of TdT in BPDC neoplasm can be mistaken for lymphoblastic lymphoma, which lacks pDC markers such as CD123 and BDCA-2. Distinction from monocytic leukemias can also be quite challenging due to their common predilection for extramedullary infiltration, especially the skin, and their shared expression of CD4 and CD56. Some myelomonocytic leukemia cases may also weakly express CD123, however expression of TCL1 in BPDC tumors, and lysozyme in monocytic leukemias distinguishes the two entities. NK/T cell lymphoma usually enters the differential diagnosis because of CD56 expression; however, these latter lymphomas show angioinvasion and necrosis and are positive for cytoplasmic CD3 and EBV, and negative for CD123, BDCA-2, and TCL1.

26.4.2.5. Prognosis and Treatment

BPDC neoplasm has an extremely poor prognosis, with a median overall survival of 12–14 months. Expression of CD7 (and BDCA-2) may identify a more aggressive subgroup. Multiagent chemotherapy is effective in majority of cases however rapid relapses are very common, as is transformation to AML. The best responses to date have been seen with intensive mixed AML-lymphoma regimens followed by stem cell transplantation.

26.5. Lymph Node Stromal Tumors

Primary LN stromal tumors represent neoplasms that arise from resident stromal cell populations. FDC sarcoma was the first type identified almost 20 years ago, with extranodal presentations of similar tumors recognized soon thereafter. The association of FDC sarcoma with pre-existing, coincident or subsequent development of hyaline-vascular Castleman's disease (HVCD), [28] their shared phenotypic features, [29] and the presence of clonal genetic changes in HVCD[37] supports an origin of FDC sarcoma from dysplastic follicular dendritic cells. FRC sarcoma presumably arises from the reticular (fibroblastic) network. The 2008 WHO classification also lists an indeterminate dendritic cell tumor type for presumed primary lymph node stromal neoplasms with unclear histogenesis, but the category is too vague to warrant further discussion.

26.5.1. Follicular Dendritic Cell (FDC) Sarcoma

26.5.1.1. Incidence, Demographics and Clinical Features

FDC sarcoma presents in lymph nodes and extranodal sites, with Waldeyer's ring tissue (tonsil and oral cavity), gastrointestinal tract, soft tissue, liver, and spleen being the most common non-nodal sites in decreasing order of frequency [38–40]. Cervical and axillary lymph nodes are most frequently involved followed by supraclavicular, para-aortic, mesenteric, hilar, and mediastinal sites. Among the approximately 200 cases reported, there is an equal

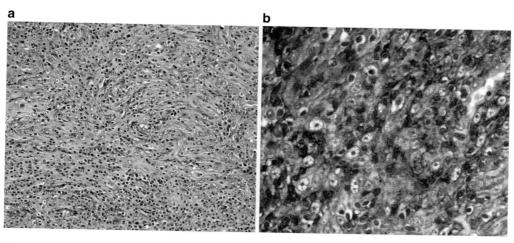

Fig. 26-10. Follicular dendritic cell sarcoma. (**a**) Spindle cell neoplasm arrayed in whorls. (**b**) CD21 immunostain

incidence among males and females, and a median age of 44 years at presentation. Patients usually present with a slow-growing, painless mass but abdominal tumors can be painful. Constitutional symptoms are rare and can include paraneoplastic pemphigus[41] or amyloidosis in cases arising from HVCD.

26.5.1.2. Pathologic Features

Both nodal and extranodal FDC sarcomas can show a variety of morphologic appearances which can complicate diagnosis. The classical appearance is that of whorls or storiform fascicles of spindle-shaped cells with abundant cytoplasm, ill-defined cell borders, and nuclear pseudoinclusions. Numerous small lymphocytes are usually sprinkled throughout the tumor (Fig. 26-10). Colonization of pre-existing germinal centers by tumor cells is common. Tumors with epithelioid, clear cell, myxoid, or anaplastic features are also commonly seen and some have bizarre or multinucleated Warthin-Finkeldey-like giant cells. Most cases will show a variety of different histologic appearances at different sites, with extranodal tumor implants often showing increased cellularity, loss of admixed lymphocytes, marked cytologic atypia, increased mitoses, or necrosis.

The inflammatory pseudotumor-like variant of FDC sarcoma, presents with abdominal symptoms and occurs almost exclusively in females. It has prominent lymphoplasmacytic cell infiltrate and the neoplastic spindle cells are difficult to identify without immunostains. Fibrin deposition can sometimes be found in the vessel walls within the tumor.

26.5.1.3. Laboratory Testing for Diagnosis

Once suspected, FDC sarcoma can be easily confirmed by immunostaining. The neoplastic cells of FDC sarcomas, like their normal counterparts, express CD21, CD23 and CD35, with two or more of these markers being positive in 90–95% of cases [9,42]. Other markers of FDC that can also be used include desmoplakin, EGFR, epithelial membrane antigen (EMA), fascin, podoplanin (D2-40 antibody), and the unclustered antibodies Ki-FDC1p, Ki-M4p, CNA 42 and R4/23. Ultrastructural studies will show interdigitating cytoplasmic processes and characteristic intercellular tight junctions or desmosomes. No defining genetic change has yet been associated with FDC sarcoma, but case reports have shown multiple clonal chromosomal aberrations [43,44].

26.5.1.4. Differential Diagnosis

The differential diagnosis of FDC sarcoma is broad, and includes melanoma and sarcomatoid carcinoma, the rare intranodal schwannoma/palisaded myofibroblastoma, and at extranodal sites, meningioma, thymoma, and gastrointestinal stromal tumor. The distinction between other nodal stromal tumors can also be difficult on morphologic grounds. FDC express HLA-DR, and are variably positive for CD68, S-100, and vimentin like other tumors in this differential, but FDC sarcomas are negative for Melan-A and HMB 45 (unlike melanoma), smooth muscle actin (unlike FRC sarcoma and IMT), and CAM5.2 cytokeratin (unlike FRC sarcoma).

Focal florid proliferations of dysplastic FDC characterize the *stromal-rich variant of HVCD* and may be the precursor lesion to FDC sarcoma. Such cases that show only small foci of dysplastic FDC but have other features of HVCD, such as vascular proliferation, regressed follicles and proliferations of reactive plasmacytoid DC, should be diagnosed as HVCD and not FDC sarcoma [45].

26.5.1.5. *Prognosis and Treatment*

The clinical behavior of FDC sarcoma has been poorly reported in the literature. In our experience, both nodal and extranodal cases have an initial behavior similar to lymphoma, with multifocal locoregional lymph node involvement and frequent relapses following surgical debulking or chemotherapy [46]. As progression occurs, FDC sarcomas usually invade into adjacent organs leading eventually to unresectable disease. Intra-abdominal location, large tumor size (greater than 6 cm), tumor cell pleomorphism, high mitotic activity, and necrosis have been reported as poor prognostic factors [38].

No standardized treatment protocol has yet been established for FDC sarcoma, and is greatly needed. Surgical excision alone is the treatment of choice for localized disease. A variety of treatment modalities including surgery, chemotherapy, and radiation, either alone or in combination have been utilized for recurrent or extensive disease. The combination of cyclophosphamide, daunorubicin, vincristine, and prednisone (CHOP) used for treatment of non-Hodgkin's lymphomas has been the most commonly employed.

26.5.2. Fibroblastic Reticular Cell (FRC) Sarcoma

FRC tumor/sarcoma has only been recently recognized as a distinct lymph node-based malignancy that morphologically resembles FDC sarcoma but lacks FDC markers [47,48]. Since a subpopulation of normal LN FRC express cytokeratin of types 18 and 8, detected by antibody CAM 5.2, it has been suggested that such cytokeratin expression in a LN stromal tumor may define the phenotype of this neoplasm. FRC sarcomas exhibit features of myofibroblasts in that they are positive for smooth muscle actin and vimentin, and variably positive for desmin and keratin 8/18, but are negative for CD21, CD23, CD35, CD1a, and S-100. Ultrastructurally, desmosomes are absent but variable myofibroblastic differentiation is seen, with fusiform densities, moderate amounts of rough endoplasmic reticulum, long cytoplasmic processes, tonofilaments, and basal lamina-like extracellular material. Cases with intermediate differentiation between FDC and FRC sarcoma have been reported. In the handful of reported cases, FRC sarcomas occurred mostly in male patients with cervical, epitrochlear, pulmonary hilar or mediastinal lymphadenopathy or splenic involvement and were associated with fever, pain, and night sweats. The clinical course has been quite variable and prognostic factors are not yet established. Surgery, either alone or in combination with adjuvant chemotherapy and/or radiation has been used.

26.5.3. Other myofibroblastic tumors presenting in lymphoid tissues

As with FDC proliferations, hyperplasia of FRC (i.e. stromal overgrowth) may be seen in Castleman's disease and can rarely produce discrete *myoid tumors*. Other spindle cell tumors with smooth muscle or myofibroblastic differentiation that have admixed lymphocytes, particularly inflammatory myofibroblastic tumor (IMT, formerly inflammatory pseudotumor) and leiomyosarcoma can present in lymphoid tissues and spleen. In IMT, the fibroblastoid tumor cells express ALK protein as a result of balanced chromosomal translocation involving the ALK gene locus on chromosome 2.

Selected Reviews

Pileri SA et al. Tumours of histiocytes and accessory dendritic cells: an immunohistochemical approach to classification from the International Lymphoma Study Group based on 61 cases. Histopathology 2002; 41:1–29.
- A comparison of the presenting features of this group of tumors.

Chan JK, et al. Follicular dendritic cell tumor. Clinicopathologic analysis of 17 cases suggesting a malignant potential higher than currently recognized. Cancer 1997; 79:294–313.
- The most complete clinicopathologic series on FDC sarcoma.

References

1. Swerdlow SH, Campo E, Harris NL, et al., eds. WHO classification of tumours of hematopoietic and lymphoid tissues. Lyon: IARC, 2008.
2. Ito T, Liu YJ, Kadowaki N. Functional diversity and plasticity of human dendritic cell subsets. Int J Hematol 2005;81:188–96.
3. Grouard G, Rissoan MC, Filgueira L, Durand I, Banchereau J, Liu YJ. The enigmatic plasmacytoid T cells develop into dendritic cells with interleukin (IL)-3 and CD40-ligand. J Exp Med 1997;185:1101–11.
4. Cella M, Jarrossay D, Facchetti F, et al. Plasmacytoid monocytes migrate to inflamed lymph nodes and produce large amounts of type I interferon. Nat Med 1999;5:919–23.
5. Angel CE, Chen CJ, Horlacher OC, et al. Distinctive localization of antigen-presenting cells in human lymph nodes. Blood 2009;113:1257–67.
6. Chu T, D'Angio GJ, Favara BE, Ladisch S, Nesbit M, Pritchard J. Histiocytosis syndromes in children. Lancet 1987;2:41–2.
7. Howarth DM, Gilchrist GS, Mullan BP, Wiseman GA, Edmonson JH, Schomberg PJ. Langerhans cell histiocytosis: diagnosis, natural history, management, and outcome. Cancer 1999;85:2278–90.
8. Yousem SA, Colby TV, Chen YY, Chen WG, Weiss LM. Pulmonary Langerhans' cell histiocytosis: molecular analysis of clonality. Am J Surg Pathol 2001;25:630–6.
9. Pileri SA, Grogan TM, Harris NL, et al. Tumours of histiocytes and accessory dendritic cells: an immunohistochemical approach to classification from the International Lymphoma Study Group based on 61 cases. Histopathology 2002;41:1–29.
10. Lau SK, Chu PG, Weiss LM. Immunohistochemical expression of Langerin in Langerhans cell histiocytosis and non-Langerhans cell histiocytic disorders. Am J Surg Pathol 2008;32:615–9.
11. Pinkus GS, Lones MA, Matsumura F, Yamashiro S, Said JW, Pinkus JL. Langerhans cell histiocytosis immunohistochemical expression of fascin, a dendritic cell marker. Am J Clin Pathol 2002;118:335–43.
12. Willman CL, Busque L, Griffith BB, et al. Langerhans'-cell histiocytosis (histiocytosis X) – a clonal proliferative disease. N Engl J Med 1994;331:154–60.
13. Murakami I, Gogusev J, Fournet JC, Glorion C, Jaubert F. Detection of molecular cytogenetic aberrations in Langerhans cell histiocytosis of bone. Hum Pathol 2002;33:555–60.
14. Rust R, Kluiver J, Visser L, et al. Gene expression analysis of dendritic/Langerhans cells and Langerhans cell histiocytosis. J Pathol 2006;209:474–83.
15. Arico M, Girschikofsky M, Genereau T, et al. Langerhans cell histiocytosis in adults. Report from the International Registry of the Histiocyte Society. Eur J Cancer 2003;39:2341–8.
16. Gadner H, Grois N, Arico M, et al. A randomized trial of treatment for multisystem Langerhans' cell histiocytosis. J Pediatr 2001;138:728–34.
17. Bohn OL, Ruiz-Arguelles G, Navarro L, Saldivar J, Sanchez-Sosa S. Cutaneous Langerhans cell sarcoma: a case report and review of the literature. Int J Hematol 2007;85:116–20.
18. Ferringer T, Banks PM, Metcalf JS. Langerhans cell sarcoma. Am J Dermatopathol 2006;28:36–9.
19. Gaertner EM, Tsokos M, Derringer GA, Neuhauser TS, Arciero C, Andriko JA. Interdigitating dendritic cell sarcoma. A report of four cases and review of the literature. Am J Clin Pathol 2001;115:589–97.
20. Pillay K, Solomon R, Daubenton JD, Sinclair-Smith CC. Interdigitating dendritic cell sarcoma: a report of four paediatric cases and review of the literature. Histopathology 2004;44:283–91.

21. Favara BE, Feller AC, Pauli M, et al. Contemporary classification of histiocytic disorders. The WHO Committee On Histiocytic/Reticulum Cell Proliferations. Reclassification Working Group of the Histiocyte Society. Med Pediatr Oncol 1997;29:157–66.

22. Weitzman S, Jaffe R. Uncommon histiocytic disorders: the non-Langerhans cell histiocytoses. Pediatr Blood Cancer 2005;45:256–64.

23. Zelger BW, Sidoroff A, Orchard G, Cerio R. Non-Langerhans cell histiocytoses. A new unifying concept. Am J Dermatopathol 1996;18:490–504.

24. Sun W, Nordberg ML, Fowler MR. Histiocytic sarcoma involving the central nervous system: clinical, immunohistochemical, and molecular genetic studies of a case with review of the literature. Am J Surg Pathol 2003;27:258–65.

25. Chen W, Lau SK, Fong D, et al. High frequency of clonal immunoglobulin receptor gene rearrangements in sporadic histiocytic/dendritic cell sarcomas. Am J Surg Pathol 2009.

26. Feldman AL, Arber DA, Pittaluga S, et al. Clonally related follicular lymphomas and histiocytic/dendritic cell sarcomas: evidence for transdifferentiation of the follicular lymphoma clone. Blood 2008;111:5433–9.

27. Rosai J, Dorfman RF. Sinus histiocytosis with massive lymphadenopathy. A newly recognized benign clinicopathological entity. Arch Pathol 1969;87:63–70.

28. Paulli M, Rosso R, Kindl S, et al. Immunophenotypic characterization of the cell infiltrate in five cases of sinus histiocytosis with massive lymphadenopathy (Rosai–Dorfman disease). Hum Pathol 1992;23:647–54.

29. Paulli M, Bergamaschi G, Tonon L, et al. Evidence for a polyclonal nature of the cell infiltrate in sinus histiocytosis with massive lymphadenopathy (Rosai–Dorfman disease). Br J Haematol 1995;91:415–8.

30. Pulsoni A, Anghel G, Falcucci P, et al. Treatment of sinus histiocytosis with massive lymphadenopathy (Rosai–Dorfman disease): report of a case and literature review. Am J Hematol 2002;69:67–71.

31. Audouin J, Comperat E, Le Tourneau A, et al. Myeloid sarcoma: clinical and morphologic criteria useful for diagnosis. Int J Surg Pathol 2003;11:271–82.

32. Pileri SA, Ascani S, Cox MC, et al. Myeloid sarcoma: clinico-pathologic, phenotypic and cytogenetic analysis of 92 adult patients. Leukemia 2007;21:340–50.

33. Jones D, Dorfman DM, Barnhill RL, Granter SR. Leukemic vasculitis: a feature of leukemia cutis in some patients. Am J Clin Pathol 1997;107:637–42.

34. Herling M, Jones D. CD4+/CD56+ hematodermic tumor: the features of an evolving entity and its relationship to dendritic cells. Am J Clin Pathol 2007;127:687–700.

35. Petrella T, Comeau MR, Maynadie M, et al. 'Agranular CD4+ CD56+ hematodermic neoplasm' (blastic NK-cell lymphoma) originates from a population of CD56+ precursor cells related to plasmacytoid monocytes. Am J Surg Pathol 2002;26:852–62.

36. Khoury JD, Medeiros LJ, Manning JT, Sulak LE, Bueso-Ramos C, Jones D. CD56(+) TdT(+) blastic natural killer cell tumor of the skin: a primitive systemic malignancy related to myelomonocytic leukemia. Cancer 2002;94:2401–8.

37. Chen WC, Jones D, Ho CL, et al. Cytogenetic anomalies in hyaline vascular Castleman disease: report of two cases with reappraisal of histogenesis. Cancer Genet Cytogenet 2006;164:110–7.

38. Chan JK, Fletcher CD, Nayler SJ, Cooper K. Follicular dendritic cell sarcoma. Clinicopathologic analysis of 17 cases suggesting a malignant potential higher than currently recognized. Cancer 1997;79:294–313.

39. Hollowood K, Stamp G, Zouvani I, Fletcher CD. Extranodal follicular dendritic cell sarcoma of the gastrointestinal tract. Morphologic, immunohistochemical and ultrastructural analysis of two cases. Am J Clin Pathol 1995;103:90–7.

40. Monda L, Warnke R, Rosai J. A primary lymph node malignancy with features suggestive of dendritic reticulum cell differentiation. A report of 4 cases. Am J Pathol 1986;122:562–72.

41. Lee IJ, Kim SC, Kim HS, et al. Paraneoplastic pemphigus associated with follicular dendritic cell sarcoma arising from Castleman's tumor. J Am Acad Dermatol 1999;40:294–7.

42. Grogg KL, Lae ME, Kurtin PJ, Macon WR. Clusterin expression distinguishes follicular dendritic cell tumors from other dendritic cell neoplasms: report of a novel follicular dendritic cell marker and clinicopathologic data on 12 additional follicular dendritic cell tumors and 6 additional interdigitating dendritic cell tumors. Am J Surg Pathol 2004;28:988–98.

43. Jones D, Amin M, Ordonez NG, Glassman AB, Hayes KJ, Medeiros LJ. Reticulum cell sarcoma of lymph node with mixed dendritic and fibroblastic features. Mod Pathol 2001;14:1059–67.

44. Sander B, Middel P, Gunawan B, et al. Follicular dendritic cell sarcoma of the spleen. Hum Pathol 2007;38:668–72.
45. Lin O, Frizzera G. Angiomyoid and follicular dendritic cell proliferative lesions in Castleman's disease of hyaline-vascular type: a study of 10 cases. Am J Surg Pathol 1997;21:1295–306.
46. Soriano AO, Thompson MA, Admirand JH, et al. Follicular dendritic cell sarcoma: a report of 14 cases and a review of the literature. Am J Hematol 2007;82:725–8.
47. Andriko JW, Kaldjian EP, Tsokos M, Abbondanzo SL, Jaffe ES. Reticulum cell neoplasms of lymph nodes: a clinicopathologic study of 11 cases with recognition of a new subtype derived from fibroblastic reticular cells. Am J Surg Pathol 1998;22:1048–58.
48. Martel M, Sarli D, Colecchia M, et al. Fibroblastic reticular cell tumor of the spleen: report of a case and review of the entity. Hum Pathol 2003;34:954–7.

Chapter 27

Extranodal Lymphomas and Tumors of the Thymus

Brian D. Stewart, John T. Manning, and Dan Jones

Abstract/Scope of Chapter This chapter provides an overview of lymphomas and related tumors presenting at extranodal locations. Commonalities and differences in the approach to diagnosis, staging, and their pathogenesis are summarized. Intrinsic tumors of the thymus are also discussed.

Keywords Extranodal lymphoma, incidence by site • Skin, lymphomas • Brain, lymphoma • Central nervous system, lymphoma • Head and neck, lymphoma • Thyroid, lymphoma • Lung, lymphoma • Small bowel, lymphoma • Liver • Lymphoma • Testes, adrenal, lymphoma • Ovary, lymphoma • Endometrium, lymphoma • Thymus, maturation • Thymus, B cells • Thymoma, classification • Thymic carcinoma • Lymphoblastic lymphoma, mediastinal • Hodgkin lymphoma, thymus • Mediastinal B-cell lymphoma, thymic origin

27.1. Overview of Extranodal Lymphomas

27.1.1. General Features

The definition of an extranodal lymphoma is usually one in which the presenting tissue site is the location of primary involvement for at least 3–6 months following diagnosis. However, some extranodal lymphomas show systemic spread much more rapidly (e.g. those in the spleen or tonsils), whereas lymphomas at other sites (e.g. the skin or stomach) can remain localized for many years even without treatment. The general demographic features of extranodal lymphomas are similar to nodal cases, with median age in the fifth to sixth decade at diagnosis, except for those cases with antigen-driven or autoimmune etiology (e.g. MALT lymphomas), which usually present at a slightly younger age.

The overall distribution of lymphomas at different extranodal sites is shown in Table 27-1. Several conclusions can be drawn: (1) there are major differences in the types of extranodal lymphomas arising in pediatric and adult patients;[1] (2) geographic differences are noted in the incidence of extranodal lymphomas related to their inciting causes; (3) lymphomas are rare in immune-privileged sites such as the central nervous system (CNS) and testes; and (4) although individual differences in histologic types occur at each site, diffuse large B-cell lymphoma (DLBCL) and marginal zone lymphoma of MALT type (MALT lymphoma) are the most common B-cell lymphomas at most extranodal sites in adult patients, with follicular lymphoma (FL) commonly involving any organ with secondary lymphoid tissue, including bowel mucosa.

From: *Neoplastic Hematopathology*: Contemporary Hematology,
Edited by: D. Jones, DOI 10.1007/978-1-60761-384-8_27,
© Humana Press, a part of Springer Science+Business Media, LLC 2010

Table 27-1. Incidence of extranodal lymphoma in adults and children.

Sites (in decreasing order of frequency)	% of all lymphomas	Most common subtype (adult)	Most common subtype (children)
Gastrointestinal tract	10–20	MALT, DLBCL	DLBCL, BL, ALCL
Skin	6	MF	DLBCL
Bone	4–5	DLBCL	Rare
Head and neck	2–3		
Salivary glands		MALT	Rare
Tonsil/Waldeyer's ring		DLBCL, FL	BL, DLBCL
Nose/oropharynx		DLBCL, NK/T (Asia)	DLBCL
Thyroid		MALT, LBCL	Rare
Thymus	2–4	PMBCL	Precursor T-LBL
CNS	1–2	DLBCL	Rare
Breast	1	DLBCL, MALT	Rare
Testes	1	DLBCL	Rare
Lung/airway	<1	MALT, DLBCL	HL
Spleen	<1	DLBCL	Rare
Heart	<1	DLBCL	Rare
GYN tract	Rare	DLBCL, BL	Rare
Adrenal	Rare	DLBCL	Rare

CNS nervous system, *GYN* gyncelogic, other abbreviations as in text

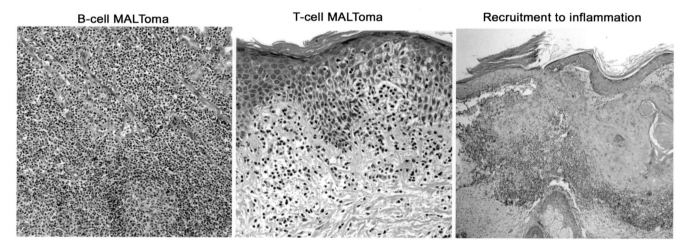

Fig. 27-1. Drivers of extranodal lymphoma. (**a**) B-cell MALT lymphoma. (**b**) T-cell "MALT" lymphoma. Mycosis fungoides represents a prototypic antigen-driven lymphoma as nearly all cases arise in patients with long-standing dermatitis, often of the hypersensitivity type. Early MF often shows infiltration into the epidermis at discrete sites with associated spongiosis consistent with response to an external antigen. (**c**) Chronic lymphocytic leukemia involving the base of a cutaneous squamous cell carcinoma, as an example of recruitment of lymphoma to sites of ongoing inflammation or immune activation

The most important insight into the development of lymphomas at extranodal sites was the observation that lymphomas sometimes develop from the nonneoplastic mucosa-associated lymphoid tissue (MALT) that arises in inflammatory states. The concept was first developed to explain the emergence of low-grade marginal zone B-cell lymphomas in the small intestine of patients with preceding bacterial infections, but Isaacson and colleagues [2] subsequently expanded the concept to explain the inflammatory-based histogenesis of MALT lymphomas at other extranodal sites (Fig. 27-1a). As summarized in Table 27-2, several additional B-cell

Table 27-2. Mechanisms of outgrowth of extranodal lymphoproliferative neoplasms.

Type	Sites	Inciting cause
MALT lymphomas		
Infection-driven	Stomach	*Helicobacter pylori* infection
	Small bowel	*Campylobacter bacter* overgrowth
	Skin	*Borrelia burgdorferi* infection
	Conjunctivae	*Chylamydia psittaci* infection
Autoimmune-driven	Thyroid	Hashimoto's thyroiditis
	Ocular, salivary gland	Sjögren syndrome
DLBCL		
Infection-driven	Effusions	HHV8 latent or lytic infection
	Implants, foreign bodies in soft tissue	Persistent inflammation with outgrowth of EBV+ B cells
	CNS, GI tract	EBV-driven B-cell proliferation due to immunodeficiency states
T-cell lymphomas		
Mycosis fungoides	Skin	Hypersensitivity dermatitis due to allergy, infection, or superantigen
EATL	Gastrointestinal tract	Autoimmune/dietary (anti-gliadin antibodies)
AILT	Lymph node, skin, GI tract	Hypersensitivity reactions (drugs)
T-LGL leukemia	Blood, bone marrow	Autoimmune attack against hematopoietic elements (myeloid granule proteins)

and T-cell lymphomas have a clear association with preceding inflammatory states, such as mycosis fungoides (MF) arising out of chronic dermatitis (Fig. 27-1b).

Another driver of the extranodal localization of lymphoproliferative disorders is the recruitment of tumor lymphocytes to sites of ongoing inflammation or immune activation. This is particularly common in follicular lymphoma (FL), which homes to germinal centers at any tissue site, and in chronic lymphocytic leukemia/small lymphocyte lymphoma (CLL/SLL), which colonizes sites of preexisting inflammation. As a result, CLL is often found incidentally in skin, prostate, and bladder biopsies done for other reasons (Fig. 27-1c). The role of differential homing of distinct lymphocyte populations to certain extranodal sites has been proposed to explain the association of particular immunophenotypes with bowel and cutaneous lymphoma subtypes (see Chap. 38) [3–5].

27.2. Staging and Prognostic Schema for Extranodal Lymphomas

The Ann Arbor classification system (Chap. 17, Table 17.2) is the primary modality used to stage lymphomas for therapy selection. However, it is not well-suited for extranodal lymphomas because most of their spread to lymph nodes occurs only late in the disease course, with distinctive patterns seen at each tissue site, making a uniform schema difficult to apply. This is particularly true for cutaneous lymphomas where the extent of disease needs other metrics (e.g. skin score in MF), and for extranodal marginal zone lymphomas, which can involve multiple MALT sites (e.g. the lung and salivary gland), but not necessarily have an adverse prognosis as would be anticipated from their high Ann Arbor stage.

In diffuse large B-cell lymphoma (DLBCL), the International Prognostic Index (IPI) which incorporates age, performance status, and serum lactate dehydrogenase (LDH) levels, works well for outcome prediction in most extranodal DLBCL types. Molecular subclassification of extranodal DLBCL into germinal center B-cell (GCB)-like and activated B-cell (ABC)-like types generally shows the same poorer outcome for the ABC group as seen for nodal tumors, although ABC-like cases are more common at extranodal sites than in lymph node. As would be expected, GCB-like DLBCLs predominate at sites with preexisting lymphoid tissues (e.g. the tonsils and intestine), whereas ABC-like cases are more common in organs that normally lack immune function.

27.3. Lymphomas Involving Specific Tissue Sites

27.3.1. Lymphomas Involving Skin and Soft Tissue

The skin is the second most common site of extranodal lymphoma, with T-cell tumors (mostly mycosis fungoides and its variants) being more than twice as common as B-cell neoplasms (Table 27-3) [6]. Among B-cell tumors, secondary involvement of the skin by systemic DLBCL or by low-grade lymphomas colonizing inflammatory infiltrates is more common than primary presentations. Specialized cutaneous types of B-cell lymphoma include the extremely indolent MALT lymphoma and follicle center lymphoma, both of which may have antigenic triggers such as Borrelia infection (Lyme disease) and persistent folliculitis, [7] and an aggressive "leg-type" of DLBCL with an ABC/post-GC immunophenotype that usually rapidly progresses and disseminates [8–10]. Other types of cutaneous DLBCL (many of the GCB immunophenotype) are much more indolent requiring only excision and localized radiotherapy.

Most lymphomas that involve the soft tissues do so secondarily, and are most commonly DLBCL or the diffuse (sclerotic) variant of follicular lymphoma. DLBCLs and anaplastic large cell lymphoma (ALCL) can also arise because of persistent soft tissue inflammation resulting from implants and foreign bodies or near joint spaces with surgical prostheses. Another example of a primary soft tissue lymphoproliferative disorder is amyloidoma, which is a localized deposition of immunoglobulin seen rarely in plasma cell neoplasms, often involving the chest wall (Fig. 27-2).

27.3.2. Lymphomas of the Central Nervous System (CNS)

Lymphomas primarily involving the CNS have increased threefold since 1970, comprising 5% of all primary brain tumors, and 1–2% of all lymphomas and are mostly DLBCL that pursue an aggressive clinical course (Table 27-4) [11,12]. Distinction is made between EBV+ DLBCL arising in patients with immunodeficiency, and EBV- cases arising in immunocompetent patients (so-called primary DLBCL) for which radiotherapy is the primary treatment modality (Fig. 27-3). In addition to IPI score, high protein concentration in the cerebrospinal fluid (CSF) and deep brain involvement are adverse prognostic factors among the EBV-negative cases [13]. Secondary CNS lymphomatous involvement is usually seen only with advanced-stage DLBCL or relapse of mediastinal B-cell lymphoma. Involvement of the CSF/meninges at presentation or relapse is relatively common in lymphoblastic lymphoma/leukemia [14].

27.3.3. Lymphomas of the Head and Neck and Thyroid

Extranodal lymphomas arising in the head and neck account for 2–3% of all lymphomas, and include MALT lymphomas of the orbit, thyroid, and salivary glands, [15] GC-derived B-cell lymphomas of the tonsils/Waldeyer's ring (i.e. DLBCL, follicular lymphoma, and Burkitt lymphoma), [16] and DLBCL and EBV+ NK/T-cell lymphomas of the nose, paranasal sinuses, and oropharynx (Table 27-5) [17]. Secondary spread of follicular lymphoma into the salivary glands from adjacent lymph nodes is also common. Although outcomes are generally good, morbidity and mortality often relate to surgically unresectable disease invading into CNS and other critical anatomic compartments.

Lymphomas comprise up to 5% of thyroid neoplasms and when confined to the thyroid are mostly MALT lymphomas arising from Hashimoto's disease or other causes of lymphocytic thyroiditis [18]. Thyroid involvement by DLBCL is also very common, but in those cases secondary extension of the lymphoma from neck lymph nodes should be considered.

27.3.4   Lymphomas of Lung and Airway

The majority of lymphoproliferative disorders involving the lung spread from adjacent lymph nodes or the mediastinum (including primary mediastinal/thymic large B-cell lymphoma

Table 27-3. Benign and neoplastic lymphocyte-rich lesions presenting in skin (Also see Chap. 24).

Type	Incidence	Pattern of infiltration	Markers	Others features
B-cell-rich lesions (CD20+, CD79a+) in dermis				
Large B-cell lymphoma	Common	Dermis, subcutis		Often primary but need to exclude systemic, indolent except leg-type
MZL lymphoma of MALT type (immunocytoma)	Common	Reactive GCs, monocytoid B cells/plasma cells	Monotypic IgK or IgL	Rare cases in US associated with chronic *Borrelia* infection
Follicle center lymphoma (FCL)	Uncommon Head/trunk	Periadnexal	CD10+ BCL2-	Indolent, likely a variant of MALT lymphoma
Systemic follicular lymphoma (FL)	Common	Colonizes reactive germinal centers & folliculitis	CD10+ BCL2+	Consider when nodular lymphoma is CD10+ BCL2+
CLL/SLL	Uncommon	Periadnexal, admixed with inflammation	CD5+CD23+	Always secondary involvement from blood or lymph node
Folliculitis, acne rosacea	Common Head, trunk	Dense, polymorphous folliculotropic	Ig polyclonal	Correlate with clinical appearance
Nodular lymphoid hyperplasia (pseudolymphoma)	Common	GC remnants, often dense polymorphous	Ig polyclonal	Light eruption, drug reaction, or infections
T-cell rich lesions (CD3+ CD5+)				
Lymphocytes in epidermis				
Mycosis fungoides	Common	Basal layer seeding of atypical lymphs	CD4+ >>CD8+	Involves sun-protected areas early in disease course
Chronic dermatitis	Very common	Spongiosis, epidermal reaction, no lymphocyte atypia	CD8≥CD4	Avoid doing molecular studies if lesion looks reactive
Dermal-based				
CD30+ LPD (lymphomatoid papulosis, ALCL)	Uncommon	Sheet-like dermal or perivascular clusters of CD30+ cells	Often with loss of pan-T-cell antigens (e.g. CD3, CD5)	Clinical history of regressing lesions
Dense lichenoid dermatitis with CD30+ cells [96]	Common	Dense, band-like, effacement of epidermal junction	Mixed B cells and T cells, variable CD30	Drug reactions, insect bites, allergic reactions
Lymphocytic vasculitis [97]	Common	Lymphocytes in and around venules with or without fibrin	CD4>CD8+	Autoimmune, infections (herpes, rickettsia) or bug bite
Subcutaneous infiltrates				
Subcutaneous panniculitis-like TCL	Rare	Limited to subcutis, polymorphic, atypical lymphs, necrosis	CD8+	Extremities and trunk, multifocal
Gamma-delta TCL	Very rare	Tumor densest in dermis, extends into subcutis/epidermis	CD4-CD8- variable CD56+	Hemophagocytic syndrome
Panniculitis	Common	Fat necrosis, minimal lymphocyte atypia	CD8+ > CD4+	Reaction to steroids, lupus, infections

GC germinal center, *TCL* T-cell lymphoma, *ALCL* anaplastic large cell lymphoma, *LPD* lymphoproliferative disorder.

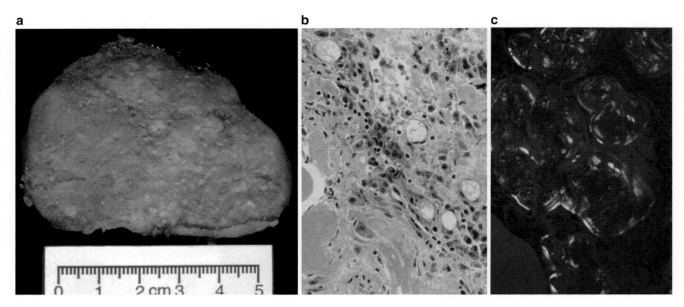

Fig. 27-2. Amyloidoma: (**a**) Poorly circumscribed chest wall mass with a waxy cut surface. (**b**) Histological examination reveals localized collections of plasma cells and eosinophilic fibrotic material. (**c**) Polarization microscopy reveals apple-green birefringence consistent with amyloid AL (light chain immunoglobulin deposition)

Table 27-4. Lymphomas presenting in the central nervous system.

Type	Histologic features	Others features
Brain [98, 99]		
Large B-cell lymphoma (LBCL)	Perivascular accentuation, necrosis and surface spread	EBV+ in primary immunodeficient cases Otherwise tumors are EBV-
Lymphomatoid granulomatosis	Polymorphous, angioinvasive mixed infiltrates EBV+ B cells but not clustered or sheet-like as in LBCL	Multinodular lesions, also involving skin, kidney, and lung, waxing and waning course, grade 3 lesions may progress to overt EBV+ LBCL
Meninges [100]		
Marginal zone (lymphoplasmacytic type)	Reactive GCs and sheets of monocytoid B cells or plasma cells	Paraprotein in urine or serum, usually IgM but can be IgG
Follicular lymphoma	Often diffuse rather than nodular growth pattern	CD10+ clonal B cells
Large B-cell lymphoma (LBCL)		Usually spread from brain or systemic origin

Abbreviations as in Table 27.3

and Hodgkin lymphoma), the pleura (DLBCL, FL), or are due to leukemic extravasation from blood vessels into the parenchyma (e.g., CLL, MCL). Primary pulmonary lymphomas are uncommon, comprising ~1% of lung tumors and ~4% of extranodal lymphomas, with MALT lymphoma and DLBCL constituting the majority of cases (Fig. 27-4, Table 27-6) [19–21]. Lymphomas of bronchial-associated lymphoid tissue ("BALTomas") have a high incidence of NF-kappa B pathway dysregulation [22] often due to chromosomal translocations,

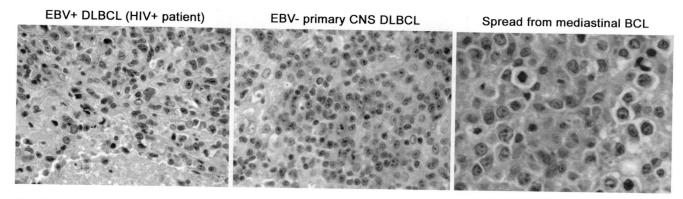

Fig. 27-3. Lymphoma, presenting in the central nervous system. (**a**) EBV+ DLBCL shows necrosis and a polymorphous infiltrate. (**b**) EBV-negative primary DLBCL of the CNS shows a monomorphous infiltrate of large lymphocytes. (**c**) Spread of mediastinal B-cell lymphoma (BCL) to the brain at relapse

Table 27-5. Extranodal lymphoid lesions presenting in the head and neck [101,102].

Type	Incidence/site	Histology	Markers	Others features
B-cell lymphoproliferative disorders (CD20+, CD79a+)				
Large B-cell lymphoma	Common Nasal, paranasal, or tonsil	Tumor masses, ulceration, necrosis		Primary presentations common, frequent necrosis and ulceration
Follicular lymphoma	Common Tonsil	Nodular infiltrates	CD10+ BCL2+	Usually systemic
Burkitt lymphoma	Uncomon Tonsil/mandible	Sheet-like, follicle colonization	CD10+ BCL2-	Usually primary presentation
MZL lymphoma of MALT type	Thyroid, salivary glands	Reactive GCs, mucosal infiltrates	Monotypic Ig in plasma cells	Spreads to other MALT sites (e.g. GI tract)
T-cell and NK-cell lymphomas (cytoplasmic CD3+)				
NK/T-cell lymphoma, nasal-type (Midline granuloma)	Uncommon in US	Polymorphous, angioinvasion, necrosis	EBV+	Can be low-grade cytology making diagnosis difficult
Reactive disorders				
Infectious mononucleosis	Common in children	Reactive GCs and mixed T-cell and B-cell immunoblasts	EBV+	Also seen with CMV and other herpesviruses
Lymphoid hyperplasia	Common in children	Large reactive GCs		Actinomycosis is common cause in tonsil
Sialoadenitis and nasal polyps	Common	Minimal lymphocyte atypia, eosinophils usually prominent	Mixed B cells and T cells	Allergic, autoimmune and infectious (viral, fungal) causes

Abbreviations as in Table 27.3

particularly the t(11;18)/API2-MALT1 which is seen in up to 50% of cases, suggesting that antigen-driven proliferation may be less important in their pathogenesis than in MALT lymphomas arising at other sites [23]. Another pattern of lung MALT lymphoma is a plasmacytic variant with extensive sclerosis and immunoglobulin deposition with only scant lymphoma cells, [24,25] with similar-appearing plasma cell-rich reactive lesions also reported [26,27].

27.3.5. Lymphomas of the Spleen

Most lymphoproliferative neoplasms that involve the bone marrow will involve the spleen to a similar degree; exceptions include the preferential splenic involvement seen in Hairy cell leukemia (HCL), splenic marginal zone lymphoma (SMZL), variants of mantle cell

Fig. 27-4. Primary DLBCL of lung. Multifocal tumor masses replace most of the lung parenchyma

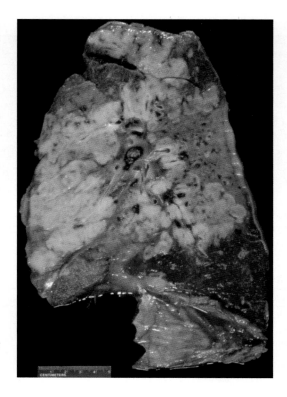

Table 27-6. Benign and neoplastic lymphocyte-rich lesions presenting in the lung and airway [19].

Type	Frequency	Pattern of infiltration	Markers, others features
B-cell-rich lesions (CD20+, CD79a+)			
MZL of MALT type	Relatively common	Loose, intra-alveolar, and nodular with infiltration into GCs, bronchial mucosa	Multinodular radiologic appearance, spreads to other MALT sites
Large B-cell lymphoma, NOS	Uncommon	Expansile masses, often necrotic	Can mimic carcinoma radiologically
Mediastinal large B-cell lymphoma	Uncommon	Dense fibrosis, often with crushed lymphoid infiltrate	Young adults/females, more often contiguous spread from mediastinum
CLL/SLL	Uncommon	Colonizes chronic inflammation (bronchitis)	Ground-glass radiologic appearance
Nodular lymphoid hyperplasia (pseudolymphoma)	Uncommon	Reactive lesion resembling MALT but less extensive, no demonstrable Ig clonality	Seen in autoimmune states
Lymphocytic interstitial pneumonia	Relatively common	Reaction pattern with mixed B-cell and T-cell diffuse interstitial lymphoid infiltrates	Seen in autoimmune disease with dysproteinemia, HIV infection (children)
T-cell rich lesions			
Bronchitis	Common	Peribronchial cuffing by mixed lymphoid infiltrates	
Hodgkin lymphoma	Relatively common	Polymorphous infiltrates with R-S cells/ mononuclear variants, expands/invades bronchial wall, and intrapulmonary nodes, intravascular growth seen at relapse	Usually spreads from mediastinum
Lymphomatoid granulomatosis	Uncommon	Polymorphous including plasma cells and histiocytes, CD4 > CD8 T cells scattered EBV+ B cells,	Sheets of large B cells favors LBCL of LyG type

Abbreviations as in Table 27-3; *HIV* human immunodeficiency virus

lymphoma (MCL) and lymphoplasmacytic lymphoma (LPL), T-cell and NK-cell large granular lymphocyte leukemia (LGLL), and hepatosplenic T-cell lymphoma (Table 27-7). In splenectomy specimens, gross appearance is highly informative in distinguishing neoplasms with involvement of the red pulp (CLL/SLL, LPL, HCL, HSTCL, and LGLL)

Table 27-7. Lymphoproliferative disorders presenting in spleen [103].

Type	Incidence	Growth pattern	Markers	Others features
B-cell lymphoproliferative disorders (CD20+, CD79a+)				
Large B-cell lymphoma	Common	Tumor masses, a red pulp-only form is also known		Primary type or with Stage IV disease, necrosis common
Hodgkin lymphoma	High stage cases	Tumor masses, can be subtle	CD15+/CD30+	Classical HL only
Follicular lymphoma	Common	White pulp	CD10+ t(14;18)	Almost always Stage IV
Splenic marginal zone lymphoma	Uncommon	Infiltration of white pulp follicles, red pulp	CD5-/CD10- del7q or +3	Perisplenic LN enlarged, intrasinusoidal in BM
Mantle cell lymphoma	Uncommon	Infiltration of follicles, red pulp	CD5+CD23- t(11;14)	Primary splenic presentations with high serum β2-microglobulin
CLL/SLL	Common	Red > white pulp	CD5+CD23+ del13q14, +12	
Lymphoplasmacytic lymphoma	Common	Red and white pulp	Monotypic Ig CD5-/CD10-	Paraprotein in serum or urine
Hairy cell leukemia	Uncommon	Red pulp only	CD11c+/CD25+ CD103+/CD123+	Blood lakes
T-cell lymphoproliferative disorders (CD3+)				
Hepatosplenic lymphoma	Very rare	Red pulp	CD8+/TIA1+ Granzyme B- Isochromosome 7q	Intrasinusoidal in BM, liver
LGL leukemia	Common	Red pulp	CD8+/TIA1+ Granzyme B+	Modest splenomegaly, cytopenias Chronic course
PTCL, NOS [104]	Uncommon	Tumor masses	Usually CD4+	Usually systemic spread

Abbreviations as in Table 27.3.

or white pulp (FL, MCL, SMZL) from those neoplasms forming discrete tumor masses (DBLCL, Hodgkin lymphoma) (Fig. 27-5). But alternate splenic presentations of each lymphoproliferative disorder have been reported, such as red pulp involvement in the leukemic variants of MCL. In one series of primary splenic presentations of lymphoma, 56% were SMZL, 13% FL, 12% DLBCL, 10% MCL, 6% CLL/SLL, and 3% LPL [28].

27.3.6. Lymphomas of the Gastrointestinal (GI) Tract

The GI tract is the most common site for extranodal lymphoma, representing 10–20% of cases and affecting the stomach, small intestine, and colon in order of decreasing frequency, with the most common types being MALT lymphoma and DLBCL (Table 27-8). Esophageal primaries are rare, with fewer than 50 cases reported [29]. For MALT lymphoma, the inciting pathogenesis has the most prognostic significance, with translocation-driven cases having a worse the outcome than antigen-driven tumors (See Chap. 15) [30]. In DLBCL, outcome is primarily influenced by the stage and IPI score. Follicular lymphomas localized to the small bowel have favorable outcome and a unique pattern of adhesion marker expression (Fig. 27-6a) [31]. The incidence of Burkitt lymphoma involving sites of Peyer's patch tissue or the appendix is increased in pediatric patients, those with immunosuppression, and in people in underdeveloped countries [32]. The rare T-cell lymphomas arising from intestinal mucosa-homing T cells generally present in the jejunum with ulceration or perforation as a result of large cell transformation (Fig. 27-6b) [33]–[35].

The type of lymphomas involving the liver are similar to those seen in the spleen, with rare primaries reported [36]. Hepatic spread of systemic DLBCL and FL are the most commonly encountered tumors, but primary liver lymphomas may be increased in patients with chronic viral hepatitis or autoimmune diseases.

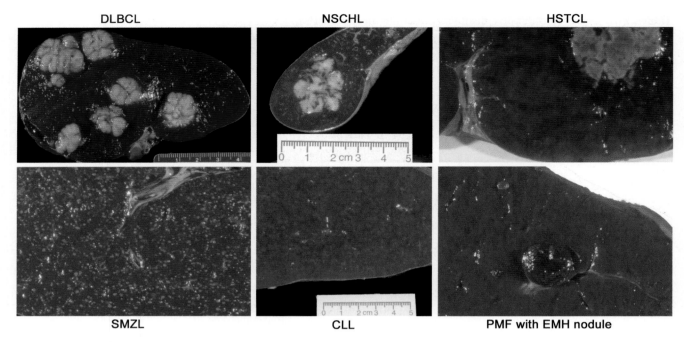

Fig. 27-5. Lymphoprolfierative disorders involving the spleen. (*Top left*) DLBCL shows multinodular tumor masses; (*Top middle*) Nodular sclerosis classical Hodgkin lymphoma (NSCHL) shows a single necrotic nodule in a normal-sized spleen; (*Top right*) Hepatosplenic T-cell lymphoma shows red pulp involvement with an infarct (yellow area at top); (*Bottom left*) Splenic marginal zone B-cell lymphoma (SMZL) shows a multinodular pattern of white pulp infiltration; (*Bottom, middle*) Red pulp expansion with splenic fibrosis in CLL. (*Bottom right*) A massively expanded spleen shows bulging, well-circumscribed red nodules representing extramedullary hematopoietic (EMH) in a patient with long standing primary myelofibrosis

Table 27-8. Lymphomas presenting in gastrointestinal tract [105,106].

	DLBCL	Follicular lymphoma	Burkitt lymphoma	MZL of MALT type[a]	MCL[b]	Enteropathy-associated TCL[c]
Esophagus	–	–	–	+ (usually S)	Rare	–
Stomach	+++ (P & S)	+ (S)	+ (usually S)	+++ (P)	+	Rare
Small bowel	++ (P & S)	+++ (P & S)	+ ileum	+ (P & S) Duodenum[d]	++	+, jejunum
Colon	+++ (P & S)	+ (S)	Rare	Rare	++	Rare

Abbreviations as in Table 27.3; –; not seen, +; uncommon, ++;occasional, +++;common, P: primary presentation, S: spread from systemic lymphoma (i.e. Stage IV), MZL; marginal zone lymphoma, MALT: mucosa-associated lymphoid tissue, MCL; mantle cell lymphoma, TCL; T-cell lymphoma
[a] MALT type lymphoma in the small bowel is often rich in plasma cells resembling a plasmacytoma, whereas in other sites the classical features of reactive follicles, lymphoepithelial lesions, and monocytoid B-cell clusters are present
[b] Involvement can be focal or densely nodular (i.e. lymphomatous polyposis)
[c] Ulceration, often transmural, with adjacent areas showing mulitfocal epithelial infiltration
[d] Variants of MALT lymphoma presenting in the duodenum include plasmacytoma and immunoproliferative small intestinal disease (IPSID) including alpha heavy chain disease and Mediterranean lymphoma. Secondary involvement of the bowel is usually from gastric MALT lymphoma

27.3.7. Bone Lymphoma vs. Bone Marrow Lymphoma

At least 50% of lymphomas presenting as discrete bone lesions will be high-stage systemic DLBCL when staging is performed. Sclerosing follicular lymphoma and Hodgkin lymphoma [37] can also present as localized bone lesions. In contrast, primary bone lymphoma (PBL) with no evidence of systemic spread at presentation is a highly-distinctive clinical entity manifesting as localized lesions within the long bones of the extremities, the jaw, or the ribs. PBL has a highly

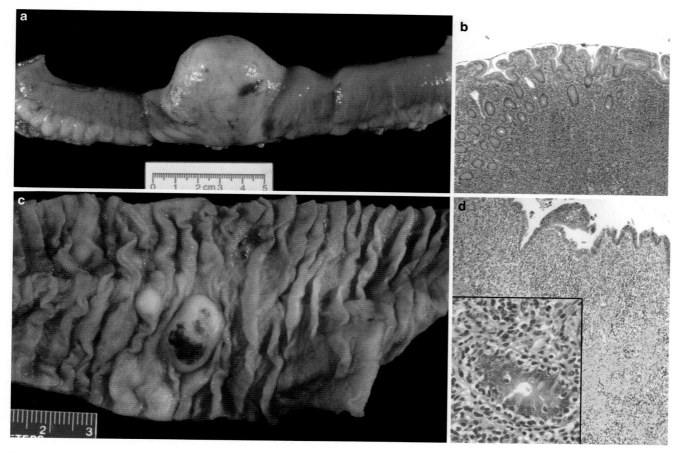

Fig. 27-6. Bowel lymphomas. (**a**) Single large tumor mass in the duodenum representing primary follicular lymphoma of the bowel; mesenteric lymph nodes were negative for tumor. (**b**) This tumor shows a diffuse and nodular transmural B-cell infiltrate positive for CD10 (not shown). (**c**) Enteropathy-associated T-cell lymphoma with multiple tumors in the jejunum, terminal ileum, and proximal colon. Areas of deep ulceration were also present. (**d**) Sections shows a transmural large cell lymphoid infiltrate with epithelial infiltration by an atypical but lower-grade lymphoid infiltrate (inset) representing the lower-grade lymphoma component

favorable prognosis, with many patients in the prechemotherapy era cured with surgical resection and/or localized radiotherapy only [38]. PBL usually presents with monostotic or grouped polyostotic destructive lesions that extend through the bone cortex into adjacent soft tissue (Fig. 27-7a). Nearly all PBL cases are DLBCL, commonly with CD10 expression; tumor cell morphology is variable but often shows a multilobate appearance (Fig. 27-7b) [39]. In contrast, lymphomas of the bone marrow space detected on nondirected biopsy (Fig. 27-7c) are highly aggressive and often associated with splenic involvement and multisystem organ dysfunction, resulting in rapid deterioration and death within weeks to months of diagnosis [40,41]. This entity may be a variant of the aggressive intravascular lymphoma.

27.3.8. Lymphomas Presenting at Other Sites

Breast: Primary breast lymphoma comprises 1% of all lymphomas and 2% of all extranodal cases, with DLBCL and MALT lymphoma being the most frequent [42,43]. MALT lymphomas of the breast (Fig. 27-8) often have a more aggressive course than similar tumors

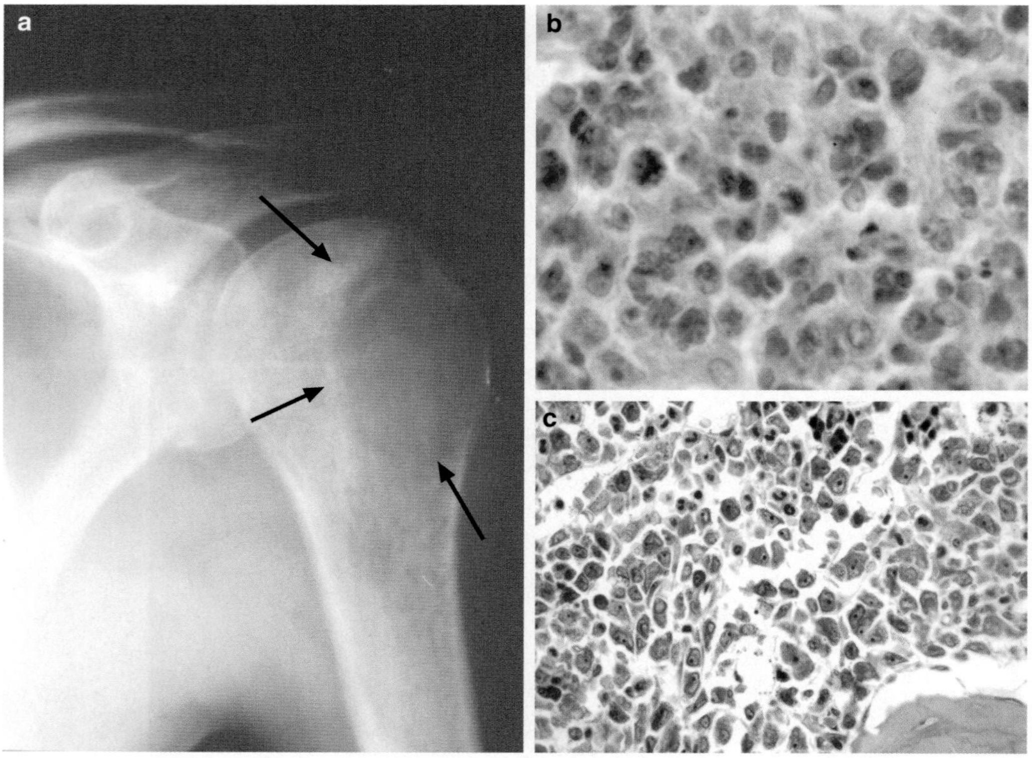

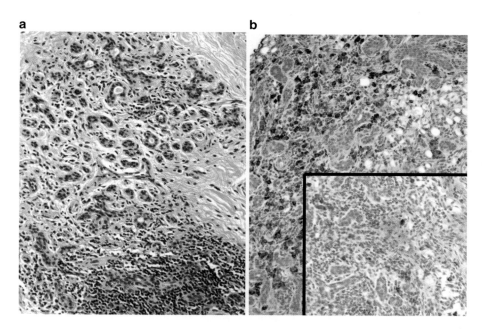

Fig. 27-7. Primary bone lymphoma (PBL) compared to primary bone marrow lymphoma. (**a**) Radiograph from PBL in a 45-year old male reveals a large, destructive, radiolucent discrete bone lesion in the left humerus. (**b**) Bone biopsy from a case of PBL with multilobate nuclear contours. This patient was alive 26 years following radiotherapy without any evidence of residual disease. (**c**) DLBCL with immunoblastic morphology detected on a non-directed bone marrow biopsy in a 56-year-old woman. Patient had hypercalcemia, but no evidence of extramedullary disease, and died of disease 3 weeks after diagnosis

Fig. 27-8. MALT lymphoma, breast. (**a**) Breast parenchyma is invaded by a small lymphocytic infiltrate with lymphoepithelial lesions. (**b**) The plasmacytic component shows monotypic immunoglobulin kappa light chain staining (lambda light staining in inset)

at other sites [42]. Secondary spread of lymphoma from adjacent axillary lymph nodes should be considered in cases of DLBCL and FL.

Heart: Primary lymphoma of the heart and great vessels comprises less than 2% of all primary cardiac tumors but carries a poor prognosis due to its disruption of the cardiac conduction system [44]. The majority of secondary cardiac lymphomas occur in the right side of the heart and are noted in up to 10% of disseminated DLBCL in autopsy series [45]–[47] Posttransplant lymphoproliferative disorders can also involve the allograft in patients with a heart transplant [48,49].

Adrenal: Less than 100 cases of primary adrenal lymphoma have been reported to date, [50] but secondary adrenal involvement in high-stage DLBCL is extremely common due to hematogenous spread or extension from adjacent lymph nodes. A well-recognized presentation of the rare intravascular lymphoma in the adrenal gland occurs because of its effects on endocrine function [51].

Gynecologic tract: Secondary involvement of the ovary in high-stage DLBCL and Burkitt lymphoma is relatively common. However, despite the presence of ovary-associated lymphoid aggregates, primary ovarian lymphoma is extremely rare and accounts for less than 0.5% of lymphomas, and 1.5% of ovarian tumors [52]. The association of lymphomatous involvement with both ascites and an elevated CA-125 can mimic the far more common epithelial types of ovarian cancer. Primary or secondary lymphomatous involvement of the uterine corpus is also extremely rare (less than 0.5% of lymphomas) with the vast majority being DBLCL of presumed cervical origin [53]. In contrast, extramedullary myeloid tumors involving the uterus are more common [54].

Testes: Primary lymphoma of the testis accounts for 1% of all lymphomas but up to 10% of all testicular tumors, being the most common testicular tumor found in men older than 50. In adults, nearly all cases are DLBCL, and have an increased incidence of relapse in the contralateral testicle and the CNS suggests preferential homing to those sites [55,56]. Overall survival at 10 years is only 20–35%, making testicular DLBCL the second most aggressive extranodal type after CNS presentations, possibly both related to the poor penetration of systemic chemotherapy at those sites [55,56]. The testis is also a common site of relapse

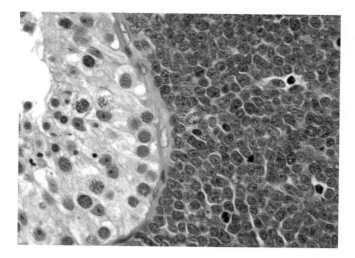

Fig. 27-9. B lymphoblastic lymphoma, testes. Blastoid lymphocytes infiltrate around seminiferous tubules in a patient with relapsed disease

of lymphoblastic leukemia and Burkitt lymphoma [57] and an occasional site of primary lymphoblastic lymphoma (Fig. 27-9).

27.4. Tumors of the Thymus

27.4.1. Biology and Function of the Thymus

The thymus is the site of T-cell maturation during late embryogenesis and early childhood. The mesenchymal portion (i.e. stromal elements) forms from the third branchial cleft and has a lobulated structure composed of a capsule, cortex, and medulla (Fig. 27-10). The medulla contains specialized lymphoepithelial structures called Hassall's corpuscles that function in lymphocyte apoptosis [58].

The initiating event in thymic T-cell (thymocyte) maturation is the movement of precursor T cells emigrating from the bone marrow into the medulla, followed by their trafficking to subcapsular cortical locations. Maturation of thymocytes in the cortex is accompanied by expression of the single chain pre-TCR, and then the intact TCR (either γ/δ or α/β chains) with testing of the functional capability of the TCR by binding MHC on the surface of

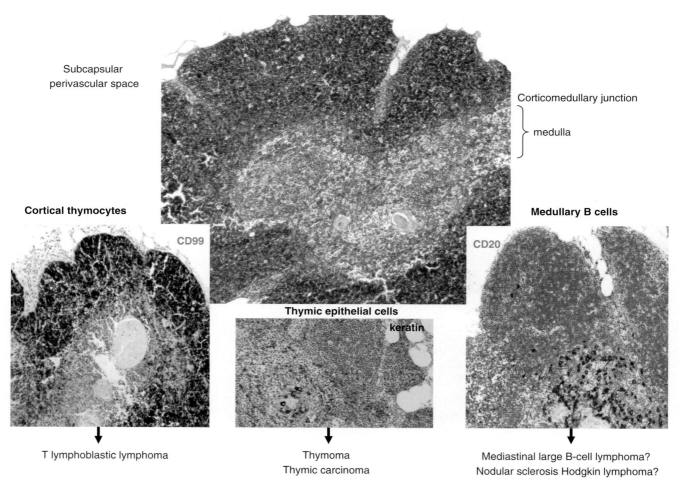

Fig. 27-10. Structure of the thymus and its tumor types

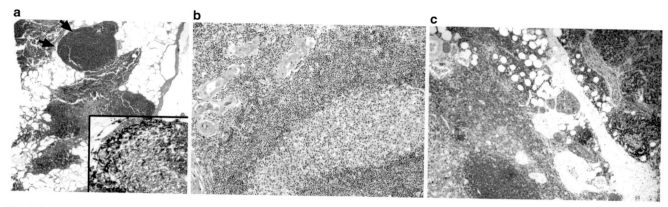

Fig. 27-11. Pre-neoplastic thymic B-cell expansions. (**a**) Thymic involution with aging is associated with contraction of the cortex and expansions of pericapsular B cells (inset is CD20 immunostain on area indicated by arrows). (**b**) Germinal center (GC) formation in the thymic medulla from a patient with myasthenia gravis. (**c**) CD20 immunostain in a thymus from a patient with myasthenia gravis shows marked increases in GCs and thymic B-cell populations

stromal cells and antigen presenting cells. TCRs that signal too strongly are eliminated by apoptosis (positive selection), as are T cells that fail to bind MHC (negative selection). By this process, T cells emerge from the thymus with an intermediate-affinity TCR, so that the autoimmune consequences of circulating autoreactive T cells can be limited.

In adults, the thymus begins to involute with replacement by adipose tissue. With the shift away from thymocyte production in early adulthood, the role of the thymus in B-cell maturation becomes more predominant (see below). In patients with certain autoimmune diseases (e.g. myasthenia gravis and acquired autoantibody syndromes), [59] the thymic immune control is defective with the production of destructive autoantibodies [60] and the thymus shows progressive replacement by reactive germinal centers, thus mimicking a secondary lymphoid organ (Fig. 27-11) [61]. Such patients have a higher risk for development of thymomas and thymic endocrine lesions, as well as lymphomas of various types, [62,63] and they can release increased numbers of immature thymic precursors, which circulate in the blood.

27.4.2. Cell Types of the Thymus

Thymocytes (precursor T cells): Precursor T cells (thymocytes) undergo step-wise maturation that is linked to TCR-mediated programmed cell death and expansion. The details of T-cell maturation are summarized in Chap. 31, with progressive states of thymus maturation ["double-negative" (DN) to "double-positive" (DP) to "single-positive" (SP)] named on the basis of the surface expression patterns of CD4 and CD8. DN thymocytes are found in the upper cortex and express only the CD2 and CD7 T-cell markers at their earliest stages. DP thymocytes, located in the mid- and lower cortex also express CD1a and CD3, as well as CD4 and CD8, and progressively acquire intact TCRs of either the α/β or the γ/δ type. SP thymocytes found in the medulla express the full range of pan-T-cell markers and either CD4 or CD8.

Thymic B cells: In adults, B cells comprise ~30% of the cells in the thymic medulla and are also found in the perivascular space (PVS) in the capsule [64,65]. They are distinct from the CD2+ thymic B cells found in young children [66]. PVS-associated B cells are positive for CD21, CD37, and CD72, and have a high rate of mutated IGH genes with nonproductive rearrangements similar to the findings in Hodgkin lymphoma tumor cells (See Chap. 20, Fig. 20-1) [64]. A small subset of thymic B cells in the medulla express the T-cell differentiation marker MAL as does a subset of mediastinal B-cell lymphoma, suggesting a possible thymic origin for this lymphoma [67]. The number of thymic B cells peaks in middle adulthood (26–49 years), and decreases slightly after 50 years of age. TNFR family members appear to be important for thymic B-cell signaling, and the chemokines CXCL13 and CCL21 may influence localization [68–70]. Whether PVS and/or medullary B cells differentiate in situ, as in mice, [71] or migrate from secondary lymphoid organs is not yet clear.

Thymic epithelium: The thymus is unique among lymphoid organs in having many different stromal subsets that express cytokeratin that have been termed "thymic epithelium". At least 6 different functional subsets have been defined, each mapping to different functional micro-environments of the thymus (e.g. subcapsular, upper cortex, mid cortex, corticomedullary junction, and medulla) [72]. Differential expression of chemokines in thymic epithelial sub-sets likely drives intrathymic migration and shifts in thymocyte maturation [73]. Thymomas and thymic carcinomas represent neoplasms of these stromal subsets and likely progress from pre-neoplastic localized proliferations of thymic epithelium.

27.4.3. Thymoma and Thymic Carcinoma

Thymomas are generally indolent neoplasms that arise sporadically, as well as at increased rates in patients with autoimmune disorders of the thymus (e.g. myasthenia gravis) [74]. Thymomas, which always contain some admixed component of nonneoplastic thymocytes, slowly expand producing a thick fibrous capsule. There have been multiple approaches to the classification of thymomas and their rare malignant counterparts (Table 27-9). The original morphologic classification of Rosai and colleagues and subsequent work by Suster and Moran have focused on the degree of cytologic atypia within the epithelial component. The Masoaka staging system highlights the clinically significant findings of micro-scopic and macroscopic capsular invasion, involvement of adjacent organs (usually the lung), and the uncommon lymph node metastasis or distant spread [75].

The morphogenetic thymoma classification of Mueller-Hermelink and colleagues focuses on the histologic appearance of both the epithelial and thymocyte component to distinguish a presumed cell of origin for each tumor type. The histogenetic features of thymomas are roughly correlated with clinical behavior. For example, lymphocyte-rich and mixed thymomas, which are

Table 27-9. Classification schemes for thymoma and thymic carcinoma.

Classification	Subtypes	Based on:	Strengths	Weaknesses
Bernatz [107]	Lymphocyte-predominant Epithelial-predominant Mixed Spindle cell thymoma	Proportion of epithelial cells to lymphocytes, shape of tumor	Good reproducibility	Not well correlated with outcome
Masaoka [75]	I: Encapsulated II: Microinvasive III: Grossly invasive IV: Disseminated	Clinical stage of disease	Outcome-based, focus on capsular invasion	Requires correlation with findings at surgery
Müller-Hermelink [108]	Medullary Mixed Organoid Cortical Well-differentiated thymic carcinoma Malignant carcinoma	Histogenetic derivation	Correlation between types and invasiveness	Complexity may limit reproducibility
Suster and Moran [109]	Thymoma Atypical thymoma Thymic carcinoma	Degree of differentiation	Simplified nomenclature	Doesn't reflect histologic differentiation type
Integrated WHO classification [110]	A: spindle-shaped, AB: mixed B1-B3: epithelioid C: carcinoma	Presumed cell of origin, degree of atypia	Translates across different schema	Complex, with multiple different goals

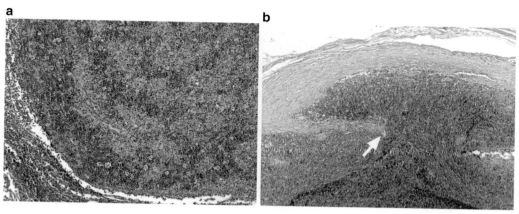

Fig. 27-12. Thymoma, cortical (lymphocytic) type. (**a**) Islands of thymic epithelium alternating with numerous thymocytes and other immune cells. (**b**) Microscopic infiltration into the capsule (*arrow*) in a cytologically bland thymoma. This thymoma would be classifed as type B2 in the WHO classification

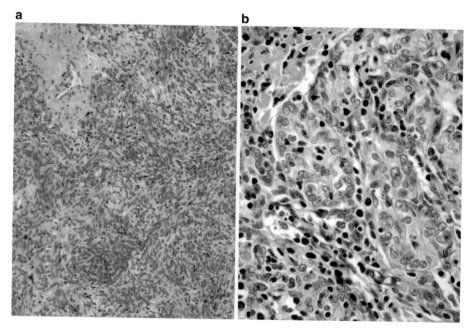

Fig. 27-13. Thymoma, medullary type. (**a**) Classical appearance with whorls of spindle cells with few admixed thymocytes. (**b**) A rosetting pattern of growth with increased numbers of admixed thymocytes is seen in some cases. This thymoma would be classified as Type A in the WHO classification

believed to arise from epithelial cells that reside in the cortex (Fig. 27-12), present at a higher stage, more frequently show capsular invasion, and have a worse prognosis [76]. In contrast, spindle cell thymomas (Fig. 27-13), which are believed to arise from epithelial cell populations that reside in the medulla or at the C-M junction, present at a lower stage and have a better prognosis [76]. The current WHO classification schema is an effort to incorporate both histogenetic and clinical predictors into a unified approach.

There has also been extensive debate about the terminology used to diagnose thymic epithelial tumors that have only a minimal lymphoid component or those with

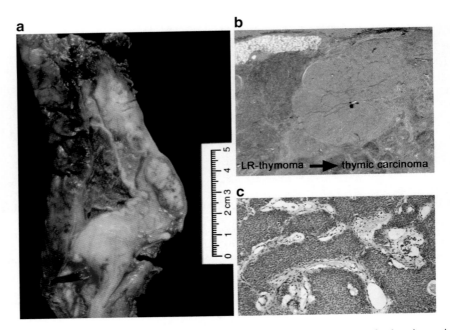

Fig. 27-14. Thymic carcinoma. (**a**) Resection by extrapleural pneumonectomy of a thymic carcinoma invading into pleura. (**b**) Areas of benign-appearing lymphocyte-rich (LR) thymoma alternating with cellular high-grade thymic carcinoma. (**c**) Typical histologic appearance of well-differentiated thymic carcinoma with lobules separated by hyalinized stroma (Type B3 thymoma, WHO)

marked cytologic atypia. Many of these tumors appear to represent progression of thymoma to thymic carcinoma in a clonal evolution pattern common to any tumor type (Fig. 27-14a/b). Evidence of clinical aggressiveness in a thymoma, such as capsular or tissue invasion (Fig. 27-14a), is often associated with histologic progression including increased tumor cell pleomorphism, increased mitosis, and necrosis. There is also often intratumoral variation in these clinically aggressive tumors, with both poorly differentiated carcinoma-like and more benign thymoma-like areas (Figure 27.14b). However, some malignant thymic carcinomas appear to arise de novo without evidence of a background thymoma. Squamous cell carcinoma and the well-differentiated thymic carcinoma (type C thymoma in the WHO schema) represent two such examples (Fig. 27-14c) [77,78].

27.4.4. T Lymphoblastic Lymphoma

T lymphoblastic lymphoma (T-LBL) is the most common mediastinal tumor in children and young adults and arises from immature thymocytes. The histologic appearance is always that of a sheet-like infiltrate of blastic lymphocytes (Fig. 27-15) that invades adjacent soft tissues in a single-file fashion. Although the majority of T-LBLs appear to arise in the thymus, most will involve the blood and bone marrow at diagnosis (30-40% in children, 15–30% in adults)[79] or at relapse. Extrathymic LBL shows phenotypic differences, and includes both primitive BM variants in younger patients[80] and lymph node-based tumors in older patients [81,82]. Expression of terminal deoxynucleotidyl transferase (TdT) separates T-LBL from more mature T-cell neoplasms. The molecular pathogenesis of T-LBL involves a number of different recurrent chromosomal translocations that activate transcriptional factors which regulate thymocyte differentiation stage (typically HOX family genes), often by juxtaposition of these genes to the TCR enhancer loci [83]. The immunophenotype of T-LBL can often be mapped, to some degree, onto the stages of thymocyte development, with the most common phenotype corresponding to the double-positive subset (CD1a+, CD2+, cytoplasmic

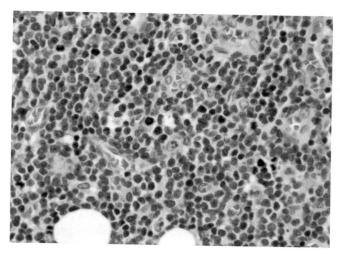

Fig. 27-15. Thymic lymphoblastic lymphoma

CD3+, CD4+, and CD8+). The stepwise pattern of TCRG, TCRD, TCRB, and TCRA gene rearrangements in these tumors also resemble the patterns seen in thymocyte development (See Chap. 31) [84]. The most primitive T-LBL will often express only CD7 and/or CD2 in association with myeloid markers such as CD13 and CD33 and may have FLT3 mutations. The small subset of mediastinal T-LBL which lacks TdT expression but shows blastic appearance and a high mitotic rate may arise from more mature medullary thymocytes.

When using flow cytometry to diagnose thymic lymphoblastic lymphoma, it is important to consider that alterations in thymocyte subpopulations can also accompany thymoma [85]. Therefore, thymoma should always be considered first when an abnormal immature T-cell population is detected in needle biopsies or aspirates of older patients with mediastinal masses. In fact, such abnormal T-cell proliferations in thymomas [86] can rarely terminate in lymphoblastic lymphoma [87].

27.4.5. Mediastinal Large B-Cell Lymphoma

Primary mediastinal large B-cell lymphoma (PMBCL), as discussed in Chap. 17, is uncommon (2–4% of lymphomas) but distinct from almost all other DLBCL types in being more common in females and young adults (median age 35 years). In advanced disease, the tumor can invade the adjacent structures of the lungs, pleura, and pericardium, and has a tendency to involve the kidneys, adrenals, liver, ovaries, and CNS parenchyma [88,89]. Although there are some molecular features in common with other DLBCL, such as BCL6 mutation, [90,91] the presence of JAK2 amplification, [92] MAL expression, [67] crippling IGH somatic mutations, and a distinct gene expression profile [93,94] supports a distinct pathogenesis, likely from resident thymic B cells (Fig. 27-16a/b).

27.4.6. Hodgkin Lymphoma

Nodular sclerosis classical Hodgkin lymphoma (NSCHL) is the most common subtype of HL, and most patients with NSCHL present with a mediastinal mass suggesting an origin from thymic tissue. Rarely, biopsy of NSCHL in the mediastinum may still show an association with thymic tissue (Fig. 27-16c-e) [95] Gene expression studies have demonstrated that tumor cells in NSCHL have phenotypic similarities with PMBCL, including defects in BCR signaling and similar mechanisms of NF-kB and JAK-STAT pathway dysregulation.

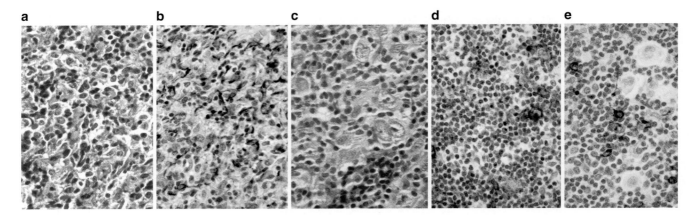

Fig. 27-16. B-cell lymphomas arising in the mediastinum. (**a**) Mediastinal large B-cell lymphoma shows tumor cells infiltrating between reticulated fibrosis. (**b**) Residual thymic epithelium detected by keratin immunostain. (**c**) Nodular sclerosis Hodgkin lymphoma presenting as a mediastinal mass shows infiltration into the thymic medulla. (**d**) Reed-Sternberg cells show CD30 immunostaining. (**e**) Intermixed medullary thymic epithelium are positive on keratin immunostain

Furthermore, molecular analyses of the expressed immunoglobulin gene sequences in NSCHL have also suggested defective BCR signaling (Chap. 20). These results may suggest a model whereby the thymic microenvironment can rescue B cells with defective BCR signaling, and thus promote tumor development of either PMBCL or NSCHL.

Suggested Readings

Suster S, Moran CA. Thymoma classification: current status and future trends. Am J Clin Pathol 2006; 125:542–54.

Kurtin PJ, Myers JL, Adlakha H, et al. Pathologic and clinical features of primary pulmonary extranodal marginal zone B-cell lymphoma of MALT type. Am J Surg Pathol 2001;25:997–1008.

Johnson PW, Davies AJ. Primary mediastinal B-cell lymphoma. Hematology Am Soc Hematol Educ Program 2008;2008:349–58.

References

1. Burkhardt B, Zimmermann M, Oschlies I, et al. The impact of age and gender on biology, clinical features and treatment outcome of non-Hodgkin lymphoma in childhood and adolescence. Br J Haematol 2005;131:39–49.
2. Jaffe ES, Harris NL, Stein H, Isaacson PG. Classification of lymphoid neoplasms: the microscope as a tool for disease discovery. Blood 2008;112:4384–99.
3. Sokolowska-Wojdylo M, Wenzel J, Gaffal E, et al. Circulating clonal CLA(+) and CD4(+) T cells in Sezary syndrome express the skin-homing chemokine receptors CCR4 and CCR10 as well as the lymph node-homing chemokine receptor CCR7. Br J Dermatol 2005;152:258–64.
4. Magro CM, Dyrsen ME. Cutaneous lymphocyte antigen expression in benign and neoplastic cutaneous B- and T-cell lymphoid infiltrates. J Cutan Pathol 2008;35:1040–9.
5. Dogan A, Du M, Koulis A, Briskin MJ, Isaacson PG. Expression of lymphocyte homing receptors and vascular addressins in low-grade gastric B-cell lymphomas of mucosa-associated lymphoid tissue. Am J Pathol 1997;151:1361–9.
6. Willemze R, Jaffe ES, Burg G, et al. WHO-EORTC classification for cutaneous lymphomas. Blood 2005;105:3768–85.
7. Bogle MA, Riddle CC, Triana EM, Jones D, Duvic M. Primary cutaneous B-cell lymphoma. J Am Acad Dermatol 2005;53:479–84.

8. Dijkman R, Tensen CP, Jordanova ES, et al. Array-based comparative genomic hybridization analysis reveals recurrent chromosomal alterations and prognostic parameters in primary cutaneous large B-cell lymphoma. J Clin Oncol 2006;24:296–305.

9. Kodama K, Massone C, Chott A, Metze D, Kerl H, Cerroni L. Primary cutaneous large B-cell lymphomas: clinicopathologic features, classification, and prognostic factors in a large series of patients. Blood 2005;106:2491–7.

10. Senff NJ, Hoefnagel JJ, Jansen PM, et al. Reclassification of 300 primary cutaneous B-Cell lymphomas according to the new WHO-EORTC classification for cutaneous lymphomas: comparison with previous classifications and identification of prognostic markers. J Clin Oncol 2007;25:1581–7.

11. Jahnke K, Korfel A, O'Neill BP, et al. International study on low-grade primary central nervous system lymphoma. Ann Neurol 2006;59:755–62.

12. Shenkier TN, Blay JY, O'Neill BP, et al. Primary CNS lymphoma of T-cell origin: a descriptive analysis from the international primary CNS lymphoma collaborative group. J Clin Oncol 2005;23:2233–9.

13. Ferreri AJ, Blay JY, Reni M, et al. Prognostic scoring system for primary CNS lymphomas: the International Extranodal Lymphoma Study Group experience. J Clin Oncol 2003;21:266–72.

14. Salzburg J, Burkhardt B, Zimmermann M, et al. Prevalence, clinical pattern, and outcome of CNS involvement in childhood and adolescent non-Hodgkin's lymphoma differ by non-Hodgkin's lymphoma subtype: a Berlin-Frankfurt-Munster Group Report. J Clin Oncol 2007;25:3915–22.

15. Ambrosetti A, Zanotti R, Pattaro C, et al. Most cases of primary salivary mucosa-associated lymphoid tissue lymphoma are associated either with Sjoegren syndrome or hepatitis C virus infection. Br J Haematol 2004;126:43–9.

16. Essadi I, Ismaili N, Tazi E, et al. Primary lymphoma of the head and neck: two case reports and review of the literature. Cases J 2008;1:426.

17. Epstein JB, Epstein JD, Le ND, Gorsky M. Characteristics of oral and paraoral malignant lymphoma: a population-based review of 361 cases. Oral Surg Oral Med Oral Pathol Oral Radiol Endod 2001;92:519–25.

18. Derringer GA, Thompson LD, Frommelt RA, Bijwaard KE, Heffess CS, Abbondanzo SL. Malignant lymphoma of the thyroid gland: a clinicopathologic study of 108 cases. Am J Surg Pathol 2000;24:623–39.

19. Koss MN. Pulmonary lymphoid disorders. Semin Diagn Pathol 1995;12:158–71.

20. Solomonov A, Zuckerman T, Goralnik L, Ben-Arieh Y, Rowe JM, Yigla M. Non-Hodgkin's lymphoma presenting as an endobronchial tumor: report of eight cases and literature review. Am J Hematol 2008;83:416–9.

21. Kurtin PJ, Myers JL, Adlakha H, et al. Pathologic and clinical features of primary pulmonary extranodal marginal zone B-cell lymphoma of MALT type. Am J Surg Pathol 2001;25:997–1008.

22. Chng WJ, Remstein ED, Fonseca R, et al. Gene expression profiling of pulmonary mucosa-associated lymphoid tissue lymphoma identifies new biologic insights with potential diagnostic and therapeutic applications. Blood 2009;113:635–45.

23. Zinzani PL, Poletti V, Zompatori M, et al. Bronchus-associated lymphoid tissue lymphomas: an update of a rare extranodal maltoma. Clin Lymphoma Myeloma 2007;7:566–72.

24. Satani T, Yokose T, Kaburagi T, Asato Y, Itabashi M, Amemiya R. Amyloid deposition in primary pulmonary marginal zone B-cell lymphoma of mucosa-associated lymphoid tissue. Pathol Int 2007;57:746–50.

25. Rawal A, Finn WG, Schnitzer B, Valdez R. Site-specific morphologic differences in extranodal marginal zone B-cell lymphomas. Arch Pathol Lab Med 2007;131:1673–8.

26. Jones D, Renshaw AA. Recurrent crystal-storing histiocytosis of the lung in a patient without a clonal lymphoproliferative disorder. Arch Pathol Lab Med 1996;120:978–80.

27. Kojima M, Nakamura N, Otuski Y, et al. Pulmonary lesion of idiopathic plasmacytic lymphadenopathy with polyclonal hyperimmunoglobulinemia appears to be a cause of lymphoplasmacytic proliferation of the lung: a report of five cases. Pathol Res Pract 2008;204:185–90.

28. Mollejo M, Rodriguez-Pinilla MS, Montes-Moreno S, et al. Splenic Follicular Lymphoma: Clinicopathologic Characteristics of a Series of 32 Cases. Am J Surg Pathol 2009;33:730–8.

29. Zhu Q, Xu B, Xu K, Li J, Jin XL. Primary non-Hodgkin's lymphoma in the esophagus. J Dig Dis 2008;9:241–4.

30. Krugmann J, Dirnhofer S, Gschwendtner A, et al. Primary gastrointestinal B-cell lymphoma. A clincopathological and immunohistochemical study of 61 cases with an evaluation of prognostic parameters. Pathol Res Pract 2001;197:385–93.

31. Bende RJ, Smit LA, Bossenbroek JG, et al. Primary follicular lymphoma of the small intestine: alpha4beta7 expression and immunoglobulin configuration suggest an origin from local antigen-experienced B cells. Am J Pathol 2003;162:105–13.

32. Afolayan EA, Anjorin AS. Incidence of primary extranodal lymphoma involving gastrointestinal tract by histological type at Ilorin. Niger J Med 2001;10:135–8.

33. Schmitt-Graff A, Hummel M, Zemlin M, et al. Intestinal T-cell lymphoma: a reassessment of cytomorphological and phenotypic features in relation to patterns of small bowel remodelling. Virchows Arch 1996;429:27–36.

34. Katoh A, Ohshima K, Kanda M, et al. Gastrointestinal T cell lymphoma: predominant cytotoxic phenotypes, including alpha/beta, gamma/delta T cell and natural killer cells. Leuk Lymphoma 2000;39:97–111.

35. Zettl A, Ott G, Makulik A, et al. Chromosomal gains at 9q characterize enteropathy-type T-cell lymphoma. Am J Pathol 2002;161:1635–45.

36. Salmon JS, Thompson MA, Arildsen RC, Greer JP. Non-Hodgkin's lymphoma involving the liver: clinical and therapeutic considerations. Clin Lymphoma Myeloma 2006;6:273–80.

37. Ostrowski ML, Inwards CY, Strickler JG, Witzig TE, Wenger DE, Unni KK. Osseous Hodgkin disease. Cancer 1999;85:1166–78.

38. Ostrowski ML, Unni KK, Banks PM, et al. Malignant lymphoma of bone. Cancer 1986;58:2646–55.

39. Jones D, Kraus MD, Dorfman DM. Lymphoma presenting as a solitary bone lesion. Am J Clin Pathol 1999;111:171–8.

40. Jones D. Large Cell lymphoma presenting in the bone marrow. Case Rev Pathol 2000;5:281–6.

41. Kajiura D, Yamashita Y, Mori N. Diffuse large B-cell lymphoma initially manifesting in the bone marrow. Am J Clin Pathol 2007;127:762–9.

42. Talwalkar SS, Miranda RN, Valbuena JR, Routbort MJ, Martin AW, Medeiros LJ. Lymphomas involving the breast: a study of 106 cases comparing localized and disseminated neoplasms. Am J Surg Pathol 2008;32:1299–309.

43. Validire P, Capovilla M, Asselain B, et al. Primary breast non-Hodgkin's lymphoma: A large single center study of initial characteristics, natural history, and prognostic factors. Am J Hematol 2009;84:133–9.

44. Ottaviani G, Matturri L, Rossi L, Jones D. Sudden death due to lymphomatous infiltration of the cardiac conduction system. Cardiovasc Pathol 2003;12:77–81.

45. Ban-Hoefen M, Zeglin MA, Bisognano JD. Diffuse large B cell lymphoma presenting as a cardiac mass and odynophagia. Cardiol J 2008;15:471–4.

46. Stakos DA, Xatseras DI, Boudoulas H. Cardiac lymphoma. Eur Heart J 2006;27:1538.

47. Fujisaki J, Tanaka T, Kato J, et al. Primary cardiac lymphoma presenting clinically as restrictive cardiomyopathy. Circ J 2005;69:249–52.

48. Schubert S, Abdul-Khaliq H, Lehmkuhl HB, et al. Diagnosis and treatment of post-transplantation lymphoproliferative disorder in pediatric heart transplant patients. Pediatr Transplant 2009;13:54–62.

49. Aversa SM, Stragliotto S, Marino D, et al. Post-transplant lymphoproliferative disorders after heart or kidney transplantation at a single centre: presentation and response to treatment. Acta Haematol 2008;120:36–46.

50. Singh D, Kumar L, Sharma A, Vijayaraghavan M, Thulkar S, Tandon N. Adrenal involvement in non-Hodgkin's lymphoma: four cases and review of literature. Leuk Lymphoma 2004;45:789–94.

51. Kraus MD, Jones D, Bartlett NL. Intravascular lymphoma associated with endocrine dysfunction: a report of four cases and a review of the literature. Am J Med 1999;107:169–76.

52. Elharroudi T, Ismaili N, Errihani H, Jalil A. Primary lymphoma of the ovary. J Cancer Res Ther 2008;4:195–6.

53. Vang R, Medeiros LJ, Ha CS, Deavers M. Non-Hodgkin's lymphomas involving the uterus: a clinicopathologic analysis of 26 cases. Mod Pathol 2000;13:19–28.

54. Garcia MG, Deavers MT, Knoblock RJ, et al. Myeloid sarcoma involving the gynecologic tract: a report of 11 cases and review of the literature. Am J Clin Pathol 2006;125:783–90.

55. Visco C, Medeiros LJ, Mesina OM, et al. Non-Hodgkin's lymphoma affecting the testis: is it curable with doxorubicin-based therapy? Clin Lymphoma 2001;2:40–6.

56. Zouhair A, Weber D, Belkacemi Y, et al. Outcome and patterns of failure in testicular lymphoma: a multicenter Rare Cancer Network study. Int J Radiat Oncol Biol Phys 2002;52:652–6.

57. Gomez Garcia I, Rodriguez Patron R, Sanz Mayayo E. et al [Primary testicular lymphoma. Report of a new case and review of the literature]. Actas Urol Esp 2004;28:141–6.

58. Mandal M, Crusio KM, Meng F, et al. Regulation of lymphocyte progenitor survival by the proapoptotic activities of Bim and Bid. Proc Natl Acad Sci U S A 2008;105:20840–5.

59. Meager A, Peterson P, Willcox N. Hypothetical review: thymic aberrations and type-I interferons; attempts to deduce autoimmunizing mechanisms from unexpected clues in monogenic and paraneoplastic syndromes. Clin Exp Immunol 2008;154:141–51.

60. Leite MI, Jones M, Strobel P, et al. Myasthenia gravis thymus: complement vulnerability of epithelial and myoid cells, complement attack on them, and correlations with autoantibody status. Am J Pathol 2007;171:893–905.

61. Roxanis I, Micklem K, McConville J, Newsom-Davis J, Willcox N. Thymic myoid cells and germinal center formation in myasthenia gravis; possible roles in pathogenesis. J Neuroimmunol 2002;125:185–97.

62. Verstandig AG, Epstein DM, Miller WT Jr, Aronchik JA, Gefter WB, Miller WT. Thymoma–report of 71 cases and a review. Crit Rev Diagn Imaging 1992;33:201–30.

63. Sperling B, Marschall J, Kennedy R, Pahwa P, Chibbar R. Thymoma: a review of the clinical and pathological findings in 65 cases. Can J Surg 2003;46:37–42.

64. Flores KG, Li J, Hale LP. B cells in epithelial and perivascular compartments of human adult thymus. Hum Pathol 2001;32:926–34.

65. Spencer J, Choy M, Hussell T, Papadaki L, Kington JP, Isaacson PG. Properties of human thymic B cells. Immunology 1992;75:596–600.

66. Punnonen J, de Vries JE. Characterization of a novel CD2+ human thymic B cell subset. J Immunol 1993;151:100–10.

67. Copie-Bergman C, Plonquet A, Alonso MA, et al. MAL expression in lymphoid cells: further evidence for MAL as a distinct molecular marker of primary mediastinal large B-cell lymphomas. Mod Pathol 2002;15:1172–80.

68. Meraouna A, Cizeron-Clairac G, Panse RL, et al. The chemokine CXCL13 is a key molecule in autoimmune myasthenia gravis. Blood 2006;108:432–40.

69. Thangarajh M, Masterman T, Helgeland L, et al. The thymus is a source of B-cell-survival factors-APRIL and BAFF-in myasthenia gravis. J Neuroimmunol 2006;178:161–6.

70. Le Panse R, Cizeron-Clairac G, Bismuth J, Berrih-Aknin S. Microarrays reveal distinct gene signatures in the thymus of seropositive and seronegative myasthenia gravis patients and the role of CC chemokine ligand 21 in thymic hyperplasia. J Immunol 2006;177:7868–79.

71. Sugihara A, Inaba M, Mori SI, et al. Differentiation from thymic B cell progenitors to mature B cells in vitro. Immunobiology 2000;201:515–26.

72. Berzi A, Ayata CK, Cavalcante P, et al. BDNF and its receptors in human myasthenic thymus: implications for cell fate in thymic pathology. J Neuroimmunol 2008;197:128–39.

73. Annunziato F, Romagnani P, Cosmi L, et al. Macrophage-derived chemokine and EBI1-ligand chemokine attract human thymocytes in different stage of development and are produced by distinct subsets of medullary epithelial cells: possible implications for negative selection. J Immunol 2000;165:238–46.

74. Hoffacker V, Schultz A, Tiesinga JJ, et al. Thymomas alter the T-cell subset composition in the blood: a potential mechanism for thymoma-associated autoimmune disease. Blood 2000;96:3872–9.

75. Masaoka A, Monden Y, Nakahara K, Tanioka T. Follow-up study of thymomas with special reference to their clinical stages. Cancer 1981;48:2485–92.

76. Engel P, Marx A, Muller-Hermelink HK. Thymic tumours in Denmark. A retrospective study of 213 cases from 1970–1993. Pathol Res Pract 1999;195:565–70.

77. Zettl A, Strobel P, Wagner K, et al. Recurrent genetic aberrations in thymoma and thymic carcinoma. Am J Pathol 2000;157:257–66.

78. Lequaglie C, Giudice G, Brega Massone PP, Conti B, Cataldo I. Clinical and pathologic predictors of survival in patients with thymic tumors. J Cardiovasc Surg (Torino) 2002;43:269–74.

79. Thomas DA, O'Brien S, Cortes J, et al. Outcome with the hyper-CVAD regimens in lymphoblastic lymphoma. Blood 2004;104:1624–30.

80. Hunault M, Truchan-Graczyk M, Caillot D, et al. Outcome of adult T-lymphoblastic lymphoma after acute lymphoblastic leukemia-type treatment: a GOELAMS trial. Haematologica 2007;92:1623–30.

81. Onciu M, Lai R, Vega F, Bueso-Ramos C, Medeiros LJ. Precursor T-cell acute lymphoblastic leukemia in adults: age-related immunophenotypic, cytogenetic, and molecular subsets. Am J Clin Pathol 2002;117:252–8.

82. Onishi Y, Matsuno Y, Tateishi U, et al. Two entities of precursor T-cell lymphoblastic leukemia/lymphoma based on radiologic and immunophenotypic findings. Int J Hematol 2004;80:43–51.

83. Ballerini P, Landman-Parker J, Cayuela JM, et al. Impact of genotype on survival of children with T-cell acute lymphoblastic leukemia treated according to the French protocol FRALLE-93: the effect of TLX3/HOX11L2 gene expression on outcome. Haematologica 2008;93:1658–65.

84. Baleydier F, Decouvelaere AV, Bergeron J, et al. T cell receptor genotyping and HOXA/TLX1 expression define three T lymphoblastic lymphoma subsets which might affect clinical outcome. Clin Cancer Res 2008;14:692–700.

85. Gorczyca W, Tugulea S, Liu Z, Li X, Wong JY, Weisberger J. Flow cytometry in the diagnosis of mediastinal tumors with emphasis on differentiating thymocytes from precursor T-lymphoblastic lymphoma/leukemia. Leuk Lymphoma 2004;45:529–38.

86. Sakuraba M, Motoji T, Nitta S, Mizoguchi H, Ohnuki T. Increased thymocyte CD4+CD8+ cells and T-cell receptor beta gene rearrangements in thymoma. Jpn J Thorac Cardiovasc Surg 2003;51:481–7.

87. Macon WR, Rynalski TH, Swerdlow SH, Cousar JB. T-cell lymphoblastic leukemia/lymphoma presenting in a recurrent thymoma. Mod Pathol 1991;4:524–8.

88. Johnson PW, Davies AJ. Primary mediastinal B-cell lymphoma. Hematology Am Soc Hematol Educ Program 2008;2008:349–58.

89. Bishop PC, Wilson WH, Pearson D, Janik J, Jaffe ES, Elwood PC. CNS involvement in primary mediastinal large B-cell lymphoma. J Clin Oncol 1999;17:2479–85.

90. Iqbal J, Greiner TC, Patel K, et al. Distinctive patterns of BCL6 molecular alterations and their functional consequences in different subgroups of diffuse large B-cell lymphoma. Leukemia 2007;21:2332–43.

91. Pileri SA, Gaidano G, Zinzani PL, et al. Primary mediastinal B-cell lymphoma: high frequency of BCL-6 mutations and consistent expression of the transcription factors OCT-2, BOB.1, and PU.1 in the absence of immunoglobulins. Am J Pathol 2003;162:243–53.

92. Meier C, Hoeller S, Bourgau C, et al. Recurrent numerical aberrations of JAK2 and deregulation of the JAK2-STAT cascade in lymphomas. Mod Pathol 2009;22:476–87.

93. Roberts RA, Wright G, Rosenwald AR, et al. Loss of major histocompatibility class II gene and protein expression in primary mediastinal large B-cell lymphoma is highly coordinated and related to poor patient survival. Blood 2006;108:311–8.

94. Rosenwald A, Wright G, Leroy K, et al. Molecular diagnosis of primary mediastinal B cell lymphoma identifies a clinically favorable subgroup of diffuse large B cell lymphoma related to Hodgkin lymphoma. J Exp Med 2003;198:851–62.

95. Krugmann J, Feichtinger H, Greil R, Fend F. Thymic Hodgkin's disease – a histological and immunohistochemical study of three cases. Pathol Res Pract 1999;195:681–7.

96. Magro CM, Crowson AN, Kovatich AJ, Burns F. Drug-induced reversible lymphoid dyscrasia: a clonal lymphomatoid dermatitis of memory and activated T cells. Hum Pathol 2003;34:119–29.

97. Carlson JA, Mihm MC Jr, LeBoit PE. Cutaneous lymphocytic vasculitis: a definition, a review, and a proposed classification. Semin Diagn Pathol 1996;13:72–90.

98. Camilleri-Broet S, Martin A, Moreau A, et al. Primary central nervous system lymphomas in 72 immunocompetent patients: pathologic findings and clinical correlations. Groupe Ouest Est d'etude des Leucenies et Autres Maladies du Sang (GOELAMS). Am J Clin Pathol 1998;110:607–12.

99. Nuckols JD, Liu K, Burchette JL, McLendon RE, Traweek ST. Primary central nervous system lymphomas: a 30-year experience at a single institution. Mod Pathol 1999;12:1167–73.

100. Iwamoto FM, Abrey LE. Primary dural lymphomas: a review. Neurosurg Focus 2006;21:E5.

101. Weber AL, Rahemtullah A, Ferry JA. Hodgkin and non-Hodgkin lymphoma of the head and neck: clinical, pathologic, and imaging evaluation. Neuroimaging Clin N Am 2003;13:371–92.

102. Papouliakos S, Karkos PD, Korres G, Karatzias G, Sastry A, Riga M. Comparison of clinical and histopathological evaluation of tonsils in pediatric and adult patients. Eur Arch Otorhinolaryngol 2008;266:1309–13.

103. Arber DA, Rappaport H, Weiss LM. Non-Hodgkin's lymphoproliferative disorders involving the spleen. Mod Pathol 1997;10:18–32.

104. Stancu M, Jones D, Vega F, Medeiros LJ. Peripheral T-cell lymphoma arising in the liver. Am J Clin Pathol 2002;118:574–81.

105. Cirillo M, Federico M, Curci G, Tamborrino E, Piccinini L, Silingardi V. Primary gastrointestinal lymphoma: a clinicopathological study of 58 cases. Haematologica 1992;77:156–61.

106. Banks PM. Gastrointestinal lymphoproliferative disorders. Histopathology 2007;50:42–54.

107. Bernatz PE, Harrison EG, Clagett OT. Thymoma: a clinicopathologic study. J Thorac Cardiovasc Surg 1961;42:424–44.

108. Muller-Hermelink HK, Marx A. Thymoma. Curr Opin Oncol 2000;12:426–33.

109. Suster S, Moran CA. Thymoma classification: current status and future trends. Am J Clin Pathol 2006;125:542–54.

110. Müller-Hermelink K, Moller P, Engel P, et al. Tumors of the thymus: Introduction. In: Travis WD, Brambilla E, Müller-Hermelink HK, Harris CC, eds. Pathology and genetics of tumours of the lung, pleura, thymus and heart (WHO classification of tumours series). Lyon, France: IARC Press, 2004:148–51.

Section 4

Stem Cell Transplantation

Chapter 28

Clinical Aspects of Hematopoietic Stem Cell Transplantation

Elizabeth J. Shpall and Marcos de Lima

Abstract/Scope of Chapter This chapter provides an overview of autologous and allogeneic hematopoietic stem cell transplantation, including indications, methods of graft preparation, and new approaches to boosting engraftment and minimizing complications.

Keywords Hematopoietic stem cell transplantation, allogeneic • hematopoietic stem cell transplantation, autologous • Hematopoietic stem cell transplantation, non-myeloablative • Hematopoietic stem cell transplantation, conditioning regimen • Stem cell, preparation • Graft-versus-host disease, grading.

28.1. Introduction

Hematopoietic stem cell transplantation (HSCT), the repopulation of bone marrow with infused hematopoietic progenitors following preparative chemoradiation to eradicate the pre-existing marrow, was first performed by E. Donnall Thomas in 1956. Since that time, there has been great progress in identifying the patients who would benefit most from HSCT, in the optimal preparative and cell harvesting regimens and in management of post-transplant complications. In the last several years, there has been a shift to less toxic non-myeloablative HSCT and use of stem cells harvested from adult blood and from umbilical cord blood. Use of products that have been extensively manipulated, purged or expanded in vitro prior to infusion has also increased. These changes have resulted in an evolution of HSCT from a relatively crude procedure with high morbidity and mortality to a sophisticated series of medical interventions with improved outcomes.

28.2. Types of Transplant: Indications and Outcomes

The types of stem cell transplants currently performed are summarized in Table 28-1. In autologous HSCT, the patient provides their own stem cell source (bone marrow, peripheral blood or cord blood) thus avoiding graft-versus-host disease. Autologous HSCT from previously procured material allows dose-escalation of chemotherapy or radiation beyond the limits of myelosuppression. The recipient is "rescued" with the autologous cells after the high-dose therapy is delivered. Common indications include treatment of plasma cell myeloma and relapsed lymphomas of all types. Syngeneic HSCT is similar, with stem cells harvested from an identical twin sibling.

From: *Neoplastic Hematopathology*: Contemporary Hematology,
Edited by: D. Jones, DOI 10.1007/978-1-60761-384-8_28,
© Humana Press, a part of Springer Science+Business Media, LLC 2010

Table 28-1. Types of hematopoietic stem cell transplants and their indications.

	Stem cell source(s)	Disease condition	Advantages	Disadvantages
Autologous	Patient is own stem cell source (bone marrow, peripheral blood or cord blood)	Myeloma, Lymphoma, Leukemia	Faster immune reconstitution, no GVHD	Potential for re-infusion of clonogenic tumor cells. Higher relapse rates than allogeneic transplants.
Allogeneic, myeloablative				
Related	Bone marrow, peripheral blood or cord blood	Lymphoma, Leukemia, Marrow failures, Myeloproliferative disorders, Storage diseases	Lower GVHD rates than unrelated transplants, easy procurement	Only approximately 30% of patients have suitable match in the U.S.
Mismatched, related (Haploidentical)	Bone marrow, peripheral blood	Lymphoma, leukemia	Speed or procurement, availability	Poor/delayed immune recovery, increased rate of graft failure
Unrelated	Bone marrow, peripheral blood or cord blood		National registry, Caucasians very likely to have a donor identified, speed of procurement	Longer duration of search/procurement Low likelihood of identifying minority donors High GVHD rates Stringent HLA matching criteria
Umbilical	Procurement and storage at birth		Non-invasive Expanded donor pool (e.g., minority populations) Speed of procurement Less stringent HLA matching (4/6, 5/6) Less GVHD	Low cell dose Delayed engraftment Delayed immune reconstitution Increased immune reconstitution
Allogeneic, non-myeloablative				
Matched or mismatched, related or unrelated	Reduced intensity conditioning using bone marrow, peripheral blood or cord blood sources	Lymphoma, Myeloma, Leukemia, Marrow failures, Myeloproliferative disorders Storage diseases	Older patients Reduced mortality Lower peritransplant mortality Greater reliance on graft-versus-tumor effects.	Higher relapse rates in some conditions

In allogeneic (allo) HSCT, donor cells reconstitute hematopoiesis and also provide an immune-mediated graft-versus-tumor (GVT) effect which results in decreased relapse rates when compared to autologous transplants [1]. Allo HSCT can be from a related donor or unrelated donor. The degree of "acceptable" matching of the donor and recipient for the major histocompatibility/human leukocyte antigen (HLA) loci is a function of stem cell source, recipient age, and other factors. Cord blood grafts are more tolerant of several mismatched HLA loci, whilst bone marrow or peripheral blood stem cell sources are not. Traditional allo-HSCT has a mortality of 5–25% with four distinct contributors to the transplant-associated mortality: graft-versus-host disease (GVHD), disseminated infection due predominantly to fungi and cytolytic viruses, graft failure, and disease recurrence.

28.3. Transplant Strategies, Including Preparative Regimens and Cell Product Production

Pre-transplant chemotherapy directed against the patient's malignancy is aimed at achieving as complete a response as possible. Since HSCT often has a role as salvage therapy, particularly in acute myeloid leukemia and aggressive lymphomas, complete elimination of disease prior to HSCT is often not possible. However, transplant outcomes are usually poor in patients transplanted with refractory disease, and disease responsiveness prior to transplant is a major prognosticator for both autologous and allogeneic transplants. In the allogeneic setting, the preparative regimen also has to induce significant degrees of immunosuppression in order to prevent donor cell rejection. Such graft rejection is more common in transplants from mismatched donors or when cord blood grafts are used.

Myeloablative preparative regimens to deplete recipient bone marrow typically involve use of the alkylating agent cyclophosphamide with busulfan and/or total body irradiation (TBI), which are given before stem cell infusion. Myeloablative regimens are usually defined as regimens that induce irreversible damage to hematopoietic elements such that autologous recovery is unlikely. To reduce morbidity and mortality in the early transplant period, there has been increasing use of nonmyeloablative or reduced intensity allo-HSCT. These transplants, accomplished with reduced intensity conditioning regimens (Figure 28-1), have been gaining in popularity, especially for treatment of older or frailer patients. These reduced intensity regimens are usually associated with persistent recipient hematopoiesis after transplant (i.e. mixed chimerism).

In patients with hematopoietic malignancies, the chimeric T-cell responses in nonmyeloablative HSCT usually produce GVT, which is likely effective in controlling residual tumor in a subset of patients. As discussed in Chap. 29, semi-quantitative molecular chimerism testing using PCR-based microsatellite analysis is critical to medical management of nonmyeloablative HSCT to ensure that the donor is proceeding to full engraftment, or to provide assessment of the effects of post-HSCT immune modulatory therapy. The introduction of intravenous busulfan with monitoring of drug levels has improved the specificity of dosing and allowed more precise ablative and nonmyeloablative protocols to be developed.

Graft harvesting can involve extraction of donor bone marrow or mobilization of stem cells into peripheral blood using growth factors. Recently, antibodies against chemokine/homing receptors, such as CXCR4, have been used to improve stem cell mobilization [2]. In vitro manipulation of such harvested samples prior to infusion varies greatly between centers. T-cell depletion of the grafts will greatly reduce the incidence of severe GVHD but also produces higher tumor relapse rates, presumably due to reduced GVT T-cell responses.

Immune manipulations in the post-transplant period comprise a whole range of techniques to manage GVHD, to shift the balance between recipient and donor chimerism, and reverse impending graft failure. These include donor lymphocyte infusion (DLI) to combat recipient T-cell attack on the graft, and shifts in the level of immunosuppression. Adjuvant therapy in the immediate post-transplant period has also increased with the advent of targeted therapies,

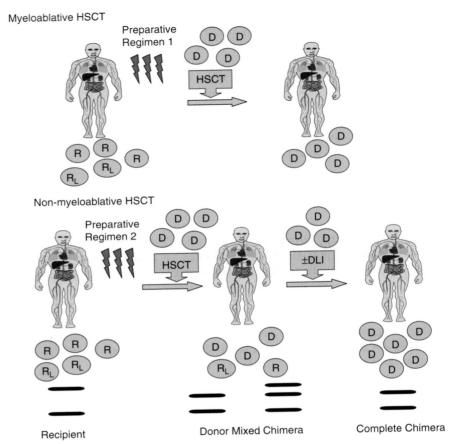

Myeloablative HSCT

Non-myeloablative HSCT

Recipient   Donor Mixed Chimera   Complete Chimera

Fig. 28-1. Preparative regimens for allogeneic transplants. Myeloablative preparative regimens are usually associated with full donor (D) chimerism and eradication of recipient (R) hematopoiesis, while non-myeloablative allogeneic hematopoietic stem cell transplants (HSCT) are frequently associated with persistent recipient cells. Such mixed chimerism may be associated with persistent disease and several strategies are employed to convert patients to full donor chimeras, such as donor lymphocyte infusions (DLI)

such as rituximab for B-cell lymphomas and imatinib for chronic myeloid leukemia. These regimens have helped reduce the incidence of relapse, especially in the nonmyeloablative HSCT setting,

28.4. Complications of HSCT

Graft-versus-host disease (GVHD) is due to the infusion of donor T cells along with the hematopoietic graft. It can cause acute symptoms and fatal cytokine responses, but more commonly shows variable and recurrent skin rash, mucositis, and inflammatory changes; long-term sequelae ("chronic GVHD") include vasculopathy and end-organ damage [3,4]. The clinical staging system for GVHD severity is shown in Table 28-2. Skin biopsy and endoscopic bowel biopsies are helpful in distinguishing GVHD from other common causes of rash including drug rash and viral exanthema. Single-cell apoptosis in the epithelium/epidermis with vacuolar interface dermatitis are the most diagnostic features of GVHD (Figure 28-2).

Therapeutic manipulations to control GVHD include use of increased immunosuppression, combination of immunosuppressants, and graft manipulation. As discussed in Chap. 29,

Table 28-2. Grading of acute graft-versus-host disease (GVHD).

Stage	Skin	Liver	Gut
1	maculopapular rash < 25%	bilirubin 2–3 mg/dL	diarrhea 500–1000 mL or persistent nausea
2	maculopapular rash 25–50%	bilirubin 3–6 mg/dL	diarrhea 1000–1500 mL
3	generalized erythroderma	bilirubin 6–15 mg/dL	diarrhea > 1500 mL
4	desquamation and bulla	bilirubin >15 mg/dL	Severe abdominal pain or ileus

Overall Grade	Severity	Skin		Liver		Gut
0	None	0		0		0
I	Mild	1–2		0		0
II	Moderate	3	or	1	or	1
III	Severe			2–3	or	2–3
IV	Life threatening	4	or	4	or	4

Criteria are those of the 1994 consensus conference on acute GVHD grading [7]

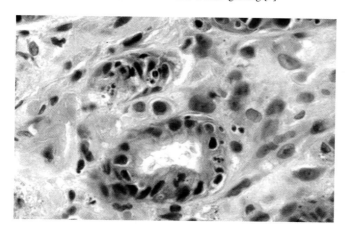

Fig. 28-2. Graft-versus-host disease in colon. Frequent apoptotic epithelial cells are noted in this post-transplant mucosal biopsy

monitoring of sorted T cells from blood using PCR-based microsatellite analysis is critical to correlating the clinically observed GVHD with the levels of T-cell chimerism.

Reactivation of latent viral infection and disseminated fungal infections: With transient loss of effective T-cell immunity in the immediate post-transplant period, patients are at great risk for a variety of serious infections. This immunosuppression is related both to the time needed for regeneration of T-cell memory and the effects of therapy. For this reason, HSCT protocols include prophylaxis for both fungal and viral infections and the use of routine monitoring for CMV and EBV viral load in plasma by quantitative PCR. A consequence of uncontrolled EBV infection is the development of post-transplant lymphoproliferative disorders, which is discussed in Chap. 30.

28.5. New Transplant Strategies

In autologous HSCT, incorporation of new drugs such as rituximab into the transplant "frame" is expected to improve results. Ex-vivo purging of tumor cells from HSC preparations has also been investigated with different degrees of success.

In allogeneic HSCT, there have been improvements in HLA matching, including combined use of serologic and molecular testing, routine use of high-resolution haplotyping methods, and better data on appropriate allelic combinations. This has led to significant improvements in the results for unrelated transplants with outcomes now similar to those obtained with sibling donors. Strategies for improving engraftment of cord blood HSCT have

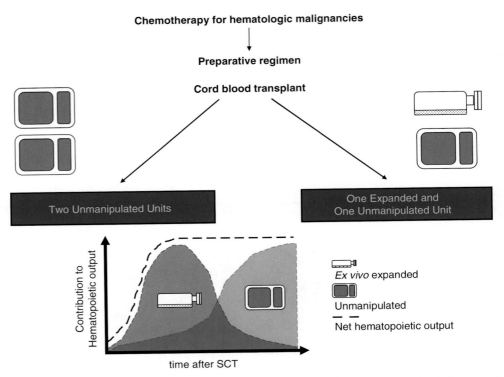

Fig. 28-3. Strategies to improve engraftment rates and speed engraftment of unrelated donor cord blood. Cell dose is a critical determinant of survival after cord blood transplantation. Ex vivo expansion and double cord blood transplants are strategies under investigation to improve engraftment following unrelated cord blood transplant. This ongoing M D Anderson Cancer Center trial investigates and compares both strategies: patients are randomized to receive a double unmanipulated cord blood transplant or a double transplant in which one unit is 100% ex-vivo expanded prior to transplant, while the other unit is unmanipulated before infusion

included the use of double cord transplantation along with ex vivo expansion (Figure 28-3), as well as strategies to increase blood stem cell homing, such as use of fucosyltransferase to change the pattern of surface selectin adhesion molecules [5].

There has also been extensive research to better define the phenotype of activated T cells which mediate GVHD versus GVT effects and to improve DLI by infusion of specific lymphocyte subsets. A parallel strategy has been the use haplo-identical natural killer (NK) cells to mediate tolerance and tumor cell killing [6]. Finally, there have been efforts to improve the bone marrow microenvironment, especially with HSCT in elderly patients, including coinfusion of mesenchymal stem cells.

Suggested Readings

Rezvani AR, Storb RF. Separation of graft-vs.-tumor effects from graft-vs.-host disease in allogeneic hematopoietic cell transplantation. J Autoimmun. 2008. 30(3):172-9.

Alousi A, de Lima M. Reduced-intensity conditioning allogeneic hematopoietic stem cell transplantation. Clin Adv Hematol Oncol. 2007. 5(7):560-70.

References

1. Kolb HJ, Schattenberg A, Goldman JM, et al. Graft-versus-leukemia effect of donor lymphocyte transfusions in marrow grafted patients. Blood 1995;86:2041–50.
2. DiPersio JF, Uy GL, Yasothan U, Kirkpatrick P. Plerixafor. Nat Rev Drug Discov 2009;8:105–6.

3. Filipovich AH, Weisdorf D, Pavletic S, et al. National Institutes of Health consensus development project on criteria for clinical trials in chronic graft-versus-host disease: I Diagnosis and staging working group report. Biol Blood Marrow Transplant 2005;11:945–56.
4. Shulman HM, Kleiner D, Lee SJ, et al. Histopathologic diagnosis of chronic graft-versus-host disease: national institutes of health consensus development project on criteria for clinical trials in chronic graft-versus-host disease: II Pathology Working Group Report. Biol Blood Marrow Transplant 2006;12:31–47.
5. Xia L, McDaniel JM, Yago T, Doeden A, McEver RP. Surface fucosylation of human cord blood cells augments binding to P-selectin and E-selectin and enhances engraftment in bone marrow. Blood 2004;104:3091–6.
6. Ruggeri L, Mancusi A, Burchielli E, Aversa F, Martelli MF, Velardi A. Natural killer cell alloreactivity in allogeneic hematopoietic transplantation. Curr Opin Oncol 2007;19:142–7.
7. Przepiorka D, Weisdorf D, Martin P, et al. 1994 Consensus Conference on Acute GVHD Grading. Bone Marrow Transplant 1995;15:825–8.

Chapter 29

Post-transplant Molecular Monitoring

Dan Jones

Abstract This chapter discusses the types of length and sequence variation encountered in the human genome that can be used to distinguish donor from recipient cells in stem cell transplantation monitoring. The development of chimerism assays based on short tandem repeats (STRs), and the recent use of single nucleotide polymorphisms (SNPs) to detect microchimerism are summarized.

Key words Stem cell transplantation, chimerism assay • Variable number of terminal repeats (VNTRs) • Short tandem repeat (STR) • Single nucleotide polymorphism (SNP), definition and uses • Copy number variation (CNV) • Human leukocyte antigen (HLA) genes • Killer inhibitory receptor (KIR) genes, typing

1. Genomic Repeats, Polymorphisms, and the Basics of Identity Testing

1.1. Types of Repeat Sequences and Polymorphic Loci in the Human Genome

The human genome shows tremendous size and sequence heterogeneity between individuals ranging from inherited single nucleotide polymorphisms (SNPs) to length variation in both short and long stretches of DNA, many of them arrayed as end-to-end tandem repeats (Table 29-1). The longest of the tandem repeats are termed *satellites* and are located in pericentromeric (alpha repeats) and subtelomeric locations [1]. The alpha satellite repeats differ in sequence between each chromosome so that they have diagnostic utility as FISH markers of specific chromosomes. As a result, they can be used in the followup of patients with hematologic malignancies that have tumor-specific aneuploidy changes.

Shorter tandem repeats [~10–100 base pairs (bps) in length] termed *minisatellites* are found throughout the genome in large numbers resulting in heterogeneity in the lengths of restriction enzyme-digested DNA that are termed variable number of tandem repeats (VNTRs). Comparison of the size of these digested DNA fragments containing VNTRs between two individuals was the first commonly used molecular identity test. Several additional types of common intermediate-sized repeats in the genome include the Alu sequence (300 bp in length, spaced every ~5,000 bases) and the long interspersed (L1) repeat, as well as many remnant endogenous retroviral sequences.

The shortest tandem repeat units in the genome include the 6-nucleotide telomere sequence present at the ends of every chromosome and the *microsatellite* repeats. Microsatellites, including di-, tri-, tetra-, and penta-nucleotide repeats are scattered at a density of one in every 15,000–30,000 bases on average, and have a variable number of 3–30 tandem repeats.

From: *Neoplastic Hematopathology*: Contemporary Hematology,
Edited by: D. Jones, DOI 10.1007/978-1-60761-384-8_29,
© Humana Press, a part of Springer Science + Business Media, LLC 2010

The number of tandem repeats in each allele for any particular microsatellite is largely inherited, but microsatellites also expand and contract by strand displacement slippage (and/or recombination) during DNA replication over the lifetime of an individual. Given their frequent expansion and contraction in the population, microsatellites are the most highly polymorphic repeats and thus have become the basis of most identity testing.

Another type of chromosomal size variation that has attracted great interest recently is *copy number variation* (CNV) [2,3]. CNVs are defined as larger segments of DNA at various chromosomal locations (often spanning multiple genes) that can become deleted or duplicated in individuals, with these expansions sometimes having subtle phenotypic effects. They likely arise from altered recombination/sister chromatid exchange. Finally, population-based sequence variation in the genome is also common and can be potentially used for identity testing. SNPs are single base pair changes present at a measurable frequency in the human population that occur every 300 bases on average, with over 10 million SNPs now reported. A number of genetic loci particularly those in the immune system have numerous polymorphisms with functional consequences including the immunoglobulin, human leukocyte antigen (HLA), and killer inhibitory receptor (KIR) genes. Some drug metabolizing enzymes (e.g. cytochrome P450 isoforms) also show frequent SNPs which have functional effects.

29.1.2. Chimerism Testing

The exploitation of variations in the size of genomic loci between individuals for hematopoietic stem cell transplantation (HSCT) monitoring has followed the development of these techniques in forensic and paternity applications (Table 29-2). The initial tests involved the detection of variations between patients in VNTRs detected by restriction fragment length polymorphism (RFLP). These techniques involve digestion of genomic DNA with several restriction enzymes followed by slab electrophoresis, blotting using a panel of minisatellite probes, and then identification of the donor and recipient patient-specific banding patterns. Like any direct genomic blotting application, this technique lacks sensitivity in mixed chimeric post-transplant samples (lower limit of 10–20%) and is technically laborious.

Beginning in the 1990s, chimerism analysis moved from the use of minisatellites to STRs. The introduction of STRs followed the routine use of capillary electrophoresis (CE) which can resolve PCR fragments that differ from each other by as little as 2 bps [4]. The work of the Federal Bureau of Investigation (FBI) and other law enforcement and forensics groups has resulted in the development of reliable multiplex STR primer sets that can detect 8–10 frequently polymorphic microsatellite loci simultaneously. These panels have been adapted for use in HSCT monitoring.

29.2. STR Chimerism Assay for Monitoring HSCT

29.2.1. Basics of the Semi-quantitative STR Chimerism Assay

Chimerism assays have two primary uses in HSCT monitoring. In the typical STR assay, genomic DNA is extracted from white blood cells (WBCs) from the peripheral blood (PB) or bone marrow (BM) obtained following HSCT ("post"-transplant sample) and its PCR amplification pattern is compared to that seen in WBCs from the donor and from the patient before transplant ("pre"-transplant sample). Since microsatellite repeats can differ by as little as 2 bps, capillary electrophoretic separation of the PCR products is required (Fig. 29-1). Several standardized primers sets have been developed that detect 8–10 loci simultaneously with primers labeled with different colored fluorochromes to improve the recognition of alleles (Fig. 29-2). Simultaneous detection of even more alleles in the same multiplex PCR reaction has been reported [5]. The ultimate limit of sensitivity of the assay is imposed by the sensitivity of peak detection in CE (usually 2% of total product) but is often less sensitive for technical and biological reasons (see below).

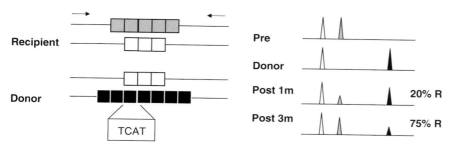

Fig. 29-1. Short tandem repeat analysis. (**a**) Illustrated is the method for PCR detection of the tetra-nucleotide microsatellite repeat THO1 on chromosome 11p15.5. One allele with 3 repeats is shared between donor and recipient, whereas the other allele has 5 repeats in the recipient and 7 in the donor. The patient had a non-myeloablative allogeneic HSCT from a sibling donor for lymphoma. (**b**) Simulated appearance of capillary electrophoretic traces from the pre, donor, and two post-transplant PCR reactions performed on total genomic DNA from blood. The increasing amount of the recipient PCR pattern in the 3-month post sample is indicative of impending graft failure

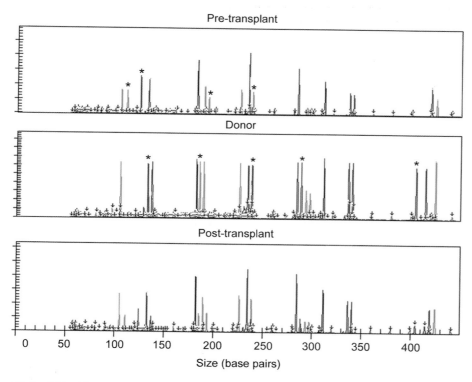

Fig. 29-2. STR chimerism study by multiplex PCR. 10 PCR sets labeled with 3 different fluoro-chromes are run together in a single PCR reaction. Asterisks indicate informative alleles that differ in size between donor and recipient. (platform is Beckman Coulter Vidiera NSD)

STR assays are designed to minimize the number of PCR amplification cycles so as to analyze samples in the logarithmic phase of the PCR reaction where quantitative levels of chimerism can be reported (Fig. 29-1). Quantitation is usually performed from the electropherogram by comparing the area under the peak(s) for informative alleles representing the donor and pre-recipient for each primer set. Some laboratories average the ratios for all informative alleles whereas others choose the most robust (or best separated) allele in calculating the percentage of chimerism. However, given its use of standard PCR, the STR chimerism assay is not strictly quantitative and the performance of the assay is difficult to standardize since the length and the sequence of each amplicon will differ between each patient and thus have different PCR amplification efficiencies.

29.2.2. Schedule for Chimerism Testing

There are not yet widely-accepted standardized protocols or schedules for the performance of post-transplant chimerism testing. Most laboratories utilize PB as the sample source, but parallel analysis of BM aspirate shows promise in detecting engraftment failure at earlier timepoints. A common evaluation schedule is 1, 3, 6, 9, and 12 months following transplant but testing is often done more frequently after prophylactic donor lymphocyte infusion (DLI). Some centers discontinue chimerism testing once engraftment has occurred. As described in Chap. 28, complex transplantation strategies involving different cell sources for multiple donors are changing the timing and needs for chimerism assays.

29.2.3. Differentiating GVH from Engraftment: Interpretation of Chimerism Assays

There are two related indications for use of the chimerism assay in HSCT monitoring, namely an assessment of the degree of donor engraftment (compared to level of recipient marrow), and an assessment of T-cell chimerism reflecting graft-versus-host disease (GVHD). To achieve these goals, most laboratories perform cell sorting of PB samples to isolate T cells to assess GVH and often use purified granulocytes as a more specific marker of engraftment. Sorting is commonly done using antibodies directed against pan-T-cell (e.g. CD3) and pan-myeloid antigens (e.g. CD33) using bead-based methods or flow cytometry activated cell sorting (FACS).

Interpretation of the results of chimerism assays involving cell sorting can be complex and is highly dependent on whether T-cell depletion of the infused donor product was done, and whether the pre-transplant conditioning was fully myeloablative or a reduced intensity regimen (See Chap. 28). Nonetheless, the finding of only donor T-cells in a post-HSCT sample may indicate an increased risk of acute GVHD, whereas mixed chimerism in the T-cell compartment usually indicates a lower degree of GVHD.

In nonmyeloablative HSCT, mixed chimerism is expected in the myeloid-sorted DNA sample, but progression to a fully donor pattern in the first six months is almost always seen with successful engraftment. An increasing amount of recipient pattern in the myeloid population is strongly indicative of graft failure or relapse of leukemia. In myeloablative HSCT done for myeloid leukemias, the finding of mixed chimerism in the myeloid compartment is indicative of relapse. Some centers also perform cell sorting on BM samples for CD34+ blasts, and in this setting, a shift towards undetectable donor CD34+ cells is usually indicative of graft rejection (or relapse in myeloid leukemias).

29.2.4. Limitations of the STR Assay

The main limitations of the STR assay for HSCT monitoring relate not only to the lower limit of sensitivity of CE (~2%) but also to technical issues related to PCR amplification of highly polymorphic short repeat sequences. These include the tendency of low-fidelity DNA polymerases, such as the *Taq* enzyme, to slip on a repetitive DNA templates giving rise to minor PCR products that are shorter than the actual STR length [6]. This "stutter" is typically one repeat length shorter than the actual STR length, but shorter and longer stutter bands can also be noted. Size variations in STRs can also reflect somatic expansion of the locus due to microsatellite instability. Also, given the instability of STR alleles, germline or somatic mutations occasionally arise in the PCR primer binding sites producing "null alleles," where amplification of one allele at a given loci is not detected.

The amount of PCR stutter observed depends on the sequence and length of a particular microsatellite locus, PCR conditions, and the particular polymerase used. The degree of stutter increases with the length of the PCR amplicon but decreases with the longer or less-than-perfect microsatellite repeat units. To minimize the effects of stutter on skewing quantitation, some laboratories utilize the informative allele with the shortest PCR amplicon and favor tetranucleotide microsatellite repeats. Finally, multiple PCR peaks can also result from non-templated addition of nucleotides by Taq polymerase that are usually one base longer than the actual target sequence.

29.3. The Effect of Genomic Sequence Variations on HSCT Outcomes

29.3.1. The Effect of the HLA Haplotype

Determinations of sequence variation in the HLA genes which comprise the major histocompatibility (MHC) complex are basis of matching donors with recipients for HSCT and solid organ transplantation (i.e. HLA matching). Typing of the alleles expressed at each of the six dominant HLA loci located at chromosome 6p21 (the "haplotype") is routinely performed on all recipients and donors to generate acceptable matches (Fig. 29-3). A compete match of the alleles at these HLA loci (A, B, C, DP, DQ, and DR) is associated with improved engraftment, reduced GVHD, and improved outcomes in HSCT. Haploidentical related or partially mismatched unrelated donors may be used, although the allo-immune responses that occur in these transplants can lead to poor engraftment and severe GVHD [7].

HLA matching has been historically done using serum antibody screens but is now largely performed using PCR-based methods, including SSO/SSP reverse blot hybridization (so-called *intermediate-resolution* haplotyping) and direct Sanger sequencing (i.e. *high resolution* typing). For common HLA alleles, the appropriate matches are well-established and the outcomes of transplant can be predicted with confidence. However, the appropriate

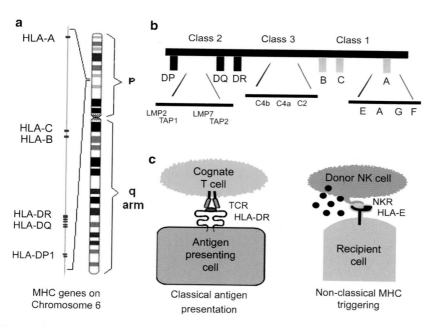

Fig. 29-3. Major histocompatibility gene complex. (**a**) A simplified schematic of the six HLA loci on chromosome 6. (**b**) The MHC gene cluster also contain other immune regulatory genes, such as complement components in the Class III cluster, TAP antigen processing genes adjacent to the Class II genes (DR, DQ, and DP), and non-classical MHC (e.g. HLA-E) adjacent to the Class I genes (HLA-A, -B, and -C). (**c**) Class II MHC expressed on antigen-presenting cells (APCs) function to present processed antigen in their binding pocket to the T-cell receptor (TCR) on cognate T cells. This is contrasted with the triggering of cytolytic attack by natural killer cells (NK) following recognition by a NK receptor/KIR of class I MHC leader peptides present on foreign (or altered host) cells in association with non-classical MHC activating ligands such as HLA-E

Table 29-1. Size and sequence variation in the human genome.

Element	Features	Detected by	Utility
Genome-wide repeat types			
Satellite	Pericentromeric and subtelomeric tandem repeats specific for each chromosome	FISH	Alpha-satellites used as chromosome–specific FISH probes
Minisatellite	10–100 bp repeat length 1 per ~3,000 bases	Southern blot following restriction digestion	Identity testing Global methylation (Alu repeat)
Microsatellite	2–7 bp repeat length 1 per ~15,000 bases	Short-cycle PCR	Identity testing Diagnosis of triplet repeat length in developmental and neuromuscular disorders
Copy number variations	Variably duplicated/deleted segments of chromosomes	SNP or CGH arrays, MLPA	Association with concurrent disease states
Single nucleotide polymorphisms (SNP)	Single base changes in genes/ intergenic regions 1 per ~300 bases	SNP arrays, allele-specific PCR	Genome-wide disease association studies, markers of uniparental disomy segments
Polymorphic genetic loci relevant to stem cell transplantation			
HLA genes	6 loci on chr 6p21 that mediate histocompatibility	Antibody panels, reverse array, DNA sequencing	Haplotype determination for SCT and solid organ donor selection
Killer inhibitor receptors (KIRs)	Mediate natural killer cell recognition	Multiplex PCR, reverse array	Predict graft rejection in haploidentical HSCT donor
Human androgen receptor gene (HUMARA)	18–20 size/sequence polymorphisms	Multiplex PCR	Alternate loci for clonality and identity testing

Abbreviations: *bp* base pair, *FISH* fluorescence in situ hybridization; *SNP* single nucleotide polymorphism; *CGH* comparative genomic hybridization; *MPLA* multiple ligation-dependent probe amplification *HLA* human leukocyte antigen

matches for rarer alleles or newly identified variants [8] is more difficult to determine, with consultation of public databases (e.g. IMGT/HLA [9] or hla/alleles.org [10]) or structure-function modeling being most helpful. In these cases, antibody testing is usually also performed as an adjunct to assist in matching.

29.3.2. KIR Typing

Besides the HLA loci, genetic polymorphisms in other immune system gene families that encode antigen-presenting molecules, antigen receptors, and cytokines and their receptors have also been shown to affect the outcome in HSCT. Among these, KIRs have attracted the most attention since they are important determinants of natural killer (NK) cell alloreactivity that can mediate graft rejection. KIRs are a moderately polymorphic family of receptors which mediate self- and nonself recognition by NK cells and other cell types of the innate immune system by detecting the presence or absence of their respective KIR ligands on the surface of other cells (Fig. 29-3c). Matching of several of the most common KIR polymorphisms correlates with decreased graft rejection in haploidentical donors [11]. Typing of the relevant polymorphisms at the KIR loci is typically done by multiplex PCR. However, as of this date, KIR typing is still considered an investigational tool at most centers.

29.3.3. SNPs Profiling as a Method of Identity Testing

The use of SNPs as markers of identity shows promise for developing much more sensitive chimerism assays since the single base pair SNP change allows use of the quantitative allele-specific PCR assays that can reliably detect as few as 1 in 10,000 chimeric cells. However, for identity testing, the low incidence of any particular polymorphism requires a large number of SNPs to be included in each screening panel to ensure that every recipient-donor pair has one or more informative SNPs. The use of SNPs profiling in forensics applications has been reported, with assays typically using 30–50 of the most polymorphic SNPs in each panel.[12] The use of SNPs in HSCT monitoring has not yet become routine, but results using quantitative PCR to detect transfusion-associated microchimerism have been reported [13].

Suggested Readings

Butler JM. Genetics and genomics of core short tandem repeat loci used in human identity testing. J Forensic Sci 2006;51(2):253-6
  • A brief discussion of the benefits and limitations of STR typing.
Velardi A. Role of KIRs and KIR ligands in hematopoietic transplantation. Curr Opin Immunol 2008;20(5):581-7.
  • A review of the data on where KIR typing may have clinical impact in HSCT.
Marsh SGE, Parham P, Barber LD. The HLA facts book, 2000, Elsevier, New York City.
  • This reference contains a series of introductory chapters on the basics of HLA matching.

Table 29-2. Methods and loci used for SCT and transfusion chimerism analysis.

Method	Current usage	Sensitivity	Application
Chimerism assessment in HSCT			
Multiple STR PCR	Common	0.4–5%	Standard STR panels in use
SNP real-time quantitative PCR	Evolving	0.01%	Can detect microchimerism
Cytogenetics/FISH	Selected uses	1–10%	Detects tumor-associated relapses
RFLP (minisatellite)	Less common	5–10%	Can be done with slab electrophoresis
Identity in sex-mismatch HSCT or other applications			
X, Y-chromosome by karyotype, FISH or PCR	Common	0.1–0.4%	For sex mismatched transplants [14]
PCR-based amelogenin genotyping	Selected uses	0.1–1%	Mostly forensic applications [15]
Proteins or functional assays			
Erythrocyte phenotyping	Less common	0.04–3%	Transfusions will preclude use [16]

References

1. Wevrick R, Willard HF. Long-range organization of tandem arrays of alpha satellite DNA at the centromeres of human chromosomes: high-frequency array-length polymorphism and meiotic stability. Proc Natl Acad Sci USA 1989;86(23):9394–8.

2. Lu X, Shaw CA, Patel A, et al. Clinical implementation of chromosomal microarray analysis: summary of 2513 postnatal cases. PLoS ONE 2007;2(3):e327.

3. Lee C, Iafrate AJ, Brothman AR. Copy number variations and clinical cytogenetic diagnosis of constitutional disorders. Nat Genet 2007;39(7 Suppl):S48–54.

4. Butler JM. Genetics and genomics of core short tandem repeat loci used in human identity testing. J Forensic Sci 2006;51(2):253–65.

5. Vallone PM, Hill CR, Butler JM. Demonstration of rapid multiplex PCR amplification involving 16 genetic loci. Forensic Sci Int Genet 2008;3(1):42–5.

6. Walsh PS, Fildes NJ, Reynolds R. Sequence analysis and characterization of stutter products at the tetranucleotide repeat locus vWA. Nucleic Acids Res 1996;24(14):2807–12.

7. Mullighan CG, Petersdorf EW. Genomic polymorphism and allogeneic hematopoietic transplantation outcome. Biol Blood Marrow Transplant 2006;12(1 Suppl 1):19–27.

8. Marsh SG (2009) Nomenclature for factors of the HLA system. Tissue Antigens 2009;74:272–275.

9. Robinson J, Waller MJ, Fail SC, Marsh SG. The IMGT/HLA and IPD databases. Hum Mutat 2006;27(12):1192–9.

10. Holdsworth R, Hurley CK, Marsh SG, et al. The HLA dictionary 2008: a summary of HLA-A, -B, -C, -DRB1/3/4/5, and -DQB1 alleles and their association with serologically defined HLA-A, -B, -C, -DR, and -DQ antigens. Tissue Antigens 2009;73(2):95–170.

11. Velardi A. Role of KIRs and KIR ligands in hematopoietic transplantation. Curr Opin Immunol 2008;20(5):581–7.

12. Sanchez JJ, Borsting C, Balogh K, et al. Forensic typing of autosomal SNPs with a 29 SNP-multiplex–results of a collaborative EDNAP exercise. Forensic Sci Int Genet 2008;2(3):176–83.

13. Utter GH, Lee TH, Rivers RM, et al. Microchimerism decades after transfusion among combat-injured US veterans from the Vietnam, Korean, and World War II conflicts. Transfusion 2008;48(8):1609–15.

14. Khan F, Agarwal A, Agrawal S. Significance of chimerism in hematopoietic stem cell transplantation: new variations on an old theme. Bone Marrow Transplant 2004;34(1):1–12.

15. Frances F, Portoles O, Gonzalez JI, et al. Amelogenin test: From forensics to quality control in clinical and biochemical genomics. Clin Chim Acta 2007;386(1–2):53–6.

16. Schaap N, Schattenberg A, Bar B, et al. Red blood cell phenotyping is a sensitive technique for monitoring chronic myeloid leukaemia patients after T-cell-depleted bone marrow transplantation and after donor leucocyte infusion. Br J Haematol 2000;108(1):116–25.

Chapter 30

Post-transplant Immune Function and the Development of Lymphoma

Deqin Ma and Dan Jones

Abstract/Scope of Chapter Both hematopoietic stem cell transplantation and solid organ transplantation are associated with short-term and long-term immune deficits that result in an increased risk of disseminated infection and malignancy. Here, we discuss these risk factors and the time-course for the development of post-transplant lymphoproliferative disorders in each transplant type.

Keywords Post-transplant lymphoproliferative disorders • Lymphoma, Epstein-Barr virus (EBV) • Epstein-Barr virus, quantitative PCR • Cytomegalovirus • Hepatosplenic T-cell lymphoma, post-transplant • Diffuse large B-cell lymphoma, post-transplant • Donor lymphocyte infusion • Post-transplant, treatment for lymphoma

30.1. Introduction

Hematopoietic stem cell transplantation (HSCT) and solid organ transplantation (SOT) lead to both transient and prolonged immune dysregulation that results in an increased incidence of malignancy. The causes of increased tumorigenesis following transplantation are complex but the most important factors are declines in immune function due to transplant conditioning regimens and the prolonged use of immunosuppressive agents that lead to the reactivation of chronic viral infections. Over time, these infections can promote outgrowth of virally-infected lymphoid populations that proceed to lymphoma. Defects in T-cell immune surveillance due to immunosuppressant therapy also lead to an increased incidence of other types of cancer. The risk factors for development of post-transplant lymphoproliferative disorders in patients following HSCT and SOT are similar but not identical.

30.2. Immune Dysregulation, Viral Reactivation and Risk of Malignancies in HSCT

HSCT is associated with transient and prolonged defects in hematopoiesis and immune function due to its myeloablative features and because of the damage done to the marrow microenvironment by conditioning regimens that include alkylating agents and total blood irradiation (TBI). Engraftment of hematopoietic elements following a myeloablative HSCT takes several weeks with the return of baseline neutrophil function within 2–4 weeks in most patients. There are however long-standing defects in T-cell immunity in nearly all patients that can last for

From: *Neoplastic Hematopathology*: Contemporary Hematology,
Edited by: D. Jones, DOI 10.1007/978-1-60761-384-8_30,
© Humana Press, a part of Springer Science+Business Media, LLC 2010

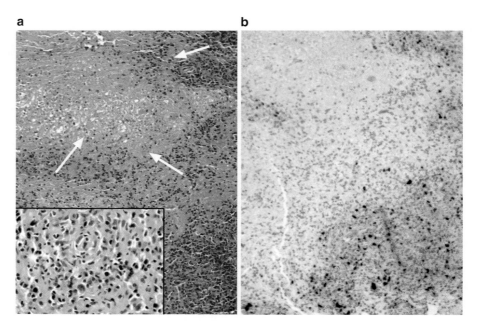

Fig. 30-1. EBV+ polymorphic PTLD. (**a**) Brain parenchyma is replaced by a polymorphous lymphoid infiltrate with a large area of necrosis (*white arrows*). Inset show scattered large nucleolated forms. (**b**) EBER ISH shows high-level EBV expression in large lymphocytes

up to 6–12 months following HSCT and defects in B-cell memory and antibody production lasting for years [1]. T-cell depletion of the graft prior to transplant, while decreasing the incidence of graft versus host disease (GVHD), results in more profound immune T-cell dysfunction. Reduced conditioning or nonmyeloablative HSCTs, which are growing in popularity, generally result in a less profound immune dysfunction (see Chap. 28).

A major risk of HSCT-related immune dysfunction is the reactivation of latent herpesvirus infection leading to disseminated cytolytic infection (particularly for cytomegalovirus), localized infections (e.g., human herpesvirus 6 in lung) and herpesvirus-associated malignancies driven by lymphotropic human herpesvirus 4 (also known as Epstein-Barr virus, EBV) and human herpesvirus 8 (HHV8, also known as the Kaposi's sarcoma-associated herpesvirus). It remains unclear whether other viruses such as hepatitis B, hepatitis C, or simian virus-40 (SV40) play a role in PTLD development [2].

Besides post-transplant lymphoproliferative disorders (PTLDs, Fig. 30-1), other malignancies that are increased following HSCT include carcinoma, melanoma, and glioblastoma [3]. Even in myeloablative HSCT, the overall incidence of PTLD is generally low, with an overall risk of approximately 1%, with PTLDs almost always of donor origin. Risk factors for PTLD development include the use of anti-thymocyte globulin or anti-CD3 monoclonal antibodies in immunosuppressive regimens, the presence of an additive underlying immunodeficiency, or T-cell depletion of the HSCT graft. When compared with matched-related HSCT donors, the risk of early-onset PTLD increases significantly in patients receiving umbilical blood transplant, and is even higher in unrelated or HLA-mismatched donors, where it can be seen in up to 20% [4].

30.3. Immune Dysregulation and Risk of Malignancies in Solid Organ Transplantation

In solid organ transplant (SOT), immune dysregulation is mainly produced by the immunosuppressant medications given to prevent graft rejection. Such agents include corticosteroids, calcineurin inhibitors (e.g., tacrolimus/FK506), and anti-cytokine monoclonal antibodies

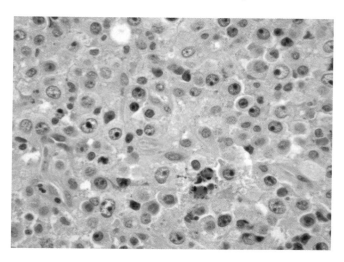

Fig. 30-2. EBV+ monomorphic B-cell PTLD. Bowel masses were detected 18 months following renal transplant. Colon resection showed diffuse transmural infiltration by a large B-cell lymphoma with immunoblastic morphology and high mitotic activity

such as against IL-2 receptor [5]. Anti-CD3 monoclonal antibodies (e.g., OKT3) are also frequently used and result in more profound T-cell dysfunction. Any significant defets in helper T-cell function will also result in a deficiency of B cells and impaired antibody production.

As with HSCT, a major risk of such SOT-related immune dysfunction is the reactivation of latent herpesvirus infection leading to the risk of disseminated cytolytic infection (particularly for cytomegalovirus) and increased risk of malignancy. Disseminated or localized infections (e.g., BK virus in bladder) which are rarely seen in HSCT can occur in SOT due to more prolonged use of immunosuppressants. Malignancies reported following SOT include both de novo malignancies such as PTLD (Fig. 30-2), and recurrence of pre-existing neoplasms since 2–5% of organ recipients have a past history of cancer. The majority of PTLDs in SOT occur within the first year post-transplant when the patients are receiving large doses of immunosuppressants. The incidence of PTLD in SOT ranges from 1 to 20%, with the highest rate in patients receiving bowel transplants, followed by heart and lung transplants; patients receiving kidney grafts have an incidence of less than 1% of developing PTLD.[3] Greater than 90% of PTLDs in SOT are of recipient origin, [6] as compared to the overwhelmingly predominance of donor PTLDs in HSCT. Overall, the risk of EBV+ PTLD depends on the type of organ transplanted, the intensity of immunosuppression, EBV serologic status at the time of transplant, age, and concomitant cytomegalovirus (CMV) infection.

HHV8-associated post-transplant malignancies are rare but more common in solid organ transplant patients, and include Kaposi's sarcoma (KS) and primary effusion lymphoma (PEL). Although exceedingly rare, T-cell and natural killer (NK) cell PTLDs more commonly arise in SOT rather than HSCT and, unlike B-cell PTLDs, are negative for EBV in the majority of cases (Table 30-1 and Fig. 30-3a). Compared with EBV+ PTLD, EBV-negative PTLDs occur at a longer interval post-transplant, are less responsive to reductions in immunotherapy, and are associated with a poor prognosis.

For SOT recipients with a prior history of malignancy, the recurrence rate of the original tumor is between 3.0 and 5.0%, [7,8] and the incidence of new malignancies other than PTLD is only 1–2% higher when compared with the general population [9]. Excluding PTLD, risk factors for other malignancies after SOT include older age, white race, male gender, past history of cancer and long-term dialysis, and are most commonly carcinomas of the skin, gastrointestinal tract and lung. First reported in the 1960s [10], tumors originating from the donor allograft are rare but can occasionally be fatal [11].

Table 30-1. Classification scheme for post-transplant lymphoproliferative disorders.

Morphologic type	Molecular/genetic	EBV present	Timing post-transplant, months (median)	Response to reduction in immuno-suppression
Plasmacytic hyperplasia	Usually polyclonal IGH	Yes	15–68 (17.5)	Yes
Polymorphic PTLD	Most are clonal IGH	Yes	3.5–96 (18)	50%
Monomorphic PTLD				
Large B-cell lymphoma	BCL6 & TP53 mutations, MGMT promoter methylation	Yes	10.5–117 (27)	No
Burkitt lymphoma	MYC-immunoglobulin translocations	Yes		No
Plasma cell myeloma, plasmacytoma	HHV8+ in a subset	Subset		No
T/NK-cell lymphomas	Karyotype showing del(6q) or trisomies	40%	1–132 (66)	No
Hepatosplenic T-cell lymphoma	Isochromosome 7q, trisomy 8	No		No
Large granular lymphocytic leukemia	Usually diploid karyotype	No		No
Classical Hodgkin lymphoma		Yes	2–3 years	No

[a]Based on references [14], [15], [17], [23], and [24]. Abbreviations are as in text

30.4. Diagnosis and Pathogenesis of Herpesvirus-Associated PTLD

EBV infects over 90% of the population with primary EBV infection, usually acquired in childhood, almost always leading to a lifelong latent infection maintained in a small number of circulating B cells or epithelial cells of the Waldeyer's ring. During such latent infection, the viral genome is maintained as an episome in the cell nucleus by a limited viral gene expression program. EBV reactivation, which represents a shift to lytic infection in B cells, is promoted by immune deficiency caused by conditioning chemotherapy, irradiation, T-cell depletion in a HSCT graft and/or iatrogenic immunosuppression [12]. This active viral production can be detected by increases in the EBV viral load in serum or plasma using quantitative PCR.

Most B-cell PTLDs emerge following EBV reactivation and contain latent or active EBV infection in the tumor cells. The range of EBV+ PTLDs are similar to those seen in immuo-deficiency-related conditions such as HIV infection, and include large B-cell lymphoma (LBCL) with immunoblastic features, Burkitt lymphoma (BL), classical Hodgkin lymphoma (CHL) and rare EBV+ T-cell malignancies (Fig. 30-3b).

This observation that PTLDs emerge quickly following EBV reactivation and tend to progress from polyclonal to oligoclonal to overt monoclonal expansions has given rise to a morphology-based PTLD classification. Immunoblastic (mononucleosis-like) proliferations and plasma cell hyperplasia are regarded as early stage or precursor lesions and may progress to polymorphous PTLD, or to monomorphous LBCL, BL, or myeloma (Table 30-1). Some PTLDs, however, present in the monomorphous stage, and PCR-detected monoclonal immunoglobulin heavy chain (IGH) gene rearrangements may be seen at any stage. Demonstration of clonal episomal EBV by Southern blot analysis can be used in the diagnosis of PTLD, but is rarely clinically useful since clonal EBV proliferation is present in both monomorphic and polymorphic variants. Instead, classification of EBV+ PTLD usually depends on combining morphologic features with the demonstration of EBV infection in the majority of tumor cells by use of in situ hybridization for the EBV-encoded small RNA (EBERs).

The morphologic progression of PTLD is correlated with stepwise accumulation of genetic changes in the tumor cells [13]. Latent EBV infection of B cells results in overexpression of virally-encoded latent membrane protein (LMP)-1 and -2 and EBV nuclear antigens (EBNAs). LMP1 and EBNA1 appear to be the viral products most directly associated with oncogenic transformation; LMP1 acts as a mimic of the tumor necrosis factor growth receptor pathway blocking apoptosis, and altering patterns of host growth factor expression, LMP2a activates Notch1 thus shifting the transcriptional program of infected cells, and EBNA1 is essential for viral replication and maintenance of latent infection. These viral genes thus drive expansion of the latently-infected and transcriptionally-reprogrammed B cells giving an opportunity for additional genetic changes to accumulate. These secondary changes include activation of microsatellite instability, rearrangement of the MYC protooncogene, mutations in BCL6, TP53, and RAS genes, and promoter hypermethylation of O6-methylguanine-DNA methyl-transferase (MGMT) (Table 30-1) [14].

Like EBV, HHV8 infection also establishes a latency state in nearly all infected patients, with production of a viral homolog of interleukin (IL)-6, and a viral homolog of cyclin D1 most important for B-cell expansion and transformation. Other viral genes, such as the transcriptional regulator K1 and a viral G protein-coupled receptor are important in driving angiogenesis and stromal expansion in Kaposi's sarcoma. HHV8-associated lymphoid trans-formation is a minor cause of PTLD producing post-transplant primary effusion lymphoma (see Chap. 17) and myeloma. HHV8 in post-transplant tumors can be demonstrated by immunostaining for the latency-associated antigen (LNA).

The initiating factor(s) and pathogenesis of EBV- HHV8- B-cell PTLDs are currently unknown but they are being more frequently reported, perhaps as prophylaxis against cur-rently known viruses improves. The median time to the development of these tumors is approximately 50 months, which is much later than for EBV+ PTLD.

30.5. Other Types of PTLD

Although the vast majority of PTLD are viral-associated B-cell malignancies, T-cell and NK-cell lymphoma makes up 15% of cases in Western countries. These have been reported to include all entities in the WHO classification, [4] but the most common types are peripheral T-cell lymphoma, not otherwise specified, followed by hepatosplenic T-cell lymphoma; true NK cell malignancies are rare [15]. Compared with B-cell cases, T/NK-cell PTLDs occur later following transplant, are usually EBV negative, and have a generally poor prognosis [4]. The morphology, immunohistochemical phenotype and genetic abnormalities are similar to those seen in immunocompetent patients. Transplant-associated Hodgkin lymphoma has rarely been reported but is usually of mixed cellularity type with EBV expression [16]. Such case may occur more commonly in renal transplant recipients [4] or in those patients with more prominent GVHD following HSCT [16,17].

30.6. Therapeutic Approaches to PTLD

In SOT, first-line therapy for PTLD is reduction of immunosuppression (Table 30-2). In HSCT, reducing immunosuppressive therapy restores EBV-specific cytotoxic T-cell (CTL) response but is associated with increased risk of GVHD. Early-stage PTLDs, such as plasma-cytic hyperplasia, can regress by this approach within several weeks [18]. Some polymorphic PTLD also respond to immunosuppression reduction but most polymorphic and nearly all monomorphic PTLDs require additional therapies. Multiagent chemotherapy and/or rituximab is usually added when reduction of immunosuppression alone is not effective in the treatment of PTLD. Rituximab is reported to have a 75% response rate when used as an adjunct to immunosuppression reduction in treatment of PTLD. However, while rituximab does deplete infected B cells, it does not restore T-cell immunity and is associated with increased risk of development of CMV reactivation. For PTLDs involving the central nervous system, radiation therapy is often used [19,20]. Although antiviral agents (e.g., acyclovir and ganciclovir) are

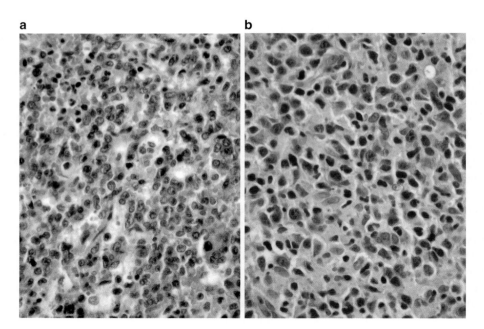

Fig. 30-3. Post-transplant T-cell lymphoproliferative disorders. (**a**) Hepatosplenic T-cell lymphoma showing splenic sinusoidal infiltration by monomorphic blastoid lymphocytes which expressed CD3 and gamma-delta T-cell receptor. Tumor arose 5 years following renal transplant. (**b**) EBV+ T-cell PTLD involving skin with a polymorphous tumor cell infiltrate resembling B-cell cases. Lesion arose 2 years following renal transplant

Table 30-2. Therapeutic strategies for PTLD.

Morphologic type	Treatment options[a]
Plasmacytic hyperplasia	Reduction of immunosuppression, antiviral agents,
Polymorphic PTLD	As above and rituximab if unresponsive
Monomorphic PTLD	
In patients with HSCT	Rituximab, immunotherapy
In patients with SOT	Reduction of immunosuppression; surgery, rituximab, IVIG, chemotherapy, radiation

[a]Based on references [18]–[22]. Abbreviations are as in text

known to block viral replication and intravenous immune globulin (IVIG) can be used to neutralize viral infectivity, both agents have limited use for treatment of established PTLD [19].

In HSCT recipients, given the more profound short-term immunodeficiency, additional approaches for controlling PTLD have been tried. Adoptive immunotherapy using donor-derived EBV-specific cytotoxic T cells (CTLs) is one such emerging approach to restoring immune competence. Infusion of such CTLs has resulted in regression of EBV-associated PTLDs in one study [21]. Infusion of the donor CTLs has also been shown to cause complete or partial remission of PTLDs in SOT recipients [22]. Ex-vivo expansion and activation of immune cells directed against viral antigens show great promise as a therapeutic tools for both EBV+ and HHV8+ post-transplant malignancies.

Suggested Reading

Knowles DM, Cesarman E, Chadburn A, *et al*. Correlative morphologic and molecular genetic analysis demonstrates three distinct categories of posttransplantation lymphoproliferative disorders. Blood 1995;85:552–65.

The initial morphogenetic classification of PTLD upon which the current WHO classification is based.

Auletta JJ, Lazaru HM. Immune restoration following hematopoietic stem cell transplantation: an evolving target. Bone Marrow Transplant 6005;35:835–85.
A comprehensive review on immune function following transplant.

References

1. Auletta JJ, Lazaru HM. Immune restoration following hematopoietic stem cell transplantation: an evolving target. Bone Marrow Transplant 2005;35:835–857.
2. Vilchez RA, Jauregui MP, Hsi ED, Novoa-Takara L, Chang C. Simian virus 40 in posttransplant lymphoproliferative disorders. Hum Pathol 2006;37:1130–36
3. Ghelani D, Saliba R, de Lima M. Secondary malignancies after hematopoietic stem cell transplantation. Crit Rev Oncol Hematol 2005;56:115–26.
4. Swerdlow SH, Webber SA, Chadburn A, Ferry JA. Post-transplant lymphoproliferative disorders In: Swerdlow SH, Campo E, Harris NL, Jaffe ES, et al., eds. WHO classification of tumours of hematopoietic and lymphoid tissues. Lyon, France: IARC, 2008:343–49
5. Villard J. Immunity after organ transplantation. Swiss Med Wkly 2006;136:71–7.
6. Dolcetti R. B lymphomas and Epstein-Barr virus: the lesson of post-transplant lymphoproliferative disorders. Autoimmun Rev 2007;7:96–101.
7. Kauffman HM, Cherikh WS, McBride MA, et al. Transplant recipients with a history of malignancy: risk of recurrent and de novo cancers. Transplant Rev 2005;19:55–64.
8. Chapman JR, Sheril AGR, Disney APS. Recurrence of cancer after renal transplantation. Transplantation Proc 2001;33:1830–1.
9. Kauffman HM. Malignancies in organ transplant recipients. J Surg Oncol 2006;94:431–3.
10. Martin DC, Rubini M, Rosen VJ. Cadaveric renal homotransplantations with inadvertent transplantation of carcinoma. JAMA 1965;192:752–4.
11. Wilson RE, Penn I. Fate of tumors transplanted with a renal allograft. Transplant Proc 1975;7: 327–31.
12. Gottschalk S, Rooney GM, Heslop HE. Post-transplant lymphoproliferative disorders. Ann Rev Med 2005;56:29–44.
13. Yin CC, Jones D. Molecular approaches towards characterization, monitoring and targeting of viral-associated hematological malignancies. Expert Rev Mol Diagn 2006;6(6):831–41.
14. Chadburn A, Cesarman E, Knowles DM. Molecular pathology of posttransplantation lymphoproliferative disorders. Semin Diagn Pathol 1997;14(1):15–26.
15. Swerdlow SH. T-cell and NK-cell post-transplantation lymphoproliferative disorders. Am J Clin Pathol 2007;127:887–895.
16. Rowlings PA, Curtis RE, Passweg PA, et al. Increased incidence of Hodgkin's disease after allogeneic bone marrow transplantation. J Clin Oncol 1999;17:3122–7.
17. Said JW. Immunodeficiency-related Hodgkin lymphoma and its mimics. Adv Anat Pathol 2007;14(3):189–94.
18. Starzl TE, Nalesnik MA, Porter KA, et al. Reversibility of lymphomas and lymphoproliferative lesions developing under cyclosporine-steroid therapy. Lancet 1984;1:583–7.
19. Cohen J, Bollard CM, Khanna R, Pittaluga S. Current understanding of the role of Epstein-Barr virus in lymphomagenesis and therapeutic approaches to EBV-associated lymphomas. Leuk Lymphoma 2008;49(S1):27–34.
20. Taylor AL, Marcus R, Bradley JA. Post-transplant lymphoproliferative disorders (PTLD) after solid organ transplantation. Crit Rev Oncol Hematol 2005;56:155–67.
21. Rooney CM, Smith CA, Ng CY, et al. Infusion of cytotoxic T cells for the prevention and treatment of Epstein-Barr virus-induced lymphoma in allogenic transplant recipients. Blood 1998;92:1549–55.
22. Haque T, Wilkie GM, Taylor C, et al. Treatment of Epstein-Barr-virus-positive post-transplantation lymphoproliferative disease with partly HLA-matched allogenic cytotoxic T cells. Lancet 2002;360:436–42.
23. Knowles DM, Cesarman A, Chadburn A, et al. Correlative morphologic and molecular genetic analysis demonstrates three distinct categories of posttranplantation lymphoproliferative disorders. Blood 1995;85:552–65.
24. Chadburn A, Chen JM, Hsu D, et al. The morphologic and molecular genetic categories of post-transplantation lymphoproliferative disorders are clinically relevant. Cancer 1998;82:1978–87.

Section 5

Experimental Hematopathology

Chapter 31

Hematopoiesis and Stem Cell Biology

Claudiu Cotta

Abstract/Scope of chapter This chapter covers hematopoiesis and the methodologies used to study maturation of bone marrow precursors into mature blood elements. The roles of particular genes and signaling pathways are highlighted.

Keywords Hematopoiesis, molecular pathways • Hematopoietic stem cell (HSC) • Hematopoiesis, yolk sac • Hematopoiesis, myeloid progenitors • Hematopoiesis, erythroid progenitors • Lymphopoiesis • Thymus, selection • Thymus, T-cell maturation • T-cell receptor, sequence of rearrangement • rag recombinase • Terminal deoxynucleotidyl transferase (TdT) • Stem cell • Self-renewal • Stem cell transplant, mouse • Methylcellulose assays • PU.1 transcription factors • PAX5 • Ikaros • Notch • JAK-STAT • Cancer stem cells

31.1. Introduction: Lineage Commitment, Epigenetics and Microenvironment

Hematopoiesis is the process of maturation of hematopoietic elements from stem cells to their mature/terminally differentiated forms. This chapter focuses on the molecular mechanisms underlying hematopoietic maturation and the experimental techniques used to study them. Chapter 5 discusses the function and localization of mature hematopoietic forms in the bone marrow, while Chap. 12 discusses the localization of mature lymphoid populations in the lymph node.

Cell lineage refers to the range of maturation states of cells that share morphologic and functional characteristics; in most circumstances, once lineage commitment has occurred it cannot be changed. In contrast, hematopoietic stem cells (HSC) are immature cells with the potential to generate all the components of the hematopoietic system. HSC have several fundamental properties: a) they can ensure the long-term reconstitution of the hematopoietic system, b) they reconstitute all lineages, and c) they self-renew through symmetrical and asymmetrical cell divisions. A "clone" is a population of cells derived from a single progenitor. Cell lineages considered here are lymphoid and myeloid (megakaryocytic, erythroid, granulocytic, macrophages). Dendritic cells (DCs) may arise from progenitors belonging to the myeloid (or possibly the lymphoid) lineage.

Many genes mediating lineage commitment in hematopoiesis encode for transcription factors. These proteins bind DNA and recruit directly, or through intermediaries, replication and transcription complexes to alter gene expression. They are also integral components of the chromatin modifying complexes that regulate the epigenetic state (e.g., acetylation or methylation of histones or DNA).

From: *Neoplastic Hematopathology*: Contemporary Hematology,
Edited by: D. Jones, DOI 10.1007/978-1-60761-384-8_31,
© Humana Press, a part of Springer Science+Business Media, LLC 2010

Hematopoiesis takes place in a specific microenvironment, defined as the localized milieu composed of stromal cells, including blood vessels, fibroblastic, myofibroblastic and DC populations, and the secreted products including cytokines (growth factors) that regulate hematopoietic growth and differentiation and chemotactic chemokines that regulate cell migration and retention.

31.2. Overview of Stages in Hematopoiesis

Currently, the most widely accepted model of hematopoiesis is a pyramidal one, with HSC at the tip and mature cells of varying lineages at the base (Fig. 31-1). Emerging data are suggesting that even relatively mature lineage-committed cells retain some limited ability to differentiate into mature elements of other lineages, but at this time, this phenomenon is poorly characterized and it is unclear how much this process contributes to mature hematopoiesis [1].

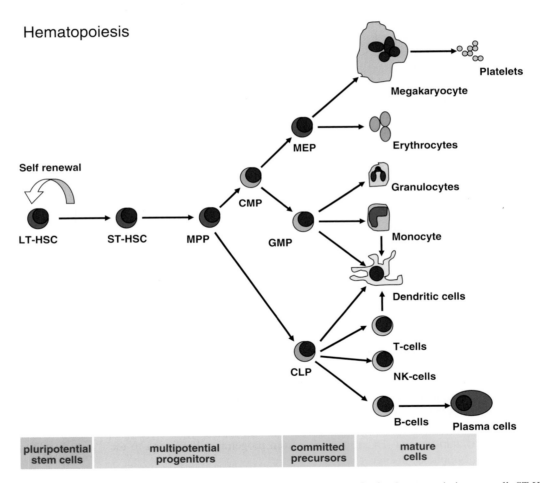

Fig. 31-1. Simplified pyramidal schema for hematopoiesis. *LT-HSC* long term reconstituting hematopoietic stem cell, *ST-HSC* short term reconstituting hematopoietic stem cell, *MPP* multipotent progenitor cell, *CLP* common lymphoid progenitor, *CMP* common myeloid progenitor, *MEP* megakaryocytic erythroid progenitor, *GMP* granulocytic monocytic progenitors

31.2.1. Hematopoiesis During Embryogenesis

During embryogenesis, the first elements with hematopoietic potential have been identified in the blood islands of the yolk sac beginning at 3 weeks post-conception (experimental evidence has also been generated in avian and murine models) [2,3]. These primitive progenitors are of mesodermic origin and have both endothelial and hematopoietic developmental potential. The next site of hematopoiesis is the aorta-gonad mesonephros system (30–37 days gestation), and is the first intra-embryonic location [2,4]. Starting at low levels in gestation week 5, fetal hematopoiesis can be identified in the liver. The numbers of erythropoietic progenitors reaches a plateau by week 9, at the time when the fetal liver is the main site of hematopoiesis [1]. In the perinatal period, the main site of hematopoiesis shifts to the bone marrow. At this stage, the spleen and the thymus become crucial sites in the development of B cells and T cells, respectively.

Several proteins have been demonstrated to be necessary for the development of normal HSC. Among these, the most important are RUNX1/AML1, SCL/TAL, GATA2, and LMO2 [5]. These genes are also activated by chromosomal translocations in different hematologic malignancies supporting their critical role [6].

31.2.2. Hematopoiesis in the Bone Marrow

In bone marrow, long-term reconstituting (LT)-HSC [7] generate short-term reconstituting (ST)-HSC, a population that still has the potential to generate all cell lineages, but only for a limited amount of time, perhaps up to 3 months [8,9]. ST-HSC then generate multipotent progenitor cells (MPP) which can reconstitute all the blood elements for only 2 weeks [10]. MPP can commit to a lymphoid or to a myeloid developmental fate. The common lymphoid progenitors (CLP) [11] are the earliest cells that have lost the ability to generate myeloid cells, while the common myeloid progenitors (CMP)[11] are their myeloid counterpart, and lack the ability to generate lymphocytes. At the CLP or CMP stages, there is very little self-renewal potential. CLP give rise to B-cell, T-cell, and natural killer (NK)-cell lineages, and possibly to subsets of DCs [12]. The megakaryocyte erythrocyte progenitors (MEP) and granulocyte monocyte progenitors (GMP) arise directly from CMP [13]. The erythroid and megakaryocytic lineages are derived from MEP, while the GMP give rise only to granulocytes and monocytes, and the related myeloid-derived DC [14]. At these developmental stages, progenitor subsets are indistinguishable by routine histologic stains and morphologic examination.

Maturation in the erythroid lineage progresses through morphologically distinct stages of proerythroblasts (pronormoblast), basophilic erythroblast (normoblast) I and II, polychromatic erythroblast (normoblast), orthochromatic erythroblast (normoblast), reticulocyte and anucleate red blood cells (erythrocytes). The least mature cells have relatively open chromatin and light blue cytoplasm. The orthochromatic normoblast is the last cell in the erythroid series with the ability to divide. As these cells mature, their nuclei become pyknotic and are finally expelled. The cytoplasm of the cells in the erythroid series becomes darker as they accumulate RNA. At the polychromatic normoblast stage, the production of cytoplasmic hemoglobin leads to changes in the color of cytoplasm and from this stage onwards hemoglobin accumulates at the expense of the nuclei acid contents. When orthochromatic normoblasts are seen in the peripheral blood, they are usually identified as nucleated red blood cells.

The stages in the development of megakaryocytes are promegakaryoblast/megakaryoblast, promegakaryocyte, and megakaryocyte. During maturation of the megakaryocytic lineage, megakaryocytes become polyploid through a process of endoreduplication (mitosis without separation of nuclear and cytoplasmic material). The nuclear maturation, as demonstrated by the lobation of the nuclei, their size and the quality of the chromatin, is not always in synchrony with the maturation of the megakaryocytic cytoplasm (quantity, granularity, and surface sloughing of platelets).

Along the granulocytic lineage, the maturation stages are promyelocyte, myelocyte, metamyelocyte, band, and mature granulocyte (neutrophil, eosinophil, or basophil). The last cell divisions usually occur at the myelocyte stage. Cytoplasmic changes consist mostly of accumulation of different types of granules. Primary, azurophilic granules are present at the promyelocyte and myelocyte stages, with generation of secondary granules predominating at the myelocyte stage. Nuclear lobation begins at the myelocyte stage, cells with notched nuclei being identified as metamyelocytes. The stages of monocytic development are more difficult to delineate, but it is accepted that morphologically-distinct stages are monoblasts, promonocytes, and monocytes. In normal adults, all the maturation steps described in the erythroid, megakaryocytic and myeloid lineages take place in the bone marrow.

31.2.3. T-Cell Maturation

T cells after the CLP stage leave the marrow and mature in the thymus. Developmental stages of immature T cells (thymocytes) are morphologically indistinguishable and require immunophenotyping to identify. T cell precursors retain the ability to proliferate which is critical to thymic selection of T-cell receptor (TCR)-responsive populations (i.e., "negative selection") and deletion of autoreactive populations (i.e., "positive selection"), both of which involve signaling through the TCR [15,16].

Immature T cells sequentially rearrange the DNA of the TCR genes to generate an expressed receptor composed of either alpha (α) and beta (β) chains (the vast majority of mature T cells) or gamma (γ) and delta (δ) chains producing a $\gamma\delta$ T cell (see Chap. 4 for summary of the structure of the TCR genes). The TCR recombination process is controlled by several enzymes, the most important being the Rag1 and Rag2 recombinases, and terminal deoxynucleotidyl transferase (TdT) [17,18]. To prevent the generation of two different TCR proteins in the same T cell, only one allele of each TCR gene rearranges at a time, termed *allelic exclusion*, and TCR rearrangement stops when a functional TCR protein is produced and begins to signal [19].

The TCRG locus rearranges first, followed by TCRD [20]. The intensity of cell signaling from the pre-TCR or TCR is crucial in the next developmental steps [21,22]. The cells with strong signaling through $\gamma\delta$ TCR become mature $\gamma\delta$ T cells, while cells with non-productive TCRG and TCRD rearrangement or having attenuated signaling switch to a $\alpha\beta$ T-cell fate [21,22]. This sequence of events explains why in most mature $\alpha\beta$ T cells, TCRG is rearranged while only a small minority of mature $\gamma\delta$ T cells have productive rearrangements of TCRB [20]. As most T cells have productive TCRG rearrangements, there is a potential for a small subset of thymocytes to develop into mature $\gamma\delta$ T cells even following TCRB rearrangement [20].

As discussed in Chap. 4, TCR rearrangement producing the TCR-$\alpha\beta$ results in a protein with a unique antigen-recognition sequence. This is due to the recombinatorial complexity of the TCRA and TCRB loci and to the process of end-joining/non-templated extension mediated by Rag1/2 and TdT, which delete and add additional nucleotides within the TCR during the recombination process. This allows each $\alpha\beta$ T-cell clone and all its progeny to recognize, with high binding affinity, a specific peptide antigen presented within the groove of Class I and Class II MHC molecules on the surface of an antigen presenting cell (APC). In contrast, the TCRG and TCRD genes have more limited combinatorial diversity which results in much more restricted (and likely lower affinity) recognition of antigen. As a result, $\gamma\delta$ T cells function in the immune system by recognition of patterned antigens, such as microbial glycoproteins and glycolipids, in association with non-classical MHC-like proteins like CD1a on APC [23]–[25]. Some $\gamma\delta$ T cells have a complete absence of non-templated additions/deletions resulting in a canonical TCR protein. Such pre-formed populations of canonical T cells can respond quickly to common microbial antigens and form a core element of the innate immune response used for surveillance at mucosal sites [26].

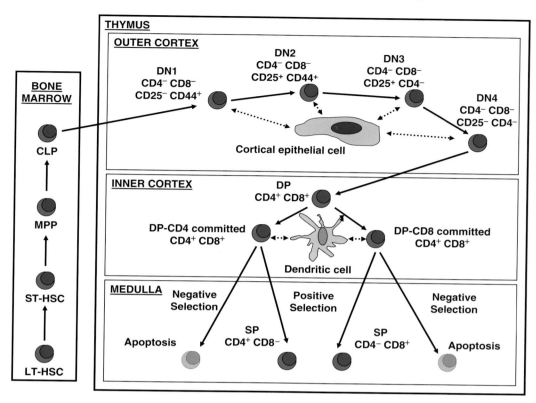

Fig. 31-2. Schematic representation of T-cell development in the bone marrow and thymus. *LT-HSC* long term reconstituting hematopoietic stem cell, *ST-HSC* short term reconstituting hematopoietic stem cell, *CLP* common lymphoid progenitor, *DN* double negative thymocyte, *DP* double positive thymocyte, *SP* single positive thymocyte (mature T cell)

Both αβ– and γδ T cells mature in the thymus, with a switch from the default γδ fate to the αβ pathway in T cells with low TCR signaling. The thymic positive selection process allows the preferential survival of immature thymocytes expressing functional TCRs that recognize the major histocompatibility complexes on APCs and transmit a growth signal. The negative selection process removes thymocytes with TCRs that bind the histocompatibility complexes (and/or self peptides) with very high affinity. Both αβ and γδ T cells undergo these processes of selection, but stringency is significantly higher for αβ T cells. These developmental steps ensure the generation of T cells that can interact with APCs, but will not proliferate so much that they trigger autoimmune processes. In parallel with the TCR rearrangement and selection, there are microanatomical and phenotype shifts from CD4– CD8– T cell progenitors located in the thymic cortex to a "double positive" stage (CD4+CD8+), and then "single-positive" CD4+CD8– or CD8+CD4– T cells located in the thymic medulla (Fig. 31-2). These intrathymic migrations bring the developing thymocytes in contact with different populations of thymic epithelial cells, (TEC) which secrete various cytokines to promote differential maturation.

31.2.4. B Cell Maturation

The initial stages in the development of B cells take place in the marrow (Fig. 31-3). Here the early B-cell progenitors, morphologically identified as small hyperchromatic lymphocytes termed *hematogones*, rearrange their immunoglobulin (Ig) genes to generate a surface bound antibody molecule, also known as the B-cell receptor (BCR), composed of heavy chain (IgH) and either the kappa or lambda light chain (IgK, IgL). The recombination process is nearly

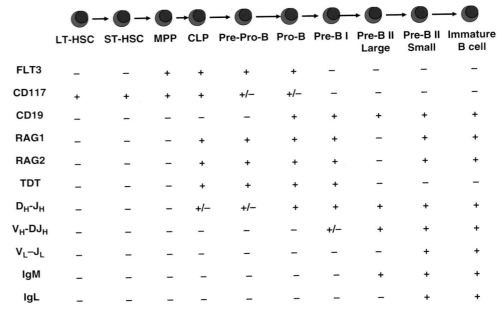

	LT-HSC	ST-HSC	MPP	CLP	Pre-Pro-B	Pro-B	Pre-B I	Pre-B II Large	Pre-B II Small	Immature B cell
FLT3	−	−	+	+	+	+	−	−	−	−
CD117	+	+	+	+	+/−	+/−	−	−	−	−
CD19	−	−	−	−	−	+	+	+	+	+
RAG1	−	−	−	+	+	+	+	−	+	+
RAG2	−	−	−	+	+	+	+	−	+	+
TDT	−	−	−	+	+	+	+	−	−	−
D_H-J_H	−	−	−	+/−	+/−	+	+	+	+	+
V_H-DJ_H	−	−	−	−	−	−	+/−	+	+	+
V_L-J_L	−	−	−	−	−	−	−	−	+	+
IgM	−	−	−	−	−	−	−	+	+	+
IgL	−	−	−	−	−	−	−	−	+	+

Fig. 31-3. Immunophenotype of B-cell maturation stages in the bone marrow. *LT-HSC* long term reconstituting hematopoietic stem cell, *ST-HSC* short term reconstituting hematopoietic stem cell, *CLP* common lymphoid progenitor, *TDT* terminal deoxynucleotidyl transferase; D_H diversity gene segment (heavy chain), J_H joining gene segment (heavy chain), V_H variable gene segment (heavy chain), V_L variable gene segment (light chain), J_L joining gene segment (light chain), *IgM* immunoglobulin M, *IgL* immunoglobulin light chain

identical to that for the TCR in T cells, controlled by the same enzymes, Rag1 and 2 and TdT and exhibiting allelic exclusion, end-joined/non-templated base pair changes and combinatorial diversity resulting in a unique BCR in each B-cell progenitor [27,28]. The earliest B-lineage cells have the Ig genes in germ-line configuration and are usually identified as pre-pro-B. Complete rearrangements of the heavy chain (IgH) define the pre-B stages (pre-B I and pre-B II large), with Ig light chain rearrangement occurring at a slightly later stage (Fig. 31-3).

Functional Ig rearrangement produces a "naïve" mature B cell, expressing surface BCR with a defined antigen specificity which is linked to a signal-transduction complex that signals at a low tonic level at rest to support survival and slow growth [29,30]. During the immune response, the BCR triggers a powerful signal when bound to MHC and an appropriate foreign antigen peptide on the surface of an adjacent APC. A poorly-understood process of selection for productive Ig rearrangements with low potential for auto-immunity also takes place similar to the thymic process. and the selected naïve B cells sequently leave the marrow, and populate the spleen and the other peripheral lymphoid organs.

B cells in extramedullary locations undergo a variety of shifts in their activation state and BCR status. As discussed in Chap. 12, following antigen binding in the interfollicular areas, B cells migrate to the germinal centers (becoming "follicular" B cells) and undergo IGH somatic hypermutation, a process mediated by the activation-induced cytosine deaminase (AICDA) protein [31,32]. During this process, base pair changes are introduced into the BCR sequence so that the affinity of the antibody for antigen is increased. B cells with the highest affinity for antigens are selected to proliferate due to hyper-responsive BCR signaling. Follicular B cells often undergo a further DNA deletion-recombination event termed class switch, that results in the change from the relatively low-affinity IgD/IgM to high-affinity IgG or specialized IgA or IgE antibodies [33]. B cells exit the germinal center to become either plasma cells, the antibody-secreting component of the humoral immune response, or long-lived pools of memory B cells, which along with memory T cells can quickly reactivate following repeated antigen exposure and form the basis of the adaptive or acquired immune response.

31.2.5. Maturation of Other Cell Types

The development of NK cells takes place in the bone marrow and their developmental stages are still poorly characterized [34]. Histiocytes and DCs are a heterogeneous group of APC and phagocytic cells with different functions and origins (see Chaps. 5 and 26). While most originate from the monocytic lineage, some DCs may derive from lymphoid progenitors [12,14,31,32].

31.3. Tools Used in the Study of the Hematopoietic Stem Cell Function

31.3.1. Animal Models

The first evidence supporting the existence of HSC originated from the observation that fraternal twin cattle that shared a placenta had the blood groups of both calves persisting for life. This indicated that mobile cells shared in embryonic development can supply a lifelong supply of mature blood cells [35]. A range of experimental approaches are now available for human and animal models to study the biology and the phenotype of HSC.

The first widely used in vivo model for HSC was the spleen colony assay [36,37]. This model, which resembles human HSC transplant, consists of a recipient animal (usually mouse) that is sublethally irradiated with a radiation dose sufficient for a complete ablation of its own bone marrow. The recipient is then injected with a cell suspension from a donor animal. The read-out is the formation in the spleens of the irradiated animals of colonies of hematopoietic cells. The composition and the size of the splenic colonies formed varies with time, so the maturation and proliferative potential of varying lineages can be assessed. The numbers of HSC in the donor bone marrow can be quantitated using sequential dilutions. Similar experiments can be used to test for the presence of CMP and CLP. The kinetics of reconstitution of the mouse thymus can also be analyzed to similarly investigate T-cell differentiation and maturation.

When human cells are used as the HSC donor source, the best results are obtained when the recipient animals are immunodeficient [38]. The identification of genetic strains of immunodeficient animals (such as NOD/SCID or RAG1/2-deficient mice) was a significant advance, allowing xenogenic HSC models using human or other non-murine donors. With the advent of flow cytometry and of in vitro functional HSC assays, the results of bone marrow transplantation in murine models could be monitored in the peripheral blood or in the bone marrow.

In mouse stem cell models, the generation of mice that differ only in certain alleles of CD45 (e.g., Ly5.1 or Ly5.2) on the surface of their hematopoietic cells allows the precise tracking of the donor cells, as well as the complete avoidance of graft rejection or of graft-versus-host reactions [39]. Purified cell populations from animals expressing either the Ly5.1 or Ly5.2 allele of CD45 are transplanted into sublethally irradiated animals expressing the other allele. Using these animal models the functions of different cell fractions or the effect of modifying agents on stem cells can be identified and quantified.

31.3.2. Improved In Vitro Stem Cell Assays

In vitro assays for HSC became possible after stromal cell lines were established [40,41]. These cell lines used in co-culture with HSC produce the supportive microenvironment that compensates for the loss of the "stem cell niche" of the bone marrow [41]. The readout in these assays are the number and types of foci of maturing hematopoietic elements that often cover the stromal cells, leading to the formation of "cobblestone areas" [42]. Currently, there are multiple stromal cell lines that allow differentiation along the myeloid, B-lymphoid, and T-lymphoid lineages.

The elucidation and production of specific colony stimulation cytokine factors lead to *methylcellulose assays*, where cells are immobilized in a methylcellulose matrix and grown in a media containing different types of cytokines [43,44]. This not only allows the identification of the developmental fate of the cultured cells and the quantification of the progenitors, but also the characterization of the biologic impact of novel cytokines and growth factors [45]. Based on the morphology of the colonies and of the cells, the progenitor cells tested by routine methylcellulose colony forming assays can be classified as colony forming units corresponding to (CFU)-granulocyte (G), erythroid (E), macrophage (M), megakaryocyte (M), CFU-E, CFU-GM (macrophage), CFU-G, CFU-M (macrophage), or burst forming unit-erythroid (BFU-E) types [44]. Using a different set of cytokines, CFU-megakaryocyte, CFU-pre-B cell can also be identified.

31.4. Functional and Immunophenotypic Definition of Stem Cells

Flow cytometric cell sorting (FACS) allows the fractionation of bone marrow cells into immunophenotypically homogeneous populations to assess the function of purified LT-HSC, ST-HSC, CLP, or CMP in experimental models [9]. A commonly-used FACS purification method is based on the dim staining of most self-renewing stem cells for vital stains such as Rhodamine 123 and Hoechst 33342. This poorly staining population, which includes most LT-HSC, has been termed the "side population" (Fig. 31-4) [46]. This method is based on the rapid efflux of some nucleic acid binding dyes from stem cells due to their over-expression of one of several ABC-type membrane transports, particularly ABCG2 [47,48].

In mice, the bone marrow population that retains the ability to reconstitute the hematopoietic system over the long-term is composed of cells that do not express classic lineage-specific markers (termed "Lin-"), including absence of B220 (mouse CD45 isoform expressed on B cells) , CD3, CD4, CD8, Mac-1– (myelomonocytic marker), Gr-1– (neutrophil marker) , or Ter119 (RBC marker). These Lin– cells are positive for the receptor tyrosine kinase KIT/CD117 and for Sca1 [7]. Peripheral blood analysis at different times shows that animals transplanted with CD34-CD38+CD117+Sca1+Thy1.1^{lo}Lin– cells have stable reconstitution of all lineages for the entire duration of an animal's life [7].

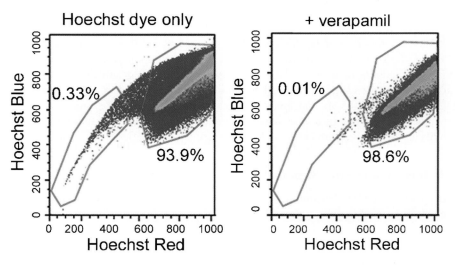

Fig. 31-4. Flow cytometric characterization of the "side population" of stem cells. *Left:* cytogram of a bone marrow sample with an encircled cell population on the left side showing low level staining (i.e., rapid efflux) for Hoechst 33342 dye. *Right:* inhibition of efflux using the channel blocker verapamil eliminates this side population (Figure courtesy of Francisco Vega, MD)

Such long-term survival of the stem cell pool implies the presence in Lin- stem cells with mechanisms capable of preserving the telomere length that would prevent genome instability. Otherwise repeated cell divisions would result in progressively shortened telomeres, limiting the ability of DNA polymerase to replicate chromosome ends. This limitless replicative property is supported by the finding of high levels of telomerase (the enzyme responsible for the regeneration of the telomeric DNA in the absence of a template) in LT-HSC [49]. Serial bone marrow transplant experiments, in which cells from the bone marrow of recipient animals are used to transplant other sublethally irradiated animals, not only show that the post-transplant bone marrow has lineage reconstituting abilities identical to those of the bone marrow in the donor, but the LT-HSC remain at a density comparable to that in the original donor. This finding points to another important characteristic of the LT-HSC: self-renewal through asymmetric cell division. The process of asymmetrical division, defined as the generation of one daughter identical to the mother (LT-HSC) and a second one that undergoes further divisions to generate differentiated cells, is poorly understood. Activation of the Wnt pathway is essential for maintaining a large stem cell pool and may control the asymmetrical cell division underlying self-renewal [50]. Activation of Wnt, in turn, leads to dephosphorylation of β-catenin, which is released from an APC/axin/GSK3β-containing cytoplasmic complex and then translocates to the nucleus, where it binds transcription regulators resulting in increased expression of genes such as Notch1 and HoxB4 [50].

Purely asymmetric cell division has the disadvantage of leaving stem cells unable to expand in number. However, stem cell pools do increase markedly during development, immediately following stem cell transplant, and after marrow injury or chemotherapy [51]. Therefore, stem cells must also be able to shift to symmetric cell division, when needed. The balance between these symmetric and asymmetric modes is likely controlled by environmental and developmental signals. The ability of HSC to self-renew through asymmetric and symmetric replication is responsible for the maintenance of a constant pool of stem cells in the bone marrow, in spite of the need for continuous generation of mature blood elements.

The usually dormant LT-HSC are induced to enter the cell cycle to generate more blood cells and ST-HSC by micro-environmental factors. The molecules or environmental clues that result only in LT-HSC renewal (without further maturation) are poorly characterized, but cytokines and growth factors that can result in maturation and lineage commitment can also induce stem cells to cycle [5]. Among the cytokines that have been proven to induce stem cells to cycle are: steel factor, [52] interleukin 11, [53] interleukin 6, [54] thrombopoietin, [55] granulocyte-macrophage colony-stimulating factor,[56] granulocyte colony-stimulating factor, and macrophage stimulating factor [56]. The loss of the ability to self renew is associated with the expression of FLT3 [57].

Human LT-HSC are less well characterized than their mouse counterparts, but are thought to have similar properties. In humans, LT-HSC have a CD38+CD90+Lin− immunophenotype with variable engraftment based on CD34 expression status [49,58,59]. Enrichment for LT-HSC can be achieved by combining purification methods using the above antibodies and vital dyes such as Hoechst 33342. In addition to these techniques, gene expression studies are now shedding light on specific patterns of gene expression in HSC that should provide more specific purification strategies in the near future. In spite of the phenotypes described for mouse and human LT-HSC, no study has yet achieved the purification of a population composed of 100% repopulating LT-HSC, an indication that some of the characteristics of stem cells are still elusive or highly dynamic.

31.5. Molecular Pathways Implicated in Lineage Specific Maturation

The ability to generate transgenic and gene-deficient (knockout) animals combined with the in-vitro HSC models described above has resulted in an increasing amount of information on the specific genes that control lineage commitment and maturation.

For example, expression of the receptor tyrosine kinase FLT3 results in the exit of progenitor cells from the LT-HSC pool [57]. Expression of several transcription factors has been shown to be important for hematopoietic maturation: the PU.1 transcription factor is involved in the myeloid-versus-lymphoid developmental decision as are HoxB4, GATA1, GATA2, FOG, and C/EBP alpha [5]. GATA1 and FOG are necessary for normal erythroid and megakaryocytic development,[60] whereas C/EBP alpha mediates the full development and maturation of the granulocytic and monocytic lineages [61].

Commitment to a lymphoid fate seems to be controlled by several parallel mechanisms. One of the most important is expression of Ikaros, a zinc finger transcription factor with multiple splice isoforms [62]. In the absence of this gene, there is no normal lymphoid development. Ikaros expression upregulates E2A, which in turn activates the expression of EBF and PAX5, transcription factors crucial for the "locking-in" of the B-cell phenotype [63,64]. Aiolos and Helios are related genes that have been shown to be crucial for the normal development of B cells and T cells, respectively (Table 31-1) [65]. In parallel with Ikaros, expression in progenitor cells of the cytokine receptor for IL-7 leads to the activation of STAT5A and STAT5B (growth factor-controlled transcription regulators), resulting in the expression of EBF [66]. These are not the only pathways that results in EBF expression, as the combined expression of E2A and PU.1 has been shown to have a similar role. In the absence of PU.1 there is no normal lymphoid, granulocytic, or macrophage development [67]. EBF upregulates the expression of PAX5 and both these transcription factors have been shown to be important in the process of Ig gene rearrangement. In normal cells, expression of PAX5 prevents cells committed to the B-developmental fate from maturing along the alternative T-lymphoid or myeloid lineages [64].

Signaling through Notch-1 is necessary for normal T cell development [68]. Binding of the Notch-1 ligands Delta and Jagged activates the Notch-1 pathway, resulting in down-regulation of IL7R (and of the B-lineage potential), and upregulation of GATA3, a transcription factor necessary for normal T-cell development [69]. Also, Notch-1 expression can result in

Table 31-1. Important genes that function in hematopoietic lineage commitment.

Transcription factor (gene symbol)	Description and role
Ikaros (IKZF1)	Zinc finger protein. At least eight isoforms described, the short ones are functionally dominant-negative. In the absence of IKZLFI there is no normal lymphoid development.
Helios (IKZF2)	Member of the Ikaros family of proteins. Necessary for normal T-cell development.
Aiolos (IKZF3)	Structure similar to Ikaros and Helios. Regulates B-cell maturation and function.
PU.1 (SPI1)	ETS family transcription factor involved in myeloid/lymphoid developmental decision. No normal lymphoid, granulocytic or monocytic development in its absence.
NOTCH1	Membrane protein. Upon ligand binding the intra-cellular portion translocates to the nucleus. Necessary for T-cell development.
E2A (TCF3)	Member of the basic helix-loop-helix family of proteins. It encodes for two proteins: E12 and E47, necessary for normal B-cell development.
GATA1	Regulates normal erythroid and megakaryocytic development
GATA2	Involved in the maintenance of stem cell potential in embryonic and adult hematopoiesis.
GATA3	Controls T-cell development
FOG (ZFPM1)	With GATA-1 regulates erythroid and megakaryocytic development.
ID2	Helix-loop-helix protein, acts as a dominant negative for basic helix-loop-helix proteins. Necessary for NK-cell development and for follicular helper T cells.
PAX5	Paired domain transcription factor, crucial for the maintenance of commitment to the B-lineage.
EBF (EBF1)	Necessary for normal B-cell development. Binds DNA through a zinc coordination domain.

increased ID3, a dominant-negative protein that inhibits E2A. In these several ways, Notch-1 not only promotes the commitment to a T-cell developmental fate, but also inhibits EBF and, consequently, development along the B-cell lineage.

The transcriptional regulator ID2 is necessary in the development of NK cells and dendritic cells [70].

31.6. The Role of the Microenvironment in Hematopoiesis

Induction of specific transcription factors in stem cells is directed by extracellular cytokines produced by stromal elements as well as by intrinsic HSC mechanisms that may be pre-programmed by a developmental clock or occur stochastically. For normal development of various lineages, cytokines such as G-CSF, thrombopoietin, GM-CSF, erythropoietin, IL-6, IL-5, IL-7 are necessary. But, while these cytokines have "lineage instructive" abilities, they are not sufficient for commitment to a certain lineage in most cases. However, they do highlight the critical role of bone marrow stroma in stem cell biology, not only in producing cytokines, but also in providing chemokines (such as CXCL13) and adhesion molecules (such as integrins) to trap maturing HSC within localized niches and in providing nutrients and essential cofactors (e.g., macrophage transfer of iron to hemoglobin in erythrocytes). The stromal-HSC interactions have recently been modeled using three-dimensional matrices or in implantable matrigel environments, but the complexity of the interactions between stroma and HSC make rigorous experiments difficult to design and interpret.

31.7. Cancer Stem Cells

The concept that only a subset of the cells within a tumor possess the ability to extensively proliferate has gained acceptance in recent years. These cancer stem cells have been operationally defined as the tumor subpopulations that share with nonneoplastic stem cells the capacity to both self-renew and differentiate. These cancer stem cells would then continuously seed the phenotypically diverse maturing subsets within the tumor. Advocates of this model have suggested that disease relapses observed following apparently effective treatment are related to this cancer stem cell pool that has HSC-like properties of relative quiescence, and resistance to conventional chemotherapy. Discovery of genetically-defined leukemia-initiating cells or leukemia stem cells in mouse models lends credence to this theory [71,72]. It has now been shown that AML samples enriched for blasts with the phenotype of HSCs (CD34+ CD38− cells) preferentially form leukemias in immunocompromised xenografts when compared with unsorted populations.

This general cancer stem cell model has been applied to a growing number of hematological and solid malignancies in which populations of cells with preferential capacity for tumorigenicity have been identified. It is clear that the immunophenotype of such stem cells will vary but that embryonic signaling pathways involved in adult stem cell maintenance, including sonic hedgehog (SHH) and Wnt are commonly dysregulated in cancer stem cells as well. Reactivation of these developmental pathways in tumors supports the hypothesis that deregulated self-renewal and proliferation of cancer stem cells are critical determinants of tumor growth, maintenance, and dissemination.

Suggested Readings

Weissman IL, Shizuru JA. The origins of the identification and isolation of hematopoietic stem cells, and their capability to induce donor-specific transplantation tolerance and treat autoimmune diseases. Blood 2008;112:3543–53.

Busslinger M. Transcriptional control of early B cell development. Annu Rev Immunol 2004;22:55–79.

Zhu J, Emerson SG. Hematopoietic cytokines, transcription factors and lineage commitment. Oncogene 2002;21:3295–303.

References

1. Migliaccio G, Migliaccio AR, Petti S, et al. Human embryonic hemopoiesis. Kinetics of progenitors and precursors underlying the yolk sac – liver transition. J Clin Invest 1986;78:51–60

2. Cumano A, Godin I. Ontogeny of the hematopoietic system. Annu Rev Immunol 2007;25:745–85.

3. Pereda J, Niimi G. Embryonic erythropoiesis in human yolk sac: two different compartments for two different processes. Microsc Res Tech 2008;71:856–62.

4. Marshall CJ, Moore RL, Thorogood P, Brickell PM, Kinnon C, Thrasher AJ. Detailed characterization of the human aorta-gonad-mesonephros region reveals morphological polarity resembling a hematopoietic stromal layer. Dev Dyn 1999;215:139–47.

5. Zhu J, Emerson SG. Hematopoietic cytokines, transcription factors and lineage commitment. Oncogene 2002;21:3295–313.

6. Rowley JD. Chromosomal translocations: revisited yet again. Blood 2008;112:2183–9.

7. Morrison SJ, Weissman IL. The long-term repopulating subset of hematopoietic stem cells is deterministic and isolatable by phenotype. Immunity 1994;1:661–73.

8. Shizuru JA, Negrin RS, Weissman IL. Hematopoietic stem and progenitor cells: clinical and pre-clinical regeneration of the hematolymphoid system. Annu Rev Med 2005;56:509–38.

9. Weissman IL, Shizuru JA. The origins of the identification and isolation of hematopoietic stem cells, and their capability to induce donor-specific transplantation tolerance and treat autoimmune diseases. Blood 2008;112:3543–53.

10. Morrison SJ, Wandycz AM, Hemmati HD, Wright DE, Weissman IL. Identification of a lineage of multipotent hematopoietic progenitors. Development 1997;124:1929–39.

11. Kondo M, Weissman IL, Akashi K. Identification of clonogenic common lymphoid progenitors in mouse bone marrow. Cell 1997;91:661–72.

12. Manz MG, Traver D, Miyamoto T, Weissman IL, Akashi K. Dendritic cell potentials of early lymphoid and myeloid progenitors. Blood 2001;97:3333–41.

13. Forsberg EC, Serwold T, Kogan S, Weissman IL, Passegue E. New evidence supporting megakaryocyte-erythrocyte potential of flk2/flt3+ multipotent hematopoietic progenitors. Cell 2006;126:415–26.

14. Manz MG, Traver D, Akashi K, et al. Dendritic cell development from common myeloid progenitors. Ann N Y Acad Sci 2001;938:167–73; discussion 73–4

15. Germain RN. T-cell development and the CD4-CD8 lineage decision. Nat Rev Immunol 2002;2:309–22.

16. Zuniga-Pflucker JC. T-cell development made simple. Nat Rev Immunol 2004;4:67–72.

17. Bollum FJ, Chang LM. Terminal transferase in normal and leukemic cells. Adv Cancer Res 1986;47:37–61.

18. Chang LM, Bollum FJ. Molecular biology of terminal transferase. CRC Crit Rev Biochem 1986;21:27–52.

19. Boucontet L, Sepulveda N, Carneiro J, Pereira P. Mechanisms controlling termination of V-J recombination at the TCRgamma locus: implications for allelic and isotypic exclusion of TCRgamma chains. J Immunol 2005;174:3912–9.

20. Joachims ML, Chain JL, Hooker SW, Knott-Craig CJ, Thompson LF. Human alpha beta and gamma delta thymocyte development: TCR gene rearrangements, intracellular TCR beta expression, and gamma delta developmental potential – differences between men and mice. J Immunol 2006;176:1543–52.

21. Lauritsen JP, Haks MC, Lefebvre JM, Kappes DJ, Wiest DL. Recent insights into the signals that control alphabeta/gammadelta-lineage fate. Immunol Rev 2006;209:176–90.

22. Terrence K, Pavlovich CP, Matechak EO, Fowlkes BJ. Premature expression of T cell receptor (TCR)alphabeta suppresses TCRgammadelta gene rearrangement but permits development of gammadelta lineage T cells. J Exp Med 2000;192:537–48.

23. Born WK, Jin N, Aydintug MK, et al. gammadelta T lymphocytes-selectable cells within the innate system? J Clin Immunol 2007;27:133–44.

24. Nanno M, Shiohara T, Yamamoto H, Kawakami K, Ishikawa H. gammadelta T cells: firefighters or fire boosters in the front lines of inflammatory responses. Immunol Rev 2007;215:103–13.

25. O'Brien RL, Roark CL, Jin N, et al. gammadelta T-cell receptors: functional correlations. Immunol Rev 2007;215:77–88.

26. Asarnow DM, Cado D, Raulet DH. Selection is not required to produce invariant T-cell receptor gamma-gene junctional sequences. Nature 1993;362:158–60.

27. Hardy RR, Kincade PW, Dorshkind K. The protean nature of cells in the B lymphocyte lineage. Immunity 2007;26:703–14.

28. Welner RS, Pelayo R, Kincade PW. Evolving views on the genealogy of B cells. Nat Rev Immunol 2008;8:95–106.

29. Hardy RR, Li YS, Allman D, Asano M, Gui M, Hayakawa K. B-cell commitment, development and selection. Immunol Rev 2000;175:23–32.

30. Hayakawa K, Asano M, Shinton SA, et al. Positive selection of natural autoreactive B cells. Science 1999;285:113–6.

31. Durandy A. Activation-induced cytidine deaminase: a dual role in class-switch recombination and somatic hypermutation. Eur J Immunol 2003;33:2069–73.

32. Neuberger MS. Antibody diversification by somatic mutation: from Burnet onwards. Immunol Cell Biol 2008;86:124–32.

33. Stavnezer J, Guikema JE, Schrader CE. Mechanism and regulation of class switch recombination. Annu Rev Immunol 2008;26:261–92.

34. Yoon SR, Chung JW, Choi I. Development of natural killer cells from hematopoietic stem cells. Mol Cells 2007;24:1–8.

35. Owen RD. Immunogenetic consequences of vascular anastomoses between bovine twins. Science 1945;102:400–1.

36. Jacobson LO, Simmons EL, Marks EK, Eldredge JH. Recovery from radiation injury. Science 1951;113:510–1.

37. Lorenz E, Uphoff D, Reid TR, Shelton E. Modification of irradiation injury in mice and guinea pigs by bone marrow injections. J Natl Cancer Inst 1951;12:197–201.

38. Lapidot T, Fajerman Y, Kollet O. Immune-deficient SCID and NOD/SCID mice models as functional assays for studying normal and malignant human hematopoiesis. J Mol Med 1997;75:664–73.

39. Shen FW, Tung JS, Boyse EA. Further definition of the Ly-5 system. Immunogenetics 1986;24:146–9.

40. Deryugina EI, Muller-Sieburg CE. Stromal cells in long-term cultures: keys to the elucidation of hematopoietic development? Crit Rev Immunol 1993;13:115–50.

41. Wineman J, Moore K, Lemischka I, Muller-Sieburg C. Functional heterogeneity of the hematopoietic microenvironment: rare stromal elements maintain long-term repopulating stem cells. Blood 1996;87:4082–90.

42. Neben S, Anklesaria P, Greenberger J, Mauch P. Quantitation of murine hematopoietic stem cells in vitro by limiting dilution analysis of cobblestone area formation on a clonal stromal cell line. Exp Hematol 1993;21:438–43.

43. Dao C, Metcalf D, Zittoun R, Bilski-Pasquier G. Normal human bone marrow cultures in vitro: cellular composition and maturation of the granulocytic colonies. Br J Haematol 1977;37:127–36.

44. Leary AG, Ogawa M. Blast cell colony assay for umbilical cord blood and adult bone marrow progenitors. Blood 1987;69:953–6.

45. Leary AG, Ikebuchi K, Hirai Y, et al. Synergism between interleukin-6 and interleukin-3 in supporting proliferation of human hematopoietic stem cells: comparison with interleukin-1 alpha. Blood 1988;71:1759–63.

46. Challen GA, Little MH. A side order of stem cells: the SP phenotype. Stem Cells 2006;24:3–12.

47. Scharenberg CW, Harkey MA, Torok-Storb B. The ABCG2 transporter is an efficient Hoechst 33342 efflux pump and is preferentially expressed by immature human hematopoietic progenitors. Blood 2002;99:507–12.

48. Zhou S, Schuetz JD, Bunting KD, et al. The ABC transporter Bcrp1/ABCG2 is expressed in a wide variety of stem cells and is a molecular determinant of the side-population phenotype. Nat Med 2001;7:1028–34.

49. Lansdorp PM. Telomeres, stem cells, and hematology. Blood 2008;111:1759–66.

50. Malhotra S, Kincade PW. Wnt-related molecules and signaling pathway equilibrium in hematopoiesis. Cell Stem Cell 2009;4:27–36.

51. Wilson A, Laurenti E, Oser G, et al. Hematopoietic stem cells reversibly switch from dormancy to self-renewal during homeostasis and repair. Cell 2008;135:1118–29.

52. Broudy VC. Stem cell factor and hematopoiesis. Blood 1997;90:1345–64.

53. Borbolla JR, Lopez-Hernandez MA, De Diego J, Gonzalez-Avante M, Trueba E, Collados MT. Use of interleukin-11 after autologous stem cell transplant: report of three cases and a very brief review of the literature. Haematologica 2001;86:891–2.

54. Kishimoto T. The biology of interleukin-6. Blood 1989;74:1–10.

55. Marcucci R, Romano M. Thrombopoietin and its splicing variants: structure and functions in thrombopoiesis and beyond. Biochim Biophys Acta 2008;1782:427–32.
56. Metcalf D. Hematopoietic cytokines. Blood 2008;111:485–91.
57. Adolfsson J, Borge OJ, Bryder D, et al. Upregulation of Flt3 expression within the bone marrow Lin(-)Sca1(+)c-kit(+) stem cell compartment is accompanied by loss of self-renewal capacity. Immunity 2001;15:659–69.
58. Baum CM, Weissman IL, Tsukamoto AS, Buckle AM, Peault B. Isolation of a candidate human hematopoietic stem-cell population. Proc Natl Acad Sci U S A 1992;89:2804–8.
59. Terstappen LW, Huang S, Safford M, Lansdorp PM, Loken MR. Sequential generations of hematopoietic colonies derived from single nonlineage-committed CD34+CD38- progenitor cells. Blood 1991;77:1218–27.
60. Chang AN, Cantor AB, Fujiwara Y, et al. GATA-factor dependence of the multitype zinc-finger protein FOG-1 for its essential role in megakaryopoiesis. Proc Natl Acad Sci U S A 2002;99:9237–42.
61. Zhang DE, Hohaus S, Voso MT, et al. Function of PU.1 (Spi-1), C/EBP, and AML1 in early myelopoiesis: regulation of multiple myeloid CSF receptor promoters. Curr Top Microbiol Immunol 1996;211:137–47.
62. Ng SY, Yoshida T, Georgopoulos K. Ikaros and chromatin regulation in early hematopoiesis. Curr Opin Immunol 2007;19:116–22.
63. Kioussis D. Aiolos: an ungrateful member of the Ikaros family. Immunity 2007;26:275–7.
64. Nutt SL, Heavey B, Rolink AG, Busslinger M. Commitment to the B-lymphoid lineage depends on the transcription factor Pax5. Nature 1999;401:556–62.
65. Pongubala JM, Northrup DL, Lancki DW, et al. Transcription factor EBF restricts alternative lineage options and promotes B cell fate commitment independently of Pax5. Nat Immunol 2008;9:203–15.
66. Roessler S, Gyory I, Imhof S, et al. Distinct promoters mediate the regulation of Ebf1 gene expression by interleukin-7 and Pax5. Mol Cell Biol 2007;27:579–94.
67. Kastner P, Chan S. PU.1: a crucial and versatile player in hematopoiesis and leukemia. Int J Biochem Cell Biol 2008;40:22–7
68. Rothenberg EV, Moore JE, Yui MA. Launching the T-cell-lineage developmental programme. Nat Rev Immunol 2008;8:9–21.
69. Hayday AC, Pennington DJ. Key factors in the organized chaos of early T cell development. Nat Immunol 2007;8:137–44.
70. Hacker C, Kirsch RD, Ju XS, et al. Transcriptional profiling identifies Id2 function in dendritic cell development. Nat Immunol 2003;4:380–6.
71. Somervaille TC, Cleary ML. Identification and characterization of leukemia stem cells in murine MLL-AF9 acute myeloid leukemia. Cancer Cell 2006;10:257–68.
72. Neering SJ, Bushnell T, Sozer S, et al. Leukemia stem cells in a genetically defined murine model of blast-crisis CML. Blood 2007;110:2578–85.

Chapter 32

Role of Host Genetics in Lymphoma

Ahmet Dogan

Abstract/Scope of Chapter This chapter covers the role of host genetic background in determining the risk of development of non-Hodgkin lymphoma (NHL) and summarizes the new developments on the relationship between the host genetic polymorphisms and clinical outcome in NHL. The technical aspects of identifying host genetic polymorphisms and potential clinical applications for risk stratification of NHL based on host genetic polymorphisms are discussed.

Keywords Lymphoma, genetics • Lymphoma, risk stratification • Diffuse large B-cell lymphoma, outcome prediction • Follicular lymphoma, outcome prediction • Genetic polymorphism • Single nucleotide polymorphisms (SNP) • Copy number variation (CNV) • Tag SNPs • Rituximab, response prediction • Genotyping • Complement-dependent cytotoxicity • C1qA • TNF • IL10, CD40 • LMO2 • TNFRSF5

32.1. Introduction

Acquired genetic changes in lymphocytes are believed to be fundamental in the development of NHL [1,2]. Environmental insults, such as chronic inflammation, lymphotropic viruses, or exposure to environmental toxins, likely cause such genetic damage. In recent years, it has become apparent that the environmental events or biological properties of neoplastic cells, including the genetic makeup of the tumor cells, cannot fully explain the pathogenesis, clinical behavior, and outcome of NHL; host genetic background also must have an important role. The evidence for this hypothesis comes from a number of sources. It has long been recognized that individuals carrying germline mutations in the ataxia telangiectasia, mutated (ATM) [3] and Nijmegen breakage syndrome (NBN/NBS1) genes have highly increased risk of developing lymphoma. Other less well-defined host genetic polymorphisms likely also play a role in lymphomagenesis.

Epidemiologic studies have shown that patients with a family history of lymphoma or other hematological malignancies have an increased risk of developing lymphoma [4,5]. More recently, gene expression profiling has identified that the signals coming from the microenvironment (i.e. belonging to the host rather than to the tumor) not only define the biological features of a neoplasm, but also may be better predictors of outcome than the tumor characteristics [6–8] Furthermore, there is no doubt that the impact of host factors on clinical outcome will increase as new biological treatment modalities using host immune mechanisms to kill tumor cells are introduced into routine practice [9].

From: *Neoplastic Hematopathology*: Contemporary Hematology,
Edited by: D. Jones, DOI 10.1007/978-1-60761-384-8_32,
© Humana Press, a part of Springer Science+Business Media, LLC 2010

32.2. Overview of Single Nucleotide Polymorphisms

32.2.1. SNPs, CNVs, and Targeted Versus Genome-wide Discovery Projects

In line with observations mentioned above, epidemiologists have started looking at ways to identify the host genetic factors that may account for the observed biological and clinical heterogeneity in cancer. This task has been helped greatly by Human Genome Project and related commercial ventures, which have identified two major types of genetic variation between individuals. Single nucleotide polymorphisms (SNPs) are single base pair changes, involving both genes and intergenic areas that are inherited and maintained in the human population. Copy number variations (CNVs) represent sub-karyotypic differences between individuals in the length of chromosomal regions (i.e. inserted or deleted DNA regions), which are often associated with repeated DNA sequences. CNVs can range up to several megabases in size, and may be inherited stably or arise de novo as a result of DNA replication errors during embryogenesis.

SNPs are the most frequent type of variation in the human genome, [10] and are believed to be the major contributors to differences in disease incidence and outcome. Recent estimates indicate that there may be over 10 million SNPs that commonly vary among individuals. These are non-randomly distributed, with 93% of genes containing at least one common SNP. Some SNPs have functional and biological consequences. International collaborations have identified and catalogued in public databases over two million such SNPs in the human genome [11].

Geneticists and epidemiologists use SNPs as markers to associate areas of the human genome to disease susceptibility; however given the sheer numbers of SNPs present in the human genome, it is not possible to type every SNP loci or to identify its disease associations. To overcome this difficulty, geneticist use tag SNPs [12]. Tag SNPs represent a region of the chromosome with high linkage disequilibrium, meaning that the tag has a tendency to be inherited with the surrounding SNPs as a group. These tags can be used as markers of genetic variation at that region without genotyping every SNP in that region. Tag SNPs are useful in whole genome SNP association studies in which hundreds of thousands of SNPs across the entire genome are genotyped. Since genome-wide SNPs studies are identifying areas of the genome that are associated with relative risk and not particular cancer-causing changes per se, such an approach is legitimate.

32.2.2. Sample Considerations for SNP Analyses

Host genetic studies utilize DNA obtained from normal tissues not from the lymphoma itself. In patients without evidence of circulating tumor, blood samples are commonly used for DNA extraction. Buccal (cheek) swabs can also be used. Given that the hazard ratios (i.e. the level of increased detection rate of a particular polymorphisms in patients with lymphoma) for any given SNP is usually not more than 2-fold, large sample sizes are needed to achieve statistical significance. Especially in studies involving selected tag SNPs or small SNP panels, it is critically important to have an appropriate normal control population that is matched to the goals of the study. Many common SNPs are in Hardy–Weinberg equilibrium in the general population, but tumor or normal patient populations that are highly selected will show great variations simply due to sampling effects. The use of rare SNPs for disease association studies is especially problematic.

32.2.3. Tools Used for SNP Genotyping and Methodologic Issues

Initial efforts to identify SNPs associated with risk of NHL development were based on a very limited number of SNPs selected on the basis of hypotheses generated by the investigators, and often used laborious polymerase chain reaction (PCR)-based methodologies.

However, in recent years, a number of high-throughput array-based technologies have emerged [13]. Some of these platforms can genotype around 1 million SNPs in one experiment. Each platform has its strengths and limitations. In general, genotyping such large numbers of SNPs is associated with higher technical complexity and cost, thus limiting the number of samples that can be studied and the statistical power of the study. It is likely that these genome-wide high-resolution scanning of SNPs will identify disease associations with previously unrecognized areas of the genome. These loci can then be investigated further to discover individual genes affected by the genetic variation and biological consequences of these variations.

32.3. Genetic Polymorphisms and Risk for Lymphoma

Early epidemiological studies have focused on identifying genetic polymorphisms associated with increased risk of developing NHL, and have shown that polymorphisms involving a number of genes affecting different biological pathways may have a role. These studies were almost exclusively hypothesis-driven, and the investigators specifically focused on a small number of genes often representing a particular biochemical pathway (Table 32-1). Some examples of the pathways reported to be associated with increased risk of development of NHL, include oxidative stress response (*NOS2A, MPO*), energy regulation (*LEP, LEPR*), detoxification genes (*GSTM1, GSTT1*), one–carbon (folate) metabolism (*CBS, FPGS*), hormone production (*CYP17A1*), DNA repair genes (*RAG1, LIG4*), and oncogenes (*BCL6, CCND1/cyclin D1*) [14].

In particular, given the associations between inflammation, the immune response and the development, biology, and clinical outcome of NHL, many studies have focused on genes such as cytokines and their receptors (*IL10, TNF, BLYS*) or innate immunity genes (*TLR4*) [15–23]. One of the largest studies, performed by the InterLymph Consortium, analyzed 3586 patients with NHL and 4018 control patients from seven centers using a PCR-based methodology to detect 12 SNPs in nine genes that have important pro-inflammatory or anti-inflammatory effects (*IL1A, IL1RN, IL1B, IL2, IL6, IL10, TNF, LTA*, and *CARD15*) [15]. The study reported that common polymorphisms in TNF and IL10, key cytokines for the inflammatory response and Th1/Th2 balance, could be susceptibility loci for NHL. Similar findings were observed in the study performed by Cerhan and colleagues at Mayo Clinic using high-throughput-array-based genotyping methodologies [19]. The study analyzed 458 patients with NHL and 484 controls and 9412 SNPs from 1253 genes. The genes were selected based on biological criteria. The study indicated that genetic variation in immune response

Table 32-1. Summary of studies linking immune gene polymorphisms with risk of lymphoma.

Study	Disease	# cases/# controls	# SNPs/# Genes	Genes identified[a]
Rothman 2006 [15]	NHL	3586/4018	12/9	TNF, IL10
Lan 2006 [16]	NHL	518/597	39/20	*IL10, IL4*
Forrest 2006 [17]	NHL	904/1442	7/6	*TLR4*
Wang 2006 [18]	NHL	982/1172	57/36	*TNF, LTA*
Cerhan 2007 [19]	NHL	458/484	9412/1253	*CREB1, FGG, MAP3K5, IPK3, LSP1, TRAF1, DUSP2, ITGB3*
Novak 2007 [20]	NHL	441/475	9/1	*TNFSF13B* (BLYS)
Cerhan 2008 [21]	NHL	441/475	54/11	TNF, LTA, NFKB1
Ansell 2008 [22]	NHL	441/475	257/50	*PRF1, CD276, TBX21, IL6*
Skibola 2008 [23]	NHL	376/801	9/2	*TNFRSF5* (CD40)

NHL non-Hodgkin lymphoma

[a] Most significant gene polymorphism associated with increased or decreased risk for NHL

(*TRAF1*, *RIPK3*, *BAT2*, and *TLR6*), mitogen activated protein kinase (MAPK) signaling (*MAP3K5*, *DUSP2*, and *CREB1*), lymphocyte traffic (*B3GNT3*, *SELPLG*, and *LSP1*), and coagulation pathways (*FGG* and *ITGB3*) may be important in the etiology of NHL. Although these findings are yet to be validated by different methodologies, or in larger cohorts of patients, they strongly suggest a link between the host polymorphisms in immunity and inflammation-associated genes and risk of NHL.

To date, larger genome-wide SNPs screening studies or analyses of CNVs have not been published in lymphoma.

32.4. Genetic Polymorphisms and Clinical Outcome in Lymphoma

Perhaps more clinically important studies have concerned the association between immunity and inflammation gene polymorphisms and the outcome of NHL after treatment,[24–33] including polymorphisms of *TNF* in diffuse large B-cell lymphoma (DLBCL); [24] *HLA Class II* and *TNF* in all types of NHL, [25] *IL10* in DLBCL, [26] *IL10* in T-cell lymphoma, [27] and multiple cytokine genes in follicular lymphoma (Table 32-2) [28]. This last study analyzed 73 SNPs from 44 immunity and inflammation-associated genes in 248 cases of follicular lymphoma with a median follow-up of 59 months. The study reported that SNPs in *IL8*, *IL2*, *IL12B*, and *IL1RN* were the most robust predictors of survival and a risk score that combined the 4 SNPs with the clinical factors was even more strongly associated with survival. (Fig. 32-1 and 32-2) A similar finding was also observed for DLBCL [32]. These results are very encouraging and suggest that risk stratification of NHL may be significantly improved by the identification of high-risk host genotypes in addition to tumor and clinical parameters.

32.5. Genetic Polymorphisms and Response to Lymphoma Therapy

Heterogeneity of response to cytotoxic chemotherapy is well documented in cancer patients, including NHL patients. There are a number of causes for such variability, and host genetic variation in drug-metabolizing enzymes has an important role [34].

Addition of antibody-based, targeted therapies such as rituximab to cytotoxic agents has become the standard for management of most B-cell lymphomas. Because the patients receiving rituximab show heterogeneity in clinical response, a number of studies have looked for genetic polymorphisms that may alter efficiency of antibody-mediated tumor cell killing. The

Table 32-2. Summary of studies linking genetic polymorphisms to clinical outcome in lymphoma.

Study	Disease	#cases	# SNPs/# genes	Genes identified[a]
Warzocha 1998[24]	NHL	273	2/2	*TNF*
Juszczynski 2002[25]	NHL	204	3/3	*TNF/HLADRB1*
Lech-Maranda 2004[26]	DLBCL	199	3/1	*IL10*
Lee 2007[27]	TCL	108	3/1	*IL10*
Cerhan 2007[28]	FL	278	73/44	*IL8, IL2, IL12B, IL1RN*
Cerhan 2007[29]	DLBCL	215	30/18	*SHMT1, BHMT, TCN1*
Habermann 2007[31]	MCL	39	682/84	*TNFSF14, NFKBIA, CASP9*
Cerhan 2008[30]	DLBCL	187	20/1	*LMO2*
Habermann 2008[32]	DLBCL	365	73/44	*IL10, IL8RB, IL1A*
Racila 2008[39]	FL	133	1/1	*C1qA*
Wang 2008[33]	DLBCL FL	407	72/37	*BRCA, XRCC4, XRCC2, SMHT1, BHMT*

NHL non-Hodgkin lymphoma, *TCL* T-cell lymphoma, *DLBCL* diffuse large B-cell lymphoma, *FL* follicular lymphoma, *MCL* mantle cell lymphoma

[a] Most significant gene polymorphism associated with clinical outcome often measured as overall survival

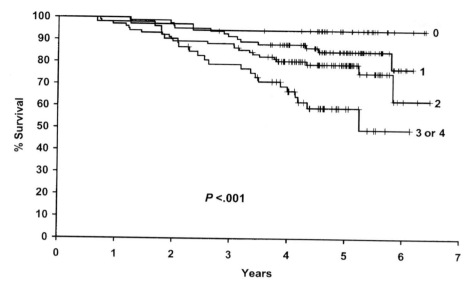

Fig. 32-1. SNPs associated with adverse outcome in lymphoma. Kaplan–Meier curves for survival in follicular lymphoma by the number of deleterious genotypes from the 4 SNP risk score based on IL8 (rs4073), IL2 (rs2069762), IL12B (rs3212227), and IL1RN (rs454078), from the study by Cerhan et al. [28]. The sum of deleterious genotypes from these 4 SNPs (0–4) was strongly associated with survival in both univariate ($P \leq .001$) and multivariate ($P \leq .001$) analyses. Patients with 3 or 4 deleterious genotypes were over 12 times more likely to die when compared with patients with zero deleterious genotypes (95% CI, 2.92–54.4), and there was a gradient in risk with the number of deleterious genotypes. This research was originally published in Blood [28]

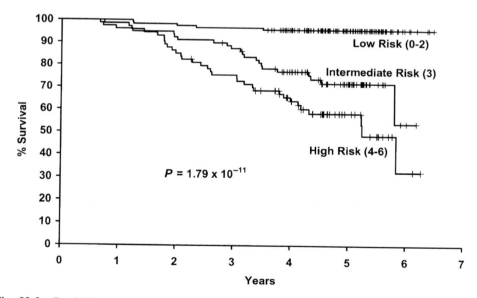

Fig. 32-2. Combining SNPs with clinical variable in lymphoma risk stratification. Kaplan–Meier curves combining the SNP and clinical and demographic risk scores, from the study by Cerhan et al.[28] The 5-year Kaplan–Meier survival estimates (95% CI) were 96% (93%–100%), 72% (62%–83%), and 58% (48%–72%) for groups at low, intermediate, and high risk, respectively. The patients with a score of 4 to 6 were more than 14 times more likely to die compared with those with a score of 0 to 2 (95% CI, 5.70–37.7). This research was originally published in Blood [28]

precise mechanism of action for rituximab in NHL is not known; however a role for antibody-dependent cellular cytotoxicity (ADCC) and complement -dependent cytotoxicity (CDC) has been proposed. In ADCC, the effector cells are required to bind the anti-CD20 antibody coating the B-cell lymphoma cells through the Fc gamma receptors (FcγR) to achieve target cell killing. A number of studies have focused on the high- and low-affinity FcγR SNPs. These early studies are retrospective and limited to small number of cases, but nevertheless suggest that FcγR SNPs may have a role in response to rituximab treatment [35–38].

More intriguing is a study on the effects of SNPs on CDC function; Racila and colleagues demonstrated that patients with a particular SNP in the complement component 1qA gene [*C1QA* (276G)] had higher C1qA serum levels and increased CDC activity but shorter remissions in follicular lymphoma [39]. This result is surprising given that CDC is believed to be one of the main mechanisms of rituximab-mediated tumor cell killing. The investigators suggested that a strong CDC at the initial phase of the immune response may reduce the chances of antigen-presenting cell maturation and function, thus preventing the development of an adaptive immune response. The lack of an adaptive immune response may lead to early relapses despite initial strong CDC response to treatment.

32.6. Integration of Environmental Factors, Host and Tumor Genetics and Phenotype in Lymphoma

As summarized above, common genetic polymorphisms in the host background are potential biomarkers for determining risk for development of NHL. However, most SNPs associated with the increased risk of NHL development have an odds ratio of less than 2.0, and therefore are unlikely to have the sufficient predictive power in isolation to justify screening and prevention programs. Additionally, the influence of different polymorphisms may be modified by environmental risk factors such as family dynamics (e.g. birth order), environmental exposures leading to autoimmune conditions, or nutritional status, [40] and may be different for different NHL subtypes [18]. To solve these issues, future studies will require large population-based cohorts and should integrate environmental risk factors as well as biological parameters, such as NHL subtype.

In contrast, early studies [28,32] suggest that common genetic polymorphisms in immunity genes may be powerful markers for the prediction of treatment response and overall survival in different subtypes of NHL with similar hazard ratios to those observed by well-established clinical parameters such as the International Prognostic Index. Additionally, it appears that a risk score that combines high-risk genotypes with the clinical and demographic factors may have even stronger predictive value [28]. These genetic polymorphisms are appealing as biomarkers because it would be relatively easy to develop high throughput clinical tests that could be performed on buccal smears or peripheral blood samples.

To interpret the mechanisms underlying correlations with the identified SNPs, better understanding of the biological consequences of risk-associated polymorphisms is needed. For example, individuals carrying *TNFRSF5* gene (CD40) polymorphisms associated with an increased risk of development of NHL, have been shown to have lower expression of CD40 on dendritic cells and lower soluble CD40 in the serum, [23] suggesting that reduced immune surveillance due to impaired CD40 signaling may be leading to increased lymphoma outgrowth. One of the promising tumor biomarkers that can predict DLBCL outcome is LMO2. LMO2 expression by the tumor cells is associated with better clinical outcome in DLBCL. A population-based study examining tag SNPs at the *LMO2* locus suggested not only that *LMO2* polymorphisms may be better predictors of clinical outcome when compared with LMO2 expression levels but also that genetic variation in *LMO2* may itself influence LMO2 expression [30]. These findings, although not yet confirmed in independent studies, raise the fascinating possibility that SNPs determine not only properties of the microenvironment but also aspects of the tumor phenotype itself.

The explosion of knowledge on the role of common genetic variations in human genes in the pathogenesis and clinical outcome of NHL has identified numerous potential biomarkers; however, the challenge of integrating this new science into robust, reproducible, and cost-effective clinical applications remains ahead.

Suggested Readings

Skibola CF, Curry JD, Nieters A. Genetic susceptibility to lymphoma. Haematologica 2007;92(7):960–9.

Syvanen AC. Toward genome-wide SNP genotyping. Nat Genet 2005;37 Suppl:S5–10.

Rothman N, Skibola CF, Wang SS, et al. Genetic variation in TNF and IL10 and risk of non-Hodgkin lymphoma: a report from the InterLymph Consortium. Lancet Oncol 2006;7(1):27–38.

- The largest study on SNP association with risk of lymphoma development.

References

1. Willis T, Dyer M. The role of immunoglobulin translocations in the pathogenesis of B-cell malignancies. Blood 2000;96(3):808–22.
2. Falini B, Mason D. Proteins encoded by genes involved in chromosomal alterations in lymphoma and leukemia: clinical value of their detection by immunocytochemistry. Blood 2002;99(2):409–26.
3. Boultwood J. Ataxia telangiectasia gene mutations in leukaemia and lymphoma. J Clin Pathol 2001;54(7):512–6.
4. Chatterjee N, Hartge P, Cerhan JR, et al. Risk of non-Hodgkin's lymphoma and family history of lymphatic, hematologic, and other cancers. Cancer Epidemiol Biomarkers Prev 2004;13(9):1415–21.
5. Wang SS, Slager SL, Brennan P, et al. Family history of hematopoietic malignancies and risk of non-Hodgkin lymphoma (NHL): a pooled analysis of 10 211 cases and 11 905 controls from the International Lymphoma Epidemiology Consortium (InterLymph). Blood 2007;109(8):3479–88.
6. Monti S, Savage KJ, Kutok JL, et al. Molecular profiling of diffuse large B-cell lymphoma identifies robust subtypes including one characterized by host inflammatory response. Blood 2005;105(5):1851–61.
7. Dave SS, Wright G, Tan B, et al. Prediction of survival in follicular lymphoma based on molecular features of tumor-infiltrating immune cells. N Engl J Med 2004;351(21):2159–69.
8. Salaverria I, Zettl A, Bea S, et al. Chromosomal alterations detected by comparative genomic hybridization in subgroups of gene expression-defined Burkitt's lymphoma. Haematologica 2008;93(9):1327–34.
9. Coiffier B, Lepage E, Briere J, et al. CHOP Chemotherapy plus Rituximab Compared with CHOP Alone in Elderly Patients with Diffuse Large-B-Cell Lymphoma. N Engl J Med 2002;346(4):235.
10. Sachidanandam R, Weissman D, Schmidt SC, et al. A map of human genome sequence variation containing 1. 42 million single nucleotide polymorphisms. Nature 2001;409(6822):928–33.
11. International HapMAp Project. 2008. (Accessed 29/12/2008, at http://www.hapmap.org/.)
12. Johnson GC, Esposito L, Barratt BJ, et al. Haplotype tagging for the identification of common disease genes. Nat Genet 2001;29(2):233–7.
13. Syvanen AC. Toward genome wide SNP genotyping. Nat Genet 2005;37:S5–10.
14. Skibola CF, Curry JD, Nieters A. Genetic susceptibility to lymphoma. Haematologica 2007;92(7):960–9.
15. Rothman N, Skibola CF, Wang SS, et al. Genetic variation in TNF and IL10 and risk of non-Hodgkin lymphoma: a report from the InterLymph Consortium. Lancet Oncol 2006;7(1):27–38.
16. Lan Q, Zheng T, Rothman N, et al. Cytokine polymorphisms in the Th1/Th2 pathway and susceptibility to non-Hodgkin lymphoma. Blood 2006;107(10):4101–8.
17. Forrest MS, Skibola CF, Lightfoot TJ, et al. Polymorphisms in innate immunity genes and risk of non-Hodgkin lymphoma. Br J Haematol 2006;134(2):180–3.
18. Wang SS, Cerhan JR, Hartge P, et al. Common genetic variants in proinflammatory and other immunoregulatory genes and risk for non-Hodgkin lymphoma. Cancer Res 2006;66(19):9771–80.
19. Cerhan JR, Ansell SM, Fredericksen ZS, et al. Genetic variation in 1253 immune and inflammation genes and risk of non-Hodgkin lymphoma. Blood 2007;110(13):4455–63.
20. Novak AJ, Slager SL, Ziesmer SC, et al. Polymorphisms in the BLyS gene are associated with an increased risk of developing B-Cell non-Hodgkin lymphoma. Blood 2007;110(11):173a.

21. Cerhan JR, Liu-Mares W, Fredericksen ZS, et al. Genetic variation in tumor necrosis factor and the nuclear factor-kappaB canonical pathway and risk of non-Hodgkin's lymphoma. Cancer Epidemiol Biomarkers Prev 2008;17(11):3161–9.

22. Ansell SM, Novak A, Yang Z-Z, et al. Genetic Variation in Genes That Regulate T-Cell Differentiation and Function Is Associated with An Increased Risk of Developing B-Cell Non- Hodgkin Lymphoma. Blood 2008;112(11):1288a–9.

23. Skibola CF, Nieters A, Bracci PM, et al. A functional TNFRSF5 gene variant is associated with risk of lymphoma. Blood 2008;111(8):4348–54.

24. Warzocha K, Ribeiro P, Bienvenu J, et al. Genetic polymorphisms in the tumor necrosis factor locus influence non-Hodgkin's lymphoma outcome. Blood 1998;91(10):3574–81.

25. Juszczynski P, Kalinka E, Bienvenu J, et al. Human leukocyte antigens class II and tumor necrosis factor genetic polymorphisms are independent predictors of non-Hodgkin lymphoma outcome. Blood 2002;100(8):3037–40.

26. Lech-Maranda E, Baseggio L, Bienvenu J, et al. Interleukin-10 gene promoter polymorphisms influence the clinical outcome of diffuse large B-cell lymphoma. Blood 2004;103(9):3529–34.

27. Lee JJ, Kim DH, Lee NY, et al. Interleukin-10 gene polymorphism influences the prognosis of T-cell non-Hodgkin lymphomas. Br J Haematol 2007;137(4):329–36.

28. Cerhan JR, Wang S, Maurer MJ, et al. Prognostic significance of host immune gene polymorphisms in follicular lymphoma survival. Blood 2007;109(12):5439–46.

29. Cerhan JR, Maurer MJ, Hartge P, et al. Polymorphisms in one-carbon metabolism genes and overall survival in diffuse large B-cell lymphoma (DLBCL). Blood 2007;110(11):469a.

30. Cerhan J, Natkunam Y, Morton L, et al. LMO2 protein expression, LMO2 germline genetic variation, and overall survival in diffuse large B-cell lymphoma (DLBCL). Ann Oncol 2008;19:107.

31. Habermann TM, Maurer MJ, Wang SS, et al. Host genetic variation in the cell cycle and NF-kappa B pathways and overall survival in mantle cell lymphoma. Blood 2007;110(11):472a–3.

32. Habermann TM, Wang SS, Maurer MJ, et al. Host immune gene polymorphisms in combination with clinical and demographic factors predict late survival in diffuse large B-cell lymphoma patients in the pre-rituximab era. Blood 2008;112(7):2694–702.

33. Wang SS, Maurer MJ, Morton LM, et al. Polymorphisms in DNA repair and one-carbon metabolism genes and overall survival in diffuse large B-cell lymphoma and follicular lymphoma. Leukemia 2008; Oct 2. [Epub ahead of print].

34. Watters JW, McLeod HL. Cancer pharmacogenomics: current and future applications. Biochim Biophys Acta 2003;1603(2):99–111.

35. Weng WK, Levy R. Two immunoglobulin G fragment C receptor polymorphisms independently predict response to rituximab in patients with follicular lymphoma. J Clin Oncol 2003;21(21):3940–7.

36. Mitrovic Z, Aurer I, Radman I, Ajdukovic R, Sertic J, Labar B. FCgammaRIIIA and FCgammaRIIA polymorphisms are not associated with response to rituximab and CHOP in patients with diffuse large B-cell lymphoma. Haematologica 2007;92(7):998–9.

37. Paiva M, Marques H, Martins A, Ferreira P, Catarino R, Medeiros R. FcgammaRIIa polymorphism and clinical response to rituximab in non-Hodgkin lymphoma patients. Cancer Genet Cytogenet 2008;183(1):35–40.

38. Kim DH, Jung HD, Kim JG, et al. FCGR3A gene polymorphisms may correlate with response to frontline R-CHOP therapy for diffuse large B-cell lymphoma. Blood 2006;108(8):2720–5.

39. Racila E, Link BK, Weng WK, et al. A polymorphism in the complement component C1qA correlates with prolonged response following rituximab therapy of follicular lymphoma. Clin Cancer Res 2008;14(20):6697–703.

40. Wang SS, Cozen W, Cerhan JR, et al. Immune mechanisms in non-Hodgkin lymphoma: joint effects of the TNF G308A and IL10 T3575A polymorphisms with non-Hodgkin lymphoma risk factors. Cancer Res 2007;67(10):5042–54.

Chapter 33

Developing Prognostic Models for Diffuse Large B-cell Lymphoma

Izidore S. Lossos

Abstract/Scope of Chapter Diffuse large B-cell lymphoma (DLBCL) is among the most common lymphomas worldwide, with variable outcome following combined chemotherapy and immunotherapy. For this reason, DLBCL has served as a prototype among lymphomas for developing gene predictors of outcome and therapy response. In this chapter, we review the use of gene expression profiling to discover and validate the outcome predictors in DLBCL. The pathway from marker discovery to routine implementation is discussed, with considerations on use of quantitative transcript profiling by real-time PCR as compared to microarray or immunohistochemistry to look at protein levels.

Keywords BCL6, prognostic marker • bortezomib, use in lymphoma • Proteasome inhibitor, use in lymphoma • Diffuse large B-cell lymphoma, prognostic markers • Diffuse large B-cell lymphoma, therapy selection • HGAL, prognostic marker • Large B-cell lymphoma, international prognostic index (IPI) • LMO2, prognostic marker • Lymphochip • NF-κB, outcome prediction in DLBCL • Rituximab, outcome predictors

33.1. The Need for Improved Prognostic Models of DLBCL

Diffuse large B-cell lymphoma (DLBCL) is the most common adult non-Hodgkin's lymphoma with more than 25,000 cases diagnosed annually in the United States. Although DLBCL has characteristic morphology, marked cytogenetic, immunophenotypic, and molecular heterogeneity underlies its variable clinical outcome. Survival is typically short in untreated cases, but a majority of patients respond to anthracycline-based combination chemotherapy, such as cyclophosphamide, adriamycin, vincristine, prednisone (CHOP). However, despite initial responses, less than half of patients with DLBCL will be cured with conventional chemotherapy regimens [1]. Recently, improvements in disease-free and overall survival has been achieved with the addition of the anti-CD20 monoclonal antibody rituximab (Rituxan) [2]. The marked variability in survival presents a challenge to physicians that not only need to search for better treatments but also need to predict outcomes either prior to or shortly after treatment initiation. Such prognostication is of utmost importance to patients and their families for them to be able to participate fully in treatment decisions and make realistic plans for their future based on the available information. Furthermore, more predictable outcomes are essential for the design and stratification of clinical trials to ensure uniform reporting, guidance for initial treatment, and the evaluation of new therapeutic approaches.

Understanding of the mechanisms underlying the predictive power of the biomarkers may form the basis for targeted therapeutic interventions. Biologic mechanisms underlying

From: *Neoplastic Hematopathology*: Contemporary Hematology,
Edited by: D. Jones, DOI 10.1007/978-1-60761-384-8_33,
© Humana Press, a part of Springer Science+Business Media, LLC 2010

DLBCL pathogenesis are complex and involve intricate relationships between multiple genes, signaling pathways, and regulatory processes [3]. Elucidation of DLBCL pathogenesis may be instrumental for the recognition of new molecular therapeutic targets, discovery of DLBCL subgroups with distinct clinical outcome, and identification of prognostic biomarkers that may more accurately predict survival of DLBCL patients. Accomplishment of these goals may form the basis for future risk-adapted treatments.

Classically, clinical surrogates, such as the International Prognostic Index (IPI), [4] have been used and found to be highly useful; however, the IPI does not adequately capture the molecular and cellular variability that underlies clinical behaviour of DLBCL. Further attempts to identify new prognostic biomarkers used a single gene approach [5]. However the latter cannot account for the multigene processes underlying DLBCL pathogenesis and thus do not accurately reflect the complex changes observed in these tumors. Consequently, new investigational tools enabling simultaneous examination of multiple components of these biologic processes might further advance our understanding of DLBCL and potentially lead to specific molecularly-targeted and patient-tailored therapies. While standard pathologic techniques do not reliably predict sensitivity to chemotherapy or outcome for individual patients, gene expression profiling has provided important insights into the biology of DLBCL, allowing a better biological classification of tumors that are more homogeneous in pathogenesis and clinical behaviour.

33.2. Overview of Previous Microarray Studies in Diffuse Large B-cell Lymphoma

DNA microarrays are a recently developed technology used to measure the expression of tens of thousands of genes simultaneously, enabling a more comprehensive evaluation of gene expression. This technique allows the comprehensive analysis of messenger RNA (mRNA) expression in tumor samples. The clinical characteristics and behavior of a tumor are determined by the specific genetic changes present in the tumor cells that are reflected in their pattern of mRNA expression creating a "molecular signature" or "fingerprint" for the tumor. The full potential of microarrays has not yet been realized, however they may be used to: (a) identify previously unrecognized disease entities with distinct biological and clinical features; (b) elucidate the key genetic profiles and lesions that define each of these new nosologic entities; (c) discover new molecular targets for future therapeutic intervention; (d) identify genes that play a potential role in determining prognosis; (e) discover previously unknown genes of major clinical relevance by exploring the function of the unassigned expressed sequence tag (EST) clones from the arrays; and (f) identify gene expression signatures correlated with response to specific therapeutic agent.

The pivotal microarray study was performed by Alizadeh et al with the use of a cDNA Lymphochip array [6]. The evaluation of 42 DLBCL tumors from patients treated with antrhacycline-based chemotherapy led to the identification of two distinct subgroups based on the expression of genes characteristic of germinal center B cells (GC) or in vitro activated peripheral blood cells (ABC). Patients with GC subtype had a significantly better overall 5-year survival (76% versus 16%, $P<0.01$), independent of the IPI score. These findings were further confirmed by the Lymphoma and Leukemia Molecular Profile Project (LLMPP) study [7] that used a similar cDNA Lymphochip array platform. Analysis of tumor samples from 240 DLBCL patients treated with anthracycline-based chemotherapy demonstrated a significant difference in the 5-year overall survival between the GC-like and ABC-like subgroups (60% versus 35% respectively). In an attempt to better understand the pathogenesis of DLBCL, Monti et al used an Affymetrix platform to profile 176 patients with treatment-naïve DLBCL [8]. By applying three unsupervised analytical methods (hierarchical clustering, self-organizing maps, and model-based probabilistic clustering, see Chap. 4) the authors identified three discrete subsets of DLBCL: oxidative phosphorylation (OxPhos), B-cell receptor (BCR) proliferation, and host response (HR). Oxidative phosphorylation tumors had increased levels of BCL2 family members, components of the 26S proteasome, and structural mitochondrial ribosomal subunits. The BCR proliferation cluster overexpressed many components of the B-cell receptor signaling cascade (immunoglobulin genes, CD19, CD79A, BLK, and SYK) and had more exuberant expression of multiple cell-cycle regulatory genes, including CDK2 and MCM family members. These tumors also had increased expression of DNA repair genes such as H2AX, PAX1P1 (PTIP), and TP53 (p53), as well as several transcription factors (including PAX5, POU2AF1 (OBF1), E2A, BCL6, STAT6, and MYC). The third gene signature was defined by the associated host responses, which were consistent with an ongoing immune inflammatory response, rather than the tumor itself, being characterized by markedly increased levels of components of the T-cell receptor and the complement cascade as well as monocyte, macrophage, and dendritic cell genes. Despite differences in the presumed pathogenetic mechanisms of each of these 3 gene patterns, the patients had similar 5-year survivals.

Although some of these early microarray expression profile studies were able to identify the presence of biologically distinct subgroups of DLBCL, they were unable to identify the relative contribution of individual genes, therefore making it difficult to build clinically useful prognostic models with a limited number of genes. To address this question, Rosenwald [7] and Shipp [9] applied supervised analytical methodologies to the Lymphochip and Affymetrix-derived gene expression profiles of 240 and 58 DLBCL patients, respectively. They constructed outcome predictors based on expression of 17 and 13 genes, respectively (Table 33-1). Interestingly, there was no overlap between the genes comprising these two outcome prediction models. This disparity in the results of two large genome-wide expression profile models has been attributed to differences in patient selection, methodology, array composition, and analytical approaches.

In an attempt to merge existing data sets, Wright et al employed a biostatistical method based on Bayes' rule of probability assignment to translate experimental results across different microarray platforms [10]. Expression data from 14 genes identified by the LLMPP [7] combined with an analysis of the Shipp study [9] was able to subdivide patients into GC-like and ABC-like types that showed significant different outcomes (Table 33.1). Nevertheless, despite these positive results, such an approach may not be clinically useful because of the complex manipulations required to rescale gene expression from Affymetrix data to match the mean and variance of the corresponding expression values from cDNA microarray data sets. In addition, this approach did not produce signatures with outcome differences in patients treated with rituximab (R) plus anthracycline-containing chemotherapy regimens that are the current gold standard of therapy.

However, in other recent work, Lenz et al [11] did demonstrate that even in patients treated with rituximab-containing regimens, patients with GC-like DLBCL had a significantly better

Table 33-1. Array-based prognostic gene expression models.

Author	Rosenwald et al. [7]	Shipp et al. [9])	Wright et al. [10]
Number of genes	17	13	14
Genes in signature	GC type	DRP2	LMO2
	BCL6	3UTR of unknown gene	BCL6
	HGAL	PRKCG	CCND2
	MHC II	MINOR	LRMP
	Proliferation signature	HTR2B	MYBL1 (A-myb)
	BMP6	PDCD4 (H731)	CD10
		TLE1	IRF4
		PDE4B	IL16
		Oviductal protein	PIM1
		ZNF212	PTPN1
			FUT8
			ITPKB
			IGHM
			CD39

outcome than patients with ABC-like tumors. Furthermore, three of the previously-developed signatures in the 17-gene model developed for CHOP-treated patients (namely, the GC B cell, lymph node stroma, and proliferation signatures) retained their significance in the R-CHOP-treated cohort, whereas the MHC class II signature did not. Consequently, the authors developed a revised prognostic model consisting of 3 signatures: GC B cell, "stromal-1," reflecting genes co-ordinately expressed in many normal mesenchymal tissues, most of which encode proteins that form or modify the extracellular matrix, and "stromal-2," which appeared to reflect the angiogenetic potential of the tumor and was associated with an adverse outcome.

33.3. Translating Microarray Studies into Prognostic Panels

In an attempt to devise a technically-simple method that could be applicable for routine clinical use, we evaluated the mRNA expression of 36 genes previously reported to predict survival [12] in tumor specimens from 66 DLCBL patients treated with anthracycline-based therapy. The top six genes ranked according to their predictive power on univariate analysis were used to construct a multivariate model. Among the selected genes, LMO2, BCL6, and FN1 predicted longer survival, whereas CCND2, CCL3 (SCYA3), and BCL2 predicted shorter survival. Based on the expression of these 6 genes, patients could be subdivided into IPI-independent risk groups with significantly different 5-year survival ranging from 65% in the low-risk to 15% in the high-risk subgroups. This model was validated in the data sets available from previously-reported studies of patients treated without rituximab (Table 33-2) [7–9,13].

This gene expression model was constructed from RNA extracted from fresh and frozen lymphoma specimens which are not routinely available. In contrast, paraffin-embedded fixed specimens, which are used routinely for immunohistochemistry (IHC), are widely available. Unfortunately, the process of formalin fixation may contribute to RNA degradation and modification that limits the extractability of high-quality RNA by routine methods. Improvements in RNA extraction protocols have allowed the extraction of short informative RNA fragments from paraffin blocks, with potential use in RNA quantification. We have recently developed an optimized methodology for RNA extraction from formalin-fixed, paraffin-embedded lymphoid tissues [14]. This method was applied to paraffin blocks of 132 DLBCL patients treated with R-CHOP regimen [15]. The paraffin-based 6-gene model predicted the outcome of DLBCL patients treated with R-CHOP (Table 33-2). Application of the 6-gene model to a recently reported array study that used frozen or fresh specimens from R-CHOP-treated DLBCL patients also confirmed its predictive power and validity in the rituximab era (Table 33-2). Furthermore, the 6-gene model also predicted the outcome of DLBCL patients in which mRNA levels were measured using multiplexed quantitative nuclease protection assay in fixed paraffin-embedded samples [16].

Table 33-2. Outcome prediction in patients with DLBCL using a 6-gene predictor applied to previously-reported data sets.

Authors	Treatment	Number of patients	RR (continuous)	P-value	RR (categorical)	P-value
Rosenwald et al. [7]	CHOP	240	1.14	0.015	1.62	0.005
Shipp et al. [9]	CHOP	58	2.84	0.004	2.20	0.047
Monti et al. [8]	CHOP	129	1.67	0.032	1.79	0.026
Hummel et al. [13]	CHOP	81	2.45	0.013	2.10	0.020
Lenz et al. [11]	CHOP	181	2.30	0.0002	1.96	0.0008
	R-CHOP	233	2.72	0.001	2.23	0.003
Malumbers et al. [15]	R-CHOP	132	1.62	0.002	3.11	0.002

The 6-gene predictor was constructed on each dataset, and then fitted with a Cox's proportional hazards model, both as a continuous and categorical score (cut at its median)

Gene expression arrays and quantitative PCR to analyze the expression of multiple genes are not routinely used in clinical practice, require fresh tumor specimens (for gene arrays), and are labor-intensive and expensive. Therefore, researchers have tried to use the information derived from RNA profiling studies to create prediction models based on more amenable techniques, such as IHC. However, IHC studies attempting to replicate the gene expression studies have yielded contradictory results [17,18] suggesting the current lack of an ideal set of IHC markers for outcome prediction in DLBCL. Hans et al. compared results of subclassification with cDNA microarrays to subtyping using a limited IHC panel [19]. They proposed an IHC model based on 3 markers: CD10, BCL6, and MUM1 (IRF4) for determination of GC-like and ABC-like DLBCL subtypes. This model was shown to have positive predictive values of 87% and 73% for correctly identifying GC-like and ABC-like DLBCL subtypes (using gene expression as the gold standard). This panel could predict outcome in that 76% of IHC-defined GC-like DLBCL OS at 5 years when compared with 34% for patients with non-GC lymphomas. However, this ~20% misclassification rate of IHC compared to gene studies suggests the need to incorporate additional IHC markers in an attempt to improve the predictive value of this model. Indeed, a recent study demonstrated that Han's model was not predictive of outcome in an independent large cohort of DLBCL patients [20].

33.4. Clinical Applicability of Prediction Models

In order for a prognostic biomarker to be useful in routine clinical practice, it must fulfill several fundamental criteria. The model must be relatively simple for clinical use and provide a high degree of discrimination among the risk groups. The ideal prognostic biomarker needs to rely on a robust and reproducible methodology using easily-accessible test samples. The predictive value must be independent from other known prognostic factors in multivariate analysis, and validated in well-designed prospective studies with a predetermined written protocol of uniform treatment and a known primary endpoint. In addition, it is important to recognize that the usefulness of prognostic factors may depend on the specific therapeutic approach and thus may undergo significant changes over time, reflecting the constant progress in the available treatments.

Therefore, introduction of new therapies requires reassessment of clinical applicability of previously-recognized prognostic factors. In addition, the usefulness of prognostic factors or models may depend on the specific clinical setting and therapeutic approach. For example, a majority of the previous expression studies were done in DLBCL patients who received anthracycline-based therapy prior to routine use of rituximab. Improved outcome with the addition of rituximab to chemotherapy might be associated with a change in the predictive value of clinical and/or biological markers resulting in the loss of prognostic power of previously-established markers or the discovery of new, previously-unidentified predictors. Therefore, the predictive value of the previously established risk factors needs to be re-evaluated and new factors identified for patients treated with rituximab-containing chemotherapy. Among the different models, only the predictive power of the GC versus ABC-like DLBCL subtypes, as well as the 6-gene model, have been confirmed to be outcome predictors in R-CHOP treated patients [11,15]. However, none of these models have been validated in prospective clinical trials but those types of studies are currently being conducted. Routine applicability of these models in daily clinical practice awaits the conclusions of these studies.

33.5. Advantages/Disadvantages of RNA Versus IHC Methods for Routine Use

Clinically-applicable prognostic tests need to be based on a widely-available, relatively simple, reproducible and robust methodology. IHC is routinely used for pathological diagnosis and consequently is considered to be an advantageous methodology on which biomarker prognostic models should be based. However, this methodology has inherent limitations that may account for the non-reproducible and conflicting results in the application of IHC-based models for prediction of outcome of patients with DLBCL. Firstly, different antibodies against the same antigen can be directed against different epitopes on the target protein. There is also marked variation between different laboratories in fixation, antigen retrieval protocols, staining methodologies, and the application of different pre-determined thresholds used to define positivity for specific antibodies. Standardization of these methodological variables is needed for universal application, but mechanisms to achieve such standardization are not currently available. In addition, IHC is a semiquantitative methodology in contrast to the RNA-based methods, and this may limit its application for prognostic factors whose level of expression correlates with clinical outcome as a continuous variable. Furthermore, antibodies are not available for many genes with potential prognostic value and thus novel monoclonal antibodies directed to newly-identified RNA-based prognostic biomarkers need to be generated and assessed in the future IHC-based prediction models.

Array-based methodologies are more quantitative and can assess expression of any gene. However, they are more expensive, labor-intensive and require good quality RNA that is usually derived from fresh or frozen specimens; the latter may limit its routine widespread applicability. Moreover, current methodologies usually simultaneously analyze multiple samples for classification. Applicability of the arrays to an individual sample may require a pre-existing dataset of well-characterized cases analyzed with the same methodology for accurate classification.

Real-time PCR-based methodologies are now widely available and may represent an optimal quantitative method that can translate laboratory discoveries from the "bench to the patient bedside" since they are easy to perform, robust, sensitive, reproducible, and economical in their RNA requirements. Furthermore, with recently developed robust methods for RNA extraction from formalin-fixed, paraffin-embedded specimens, PCR can now be applied to these widely available tissues. The process is simple and is amenable to the rapid analysis of large number of samples. Based on these characteristics, this methodology emerges as one of the optimal techniques for the design of prognostic biomarker models. However, additional work to standardize application of individual prognostic models between different laboratories and their validity in prospective studies will be needed.

33.6. Identification of Therapeutic Targets in Diffuse Large B-cell Lymphoma

Besides prognostication and identification of tumor subtypes, array studies may also be used to discover genes of clinical relevance, among ESTs with previously unknown function. The new markers may be shown to play a role in determining prognosis or in the pathophysiology of lymphoma. An example of such a discovery is cloning of HGAL that controls the migration of GC lymphocytes and GC-derived DLBCL [21,22]. In addition, identification of crucial signaling pathways for lymphoma cells may provide further insight into the mechanisms of lymphomagenesis and detect potential targets for gene-specific therapeutic developments. Hierarchical clustering of global gene expression has demonstrated that groups of genes that are abnormally activated or suppressed in the same pathway generate recognizable aberrant expression patterns. Using these distinct patterns, it is possible to generate hypotheses about the activity of signaling pathways in lymphoma cells, which could then be tested by direct experimental work (Table 33-3).

The nuclear factor kappa beta (NF-κB) family of transcription factors mediate a variety of proliferation, apoptotic, inflammatory, and immune responses and are critical for normal B-cell development and survival and operate through a characteristic set of inducible genes. In most cells, NF-κB is retained in an inactive form in the cytoplasm by binding to members of the I-κB family of proteins. In response to signaling through diverse pathways, members of the I-κB family are phosphorylated by the I-κB kinase complex (IKK) and subsequently

Table 33-3. Distinctive pathogenetic mechanisms of GC-like and ABC-like DLBCL.

Alterations	GC-like DLBCL	ABC-like DLBCL	Therapeutic intervention
Constitutive activation of NF-kB	–	++	Bortizomib
CARD11 mutations	+/–	++	Anti-NF-kB approaches
A20 (TNFAIP3) mutations	+/–	++	Anti-NF-kB approaches
BCL6 expression	++	+/–	Anti-BCL6 approaches
Constitutive activation of STAT3	–	++	JAK/STAT inhibition
Activation of protein kinase C-associated kinase (RIPK4)	+	++	
Protein kinase C beta	+/–	+	Enzastaurine
IL-4/STAT6 signaling	Normal	Dysregulated	IL-4

degraded by the ubiquitin-proteasome pathway. This leads to the release of NF-kB family members that translocate into the nucleus and activate gene transcription. High levels of expression of NF-κB target genes have been observed in ABC-like DLBCL, but not in GC-like DLBCL samples. To assess the mechanism and functional significance of NF-κB target genes in ABC-like DLBCL specimens, the activity of IKK was studied in cell line models of ABC-like DLBCL and GC-like DLBCL. The ABC-like DLBCL cell lines had constitutive activity of IKK that was absent in the GC-like DLBCL cell lines. Inhibition of IKK was cytotoxic to ABC-like but not to GC-like DLBCL cell lines [23]. Consequently, this study demonstrated that the NF-κB pathway is a potential therapeutic target in ABC-like DLBCL. In a recent study of relapsed DLBCL conducted at the National Cancer Institute, addition of the proteasome inhibitor bortezomib (which targets NF-κB) to dose-adjusted EPOCH chemotherapy markedly improved the response of ABC-like but not GC-like DLBCL.

Protein kinase C beta (*PRKCB1*) was found to be overexpressed in fatal/refractory DLBCLs based on gene expression analysis. This serine/threonine kinase is required for BCR survival signaling, including activation of NF-κB. Enzastaurin is an acyclic bisindolylmaleimide that inhibits protein kinase C beta but may also modulate the PIK3/AKT pathway. In a phase II clinical study in 55 patients with relapsed DLBCL treated with enzastaurin, four patients (7%), including three with complete remission and one patient with stable disease, demonstrated continuous freedom-from-progression 20–50 months after study entry [24].

PDE4B is a cyclic AMP phosphodiesterase associated with a poor clinical outcome that is highly expressed in ABC-like DLBCL. By inactivating cAMP, PDE4B modulates several signaling pathways and induces cell cycle arrest and apoptosis of B cells. Stimulation of the cAMP pathway in GC-like DLBCL, which expresses low levels of PDE4B, was associated with decreased phosphorylation and activity of AKT leading to mitochondrial membrane depolarization, dephosphorylation of BAD, and marked apoptosis. In contrast, stimulation of cAMP did not affect ABC-like DLBCL which highly express PDE4B [25]. These observations suggest that PDE4B inhibitors and agents that target the survival pathway controlled by AKT might be used as potential therapeutic tools.

DLBCL with a BCR proliferation signature are characterized by high expression of BCL6 and SYK proteins. With in vitro studies on DLBCL cell lines, such BCR proliferative-type tumors were preferentially highly sensitive to the BCL6 peptide inhibitor BPI, suggesting that specific targeting of BCL6 in this subtype may have therapeutic potential [26], although clinical studies have not yet been performed. Targeting of the BCR-associated kinase SYK by the specific oral inhibitor fostamatinib disodium has demonstrated some clinical activity in patients with relapsed lymphomas [27].

The finding that at least two markers of the GC-like phenotype, BCL6 and HGAL, are interleukin (IL)-4 target genes whose expression correlates independently with better OS raises the possibility that endogenous or exogenous IL-4 might differently affect DLBCL subtypes. IL-4 is a pleotrophic cytokine that regulates lymphocyte differentiation, proliferation and apoptosis. Analysis of DLBCL gene expression data revealed increased expression in GC-like DLBCL of multiple components of the IL-4 pathway suggesting its activation [28].

Evaluation of the effects of IL-4 on GC-like and ABC-like DLBCL demonstrated qualitatively different effects. In the ABC-like DLBCL, IL-4 induced activation of the AKT pathway, decreased cell proliferation, caused cell cycle arrest, and led to an aberrant and short-lived activation of STAT6 signaling.

In contrast, in GC-like DLBCL, IL-4 induced cell proliferation and prolonged STAT6 activation [28]. The differences in the IL-4-induced STAT6 signaling between GC-like and ABC-like DLBCL led to the identification of new nuclear and cytoplasmic phosphatases, TCPTP and PTP1B, respectively, which are highly expressed in the ABC-like DLBCL, and dephosphorylate STAT6 [29,30]. The different intracellular IL-4 signaling in GC and ABC-like DLBCL also translated to distinct biological effects of IL-4. In vitro, this cytokine induces cell proliferation and potentates adriamycin and rituximab cell killing of the GC-like DLBCL cell lines while inducing cell cycle arrest and protecting the ABC-like DLBCL cell lines from the cytotoxic effects of these medications. These observations suggest that DLBCL subtypes may respond differently in vivo to the cytokine milieu of the tumor. Manipulation of the different responses of DLBCL subtypes to cytokine stimulation might have therapeutic applications.

33.7. Conclusions

Microarrays are powerful tools for discovery and hypothesis generation allowing researchers to obtain an unbiased survey of gene expression in lymphoma samples. These studies have already allowed sub-classification of DLBCL into distinct subtypes with different pathogenesis and prognosis. They may now be applied to the profiling of microRNA expression that may also be useful for the sub-classification of DLBCL tumors [31]. Microarray studies have already enabled identification of new prognostic biomarkers and models in these tumors. However, the "prime-time" for their incorporation into routine clinical practice has not arrived yet. Further research will address the remaining hurdles to allow the use of prognostic biomarkers in daily oncology practice. Undoubtably, these advances will have significant implications for the design of clinical trials, development of new therapeutic approaches, and the planning of patients' treatment.

References

1. Fisher RI, Gaynor ER, Dahlberg S, et al. Comparison of a standard regimen (CHOP) with three intensive chemotherapy regimens for advanced non-Hodgkin's lymphoma. N Engl J Med 1993;328:1002–6.
2. Coiffier B, Lepage E, Briere J, et al. CHOP chemotherapy plus rituximab compared with CHOP alone in elderly patients with diffuse large-B-cell lymphoma. N Engl J Med 2002;346:235–42.
3. Lossos IS. Molecular pathogenesis of diffuse large B-cell lymphoma. J Clin Oncol 2005;23:6351–7.
4. A predictive model for aggressive non-Hodgkin's lymphoma. The International Non-Hodgkin's Lymphoma Prognostic Factors Project. N Engl J Med 1993;329:987–94.
5. Lossos IS, Morgensztern D. Prognostic biomarkers in diffuse large B-cell lymphoma. J Clin Oncol 2006;24:995–1007.
6. Alizadeh AA, Eisen MB, Davis RE, et al. Distinct types of diffuse large B-cell lymphoma identified by gene expression profiling. Nature 2000;403:503–11.
7. Rosenwald A, Wright G, Chan WC, et al. The use of molecular profiling to predict survival after chemotherapy for diffuse large-B-cell lymphoma. N Engl J Med 2002;346:1937–47.
8. Monti S, Savage KJ, Kutok JL, et al. Molecular profiling of diffuse large B-cell lymphoma identifies robust subtypes including one characterized by host inflammatory response. Blood 2005;105:1851–61.
9. Shipp MA, Ross KN, Tamayo P, et al. Diffuse large B-cell lymphoma outcome prediction by gene-expression profiling and supervised machine learning. Nat Med 2002;8:68–74.
10. Wright G, Tan B, Rosenwald A, Hurt EH, Wiestner A, Staudt LM. A gene expression-based method to diagnose clinically distinct subgroups of diffuse large B cell lymphoma. Proc Natl Acad Sci USA 2003;100:9991–6.

11. Lenz G, Wright G, Dave SS, et al. Stromal gene signatures in large-B-cell lymphomas. N Engl J Med 2008;359:2313–23.

12. Lossos IS, Czerwinski DK, Alizadeh AA, et al. Prediction of survival in diffuse large-B-cell lymphoma based on the expression of six genes. N Engl J Med 2004;350:1828–37.

13. Hummel M, Bentink S, Berger H, et al. A biologic definition of Burkitt's lymphoma from transcriptional and genomic profiling. N Engl J Med 2006;354:2419–30.

14. Chen J, Byrne GE Jr, Lossos IS. Optimization of RNA extraction from formalin-fixed, paraffin-embedded lymphoid tissues. Diagn Mol Pathol 2007;16:61–72.

15. Malumbres R, Chen J, Tibshirani R, et al. Paraffin-based 6-gene model predicts outcome in diffuse large B-cell lymphoma patients treated with R-CHOP. Blood 2008;111:5509–14.

16. Rimsza LM, Leblanc ML, Unger JM, et al. Gene expression predicts overall survival in paraffin-embedded tissues of diffuse large B-cell lymphoma treated with R-CHOP. Blood 2008;112:3425–33.

17. Colomo L, Lopez-Guillermo A, Perales M, et al. Clinical impact of the differentiation profile assessed by immunophenotyping in patients with diffuse large B-cell lymphoma. Blood 2003;101:78–84.

18. Barrans SL, Carter I, Owen RG, et al. Germinal center phenotype and bcl-2 expression combined with the International Prognostic Index improves patient risk stratification in diffuse large B-cell lymphoma. Blood 2002;99:1136–43.

19. Hans CP, Weisenburger DD, Greiner TC, et al. Confirmation of the molecular classification of diffuse large B-cell lymphoma by immunohistochemistry using a tissue microarray. Blood 2004;103:275–82.

20. Natkunam Y, Farinha P, Hsi ED, et al. LMO2 protein expression predicts survival in patients with diffuse large B-cell lymphoma treated with anthracycline-based chemotherapy with and without rituximab. J Clin Oncol 2008;26:447–54.

21. Lossos IS, Alizadeh AA, Rajapaksa R, Tibshirani R, Levy R. HGAL is a novel interleukin-4-inducible gene that strongly predicts survival in diffuse large B-cell lymphoma. Blood 2003;101:433–40.

22. Lu X, Chen J, Malumbres R, Cubedo Gil E, Helfman DM, Lossos IS. HGAL, a lymphoma prognostic biomarker, interacts with the cytoskeleton and mediates the effects of IL-6 on cell migration. Blood 2007;110:4268–77.

23. Davis RE, Brown KD, Siebenlist U, Staudt LM. Constitutive nuclear factor kappaB activity is required for survival of activated B cell-like diffuse large B cell lymphoma cells. J Exp Med 2001;194:1861–74.

24. Robertson MJ, Kahl BS, Vose JM, et al. Phase II study of enzastaurin, a protein kinase C beta inhibitor, in patients with relapsed or refractory diffuse large B-cell lymphoma. J Clin Oncol 2007;25:1741–6.

25. Smith PG, Wang F, Wilkinson KN, et al. The phosphodiesterase PDE4B limits cAMP-associated PI3K/AKT-dependent apoptosis in diffuse large B-cell lymphoma. Blood 2005;105:308–16.

26. Polo JM, Juszczynski P, Monti S, et al. Transcriptional signature with differential expression of BCL6 target genes accurately identifies BCL6-dependent diffuse large B cell lymphomas. Proc Natl Acad Sci USA 2007;104:3207–12.

27. Friedberg J, Sharman J, Schaefer-Cutillo J, et al. Tamatinib fosdium (TAMF), an oral SYK inhibitor, has significant clinical activity in B-cell non-Hodgkin's lymphoma (NHL). Ann Oncol 2008;19:116.

28. Lu X, Nechushtan H, Ding F, et al. Distinct IL-4-induced gene expression, proliferation, and intracellular signaling in germinal center B-cell-like and activated B-cell-like diffuse large-cell lymphomas. Blood 2005;105:2924–32.

29. Lu X, Chen J, Sasmono RT, et al. T-cell protein tyrosine phosphatase, distinctively expressed in activated-B-cell-like diffuse large B-cell lymphomas, is the nuclear phosphatase of STAT6. Mol Cell Biol 2007;27:2166–79.

30. Lu X, Malumbres R, Shields B, et al. PTP1B is a negative regulator of interleukin 4-induced STAT6 signaling. Blood 2008;112:4098–108.

31. Malumbres R, Sarosiek KA, Cubedo E, et al. Differentiation-stage-specific expression of microRNAs in B-lymphocytes and diffuse large B-cell lymphomas. Blood 2008.

Chapter 34

Growth Signaling and Survival Pathways in Aggressive B-cell Lymphoma

Lan V. Pham and Richard J. Ford

Abstract/Scope of Chapter The aberrations in B-cell growth signaling that characterize aggressive B-cell lymphomas, including large B-cell lymphoma and mantle cell lymphoma, are discussed. The shift from paracrine to autocrine growth factor expression and the subsequent dysregulation of multiple ligand-receptor pathways are highlighted.

Keywords B cell, maturation • Large B cell lymphoma, signaling • Mantle cell lymphoma, signaling • MALT lymphoma, signaling • BLyS (B lymphocyte stimulator) • BAFF (B cell activation factor) • CD40 • CD40 ligand (CD40L or CD154) • NF-kB, nuclear factor, kappa B • NFAT, nuclear factor of activated T cells • Signalosome • Enhanceosome

34.1. Signaling Pathways in Normal B Cells

The B (bursa- or bone marrow-derived) cell lineage, is one of several lymphocyte types in the human immune system that arise in the bone marrow from primitive progenitors and mature and differentiate in secondary lymphoid tissues, including spleen, lymph nodes, tonsils, and Peyer's patches. Humans have been estimated to maintain approximately 1×10^{12} lymphocytes in the entire immune system of which 5–15% represent B lymphocytes [1, 2]. The coordinated program of B-cell activation described below leads to the generation of a large number of short-lived, antigen-specific B cells that can clear or eliminate foreign substances through opsonization, complement activation, and macrophage- and T-cell-assisted neutralization of bacteria and viruses. Other populations of longer-lived memory B cells and plasma cells provide continuing immunologic memory and comprise the humoral portion of the adaptive immune response [2].

B cells are defined by their expression of surface immunoglobulin (IG), also known as the B-cell receptor (BCR), which is their unique signaling apparatus. After bone marrow maturation, B cells express a single clonotypic antibody with its antigen specificity primarily determined by the V (variable) region sequence selected during V-D-J recombination of the expressed IG heavy and light chains (see Chap. 4). This surface antibody/BCR recognizes a specific epitope on either soluble or membrane-associated antigen. This binding triggers a conformational shift in the BCR which leads to the formation of a multimeric protein complex with recruitment of linker/adaptor proteins and cytoplasmic tyrosine kinases such as LYN. This BCR scaffold, also known as the SMAC (supramolecular activation complex), is linked to the activation of other signaling pathways, including calcium channel signaling, that activates the NFAT transcription factors and the membrane-based phosphoinositol

From: *Neoplastic Hematopathology*: Contemporary Hematology,
Edited by: D. Jones, DOI 10.1007/978-1-60761-384-8_34,
© Humana Press, a part of Springer Science+Business Media, LLC 2010

3 kinase (PI3K), which then activates the AKT family of serine/threonine kinases further regulating cell proliferation and apoptosis.

The signals transmitted through the BCR are modulated over the lifetime of a B cell by antigen encounters, costimulatory molecules on immune accessory cells, and a set of programmed genetic changes. Circulating naïve B cells transmit a low-level survival signal through the BCR in the absence of antigen (i.e. tonic signaling), but are triggered to proliferate when the BCR binds its appropriate antigen bound to major histocompatibility complex (MHC) proteins on the surface of antigen-presenting cells (APC). These activated B cells migrate to T-B interface zones in the lymph node, where they have a high propensity to encounter antigen-primed helper T cells with a similar antigen specificity (cognate T cells), which provide costimulatory growth signals though CD40. B cells then move into the germinal center (GC) due to actions of chemotactic chemokines such as CXCL13.

This GC localization of B cells leads to exquisite regulation of the BCR signal by antigen trapped on follicular dendritic cells (FDC) and the co-stimulatory actions of APCs, follicular T cells, and FDC. The BCR itself also undergoes a genetic shift in the GC through the interrelated processes of affinity maturation (an increased affinity of the BCR for a particular antigen) and isotype switch (a shift from expression of surface IgM to soluble IgG, IgE, or IgA). The process of affinity maturation is accomplished in the GC by somatic hypermutation of the expressed Ig V-region followed by growth selection to expand only those B-cell clones that show higher affinity binding of mutated BCR to cognate antigen.

Although B cells can respond to many polysaccharide and glycolipid antigens in a T-cell-independent manner, GC-localized T cells provide essential help for effective immune response to T-cell-dependent (TD) antigens, including most peptides. These accessory signals are mediated in part by the tumor necrosis factor (TNF) family of growth and survival (G/S) receptors and ligands, particularly the receptor CD40, the B-cell survival factor BLyS/BAFF (B/B), and the proliferative factor APRIL (Table 34-1). The partner ligand/receptors are present on the surface of cognate accessory T cells (such as with CD40L) or on dendritic cells (such as for the B/B receptors).

These transient activation complexes between T cells, APCs, and B cells can be visualized in vitro as either highly-organized cell-to-cell contact points centered on the BCR known as immunologic synapses or as more dynamic signalosomes which are multi-component, macromolecular signaling complexes involving dimeric or multimeric receptor-ligand components. Signalosomes are transiently formed in dynamic lipid raft substructures within the plasma membrane primarily following activation of growth and survival pathways, particularly those involving nuclear factor kappa B (NF-kB) (Fig. 34-1). Multiple other growth and survival pathways intersect with the BCR pathway and can thus modulate the growth-versus-apoptotic effects of an antigen signal depending on the B-cell differentiation state and cellular context. In addition to PI3K and the TNF signaling family, these include the complement receptors (CD21/CD35) and the toll-like receptors (TLR) primarily utilized for microbial immunity. As described below, dysregulated BCR pathway signaling is fundamental to an understanding of B-cell lymphomagenesis.

Table 34-1. Growth and signaling receptors and their ligands implicated in B-cell lymphoma signaling.

Receptor	Receptor gene name	Chromosome location	Ligand(s)	Ligand gene name	Chromosome location	Implicated pathway (s)
CD4O	TNFRSF5	20q12-q13.2	CD4O ligand	CD4OL (CD 154, gp39)	Xq26	NF-kBl-2, AKT
BAFF-R(BR3)	TNFRSF13C	22q13.1-q13.31	BLyS (BAFF), April	TNFSF13B, TNFSF13	13q32-q34, l7p13.1	NF-kB2, P13K, AKT
BCR, B-cell antigen receptor	CD79A, CD79B	19q13.2, 17q23	Antigen at BCR	N/A	N/A	P13K, NF-kBl, NFAT

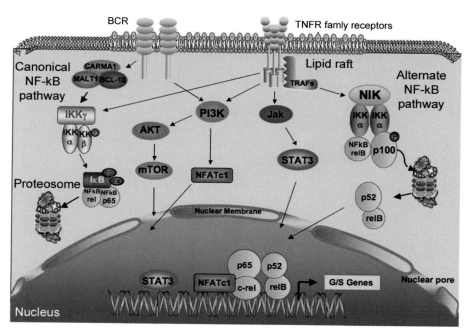

Fig. 34-1. Feed-forward growth and survival signaling pathways in large B-cell lymphoma. B-cell-associated TNFR receptors BR3 and CD40 are constitutively-activated through their cognate ligands BLyS and CD40L (CD154), respectively. Both ligands and receptors are autochthonously produced in LBCL cells providing continuous signaling stimuli that activate both the canonical NFkB1 and the alternative NFkB2 pathways. This constitutive CD40-CD40L (CD154) dyad also activates the NFAT pathway following calcium/calcineurin signaling synergizing with the PI3K/AKT pathway activated by the B-cell receptor (BCR) pathway including the CMB (Carma1, Malt-1, and BCL-10) signalosome. NF-kB and NFAT pathway transcription factors "feed-forward" in activating the CD40L (CD154), TNFSF13B (BLyS), and MYC promoters ensuring continuous tumor cell growth and survival signaling

34.2. Model Systems for B-cell Lymphoma

Dissecting the molecular pathogenesis of B-cell lymphoma requires development of appropriate in vitro cell line models and in vivo animal models. Indolent or low-grade B-cell lymphomas are very difficult to maintain for more than a week in cell culture without specific B-cell growth factors such as CD40L, interleukin (IL)-2, IL-4, IL-6, and IL-10. The poor growth of low-grade lymphomas is probably due to their strong dependence on subtle epigenetic factors such as exogenous growth stimulation in a manner similar to normal B cells. Therefore, another approach to propagate B-cell tumors is the use of bio-engineered adherent ("feeder") cell lines that can mimic some aspects of the tumor microenvironment. Low-grade B-cell lymphomas are also notoriously difficult to transfect, so attempts to improve propagation by introducing transforming genes such as telomerase have been similarly unsuccessful to date. Creation of cell lines by transformation of indolent B-cell tumor cells with Epstein-Barr virus is possible but tends to alter the phenotype of the derived lines so they are not useful as models.

In contrast, aggressive B-cell lymphomas, such as diffuse large B-cell lymphoma (DLBCL) and mantle cell lymphoma (MCL), particularly in samples obtained from effusions, blood, or pheresis products, are more amenable to in vitro culture. This is likely because they are more cell autonomous in their growth and also because their in vivo growth in fluid phase resembles the in vitro conditions more closely. Once acclimated to these in vitro conditions, such lymphoma cultures maintain many of the autocrine and paracrine signaling pathways that characterize the lymphoma in vivo. Many well characterized and validated

Table 34-2. Listing of lymphoma cells established from culture of primary tumors.

DLBCL cell lines		DLBCL cell lines		MCL cell lines	
SUDHL1	GCB	MS	GCB	Mino	cMCL
OCI-Ly19	GCB	DS	GCB	DBsp53	cMCL
OCI-Ly7	GCB	DB	GCB	Jeko-1	cMCL
HS445	GCB	JM	GCB	Granta	cMCL
HS602	GCB	FN	GCB	REC-1	cMCL
HT	GCB	EJ	GCB	NCEB-1	cMCL
OCI-Ly2	GCB	HF	GCB	Z-138	bvMCL
SUDHL10	GCB	PL	GCB	JMP-1	bvMCL
SUDHL4	GCB	MZ	GCB	BL cell lines	
OCI-Ly3	ABC	CJ	GCB	Ramos	BL
SUDHL2	ABC	SF	GCB	Raji	BL
HBL1	ABC	HB	ABC	Namalwa	BL
OCI-Ly10	ABC	LR	ABC	BJAB	BL
U2932	ABC	LP	ABC	BL2	BL

Cell lines are described in part in references 10,27,28

DLBCL, MCL, and BL cell lines have been established in our lab and many others worldwide (Table 34-2).

Translational research in lymphoma also requires the transition from in vitro culture studies to in vivo animal models. This has frequently involved injection of human lymphoma into SCID mice (xenotransplantation) or genetically-engineered (transgenic or gene knockout) mouse models (GEMMs), which are discussed in Chap. 36 in more detail. Ideally, it is best to have all of these models, as they are not redundant and offer different insights into the pathophysiology of the disease process and also provide different potential targets for experimental therapeutics. New GEMM approaches allowing conditional and lineage-specific gene expression or inducible gene deletion or rearrangement (e.g. Cre-lox system) are currently providing more tractable and valid experimental lymphoma models that should be important resources for experimental therapeutics in the near future.

34.3. Shifts in Signaling from Low-Grade to Aggressive B-cell Lymphoma

Cell culture studies have revealed that human lymphoma cells generally express similar signaling pathways and G/S receptors as their putative normal B-cell counterparts. Differences arise, however, when genetic and functional biologic characteristics are studied, with low grade (indolent) B-cell lymphoma generally showing less deviation from normal B cells in patterns of response and gene expression than aggressive lymphoma. These shared features between low-grade tumors and nonneoplastic B cells include intact BCR responses, with transient growth stimulation followed by a return to baseline, and the requirement for exogenous cytokines derived for activated immune accessory cells for continued survival.

In contrast, cultured aggressive B-cell malignancies frequently show autonomous cell growth with continuous cell cycle progression. Major differences are observed, however, in how G/S pathways are regulated, which has been shown in studies of cultured DLBCL and MCL. These explanted lymphomas can show growth that is independent of antigen, external immune cells, or exogenous/epigenetic signals and instead rely on abnormal constitutively activated G/S signaling pathways. Common mechanisms of such dysregulated autocrine signaling in DLBCL include abnormal expression of a ligand in addition to its signaling receptor, coordinate upregulation of several parallel pathways by lymphoma-associated transcriptional factors (such as anomalous upregulation by BCL6 of several NFAT and TNF family receptors and their ligands), and most interestingly abnormal subcellular localization of signaling molecules (such as CD40 and BR3 localized in the nucleus instead of the cell membrane) [3]. This altered localization of growth factor receptors turns them into transcription factors that combine with known factors such as NF-kB and NFAT to produce an enhanceosome complex (Fig. 34-2) [4].

Although many mechanisms of growth dysregulation in aggressive lymphomas have been elucidated, unresolved questions related to the sequence of events that lead to autonomous G/S signals remain. Since many components of the BCR complex are often deleted in DLBCL, growth signaling shifts instead to the costimulatory receptors TNFR, CD40, and BAFFR. It is also clear that some subsets of DLBCL also activate downstream signaling molecules such as STAT3, AKT, and the CARMA1-BCL10-MALT1 (CBM) complex. These pathways and their interactions (i.e. crosstalk) are currently under intense study, not only for elucidating pathophysiology, but also for their roles as potential therapeutic targets.

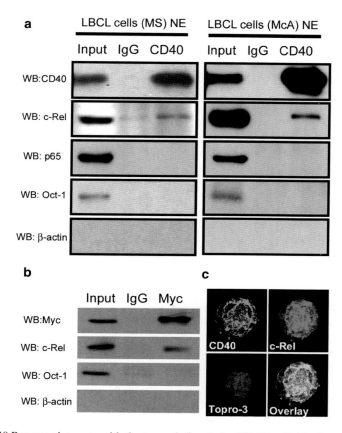

Fig. 34-2. CD40 Receptor interacts with the transcription factor NF-kB-c-Rel in the nucleus of LBCL cells. (**a**) Coimmunoprecipitation assays were performed with the nuclear extracts of LBCL-MS and LBCL-McA cells. Nuclear extracts (1 mg) from LBCL cells (MS and McA) were immunoprecipitated with a polyclonal CD40 antibody or IgG antiserum (negative control), respectively. Immunoprecipitated complexes were resolved on SDS-polyacrylamide gel electrophoresis (PAGE) and subjected to Western blotting with anti-c-Rel, anti-p65, anti-Oct-1, and anti-ß-actin antibodies. Input indicates 25 μg nuclear extract (NE). (**b**) MS cells were cotransfected with expression vectors for c-Rel (pCMV-c-Rel) and CD40wt (pcDNA3.1/myc/his-CD40). Forty-eight hours after transfection, the nuclear fraction was extracted and immunoprecipitated with monoclonal anti-Myc tag antibody. Immunoprecipitates were then Western blotted with anti-Myc (detecting recombinant CD40), anti-c-Rel, anti-Oct-1, and anti-ß-actin antibodies. Input indicates 25 μg nuclear extract. (**c**) LBCL cells (MS) were fixed with methanol and stained for CD40 (*green*), c-rel (*red*), and nuclear marker Topro-3 (*blue*) and analyzed by confocal immunofluorescence analysis. Colocalization of CD40 and c-Rel appears *yellow*. This research was originally published in Blood (see Ref. 4)

34.4. NF-kB Signaling in Diffuse Large B-cell Lymphoma (DLBCL)

Regardless of the initiating events in autonomous growth signaling in DLBCL, all eventuate in dysregulated NF-kB signaling (Fig. 34-1). NF-kB signaling plays an essential role in B-cell development, activation, proliferation, and survival by producing at least five distinct dimeric transcription factors that target specific functional classes of genes involved in cell cycle entry, apoptosis regulation, immunoregulation, and negative autoregulation of NF-kB itself. NF-kB pathways also mediate B cell proliferation and survival indirectly through cytokines such as IL-2, IL-6, and CD40L that can activate G/S receptors through either paracrine or autocrine mechanisms. The NF-kB system includes both a classic or canonical pathway (NF-kB1) and a non-classic or alternative route (NF-kB2), and perhaps a third less well-characterized "hybrid" pathway.

As discussed in Chap. 33, DLBCLs comprise a diverse group of tumors that have been extensively studied by gene expression microarray analysis and immunophenotyping and have been shown to comprise two common histogenetic subtypes with prognostic significance, although considerable overlap in phenotype and genotype clearly exist [5]. Expression of MUM1/IRF-4 and CD138 characterize the so-called activated B-cell (ABC)-like DLBCL, which appears to arise from post-GC B cells and has a more aggressive course with CHOP-type chemotherapy. In contrast, expression of BCL6 and CD10, with or without the t(14;18) chromosomal translocation involving the BCL2 locus, is characteristic of the germinal center B-cell (GCB)-like type of DLBCL. A third clinically distinct DLBCL category, primary mediastinal B-cell lymphoma (PMBL), has been shown to have a distinct genetic profile that is intermediate between those seen in GCB-like DLBCL and Hodgkin lymphoma (HL), and may arise from thymic B cells (see Chap. 17) [6]–[8].

Based on these gene expression studies, constitutive activation of the NF-kB1 pathway has been thought to distinguish the ABC-like DLBCL subtype. However, using tumor tissues and DLBCL cell lines (Fig. 34-3), we have shown that NF-kB, NFAT, and in some cases other centrally-important signaling pathways (e.g. PI3K/Akt) can be constitutively activated in both subtypes of DLBCL [9,10]. Interestingly, recent studies have demonstrated that constitutive CD40 signaling in B cells selectively activates the alternative NF-kB pathway and promotes lymphomagenesis, [11] likely accounting for the lack of association of NF-kB with any DLBCL histogenetic subtype.

Other B-cell-derived malignancies show different mechanisms of NF-kB activation from the pattern in DLBCL, such as the mutation of NFKBIA (IKBA) in Hodgkin lymphoma and the chromosomal translocations activating BCL10 and MALT1 in marginal zone lymphomas of MALT type [12,13]. As would be expected for low-grade lymphomas where the BCR signaling complex is still intact, the genetic alterations involving BCL10, CARD, and MALT1 seen in MALT lymphoma interact with the BCR and PI3K pathways directly to drive NF-kB activation (see Fig. 34-1).

34.5. Interactions Between Genetic Alterations in Lymphoma and Growth Signaling Pathways in DLBCL

As discussed in Chap. 1, B-cell malignancies have recurrent and disease-specific clonal chromosomal abnormalities which play a pivotal role in tumor development [14]. Chromosomal translocations in B-cell tumors often involve the immunoglobulin heavy chain (IGH) locus, and less commonly the IG light chains [15]. Normal B cells usually undergo a series of double-stranded DNA breaks, VDJ recombination and somatic hypermutation, to produce functional Ig proteins with high affinity for an antigen [16]. These developmentally-induced changes at the IGH loci may serve as targets for aberrant recombination with other chromosomes. The principal consequence of such translocations involving IGH is to drive transcription of gene(s) in B cells near the breakpoint on the partner chromosome due

Development of Cell Lines from Large B-cell Lymphoma Explants

Goal: Develop model cell lines that represent favorable GCB-like and the more aggressive ABC-like LBCL subtypes

Method: Tumor explants were serially passaged in culture and then characterized using conventional morphologic examination, flow cytometry, immunohistochemistry, G-banded karyotype and fluorescence in situ hybridization (FISH), and IGH gene rearrangement studies. Results were compared with those obtained from the primary tumors.

Line HF: Sample obtained from an untreated GCB-like tumor. Patient went into complete remission following the first course of chemotherapy. Reflecting its GCB-type, the cell line expresses CD10 as well as B-cell markers and is negative for MUM1. Karyotypic and FISH analyses reveal t(14;18)(q32;q21)/IGH-BCL2 rearrangement.

Line HB: ABC-like DLBCL. Patient achieved a partial response with chemotherapy, but relapsed and died of disease shortly after the sample was received. The cell lines expresses MUM1 as well as B-cell markers and is negative for CD10. Karyotypic and FISH analyses reveal t(8;14)(q24;q32)/MYC-IGH rearrangement.

Conclusion: These cell lines can be utilized as model systems to study the differential signaling pathways in DLBCL subtypes.

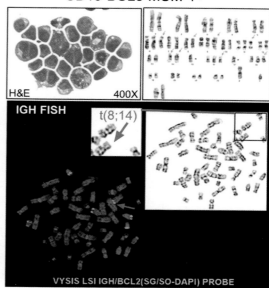

Fig. 34-3. Morphological and cytogenetic features of GCB-like and ABC-like DLBCL cell lines. The Authors thank Lynne Abruzzo, M.D., Ph.D. for cytogenetic analyses

to juxtaposition of the highly active Eμ enhancer. Therefore, the particular partner genes selected by juxtaposition to the Ig genes reveal many of the important signaling pathways implicated in lymphomagenesis [17].

DLBCL exhibits a plethora of different translocations involving the IG genes, with one or more found in about 50% of the cases [18]. Some of these are likely remnants of the earlier stages of lymphomagenesis such as the t(14;18) translocation found in 20% of DLBCL of GCB-type, but which is more characteristic of low-grade precursor follicular lymphoma. This translocation, which insertionally activates the anti-apoptotic protein BCL2, is likely important in supporting cell survival prior to the attainment of autonomous growth in DLBCL. In contrast, IG-translocations and activating mutations involving BCL6, a zinc finger transcriptional factor located at chromosome 3q27, are more specific alterations for DLBCL [19,20]. We have shown that BCL6 expression in DLBCL links growth signaling dysregulation with cell cycle alterations.

The pathways that lead to autonomous cell growth cell are also linked to unlimited DNA replication and loss of cell cycle checkpoint control. This connection can be seen in another DLBCL chromosomal translocation between IGH (or less commonly the IG light chain loci) and MYC at chromosome 8q21 [21]. Although MYC-IGH translocations are more characteristic of Burkitt lymphoma, they occur in up to 20% of DLBCL and MYC genomic amplification is found in an additional 16% of cases [22]. The Myc protein functions both as transcriptional activator and transcriptional repressor to simultaneously control genes involved in apoptosis, cell growth, and cell cycle progression [23]. Our recent studies have indicated that Myc is transcriptionally regulated by the transcription factor NFATc1 in DLBCL through a chromatin remodeling mechanism that involves the recruitment of the SWI/SNF chromatin-remodeling complex [24].

34.6. Growth Signaling in Mantle Cell Lymphoma: Similarities with DLBCL

MCL is another aggressive B-cell lymphoma which has been less well-studied than DLBCL and is more resistant to CHOP-type chemotherapy. MCL characteristically displays widespread tissue and organ involvement at clinical presentation and has a characteristic t(11:14)/CCND1-IGH chromosomal translocation in nearly all cases that drives overexpression of the cell cycle regulator cyclin D1. However, overexpression of cyclin D1 in transgenic models does not produce frank lymphoma suggesting that secondary genetic and signaling events are responsible for the aggressive behavior of MCL.

The histogenetic origin of MCL is also unclear. It lacks somatic hypermutation of IGH and tends to colonize the mantle zones of GC that are features of naïve circulating pre-GC B cells. However, it strongly coexpresses CD5 (which is not typical of the CD5-dim naïve B cells) suggesting a relationship to the B1 (CD5+) B-cell subset. In support of this, our recent studies [25] have indicated that B-cell-associated chemokine receptors (CXCR4 and CXCR5) and their cognate chemokines (CXCL12 and CXCL13) are highly expressed and functional on cultured MCL lymphomas and in mouse xenografts of MCL [26].

Because of the ability to establish MCL lines in culture, considerable progress has been recently made in establishing the reasons for the aggressive behavior of MCL. We have noted that MCL has dysregulation of G/S pathways that is more similar to DLBCL than to low-grade B-cell lymphomas. As with DLBCL, this shift to autocrine growth is primarily mediated by alterations in genes of the TNF family (CD40L, BLys/BAFF) and their receptors. In addition, similar to DLBCL, the receptors CD40 and BR3 signal with their cognate ligands not only in the plasma membrane but also in the cell nucleus, where they function as co-activators for NF-kB transcription factors such as REL. In MCL, these pathways cooperate with NFAT and AKT activation (due to PTEN deletion in some cases) to support lymphoma survival through activation of anti-apoptotic members of the BCL2 gene family such as bcl-xL and A1/bfl1. This pattern of NF-kB activation observed in MCL suggests the canonical and alternative pathways are interrelated. These signaling anomalies account, at least in part, for the autonomous cellular growth potential, immortalized tumor cell survival characteristics, and drug resistance through NF-kB-mediated upregulation of the levels of the mutidrug resistance transporter MDR1.

Interestingly, this pattern of multiple constitutively-activated growth and survival signaling cascades present in aggressive B-cell lymphoma, primarily utilizing NF-kB and AKT pathways, is similar to that seen in many solid tumors, (namely, PI3K/AKT; PKC, MAPK/Ras), suggesting that multi-hit growth factor pathway activation is a common occurrence in the pathophysiology of many human cancers. These findings also suggest that targeting multiple tumor-related pathways will likely become a strategy for "individualized therapies" in aggressive lymphoma that will be superior to use of single agents or traditional, non-selective cytotoxic chemotherapies.

References

1. LeBien TW, Tedder TF. B lymphocytes: how they develop and function. Blood 2008;112:1570–80.
2. Monroe JG, Dorshkind K. Fate decisions regulating bone marrow and peripheral B lymphocyte development. Adv Immunol 2007;95:1–50.
3. Lin-Lee YC, Pham LV, Tamayo AT, et al. Nuclear localization in the biology of the CD40 receptor in normal and neoplastic human B lymphocytes. J Biol Chem 2006;281:18878–87.
4. Zhou HJ, Pham LV, Tamayo AT, et al. Nuclear CD40 interacts with c-Rel and enhances proliferation in aggressive B-cell lymphoma. Blood 2007;110:2121–7.
5. Gilmore TD. Multiple myeloma: lusting for NF-kappaB. Cancer Cell 2007;12:95–7.
6. Alizadeh AA, Eisen MB, Davis RE, et al. Distinct types of diffuse large B-cell lymphoma identified by gene expression profiling. Nature 2000;403:503–11.
7. Rosenwald A, Staudt LM. Gene expression profiling of diffuse large B-cell lymphoma. Leuk Lymphoma 2003;44(Suppl 3):S41–7.
8. Wright G, Tan B, Rosenwald A, Hurt EH, Wiestner A, Staudt LM. A gene expression-based method to diagnose clinically distinct subgroups of diffuse large B cell lymphoma. Proc Natl Acad Sci U S A 2003;100:9991–6.
9. Pham LV, Tamayo AT, Yoshimura LC, Lin-Lee YC, Ford RJ. Constitutive NF-kappaB and NFAT activation in aggressive B-cell lymphomas synergistically activates the CD154 gene and maintains lymphoma cell survival. Blood 2005;106:3940–7.
10. Pham L, Tamayo A, Zhou H, et al. Networking modules of canonical and alternative NF-kB signaling in growth and survival regulations of large B cell lymphomas. Blood 2008:3776.
11. Homig-Holzel C, Hojer C, Rastelli J, et al. Constitutive CD40 signaling in B cells selectively activates the noncanonical NF-kappaB pathway and promotes lymphomagenesis. J Exp Med 2008;205:1317–29.
12. Sagaert X, De Wolf-Peeters C, Noels H, Baens M. The pathogenesis of MALT lymphomas: where do we stand? Leukemia 2007;21:389–96.
13. Jost PJ, Ruland J. Aberrant NF-kappaB signaling in lymphoma: mechanisms, consequences, and therapeutic implications. Blood 2007;109:2700–7.
14. Chaganti RS, Nanjangud G, Schmidt H, Teruya-Feldstein J. Recurring chromosomal abnormalities in non-Hodgkin's lymphoma: biologic and clinical significance. Semin Hematol 2000;37:396–411.
15. Kuppers R, Klein U, Hansmann ML, Rajewsky K. Cellular origin of human B-cell lymphomas. N Engl J Med 1999;341:1520–9.
16. Vanasse GJ, Halbrook J, Thomas S, et al. Genetic pathway to recurrent chromosome translocations in murine lymphoma involves V(D)J recombinase. J Clin Invest 1999;103:1669–75.
17. Seto M. Genetic and epigenetic factors involved in B-cell lymphomagenesis. Cancer Sci 2004;95:704–10.
18. Cigudosa JC, Parsa NZ, Louie DC, et al. Cytogenetic analysis of 363 consecutively ascertained diffuse large B-cell lymphomas. Genes Chromosomes Cancer 1999;25:123–33.
19. Bastard C, Tilly H, Lenormand B, et al. Translocations involving band 3q27 and Ig gene regions in non-Hodgkin's lymphoma. Blood 1992;79:2527–31.
20. Offit K, Lo Coco F, Louie DC, et al. Rearrangement of the bcl-6 gene as a prognostic marker in diffuse large-cell lymphoma. N Engl J Med 1994;331:74–80.
21. Yano T, Jaffe ES, Longo DL, Raffeld M. MYC rearrangements in histologically progressed follicular lymphomas. Blood 1992;80:758–67.
22. Rao PH, Houldsworth J, Dyomina K, et al. Chromosomal and gene amplification in diffuse large B-cell lymphoma. Blood 1998;92:234–40.
23. Eisenman RN. Deconstructing myc. Genes Dev 2001;15:2023–30.
24. Pham L, Tamayo A, Zhou H, LIn-Lee Y, Fu L, Ford R. Recruitment of the SWI/SNF chromatin remodeling complex by NFATc1 in the transcriptional regulation of the C-MYC oncogene in aggressive B-cell lymphomas. Blood 2008:3808.
25. Kurtova A, Tamayo A, Ford R, Burger J. Migratory activity and stromal cell adhesion of mantle cell lymphoma cells can be diminished by blocking of VLA-4 and CXCR4 receptors. Blood 2008:3781.

26. Bryant J, Pham L, Yoshimura L, Tamayo A, Ordonez N, Ford RJ. Development of intermediate-grade (mantle cell) and low-grade (small lymphocytic and marginal zone) human non-Hodgkin's lymphomas xenotransplanted in severe combined immunodeficiency mouse models. Lab Invest 2000;80:557–73.

27. Lam LT, Wright G, Davis RE, et al. Cooperative signaling through the signal transducer and activator of transcription 3 and nuclear factor-{kappa}B pathways in subtypes of diffuse large B-cell lymphoma. Blood 2008;111:3701–13.

28. Amin HM, McDonnell TJ, Medeiros LJ, et al. Characterization of 4 mantle cell lymphoma cell lines. Arch Pathol Lab Med 2003;127:424–31.

Chapter 35

Proteomic Profiling and Target Identification in Lymphoma

Megan S. Lim

Abstract/Scope of Chapter This chapter provides an overview of the proteomic profiling strategies that are currently in use, including mass spectrometry, protein arrays, phosphoprotein profiling, and quantitative protein analysis techniques. Examples are discussed on how these technologies can be utilized for the identification of biologic targets in human malignant lymphomas.

Keywords Anaplastic large cell lymphoma (ALCL), proteomics • ALK, (anaplastic lymphoma kinase), signaling • NPM-ALK (nucleophosmin/anaplastic lymphoma kinase fusion gene) • Kinase, proteomics • Kinase, profiling • Phosphorylation, tyrosine • Post-translational modification • Hodgkin lymphoma, proteomics • Non-Hodgkin lymphoma, proteomics • Human Proteome Organization (HUPO) • Isotope-coded affinity tag (ICAT) • Liquid chromatography with tandem mass spectrometry (LC-MS/MS), mass spectrometry (MS) • Polyacrylamide gel electrophoresis • Proteomics • Reverse phase protein array • Stable isotope labeling in cell culture (SILAC) • Proteomics, functional, antibodies, phospho-specific, subproteomics • MALDI (matrix-assisted laser desorption ionization)

35.1. Overview

Recent technologic advances in large-scale, high-throughput profiling of proteins provide exciting opportunities for biomarker discovery. These technologies will provide novel methods for early detection and diagnosis of cancer as well as classification and prognostic prediction. Proteomic profiling will also lead to better targeted therapies to enable the delivery of personalized medicine. A wide variety of proteomic profiling strategies are currently in use (Fig. 35-1). We provide an overview here of how each of these applications can be utilized for the identification of biologic targets in human malignant lymphomas.

35.2. Immunohistochemistry with Phospho/Activation Antibodies

Complex networks of signaling cascades are regulated by post-translational modifications in proteins (e.g., phosphorylation, ubiquitination, glycosylation, or proteolytic cleavage) that occur in a small subset of the total cellular pool of proteins. In contrast to (PCR-based) analysis of DNA and RNA sequences, the study of proteins is limited by the inability to amplify them. Thus, the major challenge for translational applications of protein profiling to study therapeutic targets is successfully identifying and quantifying proteins that are expressed at low

From: *Neoplastic Hematopathology*: Contemporary Hematology,
Edited by: D. Jones, DOI 10.1007/978-1-60761-384-8_35,
© Humana Press, a part of Springer Science+Business Media, LLC 2010

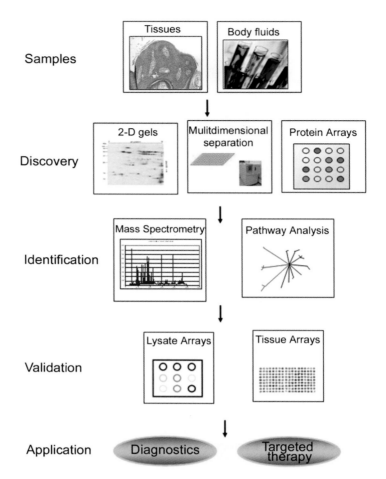

Samples

Discovery

Identification

Validation

Application

Fig. 35-1. Methods of proteomic analysis. The various techniques that can be employed to move from target discovery to validation are outlined

abundance. One strategy to improve detection is to utilize the signal amplification inherent in signaling cascades by examining the status of phosphoprotein epitopes downstream of such activated growth pathways.

Currently, there are hundreds of commercially-available antibodies that recognize the activation status of proteins via phosphorylation at either the serine/threonine or tyrosine residues. Many of these represent important signalling proteins that are deregulated in cancer. There are antibodies that recognize all tyrosine phosphorylated proteins (e.g. the pan-phospho-Tyr antibody 4G10) (Fig. 35-2a) and those that can recognize specific tyrosine phosphorylation sites (anti–phospho-STAT5A/B antisera that recognizes phosophorylation only at amino acid residues Y694/699). Obvious advantages of these latter reagents lie in the fact that particular activated proteins can be evaluated in different cellular compartments and in the context of a specific activation signal. For example, the STAT3 transcription factor migrates to the nucleus after phosphorylation so its nuclear localization can serve as a surrogate for its activation. Either routinely-processed cytology specimens or formalin-fixed paraffin-embedded tissue sections following deparaffinization and heat-induced antigen retrieval can be used for immunohistochemistry (IHC). Antibodies that recognize specific phosphorylation sites are used following standard immunostaining protocols. Antigen detection is typically performed using a peroxidase-labeled Streptavidin-biotin (ABC) method with diaminobenzidine as the chromogen substrate (see Chap. 2.1).

To ensure the specificity of phosphoprotein IHC, the immunoreactivity of the antibody should be tested in parallel by Western blot of appropriate cell lysates. For example, we performed

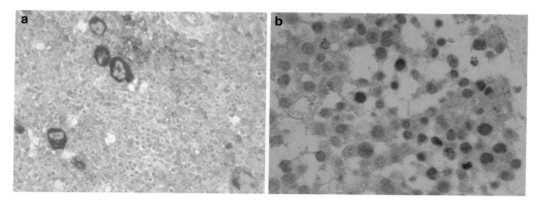

Fig. 35-2. Phosphoprotein analysis in tissues. (**a**) High levels of tyrosine phosphorylated proteins within the cytoplasm of megakaryocytes in bone marrow core biopsy of a patient with JAK2 V617F mutation positive polycythemia vera were demonstrated by immunostaining with the pan-phospho-Tyr 4G10 antibody. (**b**) Expression of phospho-p38 MAPK is seen within the nuclei of the SUDHL-4 lymphoma cell line (cell block preparation)

a study comparing the activation status of MAPK in follicular lymphoma tissue sections with activation of MAPK in lymphoma-derived cell lines [1]. To speed the analysis of a variety of targets, tissue microarrays (TMAs) composed of 40 different hematopoietic cell lines were constructed as described in Abbott et al [2]. We then established an IHC protocol to detect phosphorylated p38/MAPK (Fig. 35-2b) and confirmed assay specificity using Western blot analysis of SUDHL-4 lymphoma cells. By Western blot, these cells showed a band of the appropriate size, which could be modulated by treatment of the cells with a p38MAPK inhibitor (SB203586). To further confirm the specificity of the IHC results, formalin-fixed cell pellets of lymphoma cells showed loss of phosphop-p38 staining only after treatment with the inhibitor [1]. In a similar study, bone marrow trephine biopsy samples were used to evaluate for increased expression of phosphotyrosine proteins in megakaryocytes as a surrogate for JAK2 mutation in patients with polycythemia vera (Fig. 35-2a).

35.3. Protein Microarrays

35.3.1. Overview of Array Types

Protein microarrays are synthesized by immobilization of hundreds to thousands of peptides or proteins on a solid matrix. Protein microarray formats can be divided into two major classes: forward phase arrays and reverse phase protein arrays (RPPAs). In the forward phase array format, the analyte(s) of interest is captured from the solution phase by a variety of capture molecules, including antibody, protein, peptide or ligand that are immobilized on a substratum and act as bait molecules. Each spot contains just one type of immobilized antibody or bait protein and each array is incubated with just one test sample such as a cell lysate or serum sample. However, multiple proteins/analytes can be measured simultaneously, depending on the number of spots on the array.

In the RPPA format, each individual sample (e.g. serum sample or cell lysate) is immobilized to a different array spot such that each array is comprised of hundreds of different samples. The array is then incubated with one detection molecule (e.g., antibody) whose binding is then measured and directly compared across multiple samples [3]. Quantitation can be achieved by the use of dual-color infrared dye-labeled antibodies or with quantum dots (see Chap. 2.7). Protein microarrays have the potential to detect a protein with sensitivity that is 1,000-fold greater than an enzyme-linked immunosorbent (ELISA) assay and do not require a mass spectrometer. Finally, antibody-based microarrays enable multiplexed protein expression profiling of clinical samples in a high-throughput miniaturized format. By using recombinant single-chain

Fv (scFv) antibodies selected from a large (3×10^{10} antibody combinations) phage display library, highly-specific antibody microarrays have been used to profile pure or mixed populations of cells in blood with high sensitivity [4].

35.3.2. Using Reverse-Phase Protein Array to Probe Cytokine Signaling in Lymphoma

In a lymphoma-specific application, RPPA has been used to profile the activation state of several intracellular signaling proteins downstream of IL-4 in follicular lymphoma. Protein lysates were prepared from lymphoma samples, spotted on an array and probed with antibodies against cytokine signaling pathway components and their phospho-activated forms. Relative to follicular hyperplasia, follicular lymphoma showed basal phosphorylation levels of ERK and MEK kinases that were 4 times higher ($p < 0.001$). STAT-6, a transcriptional mediator downstream of the IL-4 receptor, showed only slight increases in lymphoma cases with basal phosphorylation levels approximately twice that of follicular hyperplasia ($p = 0.012$) [5]. This type of methodology has been expanded to evaluate the expression of 53 distinct phosphoproteins in a variety of tissue specimens [6].

35.3.3. Application of Receptor Tyrosine Kinase Arrays to Studying ALCL

Tyrosine kinases are frequently involved in neoplastic transformation [7] due to their regulation of fundamental cellular processes like proliferation, differentiation, survival and cell motility [8]. In nonneoplastic cells, receptor tyrosine kinase (RTK) activity is tightly regulated and quickly terminated by action of phosphatases or by receptor internalization and degradation. Overexpression of RTKs is common in many cancer cells and occurs via chromosomal translocations, gene mutation, amplification, or autocrine/paracrine stimulation [8,9]. The prominent role of TKs in cellular transformation is clearly demonstrated by the successful use of TK inhibitors in treatment of cancers such as imatinib in gastrointestinal stroma tumors (GISTs) with activating mutations in the KIT RTK and in BCR-ABL-expressing chronic myeloid leukemia (CML) and gefitinib in tumors with overexpression of mutationally-activated epidermal growth factor receptor [9].

In lymphoma, activation of the anaplastic large cell kinase (ALK) in anaplastic large cell lymphoma (ALCL) is one of the best examples of direct transformation due to overexpression of a RTK [10]-[12]. However, some cases of ALCL lack ALK expression. We have investigated the pathogenetic role of RTKs other than ALK in the pathogenesis of ALCL by carrying out RTK profiling. The activity of 42 RTKs was evaluated using the Proteome Profiler TM Array Kit (from R&D Systems) which is an antibody array that has both capture and control antibodies spotted in duplicate on nitrocellulose membranes. The activity of 42 RTKs was compared in an NPM-ALK-expressing ALCL line (SUDHL-1), an ALK-negative ALCL line (Mac 2A), and two Hodgkin lymphoma (HL) cell lines.

500 µg of cell lysates were diluted and incubated with the arrays to bind the extracellular domain of both phosphorylated and unphosphorylated RTKs present in the sample with unbound materials removed by washing. A pan-anti-phospho-tyrosine-antibody conjugated to horseradish peroxidase (HRP) was then used to detect the phosphorylated tyrosines on activated receptors by chemiluminescence. Chemiluminescence signals were quantitated by scanning on a transmission mode scanner and analyzed using image analysis software. Averaged background signals were subtracted from each RTK spot, using an average of the five negative control spots.

Of the 42 RTKs profiled, 12 of them including ERBB4, FGFR2A, FGFR3, MSPR/MST1R, RET, and EPHA4 were shown to be phosphorylated in the SUDHL-1 line at levels at least 5-fold higher than the background (Fig. 35-3). MET/HGFR activation was seen in the HL but not the ALCL cell lines whereas FLT3 was activated in ALCL but not in HL cell lines. These studies demonstrate the expression and activation of multiple RTKs that had

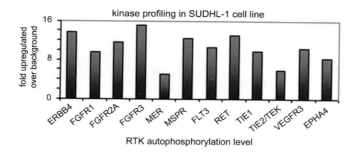

Fig. 35-3. Multiplex phospho-receptor tyrosine kinase profiling. Antibody arrays were used to demonstrate that the ALCL-derived cell line SUDHL-1 demonstrates overexpression of many receptor tyrosine kinases including ERB4, RET, and FGFR3

not been previously implicated in ALCL. Our data indicate that protein-microarray based identification of RTKs can provide important insights into the potential role of autocrine/paracrine RTK activation in the pathogenesis of ALCL.

35.4. Mass Spectrometry-Based Applications

35.4.1. Overview of Mass Spectrometry Applications in Protein Identification

Although phosphoprotein antibodies are highly useful in probing signaling, mass spectrometry (MS) remains the core methodology for definitive protein identification. MS proteomic profiling typically utilizes a bottom-up strategy in which a sample containing a complex mixture of proteins is initially digested using a proteolytic enzyme such as trypsin and then the resulting peptides are separated by liquid chromatography (LC) and analyzed by *tandem mass spectrometry* (MS/MS). The proteins are identified by matching the experimental tandem mass spectra with those from theoretical tandem mass spectra of translated genomic databases subjected to "in-silico" cleavage using specific enzymes. Figure 35-4 illustrates the components of the bottom-up proteomic analysis using LC-MS/MS.

Expression proteomics involves the large-scale identification of proteins from biological materials of interest such as specific subcellular organelles, enriched cell populations, tissues, or even an entire organ. Expression proteomics also includes the comprehensive identification of proteins in body fluids such as saliva or urine. *Quantitative proteomics* refers to global proteomic studies that monitor the shifts in the overall levels of proteins that occur in different biological states. Such quantitative analysis of the protein expression profiles of tissues or body fluids from specific disease conditions in comparison to normal states holds promise for the identification of disease biomarkers. The differential protein expression "signatures" should highlight those deregulated protein pathways central to pathogenesis. *Functional proteomics* encompasses the study of proteins in their functional environment, and the biological consequences of perturbations of the normal functional protein. This includes the analysis of protein interactions with other proteins, interactions with DNA or RNA, and post-translational modifications such as phosphorylation and glycosylation. The latter approach allows investigators to obtain information regarding the function of a protein, e.g. identifying networks of signaling pathways that are characteristic of particular physiologic and pathologic states.

35.4.2. Cellular Subproteomics

One of the major initiatives of the Human Proteome Organization (HUPO) is the comprehensive characterization of the complete subproteome of each cell type. Defining the global fingerprint of proteins expressed in a given cell type will aid in the identification of deregulated

LC-MS/MS-based proteomics

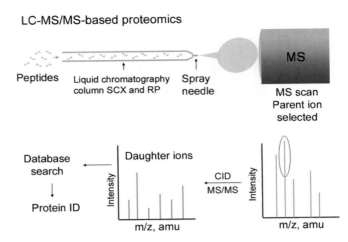

Fig. 35-4. LC-MS/MS-based proteomics. Bottom-up proteomics involves digestion of proteins into peptides, followed by liquid-chromatographic (LC) separation and tandem mass spectrometry (MS)

proteins that are characteristic of disease states and aid in the diagnosis and prognosis. Protein secretion into blood or body fluids by diseased cell types may provide a means for earlier detection of disease states including cancer. Systematic approaches to purify and identify secreted proteins from a variety of cell types have been reported and thus far include the identification of secreted proteins during differentiation of adipocytes, osteoclasts, and astrocytes. It is anticipated that these proteins represent candidate biomarkers of human disease. To that end, we have carried out global mass spectrometric analysis of the cellular proteome of cell lines derived from ALCL. Our studies identified the first comprehensive list of over 900 proteins that are expressed in ALCLs including 11 tyrosine kinases [13]. The pathogenetic roles of many of these proteins in ALCL are currently unknown.

35.4.3. Quantitative Protein Profiling

Quantitative proteomic studies are designed to determine the relative proteomic differences between one cellular state and another. In the standard method, comparison samples are electrophoresed on a 2-dimensional polyacrylamide gel, silver-stained, and then differentially-expressed protein spots are excised, eluted, and analyzed by MS. However, this is a relatively low-throughput laborious approach which requires a large amount of starting material (i.e. microgram quantities of total protein). Stable isotope labeling methods have also been used with great success for quantitative proteomics. Two major approaches include stable isotope labeling with amino acids in culture (SILAC)[14] and isotope coded affinity tags (ICAT™) [15]. Both approaches involve sample labeling with an isotope/tag that is either metabolically (SILAC), or chemically (ICAT™) incorporated into proteins in relation to their abundance and then the relative ratios of the isotopes of a particular MS-identified protein in the test and reference samples are compared. More recently, isobaric tags (iTRAQ™)[16] permitting comparison of up to 8 samples simultaneously have been developed. The proteins from each labeled sample are isolated, mixed at a 1:1 ratio and subjected to mass spectrometric analysis. Relative quantification is achieved by comparison of the peak height or areas of the isotope/tag pairs for each peptide distinguished by the mass difference of the isotope or tag.

We have utilized such an ICAT labeling strategy to characterize the proteomic consequences of rituximab treatment in cell lines derived from follicular lymphoma [17]. Our studies indicate that determination of the proteins and pathways that are regulated by antibody immunotherapy can lead to better understanding of the cellular mechanisms of drug sensitivity and resistance.

35.4.4. Interactome Analysis

Large-scale analysis of protein interactions can be performed by MS. Interacting partners in multi-protein complexes can be purified by several strategies including immunoprecipitation with specific antibodies directed against a bait protein or affinity chromatography with a tagged bait protein [18]. The purified components can then be subjected to LC-MS/MS and all proteins within the complex identified. The advantage of such co-purification protocols is that the fully-processed protein which serves as the bait can be tested in its native environment, including in several different subcellular locations. One limitation of this approach is the requirement for an antibody with specific immunoreactivity that is able to immunoprecipitate the bait protein without disrupting complex components. This drawback can be addressed by expression of the bait protein with a small epitope tag. Excellent antibodies are available for a variety of epitope tags to allow either immunoprecipitation or immunoaffinity purification. Epitope tags such as 6-histidine or GST also allow purification based on their affinity for nickel or GSH beads, respectively. Tandem affinity purification strategies have recently been employed and facilitate the analysis of highly-interacting proteins when the bait protein is expressed at lower (biologically-relevant) levels [19]. However, immunoaffinity or immunoprecipitation followed by LC-MS/MS does not readily permit determination of the stoichiometry of interacting partners. Additionally, when compared to the yeast two-hybrid method, MS/MS approaches cannot establish whether identified proteins bind directly to each other or require other linking proteins in the identified complex to stabilize their interactions.

We have used immunoprecipitation followed by MS-MS to identify interacting partners of the oncogenic chimeric fusion kinase NPM-ALK in ALCL cell lines. Proteins identified by MS were confirmed by Western blotting and reciprocal immunoprecipitation and, in some cases, their associations were examined in primary samples of ALCL. We identified a total of 46 proteins within the ALK immunocomplex, including previously-identified components of the ALK signaling pathway such as PI3K, Jak2, Jak3, Stat3, Grb2, IRS and PLCγ1. But more importantly, we also detected proteins which were not previously recognized to be associated with NPM-ALK and mapped new interaction domains on the NPM-ALK protein. These results clearly show the discovery potential of LC-MS/MS for the identification of novel proteins in a well-studied signaling pathway [20].

35.4.5. Phosphoproteomic Profiling

Post-translational modifications represent a complex set of changes that regulate protein function and influence the maintenance of cellular hemostasis. Phosphorylation is the best known modification and occurs mainly on serine, threonine, and tyrosine residues and is estimated to occur in vertebrates at a relative ratio of 1,800:200:1 for each amino acid [21]. However, there are more than 300 other described post-translational modifications of proteins including acetylation, nydroxylation, amidation, and oxidation, as well as the addition of peptides such as in ubiquitination, SUMOylation (small ubiquitin-like modifier) and ISGylation (conjugation of interferon stimulated gene 15 peptides to target proteins). Most of these modifications result in mass changes that can be detected by MS.

Recent attempts have been made to define the phosphorylation status of proteins at a global scale,[22] despite being technically challenging due to the low abundance, lability, and substoichiometric phosphorylation-site occupancy of many phosphoprotein moieties [23]. Most approaches involve the use of phospho-specific antibodies to enrich for proteins with phosphorylated residues. Due to the availability of excellent antibodies that react with phospho-tyrosines, studies focused on the analysis of tyrosine phosphoproteins far outnumber those for serine and threonine phosphoproteins. To accomplish identification of many different phophopeptides and tyrosine phosphorylation sites from complex cellular mixtures, we,[24] and others,[25] have utilized a strategy that incubates digested cellular protein lysates with a cocktail of phosphotyrosine-specific antibodies to enrich for phosphotyrosine peptides followed by standard LC-MS/MS analysis. Large-scale surveys of phosphopeptides using immunoaffinity purification of tyrosine phosphorylated peptides followed by LC-MS/MS have also been used successfully to identify the novel tyrosine kinase fusion proteins associated with lung cancer,[26] and fusions of CSF1R and RBM6 in acute myeloid leukemia [27].

35.5. Other Proteomic Techniques

Imaging mass spectrometry uses matrix-assisted laser desorption ionization (MALDI) MS to analyze tissue sections to generate an in situ protein expression profile of the specimen. Specifically, the frozen tissue sections applied to a MALDI plate are subjected to laser interrogation and analyzed at regular spatial intervals. The mass spectral data obtained at different intervals are then compared to generate a spatial distribution of masses (proteins) across the tissue section. Analyses using this approach have revealed more than 1,500 protein peaks that show correlations with histological features in just a 1 mm diameter region of a single frozen section [28]. Using this approach, investigators have been able to distinguish glial neoplasms from benign brain tissues, and differentiate tumors of different histological grades [29]. To date, this approach has only been successfully performed using frozen tissue sections.

Chemical proteomics or activity-based proteomics comprises approaches where molecular probes are used to target a selective group of functionally-related proteins in a way similar to antibody purification. For example, affinity chromatography using immobilized adenosine triphosphate, cyclic adenosine monophosphate, or cyclic guanosine monophosphate have been used to isolate a range of nucleotide-binding proteins [30]. Similarly, solid-phase extraction of glycopeptides can be used to isolate either N- or O-link glycosylated proteins even from formalin-fixed tissues,[31] or proteases specific for ubiquitin and ubiquitin-like proteins [32].

35.6. Why Proteomic Profiling May Be Better than Genomics or Gene Expression Profiling

Large-scale and high-throughput DNA and RNA profiling technologies such as array comparative genomic hybridization, gene expression microarrays, and single nucleotide polymorphism (SNP) array have contributed greatly to cancer taxonomy and classification efforts. They have also yielded important insights into coordinate gene expression and transcriptional control mechanisms. However, they are unable to define signaling events that occur at the proteomic level such as protein-protein interactions, post-translational protein modifications, or transient enzymatic activation and inhibition, except through indirect means or by bioinformatically-derived inferences, due to the differences in the time-scales of gene expression changes (many minutes to hours) and epigenetic changes in the DNA (many hours to days for CpG methylation) This compares with protein complex formation and post-translation events that change in seconds to minutes.

Proteomic methods thus have the advantage of identifying the dynamic and transient interactions (e.g. phosphorylation state or transiently forming activation complexes) that are the sum of all molecular interactions impinging on a particular cellular pathway at the moment of analysis. Such transient regulation of growth has been a major focus of laboratory studies on cancer progression and in drug screening assays. The newer generation of proteomic techniques (requiring small amounts of input material and capable of multiplex analysis) hold the promise of moving such tumor-specific proteomic studies out of the research laboratory and into the clinic to assist in rational selection of therapy.

Suggested Readings

Huang PH, White FM. Phosphoproteomics: unravelling the signalling web. Mol Cell 2008;31: 777–81.

Lim, MS, and Elenitoba-Johnson, KSJ. Mass spectrometry-based proteomic studies of human anaplastic large cell lymphoma. Mol Cell Proteomics 2006;5:1787–98.

Joubert-Caron R, Caron M. Proteome analysis in the study of lymphoma cells. Mass Spectrom Rev 2005 Jul–Aug;24(4):455–68.

Speer R, Wulfkuhle J, Espina V, Aurajo R, Edmiston KH, Liotta LA, Petricoin EF 3rd. Molecular network analysis using reverse phase protein microarrays for patient tailored therapy. Adv Exp Med Biol 2008;610:177–86.

Wingren C, Borrebaeck CA. Progress in miniaturization of protein arrays – a step closer to high-density nanoarrays. Drug Discov Today 2007 Oct;12(19–20):813–9.

References

1. Elenitoba-Johnson KS, Jenson SD, Abbott RT, et al. Involvement of multiple signaling pathways in follicular lymphoma transformation: p38-mitogen-activated protein kinase as a target for therapy. Proc Natl Acad Sci U S A 2003;100(12):7259–64.

2. Abbott RT, Tripp S, Perkins SL, Elenitoba-Johnson KS, Lim MS. Analysis of the PI-3-Kinase-PTEN-AKT pathway in human lymphoma and leukemia using a cell line microarray. Mod Pathol 2003;16(6):607–12.

3. Speer R, Wulfkuhle JD, Liotta LA, Petricoin EF III. Reverse-phase protein microarrays for tissue-based analysis. Curr Opin Mol Ther 2005;7(3):240–5.

4. Dexlin L, Ingvarsson J, Frendeus B, Borrebaeck CA, Wingren C. Design of recombinant antibody microarrays for cell surface membrane proteomics. J Proteome Res 2008;7(1):319–27.

5. Calvo KR, Dabir B, Kovach A, et al. IL-4 protein expression and basal activation of Erk in vivo in follicular lymphoma. Blood 2008;112(9):3818–26.

6. Espina V, Edmiston KH, Heiby M, et al. A portrait of tissue phosphoprotein stability in the clinical tissue procurement process. Mol Cell Proteomics 2008;7(10):1998–2018.

7. Blume-Jensen P, Hunter T. Oncogenic kinase signalling. Nature 2001;411(6835):355–65.

8. Schlessinger J. Cell signaling by receptor tyrosine kinases. Cell 2000;103(2):211–25.

9. Noble ME, Endicott JA, Johnson LN. Protein kinase inhibitors: insights into drug design from structure. Science 2004;303(5665):1800–5.

10. Morris SW, Kirstein MN, Valentine MB, et al. Fusion of a kinase gene, ALK, to a nucleolar protein gene, NPM, in non-Hodgkin's lymphoma. Science 1994;263(5151):1281–4.

11. Shiota M, Fujimoto J, Semba T, Satoh H, Yamamoto T, Mori S. Hyperphosphorylation of a novel 80 kDa protein-tyrosine kinase similar to Ltk in a human Ki-1 lymphoma cell line, AMS3. Oncogene 1994;9(6):1567–74.

12. Shiota M, Fujimoto J, Takenaga M, et al. Diagnosis of t(2;5)(p23;q35)-associated Ki-1 lymphoma with immunohistochemistry. Blood 1994;84(11):3648–52.

13. Sjostrom C, Seiler C, Crockett DK, Tripp SR, Elenitoba Johnson KS, Lim MS. Global proteome profiling of NPM/ALK-positive anaplastic large cell lymphoma. Exp Hematol 2007;35(8):1240–8.

14. Ong SE, Foster LJ, Mann M. Mass spectrometric-based approaches in quantitative proteomics. Methods 2003;29(2):124–30.

15. Gygi SP, Rist B, Gerber SA, Turecek F, Gelb MH, Aebersold R. Quantitative analysis of complex protein mixtures using isotope-coded affinity tags. Nat Biotechnol 1999;17(10):994–9.

16. Ross PL, Huang YN, Marchese JN, et al. Multiplexed protein quantitation in *Saccharomyces cerevisiae* using amine-reactive isobaric tagging reagents. Mol Cell Proteomics 2004;3(12):1154–69.

17. Everton KL, Abbott DR, Crockett DK, Elenitoba-Johnson KS, Lim MS. Quantitative proteomic analysis of follicular lymphoma cells in response to rituximab. J Chromatogr B Analyt Technol Biomed Life Sci. 2009;877(13):1335–43.

18. Kumar A, Snyder M. Protein complexes take the bait. Nature 2002;415(6868):123–4.

19. Wu F, Wang P, Young LC, Lai R, Li L. Proteome-wide identification of novel binding partners to the oncogenic fusion gene protein, NPM-ALK, using tandem affinity purification and mass spectrometry. Am J Pathol 2009;174(2):361–70.

20. Crockett DK, Lin Z, Elenitoba-Johnson KS, Lim MS. Identification of NPM-ALK interacting proteins by tandem mass spectrometry. Oncogene 2004;23(15):2617–29.

21. Hunter T. The Croonian Lecture 1997. The phosphorylation of proteins on tyrosine: its role in cell growth and disease. Philos Trans R Soc Lond B Biol Sci 1998;353(1368):583–605.

22. Mann M, Ong SE, Gronborg M, Steen H, Jensen ON, Pandey A. Analysis of protein phosphorylation using mass spectrometry: deciphering the phosphoproteome. Trends Biotechnol 2002;20(6):261–8.

23. Sachon E, Mohammed S, Bache N, Jensen ON. Phosphopeptide quantitation using amine-reactive isobaric tagging reagents and tandem mass spectrometry: application to proteins isolated by gel electrophoresis. Rapid Commun Mass Spectrom 2006;20(7):1127–34.

24. Schumacher JA, Crockett DK, Elenitoba-Johnson KS, Lim MS. Evaluation of enrichment techniques for mass spectrometry: identification of tyrosine phosphoproteins in cancer cells. J Mol Diagn 2007;9(2):169–77.

25. Rush J, Moritz A, Lee KA, et al. Immunoaffinity profiling of tyrosine phosphorylation in cancer cells. Nat Biotechnol 2005;23(1):94–101.

26. Rikova K, Guo A, Zeng Q, et al. Global survey of phosphotyrosine signaling identifies oncogenic kinases in lung cancer. Cell 2007;131(6):1190–203.

27. Bantscheff M, Schirle M, Sweetman G, Rick J, Kuster B. Quantitative mass spectrometry in proteomics: a critical review. Anal Bioanal Chem 2007;389(4):1017–31.

28. Yanagisawa K, Shyr Y, Xu BJ, et al. Proteomic patterns of tumour subsets in non-small-cell lung cancer. Lancet 2003;362(9382):433–9.

29. Schwartz SA, Weil RJ, Johnson MD, Toms SA, Caprioli RM. Protein profiling in brain tumors using mass spectrometry: feasibility of a new technique for the analysis of protein expression. Clin Cancer Res 2004;10(3):981–7.

30. Wong JW, McRedmond JP, Cagney G. Activity profiling of platelets by chemical proteomics. Proteomics 2009;9(1):40–50.

31. Tian Y, Gurley K, Meany D, Kemp C, Zhang H. N-linked glycoproteomic analysis of formalin-fixed and paraffin-embedded tissues. J Proteome Res. 2009;8(4):1657–62.

32. Hemelaar J, Galardy PJ, Borodovsky A, Kessler BM, Ploegh HL, Ovaa H. Chemistry-based functional proteomics: mechanism-based activity-profiling tools for ubiquitin and ubiquitin-like specific proteases. J Proteome Res 2004;3(2):268–76.

Chapter 36

Mouse Models of Lymphoma and Lymphoid Leukemia

M. James You

Abstract/Scope of Chapter The types and uses of mouse models of cancer are discussed. The spectrum of mouse lymphoid tumors encountered is summarized, as are the techniques used to study them.

Keywords Lymphoma, mouse models • Lymphoblastic leukemia, mouse models • Genetically engineered, mouse model • SCID mice, lymphoma • NOD/SCID mice, lymphoma • Xenograft • Knockout mice • Knockin mice • Cre/Lox

36.1. Description of Different Types of Mouse Models

36.1.1. Xenografts

The laboratory mouse is the most experimentally tractable mammalian system for advancing the basic understanding of human cancer biology and identifying new therapeutic targets. The earliest mouse models of lymphoma included inbred mouse strains that spontaneously developed lymphoid malignancies [1, 2]. For several decades, cancer drug screening was performed on these types of mice, although such models were intrinsically flawed in their ability to predict activity in human disease.

Subsequently, *xenograft* models were developed by injecting human cell lines into immunodeficient mice. Initially, xenograft models were generated in athymic *nude mice* that were homozygous for the mutant nude (nu) gene and lacked functional B cells and T cells [3]. These mice allowed human lymphomas and leukemias to be propagated in animals for testing the effects of drugs and to serially passage lymphoma explants in animals until a stable cell line emerged that could be used for both in vitro and in vivo studies.

However, many normal or neoplastic hematopoietic tissues transplanted into nude mice grow poorly. More favorable hematopoietic engraftment was obtained in severe combined immunodeficiency (SCID) mouse models. SCID mice are homozygous for an autosomal recessive mutation in the protein kinase, DNA-activated, catalytic polypeptide (PRKDC). Dysfunctional PRKDC protein in these mice prevents activation of the DNA recombinase that produces functional T-cell receptor (TCR) and immunoglobulin (Ig) proteins. Therefore, SCID mice are deficient in both humoral and cellular immunity although hematopoiesis is intact, making them suitable for xenograft propagation.

Although suitable for establishing tumors, SCID mice are prone to develop partial immune reactivity and explant rejection due to a low-level production of B cells and T cells. Moreover, SCID mice have essentially intact innate immune function, including natural

From: *Neoplastic Hematopathology*: Contemporary Hematology,
Edited by: D. Jones, DOI 10.1007/978-1-60761-384-8_36,
© Humana Press, a part of Springer Science + Business Media, LLC 2010

killer (NK) cell cytotoxicity, normal numbers of functional tissue macrophages (due to intact myelopoiesis), and normal serum complement activity, as well as having some marginal zone B cells [4]. The introduction of nonobese diabetic (NOD)/SCID mice were a further improvement since they have multiple defects in both adaptive and innate immunologic functions, an absence of mature lymphocytes (including NK cells), and deficiency of serum Ig and complement C5 [5]. These animals are widely used in drug studies and in generation of new lymphoma cell lines.

However, many investigators regard xenograft models as problematic for drug discovery and they have resulted in few clear successes and many notable failures [6]. Criticisms of this model include the fact that the profound immunodeficiency in SCID and NOD/SCID mice precludes evaluation of the effects of immunoregulatory compounds (e.g. revlimid, or antibody or cellular immunotherapies) and xenograft models do not accurately recapitulate the host-tumor interactions. Also, SCID mice are defective in DNA repair which make it difficult to assess the cytotoxic effects of DNA-damaging chemotherapy agents. But most fundamentally, since xenografts rely on injection of a limited number of established human tumors, they cannot reflect the wide genetic diversity seen in neoplastic progression.

36.1.2. Genetic Engineered Mouse Models

The use of genetically engineered mouse models (GEMMs) has enabled many important basic scientific discoveries in cancer research during the past two decades. Types of GEMMs include transgenic (gene addition), knockout (targeted gene deletion), or knockin (targeted gene addition) animals [7].

Transgenic mice are usually generated by injection of exogenous DNA into the pronucleus of fertilized zygotes which are then implanted into a (hormone-treated) pseudopregnant female mouse [8]. The transgene becomes integrated into the genome at random and is then propagated in all cells of the progeny with successful expression confirmed by protein studies. By use of transcriptional promoter and enhancer sequences that have selectivity for certain cell types (e.g. the Ig Eμ enhancer in B cells), targeted expression can be accomplished. The phenotypes, immune function, and propensity to develop tumors in the transgenic mice are then compared with the wild-type. Even more targeted expression into hematopoietic cells can be achieved by cloning a gene into a retroviral vector and transducing the gene into hematopoietic stem cells of a defined lineage, followed by stem cell transplant into an irradiated donor (See Chap. 37).

Knockin mice have genetic material inserted specifically into a particular chromosomal locus by the process of homologous recombination, whereas *knockout mice* use the same process to loop out genetic material from a particular chromosomal locus to generate germline deletion of a particular gene. The generation of germline knockin and knockout models requires homologous recombination into embryonic stem (ES) cells. This is then followed by implantation of the altered ES into a donor mouse and screening of DNA from the progeny to find one where the desired genetic change has occurred. Such heterozygote mice are then bred and backcrossed to generate mice with homozygous alterations of the gene in knockout or knockin models.

The classical knockin/knockout strategy results in expression or deletion of the gene in all cells within the animal. However, recent advances in vector design have allowed investigators to introduce gene addition/loss in only particular cell types at particular times by *inducible expression* and *inducible recombination* systems. The tetracycline (Tet)-inducible system modulates gene expression by coexpressing a transcriptional activator (TA) fused to a Tet repressor protein (TetR). A TetR responsive element (TRE) is inserted into the promoter of the transgene construct. By feeding transgene-TetR-expressing mice doxycycline, a tetracycline analogue, the transgene can be turned on or off by shifting TetR-TA binding to the TRE [9]. Other inducible systems use hormone-responsive promoter elements, such as estrogen-binding sequences.

The Cre-LoxP and FLP-frt recombinases function in somatic cells to delete DNA contained between their recognition sequences so they can be used to delete a gene flanked by these elements. The Cre recombinase, which is typically expressed in transgenic mice under cell type-specific promoters, recognizes LoxP DNA sequences and loops out any DNA between two LoxP sequences [10]. The Flp recombinase acts similarly on frt DNA sequences [11]. The Cre-Lox or FLP-frt systems are typically used to produce cell type-specific deletion of genes whose germline deletion would be lethal to the developing embryo or where lineage-specific effects are desired. Using these strategies, transgenic, knockout, or knockin alleles from multiple genes have been combined with increasing sophistication to yield more biologically relevant lineage-specific models of lymphoid neoplasia [12]–[14].

36.2. Classification Schema for Mouse Lymphoid Neoplasms and their Relationship to the Types of Human Lymphomas

The advent of GEMM requires a formal mouse tumor classification that can be mapped onto the human classification schema. The *Bethesda Proposal for Classification of Mouse Lymphoid Neoplasms in Mice* was thus proposed in 2002 by a subcommittee of the Mouse Models of Human Cancers Consortium (MMHCC) [15]. This classification combines histologic, phenotypic, and molecular features and follows the format of WHO classification of human lymphoid tumors in many respects but uses distinct terminology where appropriate. Table 36-1 lists the mouse lymphoid malignancies in the Bethesda classification and the

Table 36-1. Classification of mouse and human lymphoid neoplasms.

Cell type	2008 WHO (human)	2002 Bethesda (mice)
B-cell neoplasms		
Precursor B-cell neoplasm	B lymphoblastic leukemia/lymphoma	Precursor B-cell lymphoblastic lymphoma/leukemia (pre-B-LBL)
Mature B-cell neoplasms		
	Chronic lymphocytic leukemia/small lymphocytic lymphoma	Small B-cell lymphoma
	B-cell prolymphocytic leukemia	
	Hairy cell leukemia	
	Lymphoplasmacytic lymphoma	
	Mantle cell lymphoma	
	Splenic marginal zone lymphoma	Splenic marginal zone lymphoma
	Follicular lymphoma	Follicular B-cell lymphoma
	Diffuse large B-cell lymphoma, NOS	Diffuse large B-cell lymphoma (DLBCL)
	Common morphologic variants	DLBCL morphologic variants
	Centroblastic	Centroblastic
	Immunoblastic	Immunoblastic
	Anaplastic	
	Molecular groups	
	Germinal center B cell-like	
	Activated B cell-like	
	Immunohistochemical subgroups	
	CD5-positive DLBCL	
	Germinal center B cell-like	
	Non-germinal center-cell-like	
	Diffuse large B-cell lymphoma subtypes	
	T-cell/histiocyte rich	DLBCL, histiocyte associated (HA)
	Primary DLBCL of the CNS	
	Primary cutaneous DLBCL, leg type	
	EBV+ DLBCL of the elderly	
	Other lymphomas of large B cells	
	Primary mediastinal (thymic) Intravascular LBCL	Primary mediastinal (thymic) LBCL

(continued)

Table 36-1. (continued)

Cell type	2008 WHO (human)	2002 Bethesda (mice)
	DLBCL associated with chronic Inflammation	
	Lymphomatoid granulomatosis	
	ALK+ DLBCL	
	Plasmablastic lymphoma	
	Large B-cell lymphoma arising in HHV8-associated multicentric Castleman disease	
	Primary effusion lymphoma	
	Burkitt lymphoma	Classic Burkitt lymphoma
	Morphologic variants	Morphologic variants
		Burkitt-like lymphoma
	Plasmacytoid differentiation Extranodal MZL-MALT-type Nodal MZL	
	Plasma cell neoplasms	Plasma cell neoplasms
		Plasmacytoma
	Extraosseous plasmacytoma	Extraosseous plasmacytoma
		Anaplastic plasmacytoma
	Solitary plasmacytoma of bone	
	MGUS	
	Plasma cell myeloma	
		B-natural killer cell-like lymphoma (BNKL)
T/NK-cell neoplasms Precursor T-cell neoplasm	T lymphoblastic leukemia/ lymphoma	Precursor T-lymphoblastic lymphoma/ leukemia (pre-T-LBL)
	Blastic NK cell lymphoma	
Mature T/NK-cell neoplasms		Small T-cell lymphoma
	T-cell prolymphocytic leukemia	
	T-cell large granular lymphocytic leukemia	
		T-natural killer cell-like lymphoma
	Chronic lymphoproliferative disorder of NK cells	
	Aggressive NK cell leukemia	
	EBV+ T-cell lymphoproliferative diseases of childhood	
	Adult T-cell leukemia/lymphoma	
	Extranodal NK/T-cell lymphoma, nasal type	
	Enteropathy-associated T-cell lymphoma	
	Hepatosplenic T-cell lymphoma	
	Subcutaneous panniculitis-like T-cell lymphoma	
	Mycosis Fungoides	
	Sezary syndrome	
	Primary cutaneous anaplastic large cell lymphoma	
	Peripheral T-cell lymphoma, NOS	
	Angioimmunoblastic T-cell lymphoma	
	Anaplastic large cell lymphoma	
T-cell neoplasm, character undetermined		Large cell anaplastic lymphoma (TLCA)

"best-fit" comparisons to categories in the fourth edition of the WHO classification of human lymphoid tumors (2008) [16].

The types of mouse lymphoid malignancies are similar but not identical to those seen in humans, a fact which likely reflects differences in both overall immune dynamics and the actions of specific genes. For example, the earlier stages of lymphocytes development are similar between mice and humans, however, interleukin (IL)-7 and its receptor are essential for mouse, but not for human, early B-cell development [17]. Genes involved in immune function have diverged considerably, especially among gene families implicated in lymphomagenesis. For example, the TCL1 oncogene implicated in human T-cell prolymphocytic leukemia has six homologous mouse genes, none of which appear to exactly match the function of human TCL1.

The microarchitecture and function of primary and secondary lymphoid organs also differ between mice and humans. For example, the thymus persists well into mouse adulthood as an important site for T-cell maturation, possibly accounting for the increase in precursor T-lymphoblastic lymphoma/acute lymphoblastic leukemia (ALL) in many mouse models. In mouse lymph nodes, the follicular dendritic cell network is often more rudimentary and there are differences in the density and function of other immune accessory cells, perhaps accounting for lower incidence of germinal center-derived lymphomas such as follicular lymphoma and Hodgkin lymphoma in mice. Also, the splenic marginal zone of mice is less prominent in comparison to humans [15].

A major reason for creating GEMMs of lymphoid neoplasms is to understand the early molecular pathogenesis of these tumors in a way that would provide opportunities for prevention or early intervention in similar human cancers. In this regard, a primary goal of mouse tumor models should be to recapitulate as faithfully as possible the full range of human lymphoid neoplasms. This one-to-one mapping is also critical because it clearly indicates which human tumor types do not currently have appropriate mouse genetic models, and which are largely unique to mice. The Bethesda proposal serves as a model to recognize the similarities and differences between lymphomagenesis and is likely to be continually revised as new tumor models emerge.

36.3. Diagnostic Tools for Studying Mouse Lymphoid Neoplasms

36.3.1. Combined Modalities for Diagnosis

The starting point for all lymphoma diagnosis is microscopic examination of cytological preparations and fixed tissues, but ancillary studies now also play a critical role. In the workup of a new GEMM, close monitoring of the animals for possible signs of tumor emergence is essential, including periodic blood cell counts and blood smears, and routine flow cytometric (FC) analysis with a panel of myeloid and lymphoid antigens (Table 36-2). Whenever lymphocyte expansions are encountered, clonality determination by molecular analysis will help to establish the stage of disease.

Upon death or animal sacrifice, mouse blood samples should be immediately collected for blood cell count, differential, and smear, FC analysis, and bone marrow examination. Touch imprints of marrow from the long bones or cytospin preparation of heparizined marrow material often have the best morphology with the Wright-Giemsa stain. The methyl green pyronin (MGP) stain is particularly useful for highlighting Ig expression in plasma cells. Thin sections of paraffin-embedded formalin-fixed tumor samples should be stained with hematoxylin and eosin with additional sections cut for immunohistochemistry (IHC). Cell lines may be established from cell suspensions by passaging in culture or in NOD/SCID mice (see Chap. 34). Representative tumor samples should be kept at −80°C for molecular analysis.

36.3.2. Reagents Available for Immunophenotyping Lymphoid Malignancies

There are now quite a few antibodies that are suitable for IHC and FC (Table 36-2). However, several IHC/FC interpretative criteria are different in mice than in humans. For example, CD5 is a T-cell marker in humans that is aberrantly strongly expressed only in neoplastic B cells, including in chronic lymphocytic leukemia (CLL) and mantle cell lymphoma. In contrast, most spontaneous B-lineage lymphomas in mice exhibit expression of

Table 36-2. Immunophenotypic summary of mouse lymphoid neoplasms.[a,b]

Marker	B-LBL	SBL	MZL	FBL	DLBCL	BL	PCT	T-LBL	STL
CD45[c,d]	+	+	+	+	+	+	+	+	+
CD117[d]	−/+	−	−	−	−	−	−	−	−
IgM (cyt)[c]	+	−	−	−	−	−	+	−	−
CD79a (cyt)[c]	+	−	−	−	−	−	−	−	−
TdT (nuc)[c]	+	−	−	−	−	−	−	+	−
CD19[d]	+	+	+	+	+	+	+/−	−	−
B220[c,d]	+	+	+	+	+	+	+/−	−	−
IgM[c,d]	−	+	+	+	+/−	+	+	−	−
IgD[c,d]	−	−	−	−	−	−/+	+	+	+
Igκ[c,d]	−	+/−	+/−	+/−	+/−	+	+	−	−
Igλ[c,d]	−/+	−/+	−/+	−/+	−	+	−	−	−
CD138[c,d]	−	−	−	−	−	−	+	−	−/+
CD5[d]	−/+	−/+	−/+	−/+	−/+	−	−	+	+
CD90[d]	−	−	−	−	−	−	−	+	+
TCRα/β[d]	−	−	−	−	−	−	−	+	+
TCRγ/δ[d]	−	−	−	−	−	−	−	+	+
CD3[c,d]	−	−	−	−	−	−	−	+	+
CD4[c,d]	−	−	−	−	−	−	−	(+)	(+)
CD8[c,d]	−	−	−	−	−	−	−	(+)	(+)
CD11b/Mac-1[c,d]	−/+	−/+	−/+	−/+	−/+	−	−	−	−
Gr-1[d]	−	−	−	−	−	−	−	−	−
Ter119[d]	−	−	−	−	−	−	−	−	−

[a]Abbreviations for mouse lymphoid neoplasms: *B-LBL* precursor B-cell lymphoblastic lymphoma/leukemia, *SBL* small B-cell lymphoma, *MZL* marginal zone lymphoma, *FBL* follicular B-cell lymphoma, *DLBCL* diffuse large B-cell lymphoma, *BL* Burkitt lymphoma, *PCT* plasmacytoma, *T-LBL* precursor T-lymphoblastic lymphoma/leukemia, *STL* small T-cell lymphoma

[b]+, positive stain; −, negative stain; −/+, more frequently negative; +/−, more frequently positive; (+), strong or no expressions depending upon T-lymphoid neoplasms

[c]Detection by immunohistochemistry, *cyt* cytoplasmic staining, *nuc* nuclear staining

[d]Detection by flow cytometry

CD5, except plasmacytomas and Burkitt lymphoma. Similarly, CD38 marks human germinal center B cells but is negative in mice, and the integrin CD11b is expressed in only small subsets of human lymphoma but is expressed at low levels in up to 40% of mouse B-cell tumors [15]. Finally, while human B-cell tumor clonality is indicated by a ratio of Igκ to Igλ of greater than 4 to 1 (or 2:1 for Igλ over Igκ), the upper limit the Igκ to Igλ ratio for mice is roughly 10:1 and all mouse B-cell tumors regardless of clonotype may have detectable surface Igκ. Therefore, only Igλ restriction is usually informative in mice, and molecular studies are preferable for B-cell clonality assessment.

36.3.3. Molecular Analysis

As with human lymphoid neoplasms, demonstration of the clonality of mouse lymphoid neoplasms is extremely important for the diagnosis and classification of lymphomas and distinguishing them from pre-neoplastic oligoclonal conditions and polyclonal reactive conditions. Indeed, such early oligoclonal or low-level multiclonal lymphoid proliferations may be critical to an understanding of early stages of lymphoma initiation and they occur frequently in many GEMM models. As in humans, clonal gene rearrangements of the immunoglobulin heavy chain (IGH) locus, the TCR-gamma, or TCR-beta loci can distinguish polyclonal from neoplastic lymphoid proliferations. Southern blotting of genomic DNA digested with appropriate restriction enzymes along with probes capable of detecting the J or constant genes are most commonly used [18]. However, protocols for the use of DNA polymerase chain reaction (PCR) are also available. As in humans, lineage infidelity can occur with partial rearrangements of the TCR genes in B-cell lymphomas and vice versa. In these cases,

T-cell lymphomas may display incomplete IGH rearrangements (D→J), but usually lack the V→DJ rearrangement.

Of note, many strains of inbred mice have germline integrations of endogenous ecotropic Moloney murine leukemia virus (MuLV) that can be activated to yield an infectious virus capable of polyclonal somatic integrations in normal cells and clonal integrations in lymphomas. These can be recognized by digesting DNA with an enzyme that does not cut within the virus and hybridization with an ecotropic virus-specific probe. In such a test, oligoclonal or clonal outgrowths of cells with a newly acquired integration can be revealed by non-germline bands hybridizing with intermediate to high intensity [15].

Conventional cytogenetic studies of mouse lymphoid neoplasms using metaphase-frozen chromosome spreads can be employed to determine chromosome copy numbers and detect translocations and deletions. Karyotype analysis in mice is technically demanding because all mouse chromosomes are acrocentric (i.e. unequal p and q arms) and of similar size. An alternative approach to genomic profiling is spectral karyotyping (SKY), which uses spectral image analysis to decode the signals from multiple chromosome-specific painting probes of various colors [19]. The results from SKY are complex, but can be used to suggest gene partners in chromosomal fusions. Array comparative genomic hybridization (See Chap. 4) is a more tractable means of defining genomic gains and losses [12].

Genomic profiling has not yet been widely employed for mouse lymphoid neoplasms. Such future studies could include genome-wide expression profiling to subclassify aggressive B-cell lymphomas from mouse models into activated B-cell versus germinal types,[16] or microRNA profiling to distinguish maturation stage of B-cell neoplasms as has been done in humans [20].

36.4. Models of Lymphoid Neoplasms

36.4.1. Summary of Mouse Models of Lymphoid Malignancies

GEMMs have revealed that multiple genes are implicated in the genesis of lymphoma and leukemia. Whereas each model may shed light onto the molecular mechanisms of lymphoma and leukemia, evaluation schema for mouse tumors have not yet been standardized, which makes interpretation of the existing literature on mouse lymphoma and lymphoid leukemias models difficult to interpret with certainty. Nevertheless, Tables 36-3 and 36-4 represent the best efforts to map gene-specific models to the MMHCC categories, as appropriate.

Mouse B-cell neoplasms have been produced in GEMMs either overexpressing or deleting receptor tyrosine kinases (ERBB2, RET, ETV6/TEL-PDGFRB), other signaling kinases (BCR-ABL, BLK, BTK, PIM1), apoptosis regulators (BCL2, MCL1, BAD), cytokines (IL6, TXLNA/IL-14α), adapter molecules (TCL1, BLNK/SLP65), cytotoxic granule proteins (PRF1), kinases involved in DNA repair (ATM, XRCC5/KU80, XRCC4), transcription factors (MYC, BRD2, IKZF3/AIOLOS, HOX11), transcriptional repressors (BMI1), or cell cycle/checkpoint tumor suppressors (TP53/p53, CDKN2C/p18, and CDKN2A/p16-p14), and uracil-DNA glycosylase (UNG).

Mouse T-cell malignancies have arisen from transgenic expression or deletion of signaling molecules (ERBB2, BCR-ABL, NRAS, NOTCH3, PIM1, PIM2, AKT1, LCK, MAP3K8/TPL2, CSNK2A1/CK2α), cytokines (IFNG/interferon-γ), BCL2, early response genes (IER3/IEX-1), adapter molecules (TCL1), heat shock proteins (HSPA2/HSP70), transcription regulators (STAT5A, STAT5B, E2A, IKZF1/IKAROS, LMO1/RBTN1, LMO2/RBTN2, TAL1, POU2F1/OCT1, POU2F2/OCT2, MYC, GATA3, TP53BP1, BMI1, SMARCB1/SNF5), DNA repair proteins (AICDA/AID, ATM, MSH2, PMS2, NBS1 and XRCC6/KU70), or tumor suppressors (TP53/p53, PTEN, CDKN2A/p16, CDKN2C/p18, and BRCA2), as well as mutated T-cell receptor β-chain (δV-TCRB).

Table 36-3. Lymphoid neoplasms in transgenic mice.

Transgene[a]	Gene function	MMHCC lymphoid neoplasm[b]	Reference(s)
MT-BCR-ABL^{p210}	Chimeric oncoprotein	pre-B- and pre-T-LBL	21
TEC-BCR-ABL^{p210}	Chimeric oncoprotein	pre-T-LBL	21
tTA-BCR-ABL^{p210}	Chimeric oncoprotein	pre-B-LBL	21
MT-BCR-ABL^{p190}	Chimeric oncoprotein	pre-B-LBL	21
Eμ-TEL/PDGFRB	Chimeric oncoprotein	pre-B- and pre-T-LBL	22
MMTV-NRAS	Transmembrane oncoprotein	Mature B-cell neoplasm/pre-T-LBL	22
LCK-NOTCH3	Transmembrane receptor	Mature T-cell neoplasm/pre-T-LBL	22
LCK-TERT	Telomerase subunit	Mature T-cell neoplasm	23
LCK(prox)-TAL1	Transcription factor	pre-T-LBL	21
LCK(prox)-TAL1(R188/9G)	Transcription factor	pre-T-LBL	21
LCK-LMO1/RBTN1	Transcription factor	pre-T-LBL	22
LCK-LMO2/RBTN2	Transcription factor	pre-T-LBL	22
MT-LMO2/RBTN2	Transcription factor	pre-T-LBL	22
LCK-POU2F1/OCT1	Transcription factor	pre-T-LBL	22
LCK-POU2F2/OCT2	Transcription factor	pre-T-LBL	22
Eμ-MYC	Transcription factor	pre-B-LBL	21
CD2-c-MYC	Transcription factor	Mature T-cell neoplasm	22
Eμ-N-MYC	Transcription factor	Mature B-cell neoplasm/pre-B	22
CD2-GATA3	Transcription factor	pre-T-LBL	22
Eμ-TLX1/HOX11	Transcription factor	Mature B-cell neoplasm	22
Eμ-BRD2	Transcription factor/kinase	Mature B-cell neoplasm	22
Eμ-BMI1	Transcriptional repressor	Mature T- and B-cell neoplasms	22
Eμ-XBP1s	Stress response factor	PCT	13
Eμ-STAT5A	Signaling molecule	pre-T-LBL	22
Eμ-STAT5B	Signaling molecule	pre-T-LBL	22
H-2K^b/IgH-STAT5B	Signaling molecule	pre-T-LBL	24
H2-L^d-IL6	Cytokine	PCT-E, PCT-A	21
Eμ-IL-14α	Cytokine	SBL	25
CD4-NPM1-ALK	Fused kinase	pre-T-LBL and PCT	26
Eμ-PIM1	Serine/threonine kinase	T-cell neoplasm	22
Eμ-PIM2	Serine/threonine kinase	T-cell neoplasm	22
MMTV-ERBB2	Receptor tyrosine kinase	T-, B-, null-lymphoma	22
Eμ-RET	Receptor tyrosine kinase	pre-B-LBL	22
Eμ-CSNK2A1/CK2A1	Serine/threonine kinase	T-cell neoplasm CD4+CD8+ or CD8+	22
LCK/CD2-AKT1	Tyrosine kinase	pre-T-LBL	22
Eμ-BLK	Tyrosine kinase	pre-B-LBL	22
LCK (prox)	Tyrosine kinase	Mature T-cell neoplasm	22
LCK-TPL2 (C-terminal truncation)	Carboxy-terminal kinase	pre-T-LBL	22
Eμ-IER3/IEX-1	Early response gene	Mature T-cell neoplasm	27
INSULIN-HSP70	Heat shock protein	Mature T-cell neoplasm	22
Eμ-TCL1	Protooncogene	Mature B-cell neoplasm	28, 29
CD2-CD3ε	Protooncogene	pre-T-LBL	22
β-actin-AICDA	Activation induced cytidine deaminase	Mature T-cell neoplasm/pre-T-LBL	22
δV-TCRβ	Mutated T-cell receptor β-chain	pre-T-LBL	22
SV40-Eμ-BCL2	Anti-apoptotic factor	PCT, pre-B-LBL	21
LCK-BCL2	Anti-apoptotic factor	Mature T-cell neoplasm	30
VAV-BCL2	Anti-apoptotic factor	FL	31
MCL1	BCL-2 family member	FL, DLBCL	32

[a]Transgenes driven by various promoter/enhancer elements including those from: *MT* metallothionein, *MMTV* mouse mammary tumor virus, *TEC*, mouse tyrosine kinase, *tTA* tetracycline inducible promoter, *Eμ* enhancer of μIg gene, *LCK* T-cell kinase, *CD2* T-cell specific transmembrane glycoprotein, *H-2* histocompatibility complex class I, *CD4* T-cell surface protein, *δV-TCRβ* mutated T-cell receptor (TCR) beta chain lacking the variable domain, *VAV* lymphocyte guanine nucleotide exchange factor. MCL1 transgenic using its own promoter

[b]Types of lymphoid neoplasms are listed according to MMHCC whenever possible

Table 36-4. Lymphoid neoplasms in knockout mice.

Knockout gene	Gene function	MMHCC lymphoid neoplasm[a]	References
MSH2	DNA mismatch repair	pre-T-LBL	21
PMS2	DNA mismatch repair	pre-T-LBL	33
ATM	Checkpoint kinase/DSB DNA repair	pre-T-LBL/mature B-cell neoplasm	34
NBN/NBS1	DSB repair, Nijmegen breakage syndrome	pre-T-LBL	22
XRCC6/KU70	DNA-dependent protein kinase	pre-T-LBL	22
XRCC5/KU80 (in p53⁻/⁻)	DNA-dependent protein kinase	pre-B-LBL	22
XRCC4 (in p53⁻/⁻)	DSB repair	Mature B-cell neoplasm	35
H2AFX (in p53⁻/⁻)	Histone H2a variant	Mature B-cell neoplasm	36
PTEN	Phosphatase	T-cell lymphoma	22
p16 (INK4a)	Inhibitor of cyclin-dependent kinase	Lymphoma	37
p18 (INK4c)	Inhibitor of cyclin-dependent kinase	T- and B-cell neoplasm	22, 38
p19 (ARF)	Regulator of p53 pathway	Lymphoma	37
p16/p19 (INK4a/ARF)	Inhibitor of cyclin-dependent kinase/ regulator of p53 pathway	T and B-cell lymphoma	12
TP53	Transcription factor	SMZL, pre-T-LBL	22
TCF3/E2A	Transcription factor	T-cell lymphoma	22
SMARCB1/SNF5	Transcription factor	Mature T-cell neoplasm	22
IKZF4/Ikaros	Transcription factor	pre-T-LBL	21
IKZF3/Aiolos	Transcription factor	pre-B-LBL	21
TP53BP1	p53 binding protein	pre-T-LBL	22
NRAS	Small GTPase	pre-T-LBL	22
BTK	Cytoplasmic kinase	pre-B-LBL	22
BLNK/SLP-65	Adaptor protein	pre-B-LBL	22
PRDX1	Peroxiredoxin 1	T- and B-cell neoplasm	22
UNG	Uracil-DNA glycosylase	Mature B-cell neoplasm	22
BAD	Proapoptotic protein	DLBCL	22
IFNG (interferon-gamma)	Cytokine	T-cell neoplasm	22
PRF1 (perforin)	Pore-forming protein	Mature B-cell neoplasm	39
BRCA2	mediator of homologous Recombination	pre-T-LBL	21

[a]Types of lymphoid neoplasms are listed according to MMHCC whenever possible. See text for alternate and official gene names, *DSB* double strand DNA breaks

Only a few GEMMS have been reported that produce plasma cell neoplasms, which may reflect differences in mouse and human plasma cell differentiation. In humans, the bone-based multiple myeloma (MM) is the most common plasma cell neoplasm and is often preceded by a pre-malignant monoclonal gammopathy of undetermined significance (MGUS). A model resembling MGUS/MM models was generated in transgenic mice with Ig Eμ-directed expression of the XBP1 spliced isoform (XBP-1s), which functions normally in cellular unfolded protein/ER stress response and plasma cell development. Eμ-XBP-1s mice have elevated serum Ig and skin alterations [13]. Interleukin-6 (IL6) and NPM1-ALK transgenic mice have also yielded plasma cell neoplasms.

36.4.2. Commonly Implicated Genes in Mouse Models of Lymphoid Malignancies

In human tumorigenesis, MYC deregulation by chromosomal translocation to one of the Ig enhancers is characteristic of Burkitt lymphoma and a subset of diffuse large B-cell lymphoma (See Chap. 17). Constitutive overexpression of MYC drives cell proliferation and interferes with B-cell differentiation due to its pleotropic effects as a transcriptional and cell cycle regulator. Eμ-MYC transgenic mice develop B-cell lymphomas, but these neoplasms resemble precursor B-lymphoblastic lymphoma more than BL. Secondary translocations involving the mouse MYC locus are also frequently seen as cooperating events in B-cell lymphomas in other transgenic models. Interestingly, transgenic mice expressing MYC under the control of the T-cell-specific CD2 promoter showed the development of T-cell lymphomas only after relatively long latency, suggesting that additional cooperating genetic changes may be required for T-cell transformation. Therefore, the type of lymphomas arising in transgenic MYC mice depends not only on the gene itself but also on the tissue where it is expressed.

The CDKN2A gene encodes two distinct tumor suppressors, p16^{INK4a} and p14^{ARF} (p19^{ARF} in mice), that function as regulators of the retinoblastoma (RB1) and p53 pathways, respectively. p16^{INK4a} and other members of the INK4 family inhibit G$_1$ cyclin D-dependent kinase (CDK)-4 and CDK6, thereby preventing CDK4/6-directed RB hyperphosphorylation and blocking S phase entry. p19^{ARF} inhibits MDM2-mediated degradation of p53 and plays an important role in the apoptotic elimination of aberrantly cycling cells. p19^{ARF} also possesses p53-independent functions involving the negative regulation of Myc. Human T-ALL and B-ALL often exhibit biallelic deletions of the short arm of chromosome 9 which eliminate both copies of the CDKN2A locus. Although definitive genetic evidence is lacking, the pathogenetic relevance of p14^{ARF} is suggested by the presence of homozygous INK4a/ARF deletions in human T-ALL and B-ALL. Mice doubly null for p16^{INK4a} and p19^{ARF} are viable but succumb to lymphomas or sarcomas with a median latency of approximately 30 weeks [12]. The majority of the lymphomas from the p16^{INK4a} and p19^{ARF} deficient mice are pre-B-LBL, but pre-T-LBL can occur [18]. Although not fully characterized, specific deletion of p16^{INK4a}, p18^{INK4c}, or p19^{ARF} alone also gives rise to lymphoma, supporting the notion that all three genes play a role in transformation.

The PTEN tumor suppressor gene encodes a phosphatase that negatively regulates the phosphatidylinositol 3-kinase (PI3K) pathway. PI3K activates a variety of key signaling proteins such as the Ser/Thr kinase AKT. Activated AKT in turn phosphorylates and modulates the activity of a number of important molecules governing cell cycle control and cell survival, including forkhead transcription factors and the apoptosis regulator BAD. PTEN has a network of interactions with the p53 tumor suppressor and loss of PTEN results in p53-dependent and -independent genomic instability. Loss of PTEN function is common in human T-ALL cells, either at diagnosis or during disease progression. Loss of PTEN has been shown to promote the self-renewal of stem cells [14].

In the mouse, PTEN nullizygosity/knockout leads to early embryonic lethality, whereas PTEN heterozygotes survive and develop neoplasia in multiple organs including lymphoid tissues [12]. PTEN appears to play a particularly prominent role in the growth regulation of immunocytes as evidenced by the prevalence of autoimmune disorders in PTEN+/− mice, relating to impaired thymic negative selection and peripheral tolerance. Furthermore, PTEN deficiency has been proposed to have a role in the pathogenesis of T-cell tumors on the basis of studies in conventional (not conditional) PTEN KO mice. In constructing a mouse model to study the role PTEN in T-ALL, there are several critical limitations to the existing PTEN KO strains. One of the most significant problems is that these animals develop and die of non-hematopoietic tumors, notably carcinomas and sarcomas. The construction of a conditional allele of PTEN that permits gene deletion exclusively in lymphoid cell types at a desired time is therefore needed.

We generated such mice carrying such a conditional PTEN allele by creating a DNA vector that flanked the critical exon 5 of PTEN (encoding the phosphatase domain) with intronic LoxP sites to allow tissue-specific gene deletion using the Cre recombinase (Fig. 36-1) [14]. Following transfection of the vector and selection using the neomycin marker, ES cells containing the construct targeted to the PTEN allele were used to generate germline chimeras by blastocyst microinjection. Southern blotting of tail DNA confirmed the proper targeting and germline transmission of the altered PTEN. Mice carrying functional "floxed" alleles (PTEN^{flox}) were generated in crosses with a CAGG–Flpe transgenic strain that recognized the Flp recombination sites and deleted out the neomycin resistance gene. T-cell specific deletion of exon 5 of PTEN was then generated by crossing PTEN$^{flox/flox}$ mice with LCK-Cre transgenic mice that expressed the Cre recombinase only in T cells.

Such mice with T-cell specific deletion of the PTEN gene developed T-cell neoplasms that exhibited morphologic and immunophenotypic findings similar to human T-ALL

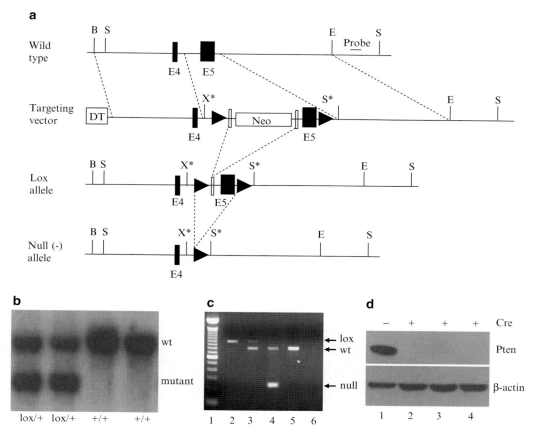

Fig. 36-1. Targeting strategy and analysis of conditional knockout of PTEN. (**a**) Mouse PTEN genomic structure and recombinant alleles. The transcript from the PTEN null allele eliminates exon 5, resulting in a translational frameshift. B, BglII; S, SacI; E, EcoRI; X, XhoI. A neomycin-resistance cassette was flanked by Flp recombination target (FRT) sites (*white bars*), and a Cre recognition LoxP site immediately upstream of the 5' FRT was placed 5' of exon 5 (arrow). A second LoxP site is placed downstream of exon 5 (*arrow*). (**b**) Southern blot analysis of mouse tail DNA digested with SacI and hybridized with the probe as indicated in the panel A. The DNA samples were prepared from the offspring of a chimera X wild type (WT, +) FVB/n mating. (**c**) PCR screen for Cre-mediated PTEN exon 5 deletion. Lane 1, molecular weight marker (1 kb ladder); lane 2, PTEN$^{lox/lox}$; lane 3, PTEN$^{lox/+}$; lane 4, PTEN$^{lox/\Delta 5}$; lane 5, PTEN$^{+/+}$ lane 6, no DNA templete control. (**d**) Western blotting analysis of PTEN expression using anti-PTEN antibody. Anti-β-actin was used for loading controls. Protein specimen was prepared from mouse embryo fibroblasts in the presence (+) or absence (−) of Cre recombinase

(Fig. 36-2 and data not shown). Onset of pre-T-LBL was seen as early as 8 weeks, and these mice typically died of leukemia by 20 weeks. This model provides an example of how tissue-targeted gene expression can result in more well-defined mouse models of lymphoma and leukemias than the non-targeted strategies. As these new technologies are increasingly used to introduce gene into specific B-cell and T-cell compartments, some of the tumor profiles reported for genes in Tables 36-3 and 36-4 may shift.

36.4.3. Summary

Genes that cause human lymphoid neoplasms when aberrantly expressed may or may not produce similar tumors in mice. Several human lymphoid neoplasms do not have defined counterparts in mice. In addition, some lymphoid neoplasms occur more frequently in mice than in humans. However, current mouse models have provided, and newer, improved

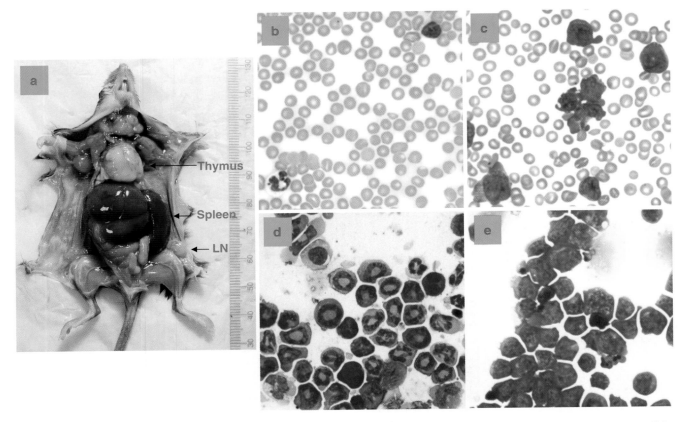

Fig. 36-2. Development of T-ALL in mice with T-cell specific deletion of the PTEN tumor suppressor gene. (**a**) Dissection of a mouse null for PTEN in the T-cell lineage, showing lymphadenopathy, splenomegaly, and a significantly enlarged thymus. (**b**) Peripheral blood smear from a control mouse. (**c**) Peripheral blood smear from PTEN-deficient mouse showing frequent lymphoid blasts. (**d**) Cytospin preparation of bone marrow from a normal control mouse. (**e**) Sheets of blasts present in a bone marrow cytospin from a PTEN-deficient animal

GEMMs will continue to provide insights on the mechanisms of human lymphoid neoplasia and serve as critical tools for preclinical testing of therapeutic agents.

Suggested Readings

Van Dyke T, Jacks T. Cancer modeling in the modern era: progress and challenges. Cell. 2002;108:135–44.
*A seminal review on the goals and problems of mouse modelling.

Sharpless NE, Depinho RA. The mighty mouse: genetically engineered mouse models in cancer drug development. Nat Rev Drug Discov 2006;5:741–54.
*The benefits and pitfalls of using the mouse for drug studies.

Morse HC 3rd, Anver MR, Fredrickson TN, Haines DC, Harris AW, Harris NL, Jaffe ES, Kogan SC, MacLennan IC, Pattengale PK, Ward JM. Bethesda proposals for classification of lymphoid neoplasms in mice. Blood 2002;100:246–58.
*The first comprehensive classification of mouse lymphoid tumors

Teitell MA, Pandolfi PP. Molecular genetics of acute lymphoblastic leukemia. Annu Rev Pathol. 2009;4:175-98.
*An overview of mouse models available in acute leukemia

References

1. Pattengale PK, Frith CH. Immunomorphologic classification of spontaneous lymphoid cell neoplasms occurring in female BALB/c mice. J Natl Cancer Inst 1983;70:169–79.
2. Huebner RJ, Gilden RV, Toni R, et al. Prevention of spontaneous leukemia in AKR mice by type-specific immunosuppression of endogenous ecotropic virogenes. Proc Natl Acad Sci U S A 1976;73:4633–5.
3. Segre JA, Nemhauser JL, Taylor BA, Nadeau JH, Lander ES. Positional cloning of the nude locus: genetic, physical, and transcription maps of the region and mutations in the mouse and rat. Genomics 1995;28:549–59.
4. Bosma MJ, Carroll AM. The SCID mouse mutant: definition, characterization, and potential uses. Annu Rev Immunol 1991;9:323–50.
5. Shultz LD, Schweitzer PA, Christianson SW, et al. Multiple defects in innate and adaptive immunologic function in NOD/LtSz-scid mice. J Immunol 1995;154:180–91.
6. Sharpless NE, Depinho RA. The mighty mouse: genetically engineered mouse models in cancer drug development. Nat Rev Drug Discov 2006;5:741–54.
7. Van Dyke T, Jacks T. Cancer modeling in the modern era: progress and challenges. Cell 2002;108:135–44.
8. Gordon JW, Ruddle FH. Gene transfer into mouse embryos: production of transgenic mice by pronuclear injection. Methods Enzymol 1983;101:411–33.
9. Gossen M, Bujard H. Tight control of gene expression in mammalian cells by tetracycline-responsive promoters. Proc Natl Acad Sci U S A 1992;89:5547–51.
10. Feil R, Brocard J, Mascrez B, LeMeur M, Metzger D, Chambon P. Ligand-activated site-specific recombination in mice. Proc Natl Acad Sci U S A 1996;93:10887–90.
11. Rodriguez CI, Buchholz F, Galloway J, et al. High-efficiency deleter mice show that FLPe is an alternative to Cre-loxP. Nat Genet 2000;25:139–40.
12. You MJ, Castrillon DH, Bastian BC, et al. Genetic analysis of Pten and Ink4a/Arf interactions in the suppression of tumorigenesis in mice. Proc Natl Acad Sci U S A 2002;99:1455–60.
13. Carrasco DR, Sukhdeo K, Protopopova M, et al. The differentiation and stress response factor XBP-1 drives multiple myeloma pathogenesis. Cancer Cell 2007;11:349–60.
14. Zheng H, Ying H, Yan H, et al. p53 and Pten control neural and glioma stem/progenitor cell renewal and differentiation. Nature 2008;455:1129–33.
15. Morse HC 3rd, Anver MR, Fredrickson TN, et al. Bethesda proposals for classification of lymphoid neoplasms in mice. Blood 2002;100:246–58.
16. Swerdlow SH, Campo E, Harris NL, et al. The WHO classification of tumors of hematopoietic and lymphoid tissues. Lyon, France: IARC Press, 2008.
17. Puel A, Ziegler SF, Buckley RH, Leonard WJ. Defective IL7R expression in T(-)B(+)NK(+) severe combined immunodeficiency. Nat Genet 1998;20:394–7.
18. Carrasco DR, Fenton T, Sukhdeo K, et al. The PTEN and INK4A/ARF tumor suppressors maintain myelolymphoid homeostasis and cooperate to constrain histiocytic sarcoma development in humans. Cancer Cell 2006;9:379–90.
19. Liyanage M, Coleman A, du Manoir S, et al. Multicolour spectral karyotyping of mouse chromosomes. Nat Genet 1996;14:312–5.
20. Calin GA, Liu CG, Sevignani C, et al. MicroRNA profiling reveals distinct signatures in B cell chronic lymphocytic leukemias. Proc Natl Acad Sci U S A 2004;101:11755–60.
21. Teitell MA, Pandolfi PP. Lymphoid Malignancies In Holland EC: Mouse Models of Cancer 1st Ed., New York, J Wiley & sons, 2004;237–259.
22. Tarantul VZ. Transgenic mice as an in vivo model of lymphomagenesis. Int Rev Cytol 2004;236:123–80.
23. Canela A, Martin-Caballero J, Flores JM, Blasco MA. Constitutive expression of tert in thymocytes leads to increased incidence and dissemination of T-cell lymphoma in Lck-Tert mice. Mol Cell Biol 2004;24:4275–93.
24. Bessette K, Lang ML, Fava RA, et al. A Stat5b transgene is capable of inducing CD8+ lymphoblastic lymphoma in the absence of normal TCR/MHC signaling. Blood 2008;111:344–50.
25. Shen L, Zhang C, Wang T, et al. Development of autoimmunity in IL-14alpha-transgenic mice. J Immunol 2006;177:5676–86.
26. Chiarle R, Gong JZ, Guasparri I, et al. NPM-ALK transgenic mice spontaneously develop T-cell lymphomas and plasma cell tumors. Blood 2003;101:1919–27.

27. Zhang Y, Finegold MJ, Porteu F, Kanteti P, Wu MX. Development of T-cell lymphomas in Emu-IEX-1 mice. Oncogene 2003;22:6845–51.

28. Hoyer KK, French SW, Turner DE, et al. Dysregulated TCL1 promotes multiple classes of mature B cell lymphoma. Proc Natl Acad Sci U S A 2002;99:14392–7.

29. Bichi R, Shinton SA, Martin ES, et al. Human chronic lymphocytic leukemia modeled in mouse by targeted TCL1 expression. Proc Natl Acad Sci U S A 2002;99:6955–60.

30. Linette GP, Hess JL, Sentman CL, Korsmeyer SJ. Peripheral T-cell lymphoma in lckpr-bcl-2 transgenic mice. Blood 1995;86:1255–60.

31. Egle A, Harris AW, Bath ML, O'Reilly L, Cory S. VavP-Bcl2 transgenic mice develop follicular lymphoma preceded by germinal center hyperplasia. Blood 2004;103:2276–83.

32. Zhou P, Levy NB, Xie H, et al. MCL1 transgenic mice exhibit a high incidence of B-cell lymphoma manifested as a spectrum of histologic subtypes. Blood 2001;97:3902–9.

33. Reitmair AH, Schmits R, Ewel A, et al. MSH2 deficient mice are viable and susceptible to lymphoid tumours. Nat Genet 1995;11:64–70.

34. Edelmann W, Yang K, Umar A, et al. Mutation in the mismatch repair gene Msh6 causes cancer susceptibility. Cell 1997;91:467–77.

35. Wang JH, Alt FW, Gostissa M, et al. Oncogenic transformation in the absence of Xrcc4 targets peripheral B cells that have undergone editing and switching. J Exp Med 2008;205:3079–90.

36. Bassing CH, Suh H, Ferguson DO, et al. Histone H2AX: a dosage-dependent suppressor of oncogenic translocations and tumors. Cell 2003;114:359–70.

37. Sharpless NE, Ramsey MR, Balasubramanian P, Castrillon DH, DePinho RA. The differential impact of p16(INK4a) or p19(ARF) deficiency on cell growth and tumorigenesis. Oncogene 2004;23:379–85.

38. Latres E, Malumbres M, Sotillo R, et al. Limited overlapping roles of P15(INK4b) and P18(INK4c) cell cycle inhibitors in proliferation and tumorigenesis. EMBO J 2000;19:3496–506.

39. Bolitho P, Street SE, Westwood JA, et al. Perforin-mediated suppression of B-cell lymphoma. Proc Natl Acad Sci U S A 2009;106:2723–28.

Chapter 37

Mouse Models of Myeloid Leukemia

Robert B. Lorsbach

Abstract/Scope of Chapter This chapter provides a broad overview of the various techniques used to model human myeloid malignancies and focuses on those areas where mouse modeling has been particularly valuable in advancing our understanding of human myeloid neoplasia. The studies in mice modeling BCR-ABL1-positive chronic myelogenous leukemia, PML–RARA-positive acute promyelocytic leukemia, and the core-binding factor acute myeloid leukemias are discussed in more detail.

Keywords Acute myeloid leukemia, mouse model • Acute promyelocytic leukemia, mouse model • Chronic myelogenous leukemia, mouse model • BCR-ABL1, mouse model • PML–RARA, mouse model • Retrovirus, murine • Viral transduction • Hematopoietic stem cell, mouse • Flow cytometry, mouse antigens • Immunohistochemistry, mouse antigens

37.1. General Considerations in Modeling Human Malignancies in the Mouse

The laboratory mouse has proven to be a powerful genetic tool for the investigation of many biologic processes given the availability of numerous inbred strains. In addition, during the past 20 years, several techniques have been developed to modify the expression of any given target gene in the laboratory mouse. These include the overexpression of a normal gene or introduction of a mutated gene using expression vectors such as retroviruses. Moreover, the development of gene targeting techniques represents perhaps the most powerful and widely used approach for investigating the function of a specific gene product. Using this methodology, numerous mouse strains have been developed in which a particular gene has been deleted (the so-called knockout mouse) or an engineered mutation introduced using either the cognate promoter of the target gene (knock-in mouse) or a heterologous promoter (transgenic mouse) (Table 37-1). These approaches have proven invaluable for the introduction into murine hematopoietic cells of many of the genetic lesions present in various human hematopoietic malignancies, resulting in useful mouse models for several human neoplasms [1,2].

The modeling of human malignancies in mice requires a significant amount of time and resources. Nevertheless, these mouse models offer a number of important advantages over conventional approaches, which typically utilize established cell lines, for the investigation of myeloid malignancy pathogenesis. First, they permit analysis of the direct role of a specific genetic alteration on the development of myeloid malignancy without the potentially confounding influence of other genetic alterations, a distinct advantage over the use of cell

From: *Neoplastic Hematopathology*: Contemporary Hematology,
Edited by: D. Jones, DOI 10.1007/978-1-60761-384-8_37,
© Humana Press, a part of Springer Science+Business Media, LLC 2010

Table 37-1. Myeloid neoplasms in genetically-modified mice.

Human disease	Gene	Method	Disease
AML with t(8;21)	*RUNX1–RUNX1T1*	Runx1 KI	EL[71,72]
		T +M	AML[36]
		Sca1 KI	Non-lethal MN[73]
		CKI + M	AML[34]
	/FLT3-LM	R +M	AML[74]
	/ICSBP–/–	R/T	AML, MS[75]
	/ETV6-PDGFRB	R	AML[76]
	Runx1 alternately spliced transcript	R/T	AML[77]
AML with inv(16)	*CBFB-MYH11*	KI +M	AML[37]
		CKI	AML[78]
APL	*PML–RARA*	T	AML[27,46]
		KI	AML[29,79]
		R	AML[40]
	PML–RARA/Pml+/– or *–/–*	T	AML[80]
	PML–RAR/KRAS[a]	T/KI	AML[81]
	PML–RARA/FLT3–ITD	T	AML[50,51]
	PLZF–RARA	T	AML[82,83]
	PLZF–RARA/RARA–PLZF	T	AML[84]
	NPM-RARA	T	AML[82]
	NUMA-RARA	T	AML[85]
AML with 11q23			
	MLL–MLLT3, t(9;11)	KI	AML, few T-ALL[39]
		TR	AML[86]
	MLL–MLLT10, t(10;11)	R	AML[87]
	MLL–GAS7, t(11;17)	R	AML/ABL/ALL[41]
	MLL–MLLT1, t(11;19)	TR	AML/TL[86]
AML with inv(3)(q21q26.2), t(3;3)(q21;q26.2)	*EVI1*	R	MDS[88]
AML with CEBPA mutation			
	CEBPA	KO p42 isoform	AML[89]
MDS			
NUP98-HOX	*NUP98*	T	MDS/AML[90]
RUNX1 point mutations		R	MDS/AML[91]
	BCL2/mutant *NRAS*	T	MDS/AML[92]
Chronic myeloid leukemia	*BCR–ABL*	T	EL[10]
		R	
CMML	*ETV6-PDGFRB*, t(5;12)	T	MN[93]
		R	MN[94]
Transient leukemia of DS	*GATA1s*	KI	Meg Proliferation[95]

CKI conditional knock-in; *CMML* chronic myelomonocytic leukemia; *DS* Down syndrome; *EL* embryonic lethal; *KI* knock-in; *M* mutagen administration also required for leukemia development; *MS* myeloid sarcoma; *R* retrovirus; *T* transgenic; *TL* T-cell lymphoma; *TR* translocator
[a]Indicates mutant gene encoding activated protein

lines which typically have acquired numerous secondary genetic abnormalities as a consequence of the selective pressures of in vitro culture. Second, genetically-modified mouse models allow for the characterization of the in vivo properties of the modeled malignancy as well as the in vivo testing of candidate therapeutics. With the advent of molecularly-targeted therapeutics, such as imatinib for chronic myelogenous leukemia (CML), the use of genetically-defined mouse models to test the bioavailability, toxicity, and efficacy of newly developed chemotherapeutic agents will undoubtedly be of great value.

Several approaches have been used for modeling myeloid malignancies in the mouse, including xenograft models, genetically modified mice, and hematopoietic stem cell (HSC) retroviral transduction. These have been discussed in detail in Chap. 36. The choice of

Table 37-2. General considerations for experimental approaches for modeling human myeloid malignancy in the mouse.

Technique	Advantages	Disadvantages
Retroviral transduction	Retroviral vectors can be rapidly generated	Requires in vitro culture and enrichment of HSCs
	Transduced cells readily identified in vectors with bicistronic fluorescent protein expression cassettes	Potential for superphysiologic expression of target protein
	Clonality of resulting neoplasm readily assessable	Potential for insertional mutagenesis
	Obviated issues related to embryonic lethality	When used to express fusion oncogenes, does not mimic haploinsufficiency of genes involved in translocation
Gene knock-in	No need for in vitro manipulation of HSCs	Long, expensive process
	Endogenous gene promoter drives physiologic level of expression of target gene	Potential for embryonic lethality
	Expression of target gene directed to appropriate cellular compartment	When used to express fusion oncogenes, mimics haploinsufficiency of only one of the genes involved in translocation
Transgenic	No need for in vitro manipulation of HSCs	May not direct expression of transgene to appropriate cellular compartment
	Wide array of well-characterized, cell-type specific promoter constructs available	Potential for superphysiologic expression of target protein
		When used to express fusion oncogenes, does not mimic haploinsufficiency of genes involved in translocation
		Inappropriately restricted expression of transgene due to promoter properties
		Silencing of transgene expression due to epigenetic phenomena or integration at transcriptionally inactive sites

which experimental technique to employ in the development of a mouse model of myeloid neoplasia depends on several factors (Table 37-2). A critical consideration is the nature of the underlying genetic lesion(s) in the malignancy being modeled. Toxicity or lethal effects of the protein of interest may mandate that its expression be maintained at physiologic levels or restricted to a specific organ or cell type. The nature of the experimental question being asked may have a significant impact on the choice of a model system. For example, a xenograft system in which human cells are transplanted into murine hosts may not be the optimal choice if one is interested in mechanisms governing leukemic cell homing to bone marrow niches, since the critical human cell surface molecules may not interact with their murine counter-receptors. Whether a mouse model will be used solely for in vitro or in vivo analyses or both should also be taken into consideration. Finally, cost and availability of animal care facilities may be an important consideration as the development of genetically-modified mouse strains typically entails several months or even years of expenses.

37.2 Classification of Murine Nonlymphoid Hematopoietic Neoplasms (the Bethesda Proposal)

With even a casual review of published studies in which mouse hematopoietic neoplasms are analyzed, it becomes readily apparent that in many instances such neoplasms are incompletely characterized and the terminology and nomenclature applied to these lesions is inconsistent at best. In an attempt to introduce some degree of uniformity, the Mouse Models of Human Cancers Consortium hematopathology subcommittee published the so-called Bethesda

Table 37-3. Bethesda classification of myeloid neoplasms in mice.

Nonlymphoid leukemias
    Myeloid leukemias
        Myeloid leukemia without maturation
        Myeloid leukemia with maturation
        Myeloproliferative disease-like myeloid leukemia
        Myelomonocytic leukemia
    Monocytic leukemia
    Erythroid leukemia
    Megakaryocytic leukemia
    Biphenotypic leukemia
    Nonlymphoid hematopoietic sarcomas
        Granulocytic sarcoma
        Histiocytic sarcoma
        Mast cell sarcoma
    Myeloid dysplasias
        Myelodysplastic syndrome
        Cytopenia with increased blasts
    Myeloid proliferations (nonreactive)
        Myeloproliferation (genetic)
        Myeloproliferative disease

Proposal, which defines and delineates the diagnostic criteria for the various types of either spontaneous or induced myeloid leukemia, myeloid neoplasia, hematopoietic sarcomas and myeloid dysplasias that may be encountered in mice (Table 37-3) [3]. Unfortunately, many published studies on mouse myeloid neoplasia continue to lack adequate morphologic and immunophenotypic characterization of the reported neoplasms and it is often unclear whether the diagnostic criteria and nomenclature included in the Bethesda proposal were employed. This lack of diagnostic standardization often makes it difficult to assess the published data and to compare the findings obtained through different experimental approaches or by independent research groups. A summary of the diagnostic groups included in the Bethesda Proposal is included in Table 37.3. Investigators involved in the characterization and investigation of myeloid neoplasia in the mouse are encouraged to read the Bethesda Proposal in its entirety, and to apply its categories in all publications related to tumors arising in their models.

37.3 Characterization of Murine Myeloid Neoplasms and Proliferations

The evaluation of murine myeloid neoplasia usually entails morphologic characterization, immunophenotyping, and in some instances molecular evaluation. Because of the anatomic peculiarities of the mouse, as described in the previous section, peripheral blood, bone marrow, spleen, liver, and other tissues as indicated must be examined histologically. As with human tissues, buffered formalin is the most commonly used fixative. Commercially-available kits for the cytochemical detection of myeloperoxidase, specific esterase, and non-specific esterase activities in mouse myelomonocytic cells are available [4]. Immunophenotyping can be achieved through either immunohistochemistry or flow cytometry (Table 37-4). Immunofluorescence is still used and can be technically less challenging since it circumvents to a large extent many of the antigen preservation concerns associated with routinely-fixed tissue. However, a major drawback of immunofluorescence is that it lacks the excellent histologic detail afforded by well-stained sections of formalin-fixed, paraffin-embedded tissue. In the past there have been fewer commercially-available, well-characterized antibodies available for the immunohistochemical detection of mouse antigens than their human counterparts in paraffin-embedded tissue. However, the availability of suitable antibodies for the immunohistochemical characterization of mouse hematopoietic neoplasms is improving

Table 37-4. Useful immunophenotypic markers in evaluation of mouse myeloid neoplasms.

Antigen	Detection method	Normal tissues[a]	Neoplasms[a]
Non-lineage/progenitor			
CD34	F, I	HSC	AML
CD117	F	HSC, MC	AML, MCN
Sca-1	F	HSC	AML
TdT	I	LyPr, BPr, TPr	MPAL
B lineage			
B220	F, I	BPr, B	MPAL
CD19	F	BPr, B	MPAL
T lineage			
CD3	F, I	TPr, T	MPAL
Myeloid			
Mac1 (CD11b)	F, I	MyPr, Mo, Ma	AML, AMoL,
Mac2	F, I	Ma, Mo, DC	AMoL, HS
Mac3 (CD107b)	F, I	Ma, DC	HS, MN
F4/80	F, I	Mo, Ma	AMoL, HS
GR-1	F	MyPr, Neu	AML, MN
Myeloperoxidase	I	MyPr, Neu	AML, MN, MS
Mast cell tryptase	I	MC	MCN
Ter119	F, I	Erythroid	Erythroleukemia
CD41	F	MK, Plt	AMKL
Factor VIII-related Ag	I	MK, Plt	AMKL

AMKL acute megakaryoblastic leukemia; *AMoL* acute monocytic/monoblastic leukemia; *B* mature B cells; *BPr* committed B cell progenitors; *DC* dendritic cell; *F* flow cytometry; *HS* histiocytic sarcoma; *I* immunohistochemistry; *LyPr* lymphoid progenitors; *Ma* macrophage; *MC* mast cell; *MCN* mast cell neoplasms; *MK* megakaryocyte; *MN* myeloproliferative neoplasia; *Mo* monocyte; *MPAL* mixed phenotype acute leukemia; *MS* myeloid sarcoma; *MyPr* myeloid progenitors; *Plt* platelets; *TPr* committed T cell progenitors; *T* mature T cells

[a] Expression within hematopoietic system and neoplasms thereof

with the availability of newly developed antibodies as well as the identification of existing antibodies directed against human antigens which also cross-react with their respective murine homologs [5]. Flow cytometry is also used extensively in the characterization of myeloid proliferations. Peripheral blood, bone marrow, and spleen are particularly amenable to flow cytometry, as single cell suspensions can be readily prepared from these organs. Cell suspensions may be difficult to obtain from other tissues and in marrow and spleen when there is coexisting fibrosis. Histologic examination should be performed in these instances to ensure that the cells evaluated by flow cytometry are representative of those actually present histologically.

Cytogenetic and molecular diagnostics can also be helpful in characterizing mouse myeloid neoplasms. Unlike the lymphoid neoplasms, where clonality can be readily assessed through the detection of clonal rearrangements of either the T-cell or B-cell antigen receptor genes, determination of clonality can be difficult in myeloid neoplasms, particularly those lacking karyotypic abnormalities. When retroviral transduction has been used, clonality of a neoplasm can readily be established through Southern blotting to evaluate proviral integration sites. Conventional cytogenetics is difficult to interpret in the mouse since all murine chromosomes are of comparable size and acrocentric. Nevertheless, techniques such as spectral karyotyping facilitate the detection of chromosomal translocations, deletions, and amplifications in metaphase preparations. Newer techniques, including array-based comparative genomic hybridization, now afford the genome-wide assessment for genomic alterations.

37.4. Modeling Chronic Myelogenous Leukemia

By definition, CML harbors a t(9;22)(q34;q11.2) chromosomal rearrangement that results in the juxtaposition of the *BCR* and *ABL1* genes, located on chromosomes 22 and 9, respectively, and in the expression of the BCR–ABL1 fusion protein [6]. This translocation was the first identified recurrent genetic abnormality in any human malignancy [7]. The chromosomal breakpoint in *ABL1* occurs within a confined region of the gene; however, there is greater variability in the location of the breakpoints within *BCR*, resulting in variable amounts of BCR being incorporated in the fusion transcript (reviewed in Ref. [8]). This variability results in 3 major BCR–ABL1 proteins, namely, the p210, p190, and p230 isoforms. The p210 is expressed most commonly in CML, whereas, the p190 BCR–ABL1 isoform is typically expressed in Ph+ ALL; the p230 isoform is expressed in rare cases. Unless otherwise noted, our discussion will be restricted to the p210 isoform of BCR–ABL1.

Mouse models have been used extensively to investigate the pathogenetic role of BCR–ABL1 in CML (Table 37-1). Initial attempts using transgenic approaches to generate a murine CML model that faithfully reflects the human disease were largely unsuccessful, due to issues relating to embryonic lethality and gene silencing [9,10]. Subsequently, retroviral-transduction and transplantation models have been developed in which mouse BM progenitors are infected with retroviruses containing the BCR–ABL1 coding sequence. Upon integration of the provirus in the genome of infected cells, the retroviral long-terminal repeat drives expression of *BCR–ABL1*. This technique is now the most widely utilized approach for modeling CML in the mouse. In early experiments, there was a low incidence of CML in recipient mice transplanted with transduced BCR–ABL1 expressing BM cells [11,12]. However, with several refinements in the experimental methodology, including the utilization of murine stem cell virus (MSCV)-based vectors, a uniformly lethal CML-like myeloproliferative neoplasm (MPN) is induced in 100% of recipient mice with a 3–4 week latency period [13–15]. Affected mice develop neutrophilic leukocytosis, splenomegaly, and ultimately pulmonary hemorrhage secondary to occlusion of the pulmonary vasculature by myeloid cells. In these animals, the disease resembles chronic phase CML with a low frequency of blasts in primary BM recipients. Interestingly, disease acceleration is observed with serial passage of BCR–ABL1 BM cells into secondary, tertiary, and quaternary recipients, presumably reflecting the need for ongoing cell division in order to acquire the necessary secondary mutations for disease progression [14].

In addition to these proof-of-principle experiments confirming its central pathogenetic role, mouse models of CML have proven invaluable in the investigation of critical motifs of BCR–ABL1 and downstream signaling pathways involved in disease development. Recipient mice transplanted with BM cells expressing a BCR–ABL1 mutant with an inactive tyrosine kinase domain failed to develop CML [15]. While consistent with in vitro data showing that ABL1 kinase activity was needed for transformation, this finding was nevertheless critical since it confirmed that ABL1 kinase activity was necessary and sufficient for leukemogenesis and thus an ideal target for therapy, a conclusion now confirmed by the therapeutic efficacy of the tyrosine kinase inhibitor imatinib in treating chronic phase CML in humans. The SRC homology 2 (SH2) domain of BCR–ABL1 binds several signaling molecules, such as SHC, resulting in markedly reduced PI3K and AKT signaling, suggesting an important pathogenetic role for this domain in CML; however, in vitro studies on the role of the SH2 domain of BCR–ABL1 in cellular transformation yielded contradictory findings [16]. Expression of a SH2 domain mutant of the p210 form of BCR–ABL1 induced leukemia with significantly prolonged latency and alteration of disease immunophenotype, with increased frequency of B lymphoblastic leukemia in recipient mice [17,18]. Interestingly, identical SH2 mutant forms of p190 BCR–ABL1 induced B lymphoblastic leukemia with a comparable latency as did wild-type p190 BCR–ABL1 [17]. These findings indicate that there is a differential requirement for signaling mediated through the SH2 domain in myeloid versus lymphoid disease in BCR–ABL1 expressing cells, and importantly, they suggest that BCR–ABL1 SH2 domain-mediated signaling may not be a suitable target for therapeutic inhibition in CML.

Mouse models have also been used to investigate the role of cytokine signaling in CML pathogenesis. BCR–ABL1 potently induces the expression of IL-3, and initial studies suggested that the growth factor-independent expansion in vitro of BCR–ABL1 expressing BM cells was attributable to autocrine effects of IL-3 [19–21]. To investigate a possible pathogenetic role for IL-3, the development of disease was assessed in mice transplanted with either IL-3 or IL-3R knockout BM cells expressing BCR–ABL1 [22,23]. Surprisingly, given this indirect evidence implicating IL-3 in CML pathogenesis, the incidence and latency of CML development was identical in mice receiving wild type cells and in those defective in IL-3 signaling. These studies highlight the utility of CML mouse models in confirming in vitro findings to identify those BCR–ABL1 mediated signaling pathways which have an obligatory role in disease development.

37.5. Modeling Acute Promyelocytic Leukemia

APL is characterized morphologically by the clonal expansion of malignant myeloid cells with differentiation arrested at the promyelocyte stage. The t(15;17)(q22;q21) chromosomal translocation is present in the preponderance of cases, resulting in the fusion between the genes for promyelocytic leukemia (*PML*) on chromosome 15 and that for the retinoic acid receptor α (*RARA*) on chromosome 17, yielding a fusion transcript which encodes PML–RARα (reviewed in Ref. [24]). Like RARα, this fusion oncoprotein binds to RA response elements (RAREs) located within the promoters of target genes. Upon exposure to RA, RARα together with associated corepressors dissociates from the RARE, thereby inducing expression of the target gene. In contrast to the native protein, PML–RARα is insensitive to physiologic levels of RA, resulting in repressed expression of RARα responsive genes. In addition, PML–RARα interferes with PML function through the dissolution of nuclear PML bodies and inhibition of the normal growth regulatory function of PML.

Several approaches to modeling APL in the mouse have been employed, including BM retroviral transduction, xenografting of human APL cells, and transgenic mice expressing *PML–RARA* under various myeloid-specific promoters (Table 37-1); [25] our discussion will focus largely on the latter. Initial attempts to model APL using the migration inhibitory factor-related protein 8 (MRP8) or the cathepsin G (CG) promoters to drive PML–RARα expression yielded myeloid leukemia with low penetrance and long latency [26–28]. Interestingly, leukemia developed with much higher penetrance in mice in which *PML–RARA* was knocked into the CG locus, a targeting strategy that yielded significantly lower levels of *PML–RARA* mRNA expression than transgenic CG mice [29]. Taken together, these observations suggest that as with several other fusion oncoproteins, PML–RARα expression alone is insufficient for leukemogenesis and that acquisition of cooperating mutations is required [30]. Furthermore, they underscore that leukemogenesis is critically sensitive to both the level at which an oncoprotein is expressed and the cellular compartment in which it is expressed.

Mouse models of APL have been used extensively in structure-function studies of PML–RARα and have provided insight into the role of oligomerization of PML–RARα in oncogenesis. In vitro studies demonstrated that several biologic properties of PML–RARα are oligomerization-dependent, including the recruitment of the transcriptional corepressors NCoR and SMRT and the abrogation of RA-induced differentiation in cell lines [31,32]. To corroborate these findings in vivo, transgenic mice were developed in which RARα was fused to a homodimerization motif (HD-RARα) [33]. While the expression of HD-RARα induced acute leukemia at a low frequency, it induced a highly-penetrant, lethal acute leukemia in cooperation with a constitutively active form of CD131, the common β chain of the receptors for IL-3, IL-5, and GM-CSF. Because HD-RARα lacks any motifs derived from PML and does not disrupt PML body formation, this oncogenic effect of HD-RARα is independent of PML and likely attributable to oligomerization alone.

37.6 Modeling "Second Hits" in Acute Myeloid Leukemia

Through the modeling of several genetically well-defined types of AML in the mouse, it is now apparent that in many instances expression of a translocation encoded fusion oncoprotein alone is insufficient for the development of AML. This has been well demonstrated for those AMLs with translocations targeting components of the core binding factor transcription complex, i.e., AML with t(8;21) and AML with inv(16)/t(16;16). The former translocation results in the juxtaposition of the *RUNX1* and *RUNX1T1* (*ETO*) genes, located on chromosomes 21 and 8, respectively, yielding expression of the RUNX1–RUNX1T1 (more commonly known as RUNX1–ETO) fusion protein. Using both knock-in and various transgenic approaches, mice engineered to express RUNX1–ETO in myeloid cells not only fail to develop leukemia but somewhat surprisingly have rather unremarkable myelopoiesis with normal peripheral blood indices [34–36]. However, a significant fraction of RUNX1–ETO expressing mice develop AML following administration of the chemical mutagen *N*-ethyl-*N*-nitrosourea (ENU), which induces point mutations [34,36]. These findings indicate that overt leukemogenesis in t(8;21) AML requires acquisition of additional mutations. Using a variety of in vivo approaches, it has similarly been established for CBFβ–MYH11 as well as several other fusion oncoproteins (including PML–RARα, PLZF–RARα, and several of the MLL fusion proteins) that leukemogenesis is a multi-step process in which one or more cooperating mutations are required for leukemia development [29,37–42]. These findings have led to the proposal that myeloid oncogenesis requires acquisition of two types of mutation [30]. The so called class I mutations represent gain-of-function alterations that confer on hematopoietic progenitors either enhanced proliferative signaling or increased resistance to apoptosis; mutations in KIT (CD117) or FLT3 which impart constitutive tyrosine kinase activity are good examples of this mutation type. The translocation-encoded fusion oncoproteins represent class II mutations. These are often considered loss-of-function mutations and block or impair myelopoiesis through their perturbation of the gene transcription cascade which underlies myeloid development.

More recent and ongoing studies have been directed at the identification of those secondary mutations which function critically in myeloid leukemogenesis. Given that all leukemic cells possess some level of genomic instability, this will prove to be a more arduous process since perhaps only a small subset of mutations will be pathogenetically "relevant" with most simply being passenger mutations. Recent advances have highlighted how the integration of data from different experimental systems can facilitate the identification of those mutations which function critically in leukemogenesis. Mouse modeling approaches have played an important role in both the identification of these cooperating mutations and analysis of candidate mutations identified through other analyses (Table 37-1).

Mouse models have proven quite valuable for the investigation of biologically-relevant cooperating mutations in APL. RARα–PML is expressed in 70–80% of all human APLs, which is in contrast to many translocation-associated AMLs where the reciprocal product is infrequently expressed [43–45]. Thus, RARα–PML may represent a cooperating mutation in APLs containing t(15;17). In support of this hypothesis, mice transgenic for both *PML–RARA* and *RARA–PML* developed leukemia with significantly greater penetrance than *PML–RARA* single transgenic mice, with no impact on the latency. Expression of RARA–PML alone neither perturbed normal hematopoiesis nor predisposed to leukemia development [46]. Precisely how RARα–PML contributes to leukemogenesis is uncertain, but may involve the perturbation of PML-mediated interactions with hyperphosphorylated RB and p53. The role of other candidate mutations in APL have also been investigated using mouse models. FLT3 is a receptor tyrosine kinase expressed in hematopoietic progenitors and in several types of AML [47]. FLT3 harbors an internal tandem duplication (FLT3–ITD) mutation, which endows it with constitutive tyrosine kinase activity, in nearly 40% of all APL cases [48,49]. In mice with transgenic *PML-RARA*, retroviral transduction of FLT3-ITD into BM cells led to a highly-penetrant APL-like disease with a very short latency compared to that control retrovirus-transduced cells in *PML-RARA* transgenic mice [50,51]. The APL-like disease induced in the P–R/FLT3–ITD animals was responsive to all trans-retinoic acid (ATRA) and transplantable to secondary recipients. These findings indicate that signaling mediated by FLT3–ITD can cooperate with PML–RARα, thus accounting for the observed reduction in disease latency.

AML with inv(16)/t(16;16) is a recognized AML subtype in the 2008 WHO classification of hematopoietic neoplasms [6]. Both the chromosomal inversion and translocation result in the juxtaposition of the *CBFB* and *MYH11* genes generating the CBFβ–MYH11 fusion oncoprotein [52]. As alluded to above, while expression of CBFβ–MYH11 is clearly a central pathogenetic event, expression of this fusion oncoprotein alone is insufficient for leukemia development [37]. Retroviral insertional mutagenesis (RIM) has been used to identify several candidate genes which may cooperate with CBFβ–MYH11 to induce leukemia [53]. RIM is based on the ability of retroviruses to integrate in a relatively random fashion throughout the genome of infected mouse cells, although integration "hot spots" do exist (technique reviewed in detail in Ref. [54]). Retroviral insertion can alter gene expression through several mechanisms. It may directly inhibit gene expression due to insertion into the coding sequence resulting in a truncated transcript or indirectly by functionally disrupting the promoter or enhancer of a given gene. Retroviral insertion may also upregulate gene expression by activating the promoter of the target gene or by mRNA stabilization through the elimination of destabilizing sequences normally located in the 3′ untranslated region of a target gene transcript. To circumvent problems related to immune clearance of virus, immunologically-naïve neonatal mice are typically inoculated with infectious virus. Through the appropriate selection and titering of a particular virus matched to a particular mouse strain, a screen can be performed in which the control mice develop leukemia at a low frequency. A distinct advantage of RIM over chemical mutagen screens is that the stably integrated provirus readily allows for determination of the integration site and identification of flanking genes using PCR-based techniques. Using RIM, 67 unique retroviral insertion sites were identified which cooperate to induce myeloid leukemia in CBFβ–MYH11 chimeric mice; similarly infected wild-type mice failed to develop AML [53]. Overexpression of two candidate genes, *Plag1* and *Plagl2*, via retroviral transduction of BM cells confirmed that both gene products efficiently cooperate with CBFβ–MYH11 to induce AML in recipient mice 3–12 weeks after transplantation. In addition, *PLAGL2* was selectively overexpressed in human AMLs containing the inv(16) [55]. The *PLAG* genes encode zinc finger-containing transcription factors [56]. Chromosomal translocations or gene amplifications targeting the *PLAG1* locus have been identified in several neoplasms, including pleomorphic adenoma, lipoblastoma, and hepatoblastoma [57–59].

Other approaches using mouse modeling have exploited data from gene expression analyses of AML to facilitate identification of CBFβ–MYH11 cooperating mutations. The meningioma 1 (*MN1*) gene was identified as the target of both the t(12;22) in rare cases of AML and the t(4;22) in menengiomas [60,61]. Furthermore, overexpression of MN1 in mouse BM cells induces a myeloproliferative neoplasm in recipient mice characterized by a neutrophilic leukocytosis [62,63]. Genome-wide gene expression profiling of large cohorts of AMLs have identified *MN1* as being significantly and selectively overexpressed in AML with inv(16) [64,65]. MN1 is a transcriptional coactivator of RAR/retinoic x receptor (RXR)-mediated transcription [66]. Given these observations, the role of MN1 in the pathogenesis of this AML subtype was investigated. Using retroviral transduction and BM transplantation, recipient mice receiving CBFβ–MYH11 knock-in BM cells coexpressing MN1 rapidly developed and succumbed to leukemia [62]. In contrast to the myeloproliferative state induced by MN1 overexpression alone, CBFβ–MYH11 and MN1 together induced an AML characterized by a blastic proliferation that expresses progenitor markers, including c-Kit (CD117), in addition to myeloid markers. These data suggest that MN1 may play an important role in the molecular pathogenesis of AML with inv(16). Interestingly, *MN1* overexpression appears to be a predictor of poor prognosis in cytogenetically normal AMLs [67]. In light of the fact that *MN1* is likewise overexpressed in AML with inv(16), an AML subtype with a relatively good prognosis, the mechanism by which MN1 contributes to leukemogenesis and the prognostic impact of its overexpression may be dependent in part on the nature of the underlying primary genetic lesions [68–70]. In summary, these studies demonstrate the important role that mouse modeling can play in the identification and analysis of cooperating mutations in AML, an area of investigation that will undoubtedly grow in importance with the development of novel small molecule inhibitors that will target the signaling pathways downstream of these secondary mutations.

37.7. Practical Considerations in the Evaluation of Myeloid Malignancies in Murine Models

Although they serve as a good experimental system for modeling human malignancies, there are several significant differences in normal hematopoiesis that must be taken into consideration when evaluating mouse models of malignancy. The turnover of hematopoietic cells is significantly higher in mice than in humans. As a result, murine bone marrow is significantly more cellular than that of humans, typically approaching 100% cellularity. Furthermore, in contrast to humans, the spleen functions as a hematopoietic organ throughout life in mice, even under homeostatic conditions. Because of these "space" limitations, leukemic processes in mice may manifest largely in extramedullary sites such as the spleen or liver. The practical impact of this is that these extramedullary sites must be routinely evaluated in any murine leukemia model.

References

1. McCormack E, Bruserud O, Gjertsen BT. Review: genetic models of acute myeloid leukaemia. Oncogene 2008;27(27):3765–79.
2. Sharpless NE, DePinho RA. The mighty mouse: genetically engineered mouse models in cancer drug development. Nat Rev Drug Discov 2006;5(9):741–54.
3. Kogan SC, Ward JM, Anver MR, et al. Bethesda proposals for classification of nonlymphoid hematopoietic neoplasms in mice. Blood 2002;100(1):238–45.
4. Cuenco GM, Nucifora G, Ren R. Human AML1/MDS1/EVI1 fusion protein induces an acute myelogenous leukemia (AML) in mice: a model for human AML. Proc Natl Acad Sci USA 2000;97(4):1760–5.
5. Kunder S, Calzada-Wack J, Holzlwimmer G, et al. A comprehensive antibody panel for immunohistochemical analysis of formalin-fixed, paraffin-embedded hematopoietic neoplasms of mice: analysis of mouse specific and human antibodies cross-reactive with murine tissue. Toxicol Pathol 2007;35(3):366–75.
6. Swerdlow SH, Campo E, Harris NL, et al. WHO classification of tumours of haematopoietic and lymphoid tissues. Lyon: IARC Press, 2008.
7. Nowell PC, Hungerford DA. A minute chromosome in human chronic granulocytic leukemia. Science 1960;132:1497.
8. Wong S, Witte ON. The BCR-ABL story: bench to bedside and back. Annu Rev Immunol 2004;22:247–306.
9. Hariharan IK, Harris AW, Crawford M, et al. A bcr-v-abl oncogene induces lymphomas in transgenic mice. Mol Cell Biol 1989;9(7):2798–805.
10. Heisterkamp N, Jenster G, Kioussis D, Pattengale PK, Groffen J. Human bcr-abl gene has a lethal effect on embryogenesis. Transgenic Res 1991;1(1):45–53.
11. Daley GQ, Van Etten RA, Baltimore D. Induction of chronic myelogenous leukemia in mice by the P210bcr/abl gene of the Philadelphia chromosome. Science 1990;247(4944):824–30.
12. Kelliher MA, McLaughlin J, Witte ON, Rosenberg N. Induction of a chronic myelogenous leukemia-like syndrome in mice with v-abl and BCR/ABL. Proc Natl Acad Sci USA 1990;87(17):6649–53.
13. Li S, Ilaria RL Jr, Million RP, Daley GQ, Van Etten RA. The P190, P210, and P230 forms of the BCR/ABL oncogene induce a similar chronic myeloid leukemia-like syndrome in mice but have different lymphoid leukemogenic activity. J Exp Med 1999;189(9):1399–412.

14. Pear WS, Miller JP, Xu L, et al. Efficient and rapid induction of a chronic myelogenous leukemia-like myeloproliferative disease in mice receiving P210 bcr/abl-transduced bone marrow. Blood 1998;92(10):3780–92.

15. Zhang X, Ren R. Bcr-Abl efficiently induces a myeloproliferative disease and production of excess interleukin-3 and granulocyte-macrophage colony-stimulating factor in mice: a novel model for chronic myelogenous leukemia. Blood 1998;92(10):3829–40.

16. Ren R. Mechanisms of BCR-ABL in the pathogenesis of chronic myelogenous leukaemia. Nat Rev Cancer 2005;5(3):172–83.

17. Roumiantsev S, de Aos IE, Varticovski L, Ilaria RL, Van Etten RA. The src homology 2 domain of Bcr/Abl is required for efficient induction of chronic myeloid leukemia-like disease in mice but not for lymphoid leukemogenesis or activation of phosphatidylinositol 3-kinase. Blood 2001;97(1):4–13.

18. Zhang X, Wong R, Hao SX, Pear WS, Ren R. The SH2 domain of bcr-Abl is not required to induce a murine myeloproliferative disease; however, SH2 signaling influences disease latency and phenotype. Blood 2001;97(1):277–87.

19. Sirard C, Laneuville P, Dick JE. Expression of bcr-abl abrogates factor-dependent growth of human hematopoietic M07E cells by an autocrine mechanism. Blood 1994;83(6):1575–85.

20. Anderson SM, Mladenovic J. The BCR-ABL oncogene requires both kinase activity and src-homology 2 domain to induce cytokine secretion. Blood 1996;87(1):238–44.

21. Hariharan IK, Adams JM, Cory S. bcr-abl oncogene renders myeloid cell line factor independent: potential autocrine mechanism in chronic myeloid leukemia. Oncogene Res 1988;3(4):387–99.

22. Li S, Gillessen S, Tomasson MH, Dranoff G, Gilliland DG, Van Etten RA. Interleukin 3 and granulocyte-macrophage colony-stimulating factor are not required for induction of chronic myeloid leukemia-like myeloproliferative disease in mice by BCR/ABL. Blood 2001;97(5):1442–50.

23. Wong S, McLaughlin J, Cheng D, Shannon K, Robb L, Witte ON. IL-3 receptor signaling is dispensable for BCR-ABL-induced myeloproliferative disease. Proc Natl Acad Sci USA 2003;100(20):11630–5.

24. Wang ZY, Chen Z. Acute promyelocytic leukemia: from highly fatal to highly curable. Blood 2008;111(5):2505–15.

25. Kogan SC. Mouse models of acute promyelocytic leukemia. Curr Top Microbiol Immunol 2007;313:3–29.

26. Brown D, Kogan S, Lagasse E, et al. A PMLRARalpha transgene initiates murine acute promyelocytic leukemia. Proc Natl Acad Sci USA 1997;94(6):2551–6.

27. Grisolano JL, Wesselschmidt RL, Pelicci PG, Ley TJ. Altered myeloid development and acute leukemia in transgenic mice expressing PML-RAR alpha under control of cathepsin G regulatory sequences. Blood 1997;89(2):376–87.

28. He LZ, Tribioli C, Rivi R, et al. Acute leukemia with promyelocytic features in PML/RARalpha transgenic mice. Proc Natl Acad Sci USA 1997;94(10):5302–7.

29. Westervelt P, Lane AA, Pollock JL, et al. High-penetrance mouse model of acute promyelocytic leukemia with very low levels of PML-RARalpha expression. Blood 2003;102(5):1857–65.

30. Speck NA, Gilliland DG. Core-binding factors in haematopoiesis and leukaemia. Nat Rev Cancer 2002;2(7):502–13.

31. Lin RJ, Evans RM. Acquisition of oncogenic potential by RAR chimeras in acute promyelocytic leukemia through formation of homodimers. Mol Cell 2000;5(5):821–30.

32. Minucci S, Maccarana M, Cioce M, et al. Oligomerization of RAR and AML1 transcription factors as a novel mechanism of oncogenic activation. Mol Cell 2000;5(5):811–20.

33. Sternsdorf T, Phan VT, Maunakea ML, et al. Forced retinoic acid receptor alpha homodimers prime mice for APL-like leukemia. Cancer Cell 2006;9(2):81–94.

34. Higuchi M, O'Brien D, Kumaravelu P, Lenny N, Yeoh EJ, Downing JR. Expression of a conditional AML1-ETO oncogene bypasses embryonic lethality and establishes a murine model of human t(8;21) acute myeloid leukemia. Cancer Cell 2002;1(1):63–74.

35. Rhoades KL, Hetherington CJ, Harakawa N, et al. Analysis of the role of AML1-ETO in leukemogenesis, using an inducible transgenic mouse model. Blood 2000;96(6):2108–15.

36. Yuan Y, Zhou L, Miyamoto T, et al. AML1-ETO expression is directly involved in the development of acute myeloid leukemia in the presence of additional mutations. Proc Natl Acad Sci USA 2001;98(18):10398–403.

37. Castilla LH, Garrett L, Adya N, et al. The fusion gene cbfb-MYH11 blocks myeloid differentiation and predisposes mice to acute myelomonocytic leukaemia. Nat Genet 1999;23(2):144–6.

38. Corral J, Lavenir I, Impey H, et al. An Mll-AF9 fusion gene made by homologous recombination causes acute leukemia in chimeric mice: a method to create fusion oncogenes. Cell 1996;85(6):853–61.

39. Dobson CL, Warren AJ, Pannell R, et al. The mll-AF9 gene fusion in mice controls myeloproliferation and specifies acute myeloid leukaemogenesis. EMBO J 1999;18(13):3564–74.

40. Minucci S, Monestiroli S, Giavara S, et al. PML-RAR induces promyelocytic leukemias with high efficiency following retroviral gene transfer into purified murine hematopoietic progenitors. Blood 2002;100(8):2989–95.

41. So CW, Karsunky H, Passegue E, Cozzio A, Weissman IL, Cleary ML. MLL-GAS7 transforms multipotent hematopoietic progenitors and induces mixed lineage leukemias in mice. Cancer Cell 2003;3(2):161–71.

42. Wong P, Iwasaki M, Somervaille TC, So CW, Cleary ML. Meis1 is an essential and rate-limiting regulator of MLL leukemia stem cell potential. Genes Dev 2007;21(21):2762–74.

43. Alcalay M, Zangrilli D, Fagioli M, et al. Expression pattern of the RAR alpha-PML fusion gene in acute promyelocytic leukemia. Proc Natl Acad Sci USA 1992;89(11):4840–4.

44. Grimwade D, Howe K, Langabeer S, et al. Establishing the presence of the t(15;17) in suspected acute promyelocytic leukaemia: cytogenetic, molecular and PML immunofluorescence assessment of patients entered into the M.R.C. ATRA trial. M.R.C. Adult Leukaemia Working Party. Br J Haematol 1996;94(3):557–73.

45. Li YP, Andersen J, Zelent A, et al. RAR alpha1/RAR alpha2-PML mRNA expression in acute promyelocytic leukemia cells: a molecular and laboratory-clinical correlative study. Blood 1997;90(1):306–12.

46. Pollock JL, Westervelt P, Kurichety AK, Pelicci PG, Grisolano JL, Ley TJ. A bcr-3 isoform of RARalpha-PML potentiates the development of PML-RARalpha-driven acute promyelocytic leukemia. Proc Natl Acad Sci USA 1999;96(26):15103–8.

47. Gilliland DG, Griffin JD. The roles of FLT3 in hematopoiesis and leukemia. Blood 2002;100(5):1532–42.

48. Callens C, Chevret S, Cayuela JM, et al. Prognostic implication of FLT3 and Ras gene mutations in patients with acute promyelocytic leukemia (APL): a retrospective study from the European APL Group. Leukemia 2005;19(7):1153–60.

49. Kottaridis PD, Gale RE, Frew ME, et al. The presence of a FLT3 internal tandem duplication in patients with acute myeloid leukemia (AML) adds important prognostic information to cytogenetic risk group and response to the first cycle of chemotherapy: analysis of 854 patients from the United Kingdom Medical Research Council AML 10 and 12 trials. Blood 2001;98(6):1752–9.

50. Kelly LM, Kutok JL, Williams IR, et al. PML/RARalpha and FLT3-ITD induce an APL-like disease in a mouse model. Proc Natl Acad Sci USA 2002;99(12):8283–8.

51. Sohal J, Phan VT, Chan PV, et al. A model of APL with FLT3 mutation is responsive to retinoic acid and a receptor tyrosine kinase inhibitor, SU11657. Blood 2003;101(8):3188–97.

52. Liu P, Tarle SA, Hajra A, et al. Fusion between transcription factor CBF beta/PEBP2 beta and a myosin heavy chain in acute myeloid leukemia. Science 1993;261(5124):1041–4.

53. Castilla LH, Perrat P, Martinez NJ, et al. Identification of genes that synergize with Cbfb-MYH11 in the pathogenesis of acute myeloid leukemia. Proc Natl Acad Sci USA 2004;101(14):4924–9.

54. Uren AG, Kool J, Berns A, van Lohuizen M. Retroviral insertional mutagenesis: past, present and future. Oncogene 2005;24(52):7656–72.

55. Landrette SF, Kuo YH, Hensen K, et al. Plag1 and Plagl2 are oncogenes that induce acute myeloid leukemia in cooperation with Cbfb-MYH11. Blood 2005;105(7):2900–7.

56. Van DF, Declercq J, Braem CV, Van de V. PLAG1, the prototype of the PLAG gene family: versatility in tumour development (review). Int J Oncol 2007;30(4):765–74.

57. Kas K, Voz ML, Roijer E, et al. Promoter swapping between the genes for a novel zinc finger protein and beta-catenin in pleiomorphic adenomas with t(3;8)(p21;q12) translocations. Nat Genet 1997;15(2):170–4.

58. Zatkova A, Rouillard JM, Hartmann W, et al. Amplification and overexpression of the IGF2 regulator PLAG1 in hepatoblastoma. Genes Chromosomes Cancer 2004;39(2):126–37.

59. Hibbard MK, Kozakewich HP, Dal CP, et al. PLAG1 fusion oncogenes in lipoblastoma. Cancer Res 2000;60(17):4869–72.

60. Buijs A, Sherr S, Van BS, et al. Translocation (12;22) (p13;q11) in myeloproliferative disorders results in fusion of the ETS-like TEL gene on 12p13 to the MN1 gene on 22q11. Oncogene 1995;10(8):1511–9.

61. Lekanne Deprez RH, Riegman PH, Groen NA, et al. Cloning and characterization of MN1, a gene from chromosome 22q11, which is disrupted by a balanced translocation in a meningioma. Oncogene 1995;10(8):1521–8.

62. Carella C, Bonten J, Sirma S, et al. MN1 overexpression is an important step in the development of inv(16) AML. Leukemia 2007;21(8):1679–90.

63. Heuser M, Argiropoulos B, Kuchenbauer F, et al. MN1 overexpression induces acute myeloid leukemia in mice and predicts ATRA resistance in patients with AML. Blood 2007;110(5):1639–47.

64. Ross ME, Mahfouz R, Onciu M, et al. Gene expression profiling of pediatric acute myelogenous leukemia. Blood 2004;104(12):3679–87.

65. Valk PJ, Verhaak RG, Beijen MA, et al. Prognostically useful gene-expression profiles in acute myeloid leukemia. N Engl J Med 2004;350(16):1617–28.

66. van Wely KH, Molijn AC, Buijs A, et al. The MN1 oncoprotein synergizes with coactivators RAC3 and p300 in RAR-RXR-mediated transcription. Oncogene 2003;22(5):699–709.

67. Heuser M, Beutel G, Krauter J, et al. High meningioma 1 (MN1) expression as a predictor for poor outcome in acute myeloid leukemia with normal cytogenetics. Blood 2006;108(12):3898–905.

68. Byrd JC, Mrozek K, Dodge RK, et al. Pretreatment cytogenetic abnormalities are predictive of induction success, cumulative incidence of relapse, and overall survival in adult patients with de novo acute myeloid leukemia: results from Cancer and Leukemia Group B (CALGB 8461). Blood 2002;100(13):4325–36.

69. Grimwade D, Walker H, Oliver F, et al. The importance of diagnostic cytogenetics on outcome in AML: analysis of 1, 612 patients enrolled into the MRC AML 10 trial. Blood 1998;92(7):2322–33.

70. Slovak ML, Kopecky KJ, Cassileth PA, et al. Karyotypic analysis predicts outcome of preremission and postremission therapy in adult acute myeloid leukemia: a Southwest Oncology Group/Eastern Cooperative Oncology Group Study. Blood 2000;96(13):4075–83.

71. Okuda T, Cai Z, Yang S, et al. Expression of a knocked-In AML1-ETO leukemia gene inhibits the establishment of normal definitive hematopoiesis and directly generates dysplastic hematopoietic progenitors [In Process Citation]. Blood 1998;91(9):3134–43.

72. Yergeau DA, Hetherington CJ, Wang Q, et al. Embryonic lethality and impairment of haematopoiesis in mice heterozygous for an AML1-ETO fusion gene. Nat Genet 1997;15(3):303–6.

73. Fenske TS, Pengue G, Mathews V, et al. Stem cell expression of the AML1/ETO fusion protein induces a myeloproliferative disorder in mice. Proc Natl Acad Sci USA 2004;101(42):15184–9.

74. Schessl C, Rawat VP, Cusan M, et al. The AML1-ETO fusion gene and the FLT3 length mutation collaborate in inducing acute leukemia in mice. J Clin Invest 2005;115(8):2159–68.

75. Schwieger M, Lohler J, Friel J, Scheller M, Horak I, Stocking C. AML1-ETO inhibits maturation of multiple lymphohematopoietic lineages and induces myeloblast transformation in synergy with ICSBP deficiency. J Exp Med 2002;196(9):1227–40.

76. Grisolano JL, O'Neal J, Cain J, Tomasson MH. An activated receptor tyrosine kinase, TEL/PDGF{beta}R, cooperates with AML1/ETO to induce acute myeloid leukemia in mice. Proc Natl Acad Sci USA 2003;100(16):9506–11.

77. Yan M, Kanbe E, Peterson LF, et al. A previously unidentified alternatively spliced isoform of t(8;21) transcript promotes leukemogenesis. Nat Med 2006;12(8):945–9.

78. Kuo YH, Landrette SF, Heilman SA, et al. Cbf beta-SMMHC induces distinct abnormal myeloid progenitors able to develop acute myeloid leukemia. Cancer Cell 2006;9(1):57–68.

79. Lane AA, Ley TJ. Neutrophil elastase cleaves PML-RARalpha and is important for the development of acute promyelocytic leukemia in mice. Cell 2003;115(3):305–18.

80. Rego EM, Wang ZG, Peruzzi D, He LZ, Cordon-Cardo C, Pandolfi PP. Role of promyelocytic leukemia (PML) protein in tumor suppression. J Exp Med 2001;193(4):521–9.

81. Chan IT, Kutok JL, Williams IR, et al. Oncogenic K-ras cooperates with PML-RAR alpha to induce an acute promyelocytic leukemia-like disease. Blood 2006;108(5):1708–15.

82. Cheng GX, Zhu XH, Men XQ, et al. Distinct leukemia phenotypes in transgenic mice and different corepressor interactions generated by promyelocytic leukemia variant fusion genes PLZF-RARalpha and NPM-RARalpha. Proc Natl Acad Sci USA 1999;96(11):6318–23.

83. He LZ, Guidez F, Triboli C, et al. Distinct interactions of PML-RARalpha and PLZF-RARalpha with co-repressors determine differential responses to RA in APL. Nat Genet 1998;18(2):126–35.

84. He LZ, Bhaumik M, Triboli C, et al. Two critical hits for promyelocytic leukemia. Mol Cell 2000;6(5):1131–41.

85. Sukhai MA, Wu X, Xuan Y, et al. Myeloid leukemia with promyelocytic features in transgenic mice expressing hCG-NuMA-RARalpha. Oncogene 2004;23(3):665–78.

86. Drynan LF, Pannell R, Forster A, et al. Mll fusions generated by Cre-loxP-mediated de novo trans-locations can induce lineage reassignment in tumorigenesis. EMBO J 2005;24(17):3136–46.

87. DiMartino JF, Ayton PM, Chen EH, Naftzger CC, Young BD, Cleary ML. The AF10 leucine zipper is required for leukemic transformation of myeloid progenitors by MLL-AF10. Blood 2002;99(10):3780–5.

88. Buonamici S, Li D, Chi Y, et al. EVI1 induces myelodysplastic syndrome in mice. J Clin Invest 2004;114(5):713–9.

89. Kirstetter P, Schuster MB, Bereshchenko O, et al. Modeling of C/EBPalpha mutant acute myeloid leukemia reveals a common expression signature of committed myeloid leukemia-initiating cells. Cancer Cell 2008;13(4):299–310.

90. Lin YW, Slape C, Zhang Z, Aplan PD. NUP98-HOXD13 transgenic mice develop a highly penetrant, severe myelodysplastic syndrome that progresses to acute leukemia. Blood 2005;106(1):287–95.

91. Watanabe-Okochi N, Kitaura J, Ono R, et al. AML1 mutations induced MDS and MDS/AML in a mouse BMT model. Blood 2008;111(8):4297–308.

92. Omidvar N, Kogan S, Beurlet S, et al. BCL-2 and mutant NRAS interact physically and function-ally in a mouse model of progressive myelodysplasia. Cancer Res 2007;67(24):11657–67.

93. Ritchie KA, Aprikyan AA, Bowen-Pope DF, et al. The Tel-PDGFRbeta fusion gene produces a chronic myeloproliferative syndrome in transgenic mice. Leukemia 1999;13(11):1790–803.

94. Tomasson MH, Sternberg DW, Williams IR, et al. Fatal myeloproliferation, induced in mice by TEL/PDGFbetaR expression, depends on PDGFbetaR tyrosines 579/581 [see comments]. J Clin Invest 2000;105(4):423–32.

95. Li Z, Godinho FJ, Klusmann JH, Garriga-Canut M, Yu C, Orkin SH. Developmental stage-selective effect of somatically mutated leukemogenic transcription factor GATA1. Nat Genet 2005;37(6):613–9.

Chapter 38

Designing Targeted Therapies for Lymphomas and Leukemias

Dan Jones

Abstract/Scope of Chapter This chapter gathers together many of the major themes of this textbook to identify shared and unique features of myeloid, T-cell, and B-cell malignancies. Therapeutic strategies that link basic immune function and cell signaling with oncogenesis are beginning to emerge and are discussed here. Considered are strategies to manipulate the microenvironment, alter tumor localization, target tumor-specific metabolic responses, and eliminate residual disease before tumor progression can occur.

Keywords Chemotherapy, classes • Immunotherapy, antibody-based • Drugs, targeting transcription factors • Kinase inhibitors • Pharmacokinetics • Pharmacodynamics • Pharmacogenomics • Cancer, models • Lymphoma, targeted therapy • Leukemia, targeted therapy • Cancer, initiation • Cancer, progression • Lymphoma, genetic syndromes, leukemia, genetic syndromes • Drugs, targeting mitochondria • Drugs, anti-apoptotic • Drugs, proteasome inhibitors • Chemokines • Integrins • Adhesion molecules, types • Mesenchymal stem cells, ex vivo manipulation

38.1. The Current State of Cancer Therapy

38.1.1. The Effectiveness and Downsides of Conventional Cytotoxic Chemotherapy

Most of the improvements in outcomes for human cancers over the last 70 years have been due to the adoption of chemotherapy regimens consisting of multiple different compounds that target general cellular metabolic processes common to all cells. Most of these drugs affect functions of DNA replication, such as DNA-crosslinking/alkylating agents (e.g., cyclophosphamide), chain-terminating nucleoside analogues/polymerase inhibitors (e.g., cytarabine), drugs which target the metabolism of nucleic acids (e.g., methotrexate), inhibitors of DNA unwinding/topoisomerases (e.g., etoposide), and mitotic spindle poisons (e.g., taxol). The effectiveness of these agents is related to their selective actions on rapidly dividing cells, which include all high-grade neoplasms. There have been vast improvements in the design of cytotoxic chemotherapy protocols since their first use by Sidney Farber in the 1940s against pediatric leukemias. In particular, the work of Emil Frei and Emil Freireich at the National Cancer Institute, and others in the 1950s and 1960s, demonstrated the effectiveness of combining different classes of agents [1]. Since that time, the development of a range of different cytotoxic agents in each drug class with different pharmacodynamic (PD) and pharmacokinetic (PK) characteristics, including some with cell-type selectivity, [2,3] have led to steady improvements in outcomes.

From: *Neoplastic Hematopathology*: Contemporary Hematology,
Edited by: D. Jones, DOI 10.1007/978-1-60761-384-8_38,
© Humana Press, a part of Springer Science+Business Media, LLC 2010

There are several obvious downsides to the use of these types of DNA-damaging agents. First, toxicities arise due to the actions of these drugs against rapidly dividing *non-neoplastic* populations (e.g., gastrointestinal mucosa, skin, and hematopoietic elements) which can lead to depressed immune function and infections, suppression of hematopoiesis, and (unpredictable) lethal multiorgan failure. Advances in supportive care, including use of prophylactic antibiotics, growth factors to overcome cytopenias, and chemoprotective agents such as Mesna, have led to improvements in the tolerability of high-dose chemotherapy. Similarly, better monitoring and drug dosing, particularly with the introduction of reduced-intensity conditioning, have dramatically reduced mortality rates for stem cell transplantation, particularly in the treatment of lymphomas.

However, nearly all classical chemotherapy drugs are also mutagenic and the newer intensive therapies for lymphomas and solid tumors have resulted in high rates of secondary malignancies. Furthermore, most standard regimens usually include several DNA-damaging drugs that capitalize on the rapidly dividing nature of tumor cells that lack a functional G1-S cell cycle checkpoint. These agents thus synergize with the tumor-associated defects in DNA repair to produce additional genetic defects in any residual tumor cells. Given the difficulties in avoiding this situation, future goals for cancer therapy should be to aggressively target low-grade tumors that have not yet developed DNA repair defects and to aim for as little residual disease as possible after initial therapy for higher-grade tumors. In this regard, the expanded use of less-toxic targeted agents for maintenance or consolidation after induction therapy is a growing trend. As more targeted therapy agents with lower toxicities become available, the potential to achieve marked reductions in residual disease is evident. This chapter will describe some of the more common classes of new agents and the pathways that they target.

38.1.2. The Challenges of New Drug Design

The task of replacing standard DNA-damaging chemotherapy with less toxic, more targeted agents is a daunting one. First, the target(s) to be attacked must be chosen based on an understanding of the underlying biology of each tumor type. Second, drugs must be developed that do not target non-neoplastic cells to the same degree as tumors and that have favorable PD and PK profiles (Table 38-1). Finally, consideration must be given to the expected patterns of secondary resistance and the methods used to detect them. In this chapter, we summarize the successes to date, and highlight the most promising approaches for the future.

Table 38-1. Parameters to be considered in drug development.

Parameter	Definitions	Parameters measured
Pharmacokinetic	Absorption, distribution, metabolism, and excretion of a drug	Formulation (oral vs. SQ vs. intravenous) and bioavailability Plasma concentration (often by mass spectrometry) Volume of distribution, half-life Total drug exposure ("area-under-the-curve" method)
Pharmacodynamic	Interactions of drug with its target or with other unintended molecules and pathways	Dose-response curves, minimum inhibitory concentration Toxicity profile
Pharmacogenomic	How a genetic polymorphism in any given patient alters response to a drug	SNP profiles (e.g., FcγR SNPs correlated with rituximab action) Genetic regulation of enzyme isoforms [e.g., expressed cytochrome 450 (CYP) or glutathione S-transferase isoforms]. Enzyme activity assays
Tumor-associated	How a given tumor responds to a given drug	In vitro response of cultured tumor to different drugs Predictive biomarkers (protein, mRNA, microRNA, genetic changes) Predicted response based on bioinformatics or in silico models Metabolomic signatures

38.1.3. Immunotherapy Directed Against Lineage-Specific Antigens

The most significant advance in therapy of lymphomas in the last decade has been the use of therapeutic antibodies directed against the pan-B-cell marker CD20. Rituximab, in particular, has resulted in improvements in outcomes for B-cell malignancies particularly diffuse large B-cell lymphoma (DLBCL), which is detailed in Chap. 33. This success with rituximab has launched the use of a large number of other therapeutic antibodies, including targeting the pan-myeloid antigen CD33 in acute myeloid leukemia (AML), other pan-B cell markers (CD19, CD22) in B-cell malignancies, and activation markers such as CD25 and CD30 in T-cell malignancies [4].

To date, none of these other antibodies have had the same therapeutic impact as anti-CD20 therapy suggesting that the specifics of the antigen to be targeted (e.g., its processing and function), the immune pathways engaged following drug binding (e.g., complement-mediated cytotoxicity versus direct toxicity), and the PD and PK of the antibody preparation are all critical. Recent improvements in therapeutic antibody design, including defucosylation to improve potency [5] and the use of bispecific reagents that target two antigens simultaneously, [6,7] may result in new successes for this type of therapy.

38.1.4. Targeting Signaling in Myeloid Neoplasms

Two different types of agents used against myeloid malignancies have shown that if a critical tumor-specific target can be found, therapy can be revolutionized. In acute promyelocytic leukemia (APL), it was discovered that all-trans retinoic acid (ATRA) was effective in maturing the neoplastic myeloid clone and achieving complete remissions in the majority of APL. It was subsequently demonstrated that this dramatic response was due to the fact that ATRA selectively binds to altered retinoid receptor transcriptional complexes produced by the t(15;17) chromosomal translocation in APL [8]. This understanding has led to a focus on developing differentiation-based targeted therapies for other acute leukemias that have altered transcription factors as initiating factors. However, dramatic responses similar to that seen with ATRA have not yet been achieved.

Similarly important was the discovery that the small molecule kinase inhibitor imatinib (Gleevec) could selectively target the kinase activity of BCR–ABL which is overproduced by the t(9;22)/BCR–ABL translocation in chronic myelogenous leukemia (CML). Daily use of this largely non-toxic compound has led to dramatic and lasting responses in nearly all patients diagnosed in the chronic phase of CML [9]. However, experience over the last 10 years using imatinib and other kinase inhibitors in other leukemias and solid tumors has shown that few tumors have a similarly strong dependency (termed "oncogene addiction") on one targetable kinase as does CML on BCR–ABL. Nonetheless, the sophisticated introduction of kinase inhibitors as part of multiagent regimens is beginning to show promising results, as with the use of FLT3 inhibitors in AML [10] and JAK2, KIT, and EGFR inhibitors in leukemias and some solid tumors (Table 38-2).

38.1.5. The Linkage Between Targeted Therapy and Personalized Medicine

In prior chapters, we have emphasized the growing importance of prognostic models that combine molecular genetic features of lymphomas and leukemias with the classical clinical and hematologic parameters. In the most sophisticated models (e.g., the molecular classification of AML), large numbers of genetic risk groups and potentially targetable genetic defects can be identified. This suggests that in the near future, molecular classification will lead to an individualized risk and therapeutic profile for every patient with leukemia. The introduction of patient-specific genetic polymorphisms in drug metabolizing and response genes (termed pharmacogenomics) will likely further individualize therapy. This level of personalized therapy poises a daunting challenge for drug design since accumulating enough patients for any given clinical trial to demonstrate effectiveness becomes a challenge even for the large cooperative oncology groups.

Table 38-2. Targetable growth factor pathway mutations in hematologic malignancies.

Tumor type	Genetic alteration/mutation	Tumor type	Effect(s)
Myeloproliferative neoplasms	BCR–ABL fusion	CML	Activation of relocalized kinase
	JAK2 kinase PM	MPNs	or ligand-independent signaling or
	MPL receptor PM	MPNs	hypersensitivity to lower levels of growth factor
	PDGFR kinase fusion	HES/MCD	
	KIT receptor kinase PM	MCD	
Acute myeloid leukemia	KIT receptor PM	CBF–AML	Ligand-independent signaling
Lymphoma	JAK2 kinase amplification	MBCL	Hypersensitivity to lower levels of growth factor
	SYK kinase activation	DLBCL	
	LCK kinase fusion/mutation	PTCL, ALL-T	

PM point mutation; *CML* chronic myelogenous leukemia; *MPNs* myeloproliferative neoplasm; *HES* hypereosinophilic syndrome; *MCD* mast cell disease; *CBF* core-binding factor leukemias; *MBCL* mediastinal B-cell lymphoma; *DLBCL* diffuse large B-cell lymphoma; *PTCL* peripheral T-cell lymphoma; *ALL-T* T-lymphoblastic leukemia/lymphoma

38.2. Shared and Non-shared Features of Transformation in Hematopoietic and Lymphoid Tumors

38.2.1. Conceptual Models of Oncogenesis

In order to improve targeted therapies, it is important to develop conceptual models of how neoplasms arise and how they progress. For many years, the development of tumors was conceptualized as a two-stage process of initiation and progression with specific environmental or genetic factors contributing more to one step or the other. A highly-influential expansion of this model was the step-wise cancer progression model developed for colorectal cancers by Bert Vogelstein and colleagues, which postulated that the certain genetic events precede others in an orderly sequence from hyperplasia to benign tumor to fully malignant transformation (i.e., the adenoma–carcinoma sequence) [11]. This model was heavily based on the observed histologic progression in many solid tumors from well-differentiated tumors resembling their normal tissue counterparts to poorly differentiated ones. While these models were conceptually important, they appear too simple to match the observed and experimentally-defined patterns of all human cancers, including many hematologic malignancies.

In their seminal review "The Hallmarks of Cancer," Hanahan and Weinberg proposed that oncogenesis is better modeled as a grouping of interrelated functional features that a cancer cell must acquire before full neoplastic transformation can occur [12]. These include:

- Limitless replicative potential
- Self-sufficiency in growth signals
- Evasion of apoptosis
- Insensitivity to anti-growth signals
- Sustained angiogenesis (or more broadly, microenvironmental conditioning)
- Tissue invasion and metastasis (or dissemination, in the case of lymphomas and leukemias)

This schema has been useful in conceptualizing the challenges for cancer therapy since it highlights features which are common to all cancers (e.g., acquisition of the "stem cell-like" binary capacity for unlimited replication) and which pathways might be unique to each tumor type. In this regard, it is important to distinguish between the problem(s) to be solved by the tumor (e.g., growth factor independence) from the method(s) that any given neoplasm employs to achieve it. For example, the acquisition of growth self-sufficiency in myeloid leukemias might be accomplished by chromosomal translocation (e.g., BCR–ABL in CML), activating mutations of signaling molecules (e.g., JAK2 in polycythemia vera), inactivating mutations in growth inhibitory pathways (e.g., SOCS1 deletion in lymphomas), or more complex patterns of epigenetic shifts and transcriptional networks (e.g., coordinate dysregulation of CD30/CD40/TNFR and their ligands in DLBCL) [13,14]. Thus, general oncogenic processes provide targets for therapy development but obtaining tumor-specific effects must be based on an understanding of the different routes to full transformation in each lymphoma and leukemia subtype.

38.2.2. Factors Related to the Initiation of Lymphomas and Leukemias

Understanding the early events in leukemia and lymphoma development is critical to the success of strategies to reduce their incidence in the population. It is clear that persistent antigen stimulation plays an important role in outgrowth of both B-cell and T-cell lymphoma subtypes. This is particularly true at extranodal sites where certain infections and autoimmune diseases are strongly linked to the development of lymphoma (see Chaps. 15 and 27). These effects may explain the dramatic differences in the incidence of particular lymphomas in different genetic populations, such as the near absence of germinal center (GC)-derived lymphomas and increases in mature T-cell lymphomas and Epstein-Barr virus (EBV) lymphomas in some Asian countries [15–17]. SNP-based genome association studies have begun to implicate population-based inherited variations in immune regulatory genes as contributors to risk for certain hematologic malignancies, but the effects are complex and difficult to summarize at this time (see Chap. 32).

However, a large percentage of lymphomas and leukemias do not have a known environmental predisposing factor. In the absence of well-defined epidemiologic risk factors, clues to the most important genetic causes for sporadic leukemias and lymphomas can be gleaned from the genes and pathways that are involved in inherited or germline syndromes that give rise to hematopoietic tumors.

As summarized in Table 38-3, genetic syndromes associated with defective DNA repair (particularly those involving inactivation of genes in the double-stranded DNA break repair pathway, such as ATM and NBS1/NBN) frequently give rise to lymphomas and lymphoid leukemias, but much less frequently to other hematopoietic tumors [18]. Lymphoid neoplasms arising in these patients can have the identical chromosomal translocations as seen in sporadic tumors of the same morphologic type (e.g., inv14(q12;q32.1)/TCL1-TCRA in ATM-associated T-cell prolymphocytic leukemia/T-PLL) [19] consistent with a role for the inherited defect in generating tumor-initiating aberrant chromosomal rearrangements.

In contrast, the functions of genes mutated in inherited syndromes that predispose to myeloid neoplasms are more diverse. Some produce bone marrow failure where stress hematopoiesis and defects in basic cellular metabolism are implicated (e.g., Shwachman–Diamond and Diamond–Blackfan anemias). Others include germline mismatch repair or p53 mutations where an increased incidence of many tumor types is noted due to the generalized mutator phenotype (e.g., Li–Fraumeni syndrome). The reasons for myeloid tumor development in other cases, such as Down syndrome (i.e., gain of chromosome 21 material), are not yet clear.

One likely explanation for differences in the propensity of certain mutations to produce lymphoid over myeloid tumors relates to the presence of the antigen receptor DNA recombination machinery that is present in lymphocytes but not in other hematopoietic cells. This recombination capacity may lead to more frequent generation of anomalous recombination events that go unrepaired in patients with pre-existing DNA repair defects. The frequent involvement of the immunoglobulin heavy chain (IGH) and T-cell receptor (TCR) gene as one partner in lymphoma-associated translocations supports a prominent role for aberrant V-D-J or class-switch recombination in tumor development.

However, there are also clear differences in the types of genes that most effectively transform lymphoid and myeloid cells. In particular, there is an increased incidence of lymphomas in patients with inherited mutations in apoptotic regulators (e.g., FAS and FAS-ligand). These syndromes produce marked pre-neoplastic expansions of lymphocytes with lymphomas usually emerging only later in early adulthood after the precursor pool has been expanded.

Table 38-3. Germline/genetic syndromes associated with lymphomas and leukemias.

Syndrome	Gene mutated	Functions of gene(s)	Hematologic phenotype	Hematologic tumor types
Syndromes with increased risk of lymphoid tumors				
Autoimmune lymphoproliferative syndrome (ALPS)	FAS (CD95), FASLG, [70] NRAS [71]	T-cell elimination following activation [72]	Defective lymphocyte apoptosis Increased CD3+CD4−CD8− and CD8+ T cells	14X ↑ in NHL 51X ↑ in NLP-HL [73]
X-linked immunodeficiency with hyper-IgM (XLP)	CD40L [74], CD40	T-cell help for B-cell class switch and GC function	Neutropenia, infections, diarrhea	EBV+ B-cell LPD
Wiscott–Aldrich syndrome (WAS)	WASP [75]	TCR/BCR signal modulator	Thrombocytopenia, eczema and recurrent infections	EBV+ LyG-like lymphomas GCB lymphomas LGL proliferation
Common variable immunodeficiency	Multigenic, including a number of cytokine genes [76]	Various	Defects in lymphocyte maturation and production	EBV+ B-cell LPD Low-grade B-cell LPD
Severe combined immunodeficiency	Many cytokine receptors, Rag1/2 [76]	Various	Defects in lymphocyte maturation and production	EBV+ LPD
Ataxia–telangiectasia (AT)	ATM	Kinase involved in DNA break repair	Defects in lymphocyte apoptosis, [77] recombinase reactivation in mature cells [78]	T-PLL, TCL1-tranlocated Other tumors [19]
Nijmingen breakage syndrome (NBS)	NBS1 (NBN) [79]	DNA break repair	Impaired DNA repair and lymphocyte apoptosis [80]	Lymphoma, particularly GI primaries [81]
Childhood cancer complex (CCC)	MLH1, [82] PMS2, [83,84] other MMR genes	DNA mismatch repair proteins	Not reported	B- and T-cell lymphomas, lymphoblastic leukemia [84,85]
Syndromes with increased risk of myeloid tumors				
Fanconi anemia	FANCA-N [86]	DNA break repair	Ineffective erythropoiesis, marrow failure	MDS, AML [86]
Diamond–Blackfan	Heme transport and ribosomal proteins [87]	Erythroid maturation and iron metabolism	Severe macrocytic anemia, defective iron transport [88]	MDS, AML [89]
Shwachman–Diamond	SBDS [90]	Cellular metabolism	Ineffective erythropoiesis, marrow failure, neutrophils migration defect [91]	MDS, AML with i(7)(q10) [92]
Kostmann syndrome (severe neutropenia)	ELA2 [93] HAX-1, unknown [94]	Neutrophil elastase Apoptotic regulator	Congenital neutropenia, bacterial infections	AML/MDS in cases with CSF3R mutation [94] Juvenile CMML
Neurofibromatosis, type 1	NF1 or NRAS	Cell proliferation and maturation		Monosomy 7 MDS [95]

Syndrome	Gene(s)	Function	Phenotype	Associated malignancy
Childhood Wilms tumor	WT1 or TP53 [96]	Transcription factors, regulators of mitosis		AML
Down syndrome	Trisomy 21 [97]	Many genes involved	Transient myeloid hyperplasia, macrocytosis, thrombocytosis, T-cell activation defects [98]	Megakaryoblastic leukemia, MPNs
Germline/genetic syndromes with increased risk of both lymphoid and myeloid tumors				
Bloom syndrome	BLM[99]	Helicase involved in DNA break repair	Impaired B-cell survival	B-cell lymphoma (most GCB-type, some EBV+)
Li-Fraumeni	TP53	Cell cycle checkpoints		AML, many other tumors
Germline/genetic syndromes involving immune genes with NO significant increased risk of hematolymphoid malignancies				
Familial hemophagocytic lymphohistiocytosis	Perforins [100] Syntaxin 11 [101] UNC13D [102]	Secretory and cytotoxic granule proteins	Uncontrolled hyperinflammation, with defective cytotoxicity	Rare AML/MDS seen with STX11 Rare T-cell lymphoma with PRF1
Leukocyte adhesion deficiency	CD18/integrin b1	Homing to granulocytes to tissues	Recurrent infections	None
IPEX[a]	FOXP3 [103]	T-cell regulation	Immunodeficiency	None

[a]Immune dysregulation, polyendocrinopathy, enteropathy, X-linked syndrome, *MMR* mismatch repair genes, *LPD* lymphoproliferative disorders, *GCB* germinal center B cell, *LyG* lymphomatoid granulomatosis, *GI* gastrointestinal tract, *CMML* chronic myelomonocytic leukemia, other abbreviations as in text

Taken together, a general model of lymphomagenesis can be proposed that combines generation of illegitimate TCR/BCR recombination events with conditions that lead to expansions of the precursor pool (e.g., antigen stimulation, lymphotropic herpesvirus infection, immune hyper-responsiveness or germline defects in apoptosis). Thus, full emergence of lymphoid malignancies becomes more likely as the pool of preneoplastic lymphocytes with translocations expands.

In contrast, the genetic defects underlying inherited and sporadic myeloid malignancies highlight the role of transcriptional reprogramming (often by whole chromosome gains/losses) in changing the patterns, sequence, or kinetics of hematopoietic maturation. This appears critical for myeloid malignancies since the normally rapid turnover of these lineages does not permit the slow stepwise development of malignancies possible in the long-lived lymphoid populations. In this model, gross dysregulation of the differentiation program would trap an increasingly large number of cells in intermediate maturation pools providing an opportunity for these cells to acquire additional genetic effects.

38.2.3. Common Mechanisms of Tumor Progression

Although the early stages of tumorigenesis are highly distinctive between mature B-cell, mature T-cell, lymphoblastic, and myeloid malignancies, the patterns of progression are depressingly similar in all. That the later stages of tumorigenesis are very similar for all tumor types has only been clarified in the molecular era often having been previously obscured by the confusing and highly idiosyncratic terminology used to describe cancer progression differently for each subtype (e.g., Richter's transformation in CLL, myeloid blast transformation in CML, acute myelofibrosis in other MPNs, or blastoid change in mantle cell or follicular lymphoma).

The morphologic features that accompany genetic progression in hematologic malignancies (i.e., poorly differentiated appearance, larger cell size, higher nucleus-to-cytoplasm ratio, and blastoid chromatin) are all largely a reflection of the increasingly rapid and abnormal progression through the cell cycle. These changes lead to accompanying failure to repair DNA damage, segregate chromosomes accurately, or fully initiate the genetic differentiation program [20]. These effects can be directly observed by the accumulation of gross chromosomal changes by cytogenetic studies (also known as clonal evolution).

Throughout this textbook, we have repeatedly returned to the common pathways that are involved in the progression of nearly all hematopoietic and lymphoid neoplasms that reflect these defects in the G1-S and G2-M checkpoints. These include loss of inhibitors of the cyclin-dependent kinases (e.g., p16/CDK2NA) and acquisition of defects in the p53-MDM2 axis [21]. It is not yet clear why the rate at which low-grade hematopoietic tumors progress to high-grade malignancy differs between histologic subtypes, but it could be related to the size of the precursor pool or the degree of immune regulatory control over expansion. In this regard, it is intriguing that the post-GC subset of CLL and T-cell LGL leukemia almost never demonstrate genetic progression possibly due to the exquisite immunoregulation of memory B cells and cytotoxic T cells, respectively.

38.2.4. Targeting General Cell Processes in Lymphoma and Leukemia

Several of the most successful new cancer therapies are directed at general cellular metabolic and catabolic processes but nonetheless show differential activity against particular leukemias or lymphomas (Table 38-4). For example, the biological response modifier (BRM) lenalidomide elicits a wide range of pharmacological effects on cancer cells including suppression of production of pro-inflammatory cytokines and pro-angiogenic factors [22]. As a single agent, lenalidomide is most active against plasma cell myeloma (which is a tumor-type heavily dependent on BM microenvironment signals), [23] and certain genetic subtypes of myelodysplastic syndromes (MDS) [24].

Table 38-4. Non-targeted biological therapies with differential effects on lymphoma/leukemia subsets.

Category	Mechanism	Example	Highest therapeutic activity
Proteasome inhibitors	Block degradation of a large number of proteins by the proteasome	Bortezomib [25]	Plasma cell myeloma, mantle cell lymphoma
Biological response modifiers	Complex, with anti-angiogenic and apoptotic effects	Lenalidomide[104]	MDS/AML with del(5q) [105] or +13 [24] Plasma cell myeloma [23]
Mitochondrial poisons	Target the dependency of tumor growth on glycolysis or influence redox state to generate reactive oxygen species	3-bromopyruvate [106] β-phenylethyl isothiocyanate [107]	Unclear
Apoptosis regulators	Shift balance between survival and apoptotic cell death	Small molecular inhibitors of BCL2 or IAP	Unclear
	Activate p53-mediated apoptosis	Nutlins [35]	
Epigenetic therapies	Histone modification;	HDAC inhibitors [36]	Cutaneous lymphoma, CML
	Inhibition of DNA methylation; Altering global transcription patterns	Decitabine/azacitidine	Low-grade MDS

There has also been great interest in targeting protein degradation in cancer cells by inhibition of the proteasome (a complex multisubunit proteolytic organelle) or the ubiquitin-conjugating enzymes which mark proteins for delivery to the proteasome. The most effective of these proteasome inhibitors, bortezomib, has preferential activity as a single agent or as part of a multiagent regimen against mantle cell lymphoma and myeloma [25]. These effects are due, at least in part, to blocking degradation of an inhibitor of the growth-promoting NF-kappa B transcriptional complex, but likely has other gene targets as well [26]. Bortezomib is synergistic with epigenetic therapies and with growth signaling blockade through the tumor necrosis factor signaling pathways, which may account for its selective tumor activity [27]. Resistance to bortezomib may result from mutations of the proteosomal subunits [28]. Other types of proteasome inhibitors which are active against other tumors are currently under evaluation.

Resistance to apoptotic cell death also likely explains why some lymphomas and leukemias are difficult to eradicate. High expression of BCL2 and other anti-apoptotic proteins has been shown to be an adverse prognostic marker in MDS, AML, DLBCL, [30] and some types of T-cell lymphoma. Therefore, manipulation of intrinsic and extrinsic apoptotic pathways have been suggested as adjuvant therapies [29]. Modulators of apoptosis, such as small molecular inhibitors of BCL2 [31] or the inhibitor of apoptosis (IAP) proteins,[32] have shown the most promise, in combination with other agents [33]. The linkage between cell cycle regulation, DNA repair, and apoptosis regulation [34] has also been exploited in the use of p53 activators such as the nutlins [35].

Epigenetic modulators, including histone deacetylase inhibitors (HDACs)[36] and DNA and histone demethylating agents, [37] are now in common use. These agents induce global transcriptional changes that have both stimulatory and inhibitory effects on tumor growth. To date, they have made the most impact in the treatment of lower-grade hematopoietic malignancies, such as early MDS for demethylating agents [37] and cutaneous T-cell lymphomas for HDACs [38]. However, additional work remains to be done on identifying biomarkers to predict response to these epigenetic therapies when used as single agents, [39] and clinical trials are underway to assess how they are best used in combination with other therapies [40].

38.3. Lymphoma/Leukemia-Specific Targeting of Signaling Pathway

38.3.1. Targeting the B-cell Receptor Pathway in B-cell Lymphoma

Normal lymphocyte signaling is complex, and involves integration of signals from the antigen receptors (BCR/antibody in B cells and TCR in T cells), src-type tyrosine kinases and TNF family receptors (e.g., CD30, CD40), and calcium signaling mediated by NFAT and lipid kinases (see Chap. 34). These signals converge ultimately on the MAP kinases which link cell proliferation, activation, and cell division [41,1]. Loss of B-cell signaling components leading to dysregulated BCR pathway activation are critical events in pathogenesis of some subtypes of plasma cell dyscrasias and DLBCL [30,42]. As a result, targeting BCR-associated kinases with small molecule inhibitors has shown promise for treatment of myeloma [43] and DLBCL [44].

A number of control pathways intersecting with the BCR signal show potential for therapeutic modulation. This is because the immune system has developed intricate mechanisms to turn off the explosive lymphocyte proliferation that follows BCR engagement by antigen. The emergence of B-cell lymphomas of MALT type following persistent antigen stimulation has highlighted the role of the CARMA1/BCL10/MALT1 complex in regulating NF-kB activation as one such control pathway (Chaps. 15 and 34) [45]. Therefore, antibody therapy directed against costimulatory receptors, or NF-kB inhibitors that directly target this pathway, are being explored for synergistic effects on inducing apoptosis in B-cell lymphomas [46–48].

38.3.2. Targeting the T-cell Receptor Pathway in T-cell Lymphoproliferative Disorders

Aberrant TCR signaling appears critical to the development of both immature [49] and mature T cell neoplasms [50]. As with B cells, engagement of costimulatory growth receptors and BCL10/CARMA1 signaling complexes [51] in T cells can influence the balance between growth and apoptosis following TCR activation. The T-cell "exhaustion" pathways, involving PD-1, LAG-3, and CTLA-4, also play a critical role in triggering T-cell senescence. These pathways appear intact in many low-grade T-cell lymphoproliferative disorders but may become deleted as tumor progress. Restoration of the function of complex regulatory networks that normally limit T-cell expansion also provides potential therapeutic approaches. These could include conventional immunotherapy (ex vivo expansion and reintroduction of regulatory T cells) or more targeted approaches with antibody immunotherapy or cytokine treatments.

38.4. Targeting Growth Signaling and the Microenvironment

38.4.1. The Potential for Microenvironmental Targeting

The early phases of most hematopoietic neoplasms are heavily dependent on trophic growth signals from surrounding antigen-presenting cells, and other non-neoplastic immune and stromal cells. Indeed, in vitro studies have demonstrated the necessity of stroma and stromal-derived chemokines and cytokines for growth of low-grade leukemias and lymphomas [52,53]. One of the most underdeveloped areas in lymphoma/leukemia drug development has been strategies to target the supportive tumor microenvironment [54]. Therapeutic approaches could be directed at altering the migration (chemotaxis) or retention of tumor cells in a particular supportive microenvironment. Targeted treatment could also focus on disrupting pathways involved in trophic stromal signals. Finally, strategies to make the microenvironment hostile to tumor growth could also be employed.

38.4.2. Targeting Chemotactic Chemokines to Influence Tumor Localization

Chemokines comprise a structurally related group of small proteins that bind to and activate G protein-coupled receptors that regulate cytoskeletal polarization and cell movement (Table 38-5). Examples include the chemokine IL-8/CXCL8, which regulates the migration of neutrophils to sites of acute inflammation, and CCL19/SLC which regulates the migration of lymphocytes across blood vessels into the lymph node [55].

The receptors for chemokines provide possible targets for immunotherapy given their preferential expression in different leukocyte (and tumor) subsets. Chemokine receptors are

Table 38-5. Classes of potentially targetable molecules involved in adhesion and cell migration.

Class	Examples	Ligands	Mechanism	Effects
Chemokine receptors	CXCR4, CCR4	Small heparin-binding chemokine proteins	G protein-coupled calcium signaling	Cytoskeletal polarization mediating migration and retention of leukocytes
Integrins	CD11a-c, CD18, CD49a-f, CD61, CD103	Extracellular matrix proteins, Ig-like CAMs on other cells	Conformational changes in integrin upon chemokine or cytokine exposure	High-affinity binding of cells to matrix or occasionally to other cells
Selectins	CD62E, CD62L, CD62P	Addressins (tissue-specific glycans) such as CD15, CLA, and HECA-452	Transient interactions to tether or slow cells in motion	Reversible low-affinity binding of leukocytes to endothelium and stromal elements
Immunoglobulin-like cell adhesion molecules (CAMs)	CD56 (NCAM), CD106 (VCAM-1)	Themselves, other CAMs, matrix proteins, and integrins	Heterotypic and homotypic interactions between CAMs and integrins	Cell-to-cell interactions, mediate extramedullary localization of leukocytes

among the most differentially expressed markers in T-cell lymphomas and myeloid leukemias subtypes and probably influence their patterns of spread. An antibody against CCR4 is now in clinical trials for treatment of T-cell lymphoma [56]. However, the rapid modulation of expression of some other chemokine receptors and their propensity for internalization (with their loss from the cell surface) may limit their utility as antigenic targets for tumor immunotherapy.

Another critical (and under-appreciated) role of chemokines is in mediating retention of hematopoietic and lymphoid precursors in specific microenvironmental niches. This is most critically seen with CXCL13 where loss of this chemokine or its receptor (CXCR4) produces early release of immature granulocytes and B cells into the blood in mouse models [57]. This property has been exploited clinically in that antibodies that disrupt CXCL13–CXCR4 interactions have been used to mobilize bone marrow elements into the blood for transplant harvesting [58,59].

38.4.3. Targeting Adhesion Molecules

Cell adhesion molecules (CAMs) of various types function to retain hematopoietic cells in a supportive microenvironment so modulation of their effects in tumor cells could potentially disrupt growth. Some families of adhesion molecules have transient effects (e.g., selectins) related to initial localization whereas others (e.g., integrins) strongly link cells to extracellular matrix and other cells (Table 38-5).

Integrins (including CD11a-c, CD18, and CD103) are differentially expressed on all leukocytes and hematolymphoid tumors, and their expression has been associated with different patterns of tumor localization in chronic lymphocytic leukemia and T-cell neoplasms. Integrins are activated by conformational change triggered by calcium flux and growth activators and then bind avidly to extracellular matrix molecules such as fibronectin or to immunoglobulin-like CAMs on other cells (so-called "inside-out" signaling). Activated integrins then participate in transmitting signals about the extracellular environment through localization of the focal adhesion kinase (FAK) and other cellular signaling complexes at sites of integrin activation. Kinase inhibitors could be employed to disrupt such "outside-in" stromal interactions. Another possible therapeutic strategy for immunotherapy applications is to engineer locked conformations of integrins, [60] or use antibodies which preferentially recognize high-affinity integrin conformations [61]. These reagents could be used to sort cell products for immunotherapy applications or to alter the localization properties of injected anti-tumor lymphocytes and antigen-presenting cells.

Therapeutic manipulations of selectins or their addressin ligands also show some promises in regulating hematopoietic stem cell migration. As described in Chap. 30, defucosylation of cell-surface selectins has already been shown to alter engraftment of infused cell products in transplant models. Such an approach may also be useful in immunotherapy applications directed at eliminating leukemias from sanctuary sites (e.g., CNS or testes) from which relapses can occur.

38.4.4. Gene-Targeted Modulation of the Microenvironment

Disrupting the growth-promoting cytokine-receptor interactions between a tumor and its microenvironment has long been a goal of targeted therapy. These include use of anti-IL-6 receptor antibodies to disrupt paracrine stromal signaling in plasma cell dyscrasia and the disruption of the osteoclastic–osteolytic activity in plasma cell myeloma by bisphosphonates [62] or antibody immunotherapy directed against RANKL [63]. However, long-term use of therapeutic antibodies is expensive, prone to development of neutralizing anti-antibodies, and difficult to target to specific niches.

To overcome these limitations, one of the most promising methods for long-term control of the tumor–stroma microenvironment has been the use of autologous or haploidentical donor mesenchymal stem cells (MSC) which can injected following ex vivo expansion and/or manipulation. In preliminary clinical trials assessing unmanipulated cells, ex vivo expanded MSC can migrate to the marrow (and other tissue sites) and integrate into the stromal network causing minimal disruptive effects [64]–[66]. Introduction of transgenic cytokines, inhibitors, or inhibitory microRNAs into MSC are now planned to allow for long-term disruption or alteration of stroma–tumor interactions [67,68]. One problem of such an approach is devising mechanisms to inactive these cells once the desired effect has been achieved since MSC can expand and shift phenotypes in vivo under influence of the tumor [69]. Although more work is needed, the principle of ex vivo expansion of genetically manipulated stromal cells holds great promise as a method for eliminating residual disease or preventing relapse of hematologic malignancies once induction therapy has reduced tumor burden.

References

1. Freireich EJ. The road to the cure of acute lymphoblastic leukemia: a personal perspective. Oncology 1997;54(4):265–9.
2. O'Connor OA. Pralatrexate: an emerging new agent with activity in T-cell lymphomas. Curr Opin Oncol 2006;18(6):591–7.
3. Larson RA. Three new drugs for acute lymphoblastic leukemia: nelarabine, clofarabine, and forodesine. Semin Oncol 2007;34(6 Suppl 5):S13–20.
4. Fanale MA, Younes A. Monoclonal antibodies in the treatment of non-Hodgkin's lymphoma. Drugs 2007;67(3):333–50.
5. Okazaki A, Shoji-Hosaka E, Nakamura K, et al. Fucose depletion from human IgG1 oligosaccharide enhances binding enthalpy and association rate between IgG1 and FcgammaRIIIa. J Mol Biol 2004;336(5):1239–49.
6. Chames P, Baty D. Bispecific antibodies for cancer therapy. Curr Opin Drug Discov Devel 2009;12(2):276–83.
7. Bargou R, Leo E, Zugmaier G, et al. Tumor regression in cancer patients by very low doses of a T cell-engaging antibody. Science 2008;321(5891):974–7.
8. Nowak D, Stewart D, Koeffler HP. Differentiation therapy of leukemia: 3 decades of development. Blood 2009;113(16):3655–65.
9. Druker BJ. Translation of the Philadelphia chromosome into therapy for CML. Blood 2008;112(13):4808–17.
10. Pratz K, Levis M. Incorporating FLT3 inhibitors into acute myeloid leukemia treatment regimens. Leuk Lymphoma 2008;49(5):852–63.
11. Cho KR, Vogelstein B. Suppressor gene alterations in the colorectal adenoma-carcinoma sequence. J Cell Biochem Suppl 1992;16G:137–41.
12. Hanahan D, Weinberg RA. The hallmarks of cancer. Cell 2000;100(1):57–70.
13. Zhou HJ, Pham LV, Tamayo AT, et al. Nuclear CD40 interacts with c-Rel and enhances proliferation in aggressive B-cell lymphoma. Blood 2007;110(6):2121–7.

14. Lossos IS. The endless complexity of lymphocyte differentiation and lymphomagenesis: IRF-4 downregulates BCL6 expression. Cancer Cell 2007;12(3):189–91.

15. Anderson JR, Armitage JO, Weisenburger DD. Epidemiology of the non-Hodgkin's lymphomas: distributions of the major subtypes differ by geographic locations. Non-Hodgkin's Lymphoma Classification Project. Ann Oncol 1998;9(7):717–20.

16. Chang KC, Huang GC, Jones D, Tsao CJ, Lee JY, Su IJ. Distribution and prognosis of WHO lymphoma subtypes in Taiwan reveals a low incidence of germinal-center derived tumors. Leuk Lymphoma 2004;45(7):1375–84.

17. Armitage J, Vose J, Weisenburger D. International peripheral T-cell and natural killer/T-cell lymphoma study: pathology findings and clinical outcomes. J Clin Oncol 2008;26(25):4124–30.

18. Friedenson B. The BRCA1/2 pathway prevents hematologic cancers in addition to breast and ovarian cancers. BMC Cancer 2007;7:152.

19. Yuille MA, Coignet LJ. The ataxia telangiectasia gene in familial and sporadic cancer. Recent Results Cancer Res 1998;154:156–73.

20. Quijano S, Lopez A, Rasillo A, et al. Association between the proliferative rate of neoplastic B cells, their maturation stage, and underlying cytogenetic abnormalities in B-cell chronic lympho-proliferative disorders: analysis of a series of 432 patients. Blood 2008;111(10):5130–41.

21. Mestre-Escorihuela C, Rubio-Moscardo F, Richter JA, et al. Homozygous deletions localize novel tumor suppressor genes in B-cell lymphomas. Blood 2007;109(1):271–80.

22. Li WW, Hutnik M, Gehr G. Antiangiogenesis in haematological malignancies. Br J Haematol 2008;143(5):622–31.

23. Blade J, Rosinol L. Advances in therapy of multiple myeloma. Curr Opin Oncol 2008;20(6): 697–704.

24. Fehniger TA, Byrd JC, Marcucci G, et al. Single-agent lenalidomide induces complete remission of acute myeloid leukemia in patients with isolated trisomy 13. Blood 2009;113(5):1002–5.

25. Tobinai K. Proteasome inhibitor, bortezomib, for myeloma and lymphoma. Int J Clin Oncol 2007;12(5):318–26.

26. Strauss SJ, Higginbottom K, Juliger S, et al. The proteasome inhibitor bortezomib acts independently of p53 and induces cell death via apoptosis and mitotic catastrophe in B-cell lymphoma cell lines. Cancer Res 2007;67(6):2783–90.

27. Boll B, Hansen H, Heuck F, et al. The fully human anti-CD30 antibody 5F11 activates NF-{kappa} B and sensitizes lymphoma cells to bortezomib-induced apoptosis. Blood 2005;106(5):1839–42.

28. Lu S, Yang J, Song X, et al. Point mutation of the proteasome beta5 subunit gene is an important mechanism of bortezomib resistance in bortezomib-selected variants of Jurkat T cell lymphoblastic lymphoma/leukemia line. J Pharmacol Exp Ther 2008;326(2):423–31.

29. Reed JC. Bcl-2-family proteins and hematologic malignancies: history and future prospects. Blood 2008;111(7):3322–30.

30. Roberts RA, Wright G, Rosenwald AR, et al. Loss of major histocompatibility class II gene and protein expression in primary mediastinal large B-cell lymphoma is highly coordinated and related to poor patient survival. Blood 2006;108(1):311–8.

31. Azmi AS, Mohammad RM. Non-peptidic small molecule inhibitors against Bcl-2 for cancer therapy. J Cell Physiol 2009;218(1):13–21.

32. Danson S, Dean E, Dive C, Ranson M. IAPs as a target for anticancer therapy. Curr Cancer Drug Targets 2007;7(8):785–94.

33. Kang MH, Reynolds CP. Bcl-2 inhibitors: targeting mitochondrial apoptotic pathways in cancer therapy. Clin Cancer Res 2009;15(4):1126–32.

34. Stagni V, di Bari MG, Cursi S, et al. ATM kinase activity modulates Fas sensitivity through the regulation of FLIP in lymphoid cells. Blood 2008;111(2):829–37.

35. Secchiero P, di Iasio MG, Gonelli A, Zauli G. The MDM2 inhibitor Nutlins as an innovative therapeutic tool for the treatment of haematological malignancies. Curr Pharm Des 2008; 14(21):2100–10.

36. Martinez-Iglesias O, Ruiz-Llorente L, Sanchez-Martinez R, Garcia L, Zambrano A, Aranda A. Histone deacetylase inhibitors: mechanism of action and therapeutic use in cancer. Clin Transl Oncol 2008;10(7):395–8.

37. Oki Y, Issa JP. Treatment options in advanced myelodysplastic syndrome, with emphasis on epigenetic therapy. Int J Hematol 2007;86(4):306–14.

38. Duvic M, Vu J. Vorinostat: a new oral histone deacetylase inhibitor approved for cutaneous T-cell lymphoma. Expert Opin Investig Drugs 2007;16(7):1111–20.

39. Stimson L, La Thangue NB. Biomarkers for predicting clinical responses to HDAC inhibitors. Cancer Lett 2009;280(2):177–83.

40. Bishton M, Kenealy M, Johnstone R, Rasheed W, Prince HM. Epigenetic targets in hematological malignancies: combination therapies with HDACis and demethylating agents. Expert Rev Anticancer Ther 2007;7(10):1439–49.

41. Dong C, Davis RJ, Flavell RA. MAP kinases in the immune response. Annu Rev Immunol 2002; 20:55–72.

42. Bea S, Zettl A, Wright G, et al. Diffuse large B-cell lymphoma subgroups have distinct genetic profiles that influence tumor biology and improve gene-expression-based survival prediction. Blood 2005;106(9):3183–90.

43. Gertz MA. New targets and treatments in multiple myeloma: Src family kinases as central regulators of disease progression. Leuk Lymphoma 2008;49(12):2240–5.

44. Chen L, Monti S, Juszczynski P, et al. SYK-dependent tonic B-cell receptor signaling is a rational treatment target in diffuse large B-cell lymphoma. Blood 2008;111(4):2230–7.

45. Lin X, Wang D. The roles of CARMA1, Bcl10, and MALT1 in antigen receptor signaling. Semin Immunol 2004;16(6):429–35.

46. Cillessen SA, Meijer CJ, Ossenkoppele GJ, et al. Human soluble TRAIL/Apo2L induces apoptosis in a subpopulation of chemotherapy refractory nodal diffuse large B-cell lymphomas, determined by a highly sensitive in vitro apoptosis assay. Br J Haematol 2006;134(3):283–93.

47. Anand P, Sundaram C, Jhurani S, Kunnumakkara AB, Aggarwal BB. Curcumin and cancer: an "old-age" disease with an "age-old" solution. Cancer Lett 2008;267(1):133–64.

48. Lam LT, Davis RE, Pierce J, et al. Small molecule inhibitors of IkappaB kinase are selectively toxic for subgroups of diffuse large B-cell lymphoma defined by gene expression profiling. Clin Cancer Res 2005;11(1):28–40.

49. Kelly JA, Spolski R, Kovanen PE, et al. Stat5 synergizes with T cell receptor/antigen stimulation in the development of lymphoblastic lymphoma. J Exp Med 2003;198(1):79–89.

50. Herling M, Patel KA, Teitell MA, et al. High TCL1 expression and intact T-cell receptor signaling define a hyperproliferative subset of T-cell prolymphocytic leukemia. Blood 2008;111(1):328–37.

51. Blonska M, Pappu BP, Matsumoto R, et al. The CARMA1-Bcl10 signaling complex selectively regulates JNK2 kinase in the T cell receptor-signaling pathway. Immunity 2007;26(1):55–66.

52. Vega F, Medeiros LJ, Lang WH, Mansoor A, Bueso-Ramos C, Jones D. The stromal composition of malignant lymphoid aggregates in bone marrow: variations in architecture and phenotype in different B-cell tumours. Br J Haematol 2002;117(3):569–76.

53. Ame-Thomas P, Maby-El Hajjami H, Monvoisin C, et al. Human mesenchymal stem cells isolated from bone marrow and lymphoid organs support tumor B-cell growth: role of stromal cells in follicular lymphoma pathogenesis. Blood 2007;109(2):693–702.

54. Podar K, Chauhan D, Anderson KC. Bone marrow microenvironment and the identification of new targets for myeloma therapy. Leukemia 2009;23(1):10–24.

55. Arai J, Yasukawa M, Yakushijin Y, Miyazaki T, Fujita S. Stromal cells in lymph nodes attract B-lymphoma cells via production of stromal cell-derived factor-1. Eur J Haematol 2000;64(5): 323–32.

56. Ishida T, Ueda R. CCR4 as a novel molecular target for immunotherapy of cancer. Cancer Sci 2006;97(11):1139–46.

57. Ma Q, Jones D, Springer TA. The chemokine receptor CXCR4 is required for the retention of B lineage and granulocytic precursors within the bone marrow microenvironment. Immunity 1999;10(4):463–71.

58. Kollet O, Petit I, Kahn J, et al. Human CD34(+)CXCR4(-) sorted cells harbor intracellular CXCR4, which can be functionally expressed and provide NOD/SCID repopulation. Blood 2002;100(8):2778–86.

59. Stiff P, Micallef I, McCarthy P, et al. Treatment with plerixafor in non-Hodgkin's lymphoma and multiple myeloma patients to increase the number of peripheral blood stem cells when given a mobilizing regimen of G-CSF: implications for the heavily pretreated patient. Biol Blood Marrow Transplant 2009;15(2):249–56.

60. Luo BH, Takagi J, Springer TA. Locking the beta3 integrin I-like domain into high and low affinity conformations with disulfides. J Biol Chem 2004;279(11):10215–21.

61. Huang L, Shimaoka M, Rondon IJ, et al. Identification and characterization of a human monoclonal antagonistic antibody AL-57 that preferentially binds the high-affinity form of lymphocyte function-associated antigen-1. J Leukoc Biol 2006;80(4):905–14.

62. Lipton A. Pathophysiology of bone metastases: how this knowledge may lead to therapeutic intervention. J Support Oncol 2004;2(3):205–13. discussion 13–4, 16–7, 19–20.

63. Terpos E, Efstathiou E, Christoulas D, Roussou M, Katodritou E, Dimopoulos MA. RANKL inhibition: clinical implications for the management of patients with multiple myeloma and solid tumors with bone metastases. Expert Opin Biol Ther 2009;9(4):465–79.

64. Ball LM, Bernardo ME, Roelofs H, et al. Cotransplantation of ex vivo expanded mesenchymal stem cells accelerates lymphocyte recovery and may reduce the risk of graft failure in haploidentical hematopoietic stem-cell transplantation. Blood 2007;110(7):2764–7.

65. Macmillan ML, Blazar BR, DeFor TE, Wagner JE. Transplantation of ex-vivo culture-expanded parental haploidentical mesenchymal stem cells to promote engraftment in pediatric recipients of unrelated donor umbilical cord blood: results of a phase I-II clinical trial. Bone Marrow Transplant 2009;43(6):447–54.

66. Garcia-Castro J, Trigueros C, Madrenas J, Perez-Simon JA, Rodriguez R, Menendez P. Mesenchymal stem cells and their use as cell replacement therapy and disease modelling tool. J Cell Mol Med 2008;12(6B):2552–65.

67. Studeny M, Marini FC, Champlin RE, Zompetta C, Fidler IJ, Andreeff M. Bone marrow-derived mesenchymal stem cells as vehicles for interferon-beta delivery into tumors. Cancer Res 2002;62(13): 3603–8.

68. Li X, Lu Y, Huang W, et al. In vitro effect of adenovirus-mediated human Gamma Interferon gene transfer into human mesenchymal stem cells for chronic myelogenous leukemia. Hematol Oncol 2006;24(3):151–8.

69. Spaeth EL, Dembinski JL, Sasser AK, et al. Mesenchymal stem cell transition to tumor-associated fibroblasts contributes to fibrovascular network expansion and tumor progression. PLoS One 2009;4(4):e4992.

70. Fisher GH, Rosenberg FJ, Straus SE, et al. Dominant interfering Fas gene mutations impair apoptosis in a human autoimmune lymphoproliferative syndrome. Cell 1995;81(6):935–46.

71. Oliveira JB, Bidere N, Niemela JE, et al. NRAS mutation causes a human autoimmune lympho-proliferative syndrome. Proc Natl Acad Sci USA 2007;104(21):8953–8.

72. Rieux-Laucat F, Le Deist F, Hivroz C, et al. Mutations in Fas associated with human lymphopro-liferative syndrome and autoimmunity. Science 1995;268(5215):1347–9.

73. Straus SE, Jaffe ES, Puck JM, et al. The development of lymphomas in families with autoimmune lymphoproliferative syndrome with germline Fas mutations and defective lymphocyte apoptosis. Blood 2001;98(1):194–200.

74. Allen RC, Armitage RJ, Conley ME, et al. CD40 ligand gene defects responsible for X-linked hyper-IgM syndrome. Science 1993;259(5097):990–3.

75. Shcherbina A, Candotti F, Rosen FS, Remold-O'Donnell E. High incidence of lymphomas in a subgroup of Wiskott-Aldrich syndrome patients. Br J Haematol 2003;121(3):529–30.

76. Okano M, Gross TG. A review of Epstein-Barr virus infection in patients with immunodeficiency disorders. Am J Med Sci 2000;319(6):392–6.

77. Gabellini C, Antonelli A, Petrinelli P, et al. Telomerase activity, apoptosis and cell cycle progression in ataxia telangiectasia lymphocytes expressing TCL1. Br J Cancer 2003;89(6):1091–5.

78. Lantelme E, Turinetto V, Mantovani S, et al. Analysis of secondary V(D)J rearrangements in mature, peripheral T cells of ataxia-telangiectasia heterozygotes. Lab Invest 2003;83(10): 1467–75.

79. Matsuura S, Tauchi H, Nakamura A, et al. Positional cloning of the gene for Nijmegen breakage syndrome. Nat Genet 1998;19(2):179–81.

80. Thierfelder N, Demuth I, Burghardt N, et al. Extreme variation in apoptosis capacity amongst lymphoid cells of Nijmegen breakage syndrome patients. Eur J Cell Biol 2008;87(2):111–21.

81. Steffen J, Maneva G, Poplawska L, Varon R, Mioduszewska O, Sperling K. Increased risk of gastrointestinal lymphoma in carriers of the 657del5 NBS1 gene mutation. Int J Cancer 2006; 119(12):2970–3.

82. Ricciardone MD, Ozcelik T, Cevher B, et al. Human MLH1 deficiency predisposes to hematological malignancy and neurofibromatosis type 1. Cancer Res 1999;59(2):290–3.

83. Kruger S, Kinzel M, Walldorf C, et al. Homozygous PMS2 germline mutations in two families with early-onset haematological malignancy, brain tumours, HNPCC-associated tumours, and signs of neurofibromatosis type 1. Eur J Hum Genet 2008;16(1):62–72.

84. De Vos M, Hayward BE, Charlton R, et al. PMS2 mutations in childhood cancer. J Natl Cancer Inst 2006;98(5):358–61.

85. Bandipalliam P. Syndrome of early onset colon cancers, hematologic malignancies & features of neurofibromatosis in HNPCC families with homozygous mismatch repair gene mutations. Fam Cancer 2005;4(4):323–33.

86. Dokal I. Fanconi anemia is a highly penetrant cancer susceptibility syndrome. Haematologica 2008;93(4):486–8.

87. Flygare J, Kiefer T, Miyake K, et al. Deficiency of ribosomal protein S19 in CD34+ cells generated by siRNA blocks erythroid development and mimics defects seen in Diamond-Blackfan anemia. Blood 2005;105(12):4627–34.

88. Keel SB, Doty RT, Yang Z, et al. A heme export protein is required for red blood cell differentiation and iron homeostasis. Science 2008;319(5864):825–8.

89. Janov AJ, Leong T, Nathan DG, Guinan EC. Diamond-Blackfan anemia. Natural history and sequelae of treatment. Medicine (Baltimore) 1996;75(2):77–8.

90. Ganapathi KA, Austin KM, Lee CS, et al. The human Shwachman-Diamond syndrome protein, SBDS, associates with ribosomal RNA. Blood 2007;110(5):1458–65.

91. Orelio C, Kuijpers TW. Shwachman-Diamond syndrome neutrophils have altered chemoattractant-induced F-actin polymerization and polarization characteristics. Haematologica 2009;94(3):409–13.

92. Maserati E, Pressato B, Valli R, et al. The route to development of myelodysplastic syndrome/acute myeloid leukaemia in Shwachman-Diamond syndrome: the role of ageing, karyotype instability, and acquired chromosome anomalies. Br J Haematol 2009;145(2):190–7.

93. Carlsson G, Aprikyan AA, Ericson KG, et al. Neutrophil elastase and granulocyte colony-stimulating factor receptor mutation analyses and leukemia evolution in severe congenital neutropenia patients belonging to the original Kostmann family in northern Sweden. Haematologica 2006;91(5):589–95.

94. Carlsson G, Melin M, Dahl N, et al. Kostmann syndrome or infantile genetic agranulocytosis, part two: Understanding the underlying genetic defects in severe congenital neutropenia. Acta Paediatr 2007;96(6):813–9.

95. Maris JM, Wiersma SR, Mahgoub N, et al. Monosomy 7 myelodysplastic syndrome and other second malignant neoplasms in children with neurofibromatosis type 1. Cancer 1997;79(7):1438–46.

96. Hartley AL, Birch JM, Harris M, et al. Leukemia, lymphoma, and related disorders in families of children diagnosed with Wilms' tumor. Cancer Genet Cytogenet 1994;77(2):129–33.

97. Malinge S, Izraeli S, Crispino JD. Insights into the manifestations, outcomes, and mechanisms of leukemogenesis in Down syndrome. Blood 2009;113(12):2619–28.

98. Scotese I, Gaetaniello L, Matarese G, Lecora M, Racioppi L, Pignata C. T cell activation deficiency associated with an aberrant pattern of protein tyrosine phosphorylation after CD3 perturbation in Down's syndrome. Pediatr Res 1998;44(2):252–8.

99. Babbe H, McMenamin J, Hobeika E, et al. Genomic instability resulting from Blm deficiency compromises development, maintenance, and function of the B cell lineage. J Immunol 2009;182(1):347–60.

100. Trizzino A, zur Stadt U, Ueda I, et al. Genotype-phenotype study of familial haemophagocytic lymphohistiocytosis due to perforin mutations. J Med Genet 2008;45(1):15–21.

101. Rudd E, Goransdotter Ericson K, Zheng C, et al. Spectrum and clinical implications of syntaxin 11 gene mutations in familial haemophagocytic lymphohistiocytosis: association with disease-free remissions and haematopoietic malignancies. J Med Genet 2006;43(4):e14.

102. Nakao T, Shimizu T, Fukushima T, et al. Fatal sibling cases of familial hemophagocytic lymphohistiocytosis (FHL) with MUNC13-4 mutations: case reports. Pediatr Hematol Oncol 2008;25(3):171–80.

103. Chang X, Zheng P, Liu Y. Homeostatic proliferation in the mice with germline FoxP3 mutation and its contribution to fatal autoimmunity. J Immunol 2008;181(4):2399–406.

104. Galustian C, Dalgleish A. Lenalidomide: a novel anticancer drug with multiple modalities. Expert Opin Pharmacother 2009;10(1):125–33.

105. List A, Dewald G, Bennett J, et al. Lenalidomide in the myelodysplastic syndrome with chromosome 5q deletion. N Engl J Med 2006;355(14):1456–65.

106. Xu RH, Pelicano H, Zhou Y, et al. Inhibition of glycolysis in cancer cells: a novel strategy to overcome drug resistance associated with mitochondrial respiratory defect and hypoxia. Cancer Res 2005;65(2):613–21.

107. Trachootham D, Zhou Y, Zhang H, et al. Selective killing of oncogenically transformed cells through a ROS-mediated mechanism by beta-phenylethyl isothiocyanate. Cancer Cell 2006;10(3):241–52.

Study Guide

These questions are intended to highlight some key concepts and technical issues covered in the text. They are not intended to be comprehensive but can be used by trainees to assess their knowledge base and to indicate which topics require further study. A discussion of each question can be found in the chapter section indicated in parentheses.

Chapter 1 (Classification of Lymphoma and Leukemias)

What organizing principle is the Working Formulation classification of lymphomas based upon? The WHO classification for lymphomas? (1.1.1)

What organizing principle is the French-American-British (FAB) classification of myeloid leukemia and myelodysplasia based upon? The WHO classification for myeloid leukemias? (1.1.2)

Which molecular mechanisms in lymphocytes are responsible for generating chromosomal translocations in lymphomas and lymphoid leukemias? (1.2)

What is the two-step model of leukemogenesis? (1.2)

Which laboratory test(s) are most commonly used to define risk groups for AML and MDS? (1.3.2)

Which B-cell differentiation stages correlate with which lymphoma types in the histogenetic classification of B-cell neoplasms? (1.3.3)

How is the classification of T-cell and NK-cell malignancies different from that used for B-cell neoplasms? (1.3.4)

Which lymphoma types are related to Epstein-Barr virus infection? Human T-cell lymphotropic virus (HTLV)? Chronic bacterial infections? (Table 1-5)

Chapter 2 (Immunostaining)

What are the postulated mechanism(s) for the effects of heat-induced antigen retrieval in immunohistochemistry (IHC)? (2.2.1)

What are the comparative benefits of monoclonal versus polyclonal antibodies for IHC? (2.2.3)

How do the PAP and ABC IHC detection methods differ? (2.3.4)

What are first-line and second-line markers for germinal center B cells? (2.3)

Give two examples where subcellular localization of a protein by IHC can provide diagnostic information (2.4.1)

What are the most important considerations when selecting particular genes from whole genome studies to use as protein biomarkers in IHC? (2.4.2)

What are some newer methods for quantitative protein profiling in tissues? (2.7)

Chapter 3 (Flow Cytometry)

What are the steps in routine flow cytometry on a blood sample? (Fig. 3.2)

What are two reasons why clinical reporting has moved away from numerical threshold reporting (3.2)

Name three markers for blasts in routine diagnostic use in flow cytometry panels (Table 3.1)

What is the average minimum number of abnormal cells required to accurately detect residual disease by flow cytometry? (3.3)

Chapter 4 (Molecular Diagnostics)

What is the central dogma of molecular biology? (4.1)

What are two mechanisms of epigenetic regulation of gene expression and how do they change the central dogma? (4.1)

At what temperatures should RNA and DNA be kept for long-term storage (Table 4-1)

Name two methods by which the quality of RNA is assessed (4.2.3)

What are two common clinical laboratory applications for reverse hybridization? (4.3.1)

Name some common inhibitors of PCR amplification of DNA and how can they be overcome (4.3.2)

How does bisulfite treatment of DNA distinguish between methylated and unmethylated cytosine? (4.3.6)

Which gene rearrangements are usually detected using a breakapart FISH probe strategy? (4.4.2)

What is the developmental sequence of rearrangement at the immunoglobulin loci? The T-cell receptor loci? (4.6.1)

Why can monoclonality in IGH or TCR PCR assays be represented by either one or two prominent amplicons? (4.6.3/5)

Why are most leukemia translocations detected using RNA (reverse transcription PCR) whereas most lymphoma translocations are detected using DNA (conventional PCR) or FISH? (4.7/4.8)

What percentage of base pair changes is used for defining mutated versus unmutated IGH genes in somatic hypermutation analysis? (4.10)

How is a heat map created from gene expression profiling data? (4.11.2)

What is the difference between an IVD and an ASR? (4.12.1)

Which types of controls are required for quantitative PCR assays? (4.12.3)

Chapter 5 (Introduction to the Bone Marrow)

What are the lifespan and bone marrow production times of neutrophils? Lymphocytes? (5.2.1 and 5.2.5)

What are common causes of hypereosinophilia? (Table 5-2)

How does the KIR system function in NK cell recognition of foreign or virally-infected cells? (5.2.2)

Which intracellular signaling pathway do the growth factors erythropoietin (EPO) and thrombopoietin (TPO) utilize? (5.2.3)

What are morphological features of myelodysplasia in the erythroid, myeloid, and megakaryocytic lineages? (5.2.6)

What do PAS-positive cytoplasmic inclusions in erythroid precursors signify? (5.2.7)

Where in the bone marrow do myeloid elements normally mature? Megakaryocytes? (5.3.1)

Which features favor a benign lymphoid aggregate over a malignant one? (5.5)

Chapter 6 (Myelodysplastic Syndromes)

What are the hematologic criteria for cytopenia in MDS? (6.1.2)

Which are some genetic syndromes predisposing to MDS? (6.1.5)

What are the bone marrow and blood diagnostic criteria for RA? RCMD? RAEB? (Table 6-2)

What are flow cytometric criteria for MDS in granulocytes? Monocytes? (6.1.8)

By IPSS criteria, what are good, intermediate, and poor risk cytogenetic changes? (6.1.9)

Which term should be used to diagnose cases with persistent cytopenia but minimal dysplasia? (6.2.1)

Why is it important to recognize hypocellular variants of MDS? (6.2.3)

What is subclinical PNH and what flow cytometric criteria can be used to diagnose it? (6.2.5)

Which molecular aberration is present in approximately 50% of CMML? (6.6.3)

Chapter 7 (Acute Myeloid Leukemia)

What are the four general classes of AML in the 2008 WHO classification? (7.3)

What are the criteria for diagnosis of AML in erythroid-predominant marrow? (7.4)

What are the consequences of demonstration of t(15;17) for treatment of AML? Of a core-binding factor translocation? (Table 7.2)

Which markers are used to demonstrate monocytic differentiation in blasts by flow cytometry, by IHC? (Table 7.5)

Chapter 8 (Treatment of Acute Myeloid Leukemia and Myelodysplastic Syndromes)

What are the standard drugs for AML therapy? How are they administered? (8.2)

In which AML subtypes is high-dose cytarabine most helpful? (8.2)

What is the impact of a FLT3 mutation on outcome in AML? An NPM1 mutation? (8.3, 8.4)

How are hypomethylating agents postulated to work in treatment of MDS? (8.9)

In which types of MDS is immunomodulatory therapy most helpful? (8.10)

Chapter 9 (Myeloproliferative Neoplasms)

Which shared features characterize (chronic) myeloproliferative neoplasms? (9.1)

Which MPN in the JAK2/MPL-mutated group has the highest rate of progression to blast phase? (9.2.2)

What is the functional consequence of the JAK2 V617F mutation? (9.2.5)

What is the most common cytogenetic change in PV? ET? PMF? (9.2.6)

What are the markers used to diagnose mastocytosis by flow cytometry? By IHC? (9.3)

Which molecular aberration producing hypereosinophilia has the highest rate of progression to AML? (9.4)

Chapter 10 (Chronic Myelogenous Leukemia)

What is the most common morphologic appearance of megakaryocytes in CML? (10.3)

Which are the BCR and ABL exons involved in the major breakpoint cluster region associated with CML? What is the size of the produced chimeric kinase? (Table 10.2)

What are the WHO criteria for accelerated phase of CML? (10.5)

How is major molecular response to imatiinib treatment defined? (10.6)

What features are incorporated in the Sokal risk score for CML? (10.7)

Chapter 11 (Therapy of Myeloproliferative Neoplasms)

What is standard therapy for CML in chronic phase? Accelerated phase? (11.2.1)

When is drug therapy indicated in PV? (11.2.2)

Chapter 12 (Lymph Node Biology and Lymphadenitis)

Where do lymphocytes enter the lymph node from the blood? (12.2)

Trace the movement within the lymph node of a B-cell following antigen activation to plasma cell formation (12.3)

Name three infections and two autoimmune diseases that produce marked follicular hyperplasia (12.5)

What produces dermatopathic lymphadenitis? (12.7)

How is bacillary angiomatosis distinguished from Kaposi's sarcoma? (12.8)

Chapter 13 (Lymphoblastic Leukemia and Lymphoma)

How does the presentation of precursor-B lymphoblastic tumors differ in children and the elderly? (13.2)

What is the most common cytogenetic finding in B lymphoblastic leukemia in children? In adults? (Table 13.1)

Name three methods to detect minimal residual disease in lymphoblastic leukemias (13.7)

What is the most common mutation detected in T lymphoblastic lymphoma? (13.8)

Chapter 14 (Chronic Lymphocytic Leukemia and Small Lymphocytic Lymphoma)

How is CLL distinguished from SLL? (14.2)

What is the basis for the Rai and Binet staging system for CLL? (14.6)

What are the two common genomic alterations that are clearly associated with adverse outcome in CLL/SLL? (14.6)

Which markers correlate with unmutated IGH genes in CLL/SLL? (Table 14.3)

Chapter 15 (Marginal Zone Lymphomas)

What are the three types of MZL and what features do they share? (15.1)

What are the three most common tissue sites for MZL of MALT type and what conditions predispose to lymphoma at each site? (15.2.2)

How do the treatments differ for gastric MALT lymphomas with or without reciprocal chromosomal translocations? (15.2.6)

Which two lymphoproliferative disorders are most commonly confused with nodal MZL on histological features? (15.3.4)

What is the most common cytogenetic/genomic change in splenic marginal zone lymphoma? (15.4.3)

Chapter 16 (Follicular Lymphoma and Mantle Cell Lymphoma)

How does the incidence of follicular lymphoma differ across the world? (16.2.1)

What are the common patterns of bone marrow involvement in follicular lymphoma? (16.2.2)

What markers and cytogenetic features distinguish follicular lymphoma and mantle cell lymphoma? (16.2.3)

Where does pediatric follicular lymphoma present and how does it differ from the much more common adult type? (16.2.4)

What is the gastrointestinal tract presentation of mantle cell lymphoma called? (16.3.1)

What gene(s) are commonly dysregulated in mantle cell lymphomas that lack t(11;14) translocation? (16.3.4)

Chapter 17 (Aggressive B-Cell Lymphoma: Large B-Cell Lymphoma and Burkitt Lymphoma)

What elements comprise the International Prognostic Index (IPI) for DLBCL? (17.1.2)

Which DLBCL morphologic variants have been commonly recognized (17.1.3)

Why is reliance on flow cytometry problematic in the diagnosis of DLBCL (17.1.4)

How frequently are t(14;18) and MYC translocations detected in DLBCL? (17.1.5)

Which two signaling pathways are commonly dysregulated in mediastinal B-cell lymphoma (17.2.1)

Which tissue sites are commonly involved in T-cell/histiocyte-rich large B-cell lymphoma? (17.2.2)

Name five different presentations of EBV-positive large B-cell lymphoma (17.4)

Which presentations of Burkitt lymphoma have a lower incidence of EBV association? (17.5.2)

What immunophenotypic features are characteristic of Burkitt lymphoma? (17.5.4)

Chapter 18 (Therapy of B-Cell Lymphoproliferative Disorders)

For which lymphoma types is CSF sampling performed during staging? (18.2)

Which lymphoma types may be observed without treatment? (18.3.1)

What is the mechanism of action of each of the five drugs in R-CHOP? (Table 18.3)

Chapter 19 (Myeloma and Other Plasma Cell Disorders)

What are the three required components for the diagnosis of plasma cell myeloma (as opposed to other plasma cell neoplasms)? (19.2.2)

What are the diagnostic criteria for plasma cell leukemia? (19.2.2)

What are the four most common genes involved in chromosomal translocations with IGH and how do they relate to prognosis? (Table 19-2)

How is lymphoplasmacytic lymphoma distinguished from myeloma? From marginal zone lymphoma? (19.3.4)

Chapter 20 (Hodgkin Lymphoma)

What are the most common sites of presentation of lymphocyte predominant HL, nodular sclerosis classical (C)HL? Mixed cellularity CHL? (20.3.1, 20.4.1)

What is the immunophenotype of tumor cells in lymphocyte predominant HL as compared to CHL? (20.3.2)

How does the localization of tumor cells in the lymph node differ between lymphocyte predominant HL and lymphocyte-rich CHL? (20.4.2)

What evidence supports the origin of HL from germinal center B-cells? (20.4.3)

Expression of which markers would favor ALCL over CHL in a CD30+ lymphoma? HL over ALCL? (20.4.4)

Chapter 21 (Treatment of Hodgkin Lymphoma)

How does the Ann Arbor system for HL stage sites of disease and which systemic symptoms are included? (Table 21.1)

How does the cure rate compare for early stage and advanced stage HL following standard chemotherapy? (21.3.1)

When should radiation therapy be used in addition to chemotherapy for CHL? (21.3.4)

What is the evidence that mid-treatment PET scans are effective in predicting progression/relapse? (21.3.3 and 21.3.4.)

What is the currently optimal therapy for relapsed CHL? (21.5.4)

Which patients with lymphocyte predominant HL can be observed without treatment following surgery? (21.3.3)

Chapter 22 (Classification of T-Cell and NK-Cell Malignances)

Which features distinguish angioimmunoblastic T-cell lymphoma from peripheral T-cell lymphoma in lymph node? (22.3)

Which morphologic variants of anaplastic large cell lymphoma have been most often recognized? (22.3)

What is the most common immunophenotype for enteropathy-associated T-cell lymphoma? (22.3)

Which mature T-cell leukemia has the best outcome? The worst outcome? (22.4)

What are the only two common reciprocal chromosomal translocations in mature T-cell malignancies? (22.5)

Which immunophenotypic features distinguish NK-cell malignancies from T-cell tumors? (22.9.3)

Chapter 23 (Treatment of Non-Cutaneous T-Cell and NK-Cell malignancies)

How do the responses to chemotherapy and radiation compare for T-cell and NK-cell malignancies? (23.4)

How does the utility of the IPI prognostic system compare in T-cell malignancies with its value in B-cell tumors? (23.5)

Chapter 24 (Cutaneous T-Cell Lymphomas)

How is disease progression in mycosis fungoides manifested clinically? Histologically? Immunophenotypically? (24.2)

Does either loss of CD3 expression in tumor cells or TCR clonality studies distinguish cutaneous ALCL from lymphomatoid papulosis? (24.3.2)

Which two rare CTCL types most resemble epidermotropic MF? (Table 24.7)

How does the immunophenotype differ between cutaneous gamma-delta T-cell lymphoma and subcutaneous panniculitis-like T-cell lymphoma? (Table 24.7)

Chapter 25 (Therapy of Cutaneous T-Cell Lymphomas)

Which size lymph nodes should be evaluated by biopsy or needle aspiration in a patient with MF? (25.2)

What are the four most common skin-directed therapies for early MF? (25.3)

What are therapeutic options for Sézary syndrome? (Fig. 25.2)

Chapter 26 (Histiocytic and Dendritic Cell Neoplasms)

What are the definitive ultrastructural and immunophenotypic features of Langerhan cells? (26.3.1)

What is the best predictor of outcome in Langerhans cell histiocytosis (26.3.1)

How is IDC sarcoma distinguished immunophenotypically from FDC sarcoma? Ultrastructurally? (Table 26.1)

What is the evidence that blastic plasmacytoid dendritic cell neoplasm is derived from immature dendritic cells? (26.4)

Chapter 27 (Extranodal Lymphomas and Tumors of the Thymus)

Which T-cell neoplasms have an association with preceding T-cell inflammatory states? (27.1)

What are the patterns of splenic involvement in different B-cell lymphoproliferative disorders? (27.3.5)

Which lymphomas most commonly involve the stomach? The duodenum? The jejunum? (27.3.6 and Table 27.8)

How does the outcome of primary bone lymphoma (discrete mass) differ from bone marrow lymphoma detected on non-directed biopsy? (27.3.7)

What are three different approaches to classifying thymomas/thymic carcinomas? (Table 27.9)

How can immature thymocytes associated with a thymoma be distinguished from thymic lymphoblastic lymphoma? (27.4.4)

Index

A

ABCG2 (stem cell marker), 538
Abnormal localization of immature precursors (ALIP), 127, 128, 131
Acute lymphoblastic leukemia (ALL), *See* also lymphoblastic
    leukemia
    B cell, 240
    differential diagnosis with AML, 148
    gene expression profiling, 248
    molecular pathogenesis 248
    T cell, 245
Acute myeloid leukemia (AML)
    blast morphology, 129, 151
    cytogenetics, 149–150
    diagnostic algorithm, 148, 160
    epigenetic changes, 157, 160
    immunophenotypic markers, 154
    induction therapy, 165–167
    mouse model, 604, 605
    mutation analysis, 158
    pathogenesis, 156, 159
    personalized risk assessment, 160, 168
    risk stratification, 167–170
    secondary, 157–158
    stem cell transplant, 172
    subtypes, 149
    targeted therapies, 171
Acute promyelocytic leukemia (APL)
    features, 149
    morphology, 151
    mouse model, 603
Adhesion molecules, types, 621
Adrenal lymphoma, 489
    intravascular lymphoma, 312
Adult T-cell leukemia/lymphoma (ATLL), 392, 399, 401, 402
    treatment, 416–418, 420
Adventitial reticular cell (ARC), bone marrow, 111
Affinity maturation (germinal center), 226, 227
Aggressive NK-cell leukemia, 404, 406, 408
AICDA, 288
ALK, oncogene
    ALCL, ALK+, 395–397, 414–415
    ALCL, ALK+, involving skin, 440
    immunohistochemistry (subcellular localization), 33

    large cell lymphoma, 27, 311–312
    proteomics (interacting proteins), 579
    signaling, 579
Alkylating agents
    AML, use in, 166
    lymphoma, use in, 327
    mechanism, 326
    risk of secondary AML, 158
All-trans retinoic acid (ATRA), use in APL 166, 168
Amyloidoma, 480–481
Amyloidosis, primary, 333
Anaplastic large cell lymphoma (ALCL), 392, 395, 397, 398, 402–404
    ALK negative, 397, 404
    ALK-positive, 397
    bone marrow, 116
    cutaneous (cALCL), 436, 437, 439, 440
    differential with Hodgkin lymphoma, 360, 362
    Hallmark cell, 397
    leukemic, 399
    lymphohistiocytic type, 397
    neutrophil-rich, 397
    null type, 395
    proteomics, 576–579
    skin involvement, systemic, 440
    small cell type, 397
    treatment, 414–416, 418, 419, 422–424
Angioimmunoblastic T-cell lymphoma (AITL), 392–395, 398,
    402–404
    treatment, 414–416, 418, 422, 423
Angiotropic lymphoma, 312–313
Ann Arbor staging system, 325
    modification for Hodgkin lymphoma, 368
Anthracyclines
    AML, use in, 165, 167
    lymphoma, use in, 327
    mechanism, 326
Antibodies, monoclonal, 23
Antibodies, phosphoprotein, 56
Antibody immunotherapy, lymphoma, 326, 328
    limitations, 327
Antigen-presenting cell (APC), 224, 227, 232
Aplastic anemia, 135–137
ASR (analyte-specific reagent), 91

Ataxia-telangiectasia syndrome, 616
Autoimmune lymphoproliferative syndrome (ALPS), 229, 616

B
Basophilia, 101, 103
BAFF (B cell activation factor), 564, 570
B-cell lymphoma,
    bone marrow, 115
    treatment, 323–332
    unclassifiable, 319–321
B cell, maturation, 535–537, 563–564
B-cell receptor (BCR), 227
    gene expression correlates, 555
    signaling, 563–565, 566–567
    supramolecular activation complex, 563
    targeting, in lymphoma, 619
BCL2
    Burkitt lymphoma, 318, 320
    effects on gene expression (FL), 288
    gene amplification in DLBCL, 308
    gene rearrangement in DLBCL, 307
    mouse models, 288, 590
    PCR, detection by, 85
    prognostic markers, DLBCL, 556
    targeting, 619
BCL6
    prognostic marker, DLBCL, 557, 559
    rearrangement, DLBCL, 307
    rearrangement, follicular lymphoma, 284
    T-cell lymphoma, expression, 394
BCL10, MALT lymphoma, 267, 268
BCR–ABL
    ALL, 240
    CRKL, substrate, 56
    mouse model, 602
    signaling, 601–602
    splice variants, 197
Bethesda proposal for classification of mouse hematolymphoid
        neoplasms, 585–586, 600
Birbeck granule (LCH), 463
Bioinformatics techniques, 87–90
Blastic plasmacytoid dendritic cell (BPDC) neoplasm, 469–470
BLyS (B lymphocyte stimulator), 564, 565
Bone lymphoma
    bone marrow/liver/spleen (BLS) lymphoma, 487
    primary bone lymphoma, 486
    systemic spread, patterns, 114–115
Bone marrow
    anaplastic large cell lymphoma, 116
    aspiration, 99, 100
    carcinoma, 118
    differential count/normal ranges, 105–106
    dysplastic changes, 105, 107, 113, 128, 140
    fibrosis grading, 100, 108, 110, 112, 113, 118
    iron stain, 108, 109
    lymphoid aggregates, benign, 115, 117
    lymphoma patterns, 113–117
    microanatomy, 108–110
    necrosis, 117
    touch preparation, 100
    trephine biopsy, 105
Bortezomib, use in lymphoma, 559
Brain, lymphoma, 480, 483

Breast lymphoma, 487
Burkitt lymphoma (BL), 303–321
    Murphy staging system, 305

C
Cancer
    initiation, 614
    genetic predisposition, 616
    models, 614
    progression, 614
    stem cells, 541
CAP (College of American Pathologists, checklists, 91
CAP inspection/proficiency testing rules, 93
Castleman disease
    hyaline vascular type, 229–231, 470
    multicentric (HHV8+), 314, 316–317
    myoid tumor/stromal-rich, 472
    plasma cell, localized, 230, 363
    relationship to FDC sarcoma, 470
CBL, mutation, MPNs, 185
CD antigens
    used in flow cytometry panels, 47
    used for immunostaining, 25
CD11c
    diagnosis of B-cell lymphomas, 274, 283
    monocytic and dendritic cell marker, 460
CD117, See KIT
CD25, immunotherapy, 452
CD30, antibody immunotherapy, 380, 422, 613
CD30 ligand, regression in lymphomatoid papulosis, 439
CD30-positive T-cell lymphoproliferative disorders, primary
        cutaneous, 436–440
    MF-ALCL-HL, overall syndrome, 11
CD34, stem cell enumeration, 57
CD38
    blast marker, 154
    CLL, 52, 256
    plasma cell neoplasms, 338
    stem cells, 538
    T-cell-rich B-cell lymphoma, 355, 356
CD40, 564–568, 570
    polymorphisms, 550
CD40 ligand (CD40L or CD154), 564, 565, 568, 570
CDK, gene amplification, 285
Cell cycle analysis, flow cytometry, 57
Central dogma, 61–63
Centroblast, 228
Centrocyte, 228
CEBPA, mutation, AML, 169
CFSE, 58
Chemokines, 620–621
    CCL17/TARC, in Hodgkin lymphoma, 361
    CCL19/SLC, lymph node entry, 620
    CCR4, immunotherapy, 422
    CXCL13, in AITL, 28, 395
    CXCR3, T-cell lymphoma, 420, 436
    CXCR4, antibody, stem cell mobilization, 507, 621
    thymic migration, 492
Chemotherapy, cytotoxic
    classes of drugs, 326, 611
    mutagenic risk, 15, 158, 612
    toxicities, 329, 612
Chimerism assay, 514–517

Chloroma, 468
CHOP chemotherapy, 327, 556
Chromosome translocations, lymphoma/leukemia, lists, 7, 8, 84, 146, 240
Chronic lymphocytic leukemia, 251–260
    chronic inflammation, involving, 478
    EBV+ transformation, 260
    hemolytic anemia, 252
    large cell transformation, 259–260
    prognostic factors, 256–258
    Rai/Binet stages, 255
    variants, 253
Chronic myeloid leukemia, atypical (aCML), 138–140, 185
Chronic myelogenous leukemia (CML), 193–206
    accelerated phase (definition), 198–199
    BCR-ABL point mutation, 198, 200, 201, 203
    blast phase/crisis, 193, 195, 198–201, 206
    genetic progression, 199, 200
    imatinib (Gleevec) resistance, 201–204
    mouse model, 602, 603
    prognostic models (Sokol score), 204–205
    therapy milestones, 201
    treatment, 215–217
    use of FISH, 197, 198, 202, 204, 205
    use of PCR, 198, 202
Chronic myelomonocytic leukemia (CMML), 138–140
    JAK2 mutation, 139
    RAS mutation, 139
Chronic neutrophilic leukemia, 206
CNS, lymphoma, 480, 483
Comparative genomic hybridization, array-based, 78–79
Complement-dependent cytotoxicity (CDC), 550
Copy number variation (CNV), human genome, 78, 514, 546
Core binding factor leukemias, inv16/t(8;21) AML
    features, 149
    mouse models, 604
    treatment, 167, 168
C1qA, polymorphisms in lymphoma, 550
Cre-Lox, in mouse models 585
Cutaneous B-cell lymphoma, 481
Cutaneous T-cell lymphoma
    CD8+ aggressive epidermotropic cytotoxic T-cell lymphoma, 443
    CD4+ small/medium-sized pleomorphic T-cell lymphoma, 428, 444
    classification, 428, 429, 431, 444
    gamma-delta, 444
    NK/T-cell lymphoma, 441–442
    treatment, 449–456
CXCL13, in AITL 395
Cyclin D1 (CCND1)
    mantle cell lymphoma 291–295
    myeloma, 343
    PCR, detection by, 85
Cyclin D3, role in myeloma 294
Cytarabine (ara-C), use in AML, 165
Cytogenetics, *See* Karyotype
Cytokines, *See* growth factors
Cytomegalovirus (CMV), infection in transplant, 523, 525

D

Demethylating (hypomethylating) agents, decitabine and azacitidine, use in MDS, 173, 619

Dendritic cell maturation/plasticity, 103, 460
Dermatopathic lymphadenitis, 232, 233
Diffuse large B-cell lymphoma (DLBCL)
    ALK+, 311, 312
    arising in T-cell lymphomas, 404
    CHOP/R-CHOP, response predictors, 555–556
    classification strategies, 304
    Epstein-Barr virus (EBV), 313
    GC versus ABC types, 35, 37, 307, 554
    immune response/stroma, outcome predictors, 309, 556
    immune system gene polymorphisms, risk/outcome, 547–549
    International Prognostic Index (IPI), 305
    leg type, skin, 312
    outcome prediction, 548
    multidimensional model, 308
    post-transplant, 523
    primary CNS, 312
    prognostic markers, 554, 558
    T-cell/histiocyte-rich, 310–313
    therapy selection, 553, 554, 556, 557
DNA
    quantitation, 65
    sequencing, 72–74
    Southern blot, 67
DNA recombination
    chromosome translocations, mechanism, 6, 287, 615
    immunoglobulin class switch, 227–228
    V-D-J, IGH/TCR production, 79–83
Donor lymphocyte infusion, 526
Drugs
    anti-apoptotic, 619
    general mechanisms/chemotherapy, 326, 611
    proteasome inhibitors, 619
    targeting metabolic pathways 618
    targeting transcription factors, 613

E

ECOG performance status criteria, 305
Emperipolesis (Rosai-Dorfman), 31, 463, 467
Endometrium, lymphoma, 489
Enhanceosome, signaling in lymphoma, 567
Enteropathy associated T-cell lymphoma
    gross appearance, 487
    low-grade component, 398
    treatment, 415, 416, 422, 423
Eosinophilia, 101
Eosinophilic granuloma (localized LCH), 462
Epigenetics, 62
Epstein-Barr virus (EBV)
    brain lymphoma, 480
    Burkitt lymphoma, 317
    EBER, 27, 314, 360, 395, 405
    EBNA1, 14, 318, 525
    Hodgkin lymphoma, 351, 355–364
    LMP1, 14, 359–360, 407, 525
    post-transplant lymphoproliferative disorders, 521–525
    R-S cells in lymphoma/CLL, 260
    role in B-cell lymphoma, 313–316
    role in NK-cell tumors, 404
    role in T-cell lymphomas, 395
    viral load, plasma, 524
Erythroleukemia, 152
Erythropoiesis, dysplastic, 131

Erdheim–Chester disease, 466
Essential thrombocythemia (ET), 177–185
    treatment, 217–218
Extramedullary myeloid tumor (EMT), 468
Extranodal lymphoma, overview, 477
Extranodal marginal zone lymphoma, mucosa-associated lymphoid,
    264–270
    incidence by site, 478, 485
    pathogenesis, 479
Extranodal NK/T-cell lymphoma
    morphology, 405
    nasal, clinical features, 415, 418, 483
    non-nasal sites, clinical features, 418, 441
    treatment, 419, 422

F
FAB (French-American-British) classification, MDS/leukemia, 5,
    125, 127, 147–148
FGFR1, rearrangements in MPNs, 180, 189–190
Fibroblastic reticular cell (FRC), 224–226
FLIPI staging system (follicular lymphoma), 280, 290
Flow cytometry
    DNA content/ploidy analysis, 339
    gating strategies, 50
    mouse antigens, 600
    panels for acute leukemia, 48
    problems in large cell lymphoma, 306
    procedure, 45–58
    quality control, 51
    quantitative marker assessment, 51
    sample report, 52
    stem cell enumeration, 57
    T-cell subset analysis, 50
FLT3
    kinase inhibitors, impact, 171
    ITD mutations, outcome, 169
    mutations, in ALL, 495
    overexpression, in ALL, 249
    role in hematopoiesis, 536, 539
Fluorescence in situ hybridization (FISH), 63, 69, 76–78, 83, 85
Follicle center lymphoma, primary skin, 285, 287, 480–481
Follicle lysis (lymph node), 232
Follicular dendritic cells (FDCs), 227, 228, 231, 232, 460, 461, 463,
    465, 470–472
Follicular dendritic cell (FDC) sarcoma, 465, 470–472
Follicular hyperplasia (lymph node), 229–234
Follicular lymphoma (FL), 279–296
    Castlemanoid variant, 285, 286
    floral variant, 285–286
    diffuse, 282
    gene expression, 288
    grading, 280–281, 291
    in situ, 285–286
    marginal zone differentiation, 284
    outcome prediction, 548
    pediatric, 285
    primary skin, 287
    prognostic models, 290
FOXP1, lymphoma, 268, 311, 312
FOXP3
    ATLL, 394, 401–402
    IPEX, 617

lymphoma-associated T-regs, prognostic impact, 290, 364, 403
    regulatory T cells, 225, 228

G
Gamma-delta T-cell lymphoma, 444
Gaucher disease, 118
Gene rearrangements, 287
Genetically engineered, mouse model (knockin/knockout), 584–585
Genetic cancer syndromes, 616
Genetic polymorphisms (SNPs), 545, 547–550
Genotyping (SNPs), 546–547
Germinal centers (GCs), 224–229, 231, 232
Graft-*versus*-host disease, grading, 509
Granulocytosis, 101, 112
Granulomatous slack skin disease, 433, 435
Grey zone lymphoma, 362
Growth factors (cytokines)
    bone marrow microenvironment, 539
    dendritic cell maturation, 460
    morphologic effects, bone marrow, 113
    role in CLL, 257
    role in follicular lymphoma, 289
    role in Hodgkin lymphoma, 361
    role in MDS treatment, 172, 174
    role in MPNs, 184
    therapeutic uses for cytopenias, 104

H
Hairy cell leukemia, 274–275
Hairy cell leukemia-variant, 274
Hashimoto's thyroiditis, 264
Head and neck, lymphoma, 480
Helicobacter pylori, role in lymphoma, 268, 479
Hematodermic tumor, 469, *See* blastic plasmacytoid dendritic cell
    neoplasm
Hematopathology
    future directions in classification, 10–15
    sample report, 16
Hematopoiesis, 531–541
    bone marrow, ranges/lifespans, 100
    erythroid progenitors, 103, 532
    megakaryocytes, 103
    molecular pathways, 539–541
    monocytes/dendritic cells, 102–103
    myeloid progenitors, 101, 532, 533
    stem/precursor, self-renewal mechanism, 533
    yolk sac, 533
Hematopoietic stem cell (HSC), 531–533, 535–539, 541
    mouse, 597, 598
Hematopoietic stem cell transplantation
    AML, use in, 172
    chimerism assay, 514–517
    conditioning regimen, 507–508
    GVH, grading, 509
    Hodgkin lymphoma, 379
    mantle cell lymphoma, 330
    stem cell preparations, 507, 510
    T-cell lymphoma, 424, 456
    types of transplant, 506–507
Hemophagocytic syndrome, 463
    T/NK-cell lymphoma, association, 414, 418, 441, 443–444

Hepatosplenic T-cell lymphoma (HSTCL), 392, 398–399, 402, 403
  alpha-beta type, 402
  post-transplant, 525, 526
  treatment, 415, 416, 418, 420, 423
HGAL, prognostic marker, 28, 559
High endothelial venule (HEV), 224, 226
High-throughput sequencing/profiling, 69, 87
Histiocyte, 460–467
Histiocytic sarcoma (HS), 466
Histiocytosis, non-LC, 465–466
Histone deacetylase inhibitors (T-cell lymphoma), 453, 456
HLA typing, 517
Hodgkin lymphoma
  ABVD, 371, 373–375
  autologous stem cell transplant (ASCT), 375, 379, 380
  CD30, 353, 355, 357–362, 364
  classical type (CHL), 349–351, 355–363
  Differential diagnosis with ALCL, 362
  L&H (lymphocytic/histiocytic) cell, 350, 352–354, 360
  lymphocyte depleted (LDHL), 349, 356–358
  lymphocyte rich (LRHL), 349, 358, 360
  mixed cellularity (MCCHL), 349, 351, 355, 356, 358–360
  nodular sclerosis type (NSCHL), 351, 355, 357–364
  nodular lymphocyte predominant, 350–356
  progressive transformation of germinal centers (PTGC), 352, 354
  prognostic models, 370, 373
  proteomics, 576
  response criteria, 377
  rituximab, use of, 376, 380
  thymus, 495
  treatment, 367–380
HOX genes, 242, 247, 248, 392
Human herpesvirus 8, 14, 308
  Kaposi's sarcoma, 235
  LNA-1, 235
  multicentric Castleman disease, 230, 314, 317
  primary effusion lymphoma, 314
Human immunodeficiency virus (HIV),
  AIDS-associated, lymphoma, 313
  Lymphadenopathy/follicular hyperplasia, 229
  lymphocyte depleted Hodgkin lymphoma, 367
Human leukocyte antigen (HLA) genes, 514
Human Proteome Organization (HUPO), 577
Human T-cell lymphotropic virus (HTLV)-1, 14, 393, 401–402, 417, 440–441
Hypereosinophilic syndromes, 188–190

I
Idiopathic cytopenia with uncertain (undetermined) significance (ICUS), 135–136
IGH (immunoglobulin heavy chain)
  clonality assays, 81
  PCR, interpretation/pitfalls, 82
Ikaros (IKZF1)
  CML blast transformation, 6
  mouse models, ALL, 591
  role in ALL, 242
  role in hematopoiesis, 540
Imatinib (Gleevec)
  BCR-ABL mutations, 203
  milestones for CML treatment, 201, 216
  resistance (definitions), 201–204, 216

Immune response modulators, also See lenalidomide, 174
Immunoblast (lymph node), 228, 231–234
Immunoblastic lymphoma, 303
Immunoblastic proliferation, viral, 232
Immunocytoma, B-cell lymphoma, skin, 265, 267
Immunodeficiency
  Burkitt lymphoma, 317
  flow cytometry, monitoring, 56
  genetic syndromes, 616
  lymphoma, B-cell, 313
  lymphoma, T-cell, 418
  post-transplant, 521–522
  viral reactivation (EBV), 522
Immunoglobulin class switch, 226–228
Immunohistochemistry
  antigen retrieval, 22–23
  basic technique, 22–24
  mouse antigens, 600
  multispectral, 40
  quantitative, 40
Immunotherapy, 323, 325, 327
  adoptive immunotherapy, transplant, 526
  antibody-based, 620–622
  cellular immunotherapy, EBV+ neoplasms, 407
Inflammatory myofibroblastic tumor (IMT), 472
Integrins, 621
Interdigitating dendritic cell (IDC), 460, 461
Interdigitating dendritic cell (IDC) sarcoma, 465
Interferon(s)
  production by pDCs, 103
  role in mycosis fungoides, 436
  use in MPNs, 217
International Prognostic Index (IPI), 305, 554
Intravascular DLBCL, 312–313
IPSID (immunoproliferative disease of the small bowel) 265
IVD (in vitro diagnostic), 91

J
JAK2
  algorithm for testing in MPNs, 215
  amplification, mediastinal lymphoma, 310
  inhibitors, 218
  molecular analysis, 182
JAK-STAT pathway
  CML, 198
  hematopoiesis, 103
  Hodgkin lymphoma, 361, 495
  mantle cell lymphoma, 294
  MPNs, 184
Juvenile xanthogranuloma (JXG), 466

K
Kaposi's sarcoma, 235
Karyotype, G-banded, 63, 75–76
  reporting terminology, 76
Kikuchi-Fujimoto disease, 463
Killer inhibitory receptor (KIR) genes, typing/transplant, 519
Kinases
  B-cell receptor pathway, 555, 563
  BCR-ABL, 601
  JAK2, 183

Kinases (*Continued*)
  profiling, 576, 579
  proteomics, 574, 576, 577, 579
  role in hematopoiesis, 539
  serine and threonine, 574, 579
  T-cell receptor pathway, 403
  tyrosine, antibody detection, 574, 576
Kinase inhibitors, 613–614
  BCR-ABL, maintenance in ALL, 246
  BCR-ABL, second-generation (dasatinib, nilotinib), 216
  FLT3, 171
  KIT, 188
  SYK, 559, 614
KIR typing, 519
KIT (CD117)
  mutation, AML, 156, 158, 169–170
  mutation, mastocytosis, 188
  staining pattern,131
  stem cells, 538
Knockin mice, 584
Knockout mice, 584, 591

L
Langerhans cell (LCs), 460–463, 465
Langerhans cell histiocytosis (LCH), 462–466
Langerhans cell sarcoma (LCS), 465
Large B-cell lymphoma, *See* also diffuse large B-cell lymphoma
  International Prognostic Index (IPI), 305, 554
  signaling, 565, 568
Large granular lymphocyte leukemia, 392, 399
Lenalidomide
  lymphoma, 331
  MDS, 125, 174
  MPNs, 217
  myeloma, 618
Lennert lymphoma, 395
Leukemia
  classification, 3–18
  genetic syndromes, 615–617
  stem cells, 145
  targeted therapy, 613–614
Leukoerythroblastosis, 214
Levey-Jennings rules, 93
Liver, lymphomas, 485, 495
LMO2
  germinal center marker, 24
  polymorphisms, 548, 550
  prognostic marker, 555–556
  T-ALL, translocation, 7
Lung, lymphoma, 480–483
Lung, inflammatory conditions, 484
Lymph node, 223–236, 264, 269, 270, 272, 275, 276
  anatomy, 225
  cortex, 224–226, 229, 236
  infarction, follicular lymphoma, 280
  medulla, 224, 234–236
  paracortex, 224–227, 232
  perifollicular sinus, 226
  primary follicles, 226
  secondary follicle, 226
Lymphoblastic leukemia/lymphoma, 239–249
  differential diagnosis, 245
  mediastinal, 480, 494, 495

mouse models, 583–594
monitoring, post-treatment, 84, 246
NOTCH1, role of, 249, 391
pathogenesis, B-cell, 240
pathogenesis, T cell, 391
prognosis, 245–246
treatment, 416–418
Lymphochip, 554, 555
Lymphoid follicle, 224, 227, 229–232
Lymphoma, 263–276, 477–496
  B-cell, 325
  classification, 3–18
  Epstein-Barr virus (EBV), 524
  genetics, 545–551
  genetic syndromes, 615–617
  mouse models, 583–594
  progression patterns, 12
  risk factors, 15
  risk stratification, 548, 549
  targeted therapy, 612
  therapy, 325–329
Lymphomatoid granulomatosis (LyG), 308, 314, 444 (skin)
  grading, 315
Lymphomatoid papulosis (LyP), 436, 438, 439
  model for regression, 440
  treatment, 453
  types A, B and C, 437–439
Lymphomatous polyposis, 291, 293
Lymphoplasmacytic lymphoma (LPL)
  autoimmune features, 344
  bone marrow, 114, 344–347
  differential diagnosis, 253 (CLL), 267, 272 (MZL)
  immunophenotype, 283
  spleen, 485
  Waldenström macroglobulinemia, 344–347
Lymphopoiesis, 105, 533
Lysosomal storage disease, 118

M
MALT1, translocation 7, 84, 265, 268
MALT lymphoma, 263–272, 274–276
  aneuploid subgroup, 265
  gastrointestinal tract, 264, 486
  lung, 266
  signaling (BCL10, CARMA), 268, 568
  skin, 267
  prognostic factors 269
  therapy 269
Mantle cell lymphoma (MCL), 290–296
  bortezimib, 619
  cell cycle alterations, 295
  cyclin D1 detection, 292–293
  lymphomatous polyposis, 293, 486
  prognostic models, 295–296
  signaling, 570–571
  splenic variant (high B2M), 485
Marginal zone lymphoma, 263–276
Mast cell leukemia, 187
Mast cells
  function, 101
  in LPL, 345–346
  in MDS, 131
  markers, 30

Mastocytosis, 186–189
  diagnostic criteria, 186
  enumeration by flow cytometry, 55
  KIT mutation, 188
Mass spectrometry (MS)
  liquid chromatography with tandem MS (LC-MS/MS) 577, 578
  matrix-assisted laser desorption ionization (MALDI), 580
Mediastinal large cell lymphoma (PMBL), 307–310, 312, 319, 321
  differential with Hodgkin lymphoma, 362
  thymic origin, 495
Mediterranean lymphoma, 265
Megaloblastic anemia, 105
Megaloblastoid erythroid maturation, 106
Mesenchymal stem cells, ex vivo manipulation, 622
Methylation, DNA, 62, 63, 65, 74–75, 87
Methylcellulose assays, stem cells, 538
MGUS (monoclonal gammopathy of undetermined significance), 334
Microarray
  analysis methods, 88
  gene expression, 62, 63, 70, 79, 86, 89, 90
  genomic, 75–79
  heat-map, 89, 90
MicroRNA (miR), 62
  AML subtyping, 145, 157, 170
  MYC overexpression, BL, 319
  profiling, 18
MLL (mixed lineage leukemia gene)
  detection by break-apart FISH, 77
  leukemia, mixed morphology, 243
  mouse models, 598
  partial tandem duplication in AML, 169
  translocations, in AML, 146, 149, 158
  translocations, in ALL, 240
Molecular Diagnostics
  assay validation requirements, 91
  cost-benefit considerations, 18
  quality control measures, 92
  sample handling, 63
Monoclonal B-lymphocytosis (MBL), 252
Monocyte, 460, 467, 468
Monocytoid B cells
  AITL, 395
  MALT lymphoma, 263, 266
  Reactive proliferations (Toxoplasmosis), 230
Monocytoid B-cell lymphoma, 270
Monocytopenia, 102
Monocytosis, 101–103
Mouse, hematolymphoid neoplasms, immunophenotyping, 588, 601
Mouse, hematolymphoid neoplasms, transgenic and GEMM models, 590–591, 598
Mouse, lymphoma, classification, 585–586
Mouse, myeloid neoplasms, classification, 600
MPL (thrombopoietin receptor), mutation, 214, 215, 218
M-protein, 333, 335, 336, 338, 341, 343, 344, 347
mTOR inhibitors, 331
Multicentric Castleman disease (MCD), 308, 316–317
Multiple myeloma, 333–344, also *See* myeloma
Mutagens, risk of lymphoma and leukemia, 14
Mutation, reporting terminology, 74
MYC, 307, 309, 310, 312, 317–320
  Burkitt lymphoma, 317–320
  detection of translocations, 85
  large B-cell lymphoma, 309, 320
  lymphoma cell lines, 569–570

mouse models, ALL/LBL, 590–592
post-transplant lymphoproliferative disorders, 524
signaling in lymphoma, 565
transformation of low-grade B-cell lymphoma, 11, 288, 296
Mycosis fungoides (MF), 428–436
  CD8+, 430
  dermatopathic changes (lymph node), 232–233, 401, 432
  differential diagnosis with dermatitis, 481
  differential diagnosis with other T-cell tumors, 29, 428, 441
  folliculotropic, 432, 434
  pathogenesis, 432–434, 478
  response criteria, 454–455
  Sézary syndrome, 401
  staging, 428–429, 450
  SWAT score, 450
  T-cell "MALT" hypothesis, 478
  transformation, 12, 430
  treatment, 454–455
Myelodysplastic/myeloproliferative neoplasms (MDS/MPN), 136, 138, 140
Myelodysplastic syndrome (MDS)
  diagnostic criteria, 124, 126
  erythroid-predominant vs erythroleukemia, 137
  epigenetic therapy, 173
  fibrotic, 130, 131
  flow cytometry, 131–133, 139
  hypocellular, 130, 135
  idiopathic cytopenia of uncertain significance (ICSU), 134
  immune-mediated, 135–137, 174
  International Prognostic Scoring System (IPSS), 129
  International Working Group, 124, 130, 137
  minimal diagnostic criteria, 124
  minor PNH clone, 136
  treatment, 173–174
Myelofibrosis, *See* Primary myelofibrosis
Myeloid neoplasms, with eosinophilia, 189
Myeloid sarcoma, 468
Myeloma
  aneuploidy, 339
  cyclin group, 342–343
  MAF group, 343
  classification, 8, 334
  gene expression profiling, 342
  IGH translocations, 342
  minimal residual disease (MRD), 338, 343
  non-secretory, 336, 338
  smoldering, 336, 342
  staging systems, 341, 342
Myeloproliferative neoplasms
  classification, 178–179, 214
  cytogenetic changes, 185
  JAK2 mutation, 182–185
  MPL mutation, 183–185
  TET2 mutation, 183
  thrombotic risk, 217, 218
  workup, 213–215

N
Natural killer (NK)-cell lymphoma,
  extranasal (skin), 441
  nasal, 393, 405, 483
  outcome, 416
  treatment, 418, 420

Natural killer-cell (NK) leukemia,
    aggressive, 406
    chronic, 406
    clinical features, 417
Neutropenia, 102, 104
    congenital syndromes, 616
    risk of MDS/AML 618
NK receptors, function, 103, 517
NK receptors, use in diagnosis/flow cytometry, 407
Nodal marginal zone lymphoma (NMZL), 263–272, 275
NOD/SCID mice, lymphoma, 584
Nodular lymphocyte predominant Hodgkin lymphoma (NLPHL),
    351–356
    differential diagnosis with T-cell-rich lymphoma, 313, 354
    diffuse, 355
    relationship to progressive transformation of GC, 231, 354–355
Non-Hodgkin lymphoma (NHL)
    genetics, 545
    treatment, 323
NOTCH
    EBV, interactions, 14, 525
    mutation in T-ALL, 249, 392
    role in lymphoiesis, 539–541
NPM1
    function, 170
    detection of mutation by electrophoresis, 70
    immunostaining to detect mutation, 35
    mutation/duplication, impact in AML, 169
    incidence of mutation in AML, 158
Nuclear factor kappa B (NF-kB), 264, 268, 276
    Hodgkin lymphoma, 361
    outcome prediction in DLBCL, 558–559
    REL amplification, 289
NFAT (Nuclear factor of activated T cells), 563, 565–568, 570

O
Ovary, lymphoma, 489

P
PageRank algorithm, 15
Pagetoid reticulosis, 433, 441
Paget's disease, 119
Paracortical hyperplasia (lymph node), 232–234
Paraprotein, 333, 334, 340, 344, 346
Paroxysmal nocturnal hemoglobinuria (PNH), 136–137
Parvovirus B19, 105
PAX5, 540
PD-1 (GC T-cell marker), uses of, 33, 395
PDGFRA, gene rearrangements in MPN, 180, 188–190
PDGFRB, gene rearrangements in MPN, 180, 188–190
Pediatric follicular lymphoma, 285
Peripheral T-cell lymphoma (PTCL)
    NOS, 391, 395
    treatment, 414–423
Pharmacodynamics (PD), 329, 611
Pharmacogenomics
    C1qA, lymphoma, 550
    cytokines/receptors, lymphoma, 548
    definition, 613
    large cell lymphoma, 547
    lymphoblastic leukemia, 246

Pharmacokinetics (PK)
    chemotherapy, 329
    definition, 611
    Philadelphia chromosome, BCR-ABL, 197, 206
Phosphorylation, tyrosine, 574–576, 579
Plasmablastic lymphoma (PBL), 308, 311, 315–317
Plasma cell leukemia (PCL), 333, 336, 338, 339, 342
Plasma cell myeloma, 333–347, also See myeloma
Plasma cell neoplasm, classification, 4–5, 334–335
Plasmacytoid dendritic cell (pDC)
    biology, 103, 460
    neoplasms, 461, 469–470
Plasmacytoma, 333, 336
Platelets
    function, 103
    granules, 101, 109
Platelet-derived growth factor receptor, chromosomal translocation,
    189, 190
PML–RARA. See Promyelocytic leukemia–Retinoic acid receptor
Polyacrylamide gel electrophoresis, 2-D, proteomics, 578
Polycythemia vera (PV)
    diagnosis, 177–185, 215
    clinical features, 214
    treatment, 217–218
Polymerase chain reaction (PCR), 62, 67–72, 74, 75, 82–84, 86
    inhibitors, 71
    quantitative, 63, 68, 70–71
    real-time, 69, 70
    reverse transcription, 64–66
Post-transplant lymphoproliferative disorders (PTLD),
    522–526
    treatment, 525–526
Primary effusion lymphoma, 308, 315, 316
Primary mediastinal large B-cell lymphoma, See mediastinal large
    B-cell lymphoma
Primary myelofibrosis (PMF)
    diagnosis, 177–185, 215
    clinical features, 214
    treatment, 217–218
Progressive transformation of germinal center (PTGC), 231, 354
Proliferation center (CLL), 254
Prolymphocytes (CLL), 252–254, 260
Promyelocytic leukemia (PML)–retinoic acid receptor alpha (RARA),
    603, 604
Promyelocytic leukemia, treatment, 168, 171
Proteasome inhibitor, use in lymphoma, 559
Proteomics, 573–580
    antibodies, 574
    functional, 577
    isotope-coded affinity tag (ICAT), 578
    phospho-specific, 574, 575, 579
    post-translational modification, 573, 577, 579
    reverse phase protein array (RPPA), 575–576
    stable isotope labeling in cell culture (SILAC), 578
    subproteomics, 577–578
PTEN, mouse model, 592–594
PU.1 and other B-cell transcription factors, including BOB1, OCT2
    myelopoiesis, 540
    lymphoma versus Hodgkin lymphoma, 34, 360

Q
Quantum dots, 39

R

Rag recombinases, role in Ig and TCR recombination, 6, 534
RAS mutation
 ALPS, 616
 AML, 158, 169
 CMML, 139
 mouse models, lymphoma, 589–591
 mouse models, MDS, 598
 myeloma, 341
Receptor tyrosine kinase, mutations in MPNs, 178
Reed–Sternberg (R–S) cell, 357, 363
Refractory anemia with ring sideroblasts and marked thrombocytosis
 (RARS-T), 138, 140
REL, gene amplification, 290
Reticular cell (lymph node), 459–461, 472
Reticular cell sarcoma, 459, 472
Retrovirus, murine, 597, 602
Reverse phase protein array (RPPA), 575–576
Richter's transformation (CLL), 259–260
Ring sideroblasts, definition, 109, 124, 126
Rituximab
 combination therapy, 326, 327
 impact on DLBCL outcome, 304, 553
 loss of expression at relapse, 327
 NLPHL, use in, 371, 376
 outcome predictors, 555
 response prediction, FC gamma receptors, 548–550
 transplant regimen, use in, 509
RNA
 Northern blot, 67
 quantitation, 65
 reverse transcriptase PCR, 68
Rosai–Dorfman disease, 463, 467

S

Sarcoma, lymph node, 465, 470, 472
SCID mice, lymphoma, 583, 584
Self-renewal (stem/precursor cell), 531, 533, 538, 539, 541
Sézary syndrome (SS), 399, 401
 primary, 433, 435
 staging, 429–431
 transformation of MF, 430–432
 treatment, 452
Short tandem repeat (STR), use in chimerism, 514–517
Side population (stem cell), 538
Signalosome, 564, 565
Single nucleotide polymorphism (SNP), 546–550
 definition and uses, 513, 514, 519
 Tag SNPs, 546, 550
Sinus histiocytosis with massive lymphadenopathy (SHML),
 463, 467
Sjogren's syndrome, 264
Skin, lymphomas, 480
Small bowel, lymphoma, 485
Small lymphocytic leukemia, 251–260
Somatic hypermutation (IGH), 86 (technique), 226–228, 256 (CLL)
Sonic hedgehog signaling
 cancer stem cells, 541
 splenic marginal zone lymphoma, 276
Splenic B-cell lymphoma/leukemia, variants, 274, 275
Splenic B-cell marginal zone lymphoma (SMZL), 264, 271–276
Splenic lymphoma with villous lymphocytes, 273

Splenic lymphomas, gross appearances, 485–486
 Stem cell transplant, *See* hematopoietic stem cell transplant
Subacute necrotizing lymphadenitis (Kikuchi's disease), 463
Subcutaneous panniculitis-like T-cell lymphoma, 442–443

T

Targeted therapy, 326–328
T cells
 autoimmune-mediated disease/risk for neoplasia, 229, 392, 615
 maturation, 490–492, 534–535
 regulatory subset, 225, 228
 thymic selection, 491, 534
T-cell/histiocyte-rich B-cell lymphoma (TCHRBCL), differential with
 Hodgkin lymphoma, 354, 355
T-cell/histiocyte-rich large B-cell lymphoma (TCHRLBCL), 310, 311, 313
T-cell large granular lymphocytic (T-LGL) leukemia
 features, 394, 400
 treatment, 420
T-cell leukemia, treatment, 416, 417, 419, 420, 422
T-cell lymphoma
 alternate classification, 403
 bone marrow, 101, 116
 bone marrow involvement, 398
 central memory type, 395
 follicular variant, 394, 395
 interfollicular, 396
 paracortical, 396
 subcutaneous panniculitits-like, 441, 443
 treatment, 413–421, 423
T-cell malignancies
 management algorithm, risk-adapted, 423
 pathogenesis, 404
 prognosis, 414, 417–420, 424
 staging, 414–416, 418, 419
T-cell prolymphocytic leukemia (T-PLL), 399–403
 skin, involvement, 401
 TCL1 expression, 399
 treatment, 416, 417, 420
T-cell receptor
 PCR, interpretation/problems, 83
 signaling in lymphoma, 403
 targeting, in lymphoma, 620
 temporal sequence of TCR recombination, 534
 Vbeta typing, flow cytometry, 400
TCL1, oncogene
 ataxia telangiectasia, 616
 AKT modulation, 403
 chronic lymphocytic leukemia, 256
 plasmacytoid dendritic cells, 461
 T-cell prolymphocytic leukemia, 7, 400–402
TCR, *See* T-cell receptor
Terminal deoxynucleotidyl transferase (TdT), 534, 536
Testicular lymphoma, 489
Therapy response predictors
 strengths and weaknesses, 10
Thymic carcinoma, 490, 492, 494
Thymoma, classification, 492
Thymus
 B cells, 491
 maturation, 490, 491
 selection, 534
 T-cell maturation, 534

Thyroid, lymphoma, 480
Tingible body macrophage, 227, 231
Tissue arrays, 37–38
TNF (tumor necrosis factor) pathway
    follicular lymphoma, 288
    germinal center function, 227
    Hodgkin lymphoma, 361
    signaling, B-cell lymphoma, 564
    SNPs, risk for lymphoma, 547
Topoisomerase inhibitors, risk of AML, 147
Toxoplasmosis, 230
Transplant, *See* hematopoietic stem cell transplant
Trisomy 3, marginal zone lymphoma, 274
Tyrosine kinase inhibitors (TKIs)
    imatinib and next generation compounds, 216
    polycythemia vera (PV), 217, 218
    treatment, 218

U
Uniparental disomy
    AML, 155
    JAK2 in MPNs, 183
Use of cytogenetics, 195–198, 202, 206

V
Variable number of terminal repeats (VNTRs), use in chimerism, 513
Vascular transformation of lymph node sinuses, 234
Viral transduction, 598, 601–603, 605

W
Waldenström macroglobulinemia (WM), 334, 344–346
World Health Organization, lymphoma/leukemia classification
    AML, 146
    lymphomas, B-cell, 9
    lymphomas, T-cell, 9
    MDS, 126
    myeloid neoplasms, 8
    problems, in AML classification, 147
    problems, in mast cell classification, 186

X
Xenograft, 583–584

Z
ZAP70 (CLL), 256